Target Organ Toxicology Series

Carcinogenesis

Target Organ Toxicology Series

Series Editors
A. Wallace Hayes, John A. Thomas, and Donald E. Gardner

Carcinogenesis
Michael P. Waalkes and Jerrold M. Ward, editors, 496 pp., 1994

Toxicology of the Lung, Second Edition
Donald E. Gardner, James D. Crapo, and Roger O. McClellan, editors, 688 pp., 1993

Cardiovascular Toxicology, Second Edition
Daniel Acosta, Jr., editor, 576 pp., 1992

Ophthalmic Toxicology
George C. Y. Chiou, editor, 352 pp., 1992

Neurotoxicology
Hugh A. Tilson and Clifford L. Mitchell, editors, 416 pp., 1992

Toxicology of the Lung
Donald E. Gardner, James D. Crapo, and Edward J. Massaro, editors, 540 pp., 1988

Endocrine Toxicology
John A. Thomas, Kenneth S. Korach, and John A. McLachlan, editors, 414 pp., 1985

Immunotoxicology and Immunopharmacology
Jack H. Dean, Michael I. Luster, Albert E. Munson, and Harry Amos, editors, 528 pp., 1985

*Reproductive Toxicology
Robert L. Dixon, editor, 368 pp., 1985

Toxicology of the Blood and Bone Marrow
Richard D. Irons, editor, 192 pp., 1985

Toxicology of the Eye, Ear, and Other Special Senses
A. Wallace Hayes, editor, 264 pp., 1985

*Toxicology of the Immune System
Jack H. Dean and Albert E. Munson, editors, 528 pp., 1985

Cutaneous Toxicity
Victor A. Drill and Paul Lazar, editors, 288 pp., 1984

Intestinal Toxicology
Carol M. Schiller, editor, 252 pp., 1984

Cardiovascular Toxicology
Ethard W. Van Stee, editor, 400 pp., 1982

*Out of print.

Target Organ Toxicology Series

Carcinogenesis

Editors

Michael P. Waalkes, Ph.D.
*Chief, Inorganic Carcinogenesis Section
Laboratory of Comparative Carcinogenesis
National Cancer Institute
Frederick Cancer Research and Development Center
Frederick, Maryland*

Jerrold M. Ward, D.V.M., Ph.D.
*Chief, Veterinary and Tumor Pathology Section
Office of Laboratory Animal Science
National Cancer Institute
Frederick Cancer Research and Development Center
Frederick, Maryland*

Raven Press New York

Raven Press, Ltd., 1185 Avenue of the Americas, New York, New York 10036

© 1994 by Raven Press, Ltd. All rights reserved. This book is protected by copyright. No part of it may be reproduced, stored in a retrieval system, or transmitted, in any form or by any means, electronical, mechanical, photocopying, or recording, or otherwise, without the prior written permission of the publisher.

Made in the United States of America

Library of Congress Cataloging-in-Publication Data

Carcinogenesis / editors, Michael P. Waalkes, Jerrold M. Ward.
    p.   cm. — (Target organ toxicology series)
  Includes bibliographical references and index.
  ISBN 0-7817-0124-4
  1. Carcinogenesis. I. Waalkes, Michael Phillip, 1953– II. Ward, Jerrold Michael, 1942– . III. Series.
  [DNLM: 1. Neoplasms—chemically induced. 2. Neoplasms—physiopathology.   QZ 202 C26423   1993]
RC268.5.C342   1993
616.99′4071—dc20
DNLM/DLC
for Library of Congress   93-28927
                                                                   CIP

    The material contained in this volume was submitted as previously unpublished material, except in the instances in which credit has been given to the source from which some of the illustrative material was derived.
    Great care has been taken to maintain the accuracy of the information contained in the volume. However, neither Raven Press nor the editors can be held responsible for errors or for any consequences arising from the use of the information contained herein.
    Materials appearing in this book prepared by individuals as part of their official duties as U.S. Government employees are not covered by the above-mentioned copyright.

9 8 7 6 5 4 3 2 1

Contents

Contributing Authors		vii
Preface		xi
1.	General Principles of Chemical Carcinogenesis *Elizabeth K. Weisburger*	1
2.	Chemicals Causally Associated with Cancers in Humans and in Laboratory Animals: A Perfect Concordance *James Huff*	25
3.	Hepatocarcinogenesis in the Rat *Ryohei Hasegawa and Nobuyuki Ito*	39
4.	Susceptibility Factors of Gastrointestinal Tract Carcinogenesis *Kosaku Sakamoto, Huimian Xu, and Abulkalam M. Shamsuddin*	67
5.	Renal Carcinogenesis *Noboru Konishi and Yoshio Hiasa*	123
6.	Urinary Bladder Carcinogenesis in the Rodent *Charles H. Frith, David L. Greenman, and Samuel M. Cohen*	161
7.	Chemically Associated Respiratory Carcinogenesis in Rodents and in Humans *James Huff*	199
8.	Upper Respiratory Tract Carcinogenesis in Experimental Animals and in Humans *R. A. Woutersen, A. van Garderen-Hoetmer, P. J. Slootweg, and Victor J. Feron*	215
9.	Multistage Skin Carcinogenesis in Mice *John DiGiovanni*	265
10.	Neurocarcinogenesis *Adalbert Koestner and Keiji Marushige*	301
11.	Male Reproductive System *Maarten C. Bosland*	339

12.	Carcinogenesis of the Hematopoietic System *J. H. Harleman, H. J. Schuurman, and C. Frieke Kuper*	403
13.	Pathology Procedures in Laboratory Animal Carcinogenesis Studies *Deborah E. Devor, John R. Henneman, Yasushi Kurata, Sabine Rehm, Christopher M. Weghorst, and Jerrold M. Ward*	429
Subject Index		467

Contributing Authors

Maarten C. Bosland, D.V.Sc., Ph.D.
Institute of Environmental Medicine
New York University Medical Center
Long Meadow Road
Tuxedo, New York 10987

Samuel M. Cohen, M.D., Ph.D.
Departments of Pathology and
  Microbiology
University of Nebraska Medical Center
600 South 42nd Street
Omaha, Nebraska 68198

Deborah E. Devor, B.S., L.A.T.G.
Laboratory of Comparative
  Carcinogenesis
National Cancer Institute
Frederick Cancer Research and
  Development Center
Building 538
Frederick, Maryland 21702

John DiGiovanni, Ph.D.
Department of Carcinogenesis
University of Texas
M. D. Anderson Cancer Center
Science Park-Research Division
P.O. Box 389, Park Road 1
Smithville, Texas 78957

Victor J. Feron, M.D., Ph.D.
Department of Biological Toxicology
TNO-Toxicology and Nutrition Institute
Utrechtseweg 48
3704 HE, Zeist, The Netherlands

Charles H. Frith, D.V.M., Ph.D.
Toxicology Pathology Associates
1102 Briar Creek Road
Little Rock, Arkansas 72211

David L. Greenman, Ph.D.
Office of Director and Scientific
  Coordination
National Center for Toxicology Research
3900 NCTR Road
Jefferson, Arkansas 72079

J. H. Harleman, D.V.S., Ph.D.
Department of Experimental Pathology
ASTA Medica AG
Kantstrape 2
Halle Westphalen, Germany 33790

Ryohei Hasegawa, M.D.
First Department of Pathology
Nagoya City University Medical School
1-Kawasumi, Mizuho-cho, Mizuho-ku
Nagoya, 467 Japan

John R. Henneman, M.S.
Carcinogenesis Studies Section
Biological Carcinogenesis and
  Development Program
Program Resources Inc./DynCorp
National Cancer Institute
Frederick Cancer Research and
  Development Center
P.O. Box B, Building 538, Room 241
Frederick, Maryland 21702

Yoshio Hiasa, M.D., Ph.D.
Second Department of Pathology
Nara Medical University
840 Shijo-cho
Kashihara, Nara, 634 Japan

James Huff, Ph.D.
Environmental Carcinogenesis Program
National Institute of Environmental Health
  Sciences
P.O. Box 12233
Research Triangle Park, North
  Carolina 27709

CONTRIBUTING AUTHORS

Nobuyuki Ito, M.D.
First Department of Pathology
Nagoya City University Medical School
1-Kawasumi, Mizuho-cho, Mizuho-ku
Nagoya, 467 Japan

Adalbert Koestner, D.V.M., M.Sc., Ph.D.
Department of Veterinary Pathobiology
Ohio State University
1925 Coffey Road
Columbus, Ohio 43210

Noboru Konishi, M.D., Ph.D.
Second Department of Pathology
Nara Medical University
840 Shijo-cho
Kashihara, Nara, 634 Japan

C. Frieke Kuper, Ph.D.
TNO-Toxicology and Nutrition Institute
Utrechtseweg 48
P.O. Box 360
3700 AJ, Zeist, The Netherlands

Yasushi Kurata, Ph.D.
First Department of Pathology
Nagoya City University Medical School
1 Kawasumi Mizuho-cho, Mizuho-ku
Nagoya, 467 Japan

Keiji Marushige, Ph.D.
Department of Pathology
Michigan State University
A620 East Fee Hall
East Lansing, Michigan 48824

Sabine Rehm, Dr., Med., Vet.
Division of Pharmaceuticals
Toxicology U.S.
SmithKline Beecham Pharmaceuticals
709 Swedeland Road
P.O. Box 1539
King of Prussia, Pennsylvania 19406

Kosaku Sakamoto, M.D., D.M.Sc.
Department of Surgery
Maki Hospital
71-1 Tsukunawa-cho
Takasaki, Gunma, T370 Japan

H. J. Schuurman, Ph.D.
Pharma Preclinical Research
Sandoz AG
CH-4002, Basel, Switzerland

Abulkalam M. Shamsuddin, M.D., Ph.D.
Department of Pathology
University of Maryland School of
  Medicine
10 South Pine Street
Baltimore, Maryland 21201

P. J. Slootweg, M.D., D.M.D., Ph.D.
Department of Pathology
University Hospital
Heidelberg Laan 100
3508 GA, Utrecht, The Netherlands

A. van Garderen-Hoetmer
Department of Biological Toxicology
TNO-Toxicology and Nutrition Institute
Utrechtseweg 48
3704 HE, Zeist, The Netherlands

Michael P. Waalkes, Ph.D.
Inorganic Carcinogenesis Section
Laboratory of Comparative
  Carcinogenesis
National Cancer Institute
Frederick Cancer Research and
  Development Center
Building 538, Room 205E
Frederick, Maryland 21702

Jerrold M. Ward, D.V.M., Ph.D.
Veterinary and Tumor Pathology Section
Office of Laboratory Animal Science
National Cancer Institute
Frederick Cancer Research and
  Development Center
Frederick, Maryland 21702

Elizabeth K. Weisburger, Ph.D., D.Sc.
5309 McKinley Street
Bethesda, Maryland 20814

Christopher M. Weghorst, Ph.D.
Laboratory of Comparative
  Carcinogenesis
National Cancer Institute
Frederick Cancer Research and
  Development Center
Building 538, Room 206
Frederick, Maryland 21702

R. A. Woutersen, M.Sc., Ph.D.
Department of Biological Toxicology
TNO-Toxicology and Nutrition Institute
Utrechtseweg 48
3704 HE, Zeist, The Netherlands

Huimian Xu, M.D.
Department of Oncology
First Affiliated Hospital
China Medical University
Shenyang, China 110001

Preface

Carcinogenesis is a multifaceted and multistaged disease that can be viewed as a form of chemical toxicity. As is the case with toxic chemicals, the effects of carcinogens are often produced only within specific target sites or tissues. This target-site specificity can involve various facets ranging from simple toxicokinetics to more complex causation factors such as expression or lack of expression of specific genes. Neoplasms are one of the most important endpoints in safety assessment of chemicals, whether they are used as drugs or food additives, or in agriculture or industry. Thus, defining the mechanisms of target-site specificity of chemical carcinogens and determining relevance of such mechanisms in humans is of clear importance. This volume offers a variety of reviews that focus on the factors that are involved in tissue-specific induction of cancers by chemicals. These reviews include information on chemical carcinogenesis, mechanisms of carcinogenesis, and pathophysiology of induced tumors. Although all aspects of carcinogenesis in each organ system could not be addressed, we provide some current information on important processes dictating sensitivity in these organs.

Michael P. Waalkes
Jerrold M. Ward

Target Organ Toxicology Series

Carcinogenesis

Carcinogenesis, edited by
M.P. Waalkes and J.M. Ward.
Raven Press, Ltd., New York © 1994.

1

General Principles of Chemical Carcinogenesis

Elizabeth K. Weisburger

Bethesda, Maryland 20814

For a book such as this, devoted generally to carcinogenesis in specific organ systems of animals, it may represent an anomaly to recall that the carcinogenic effects of a sizable number of environmental or industrial materials were first noted in humans. One of the first was the "Bergkrankheiten" of the miners in the Schneeberg and Joachimstal regions of Europe, as described by Paracelsus and Agricola in the sixteenth century. Three hundred years later a more scientific investigation of Bergkrankheiten led to the conclusion that it was lung cancer. The probable cause was the uranium (and its decay products such as radon) which coexisted with silver and cobalt in the mines (1). More recently, a similar situation has been reported among uranium miners in the Colorado plateau (2).

Other internal cancers, first noted in exposed individuals, were the bladder tumors of the dyestuff workers. Approximately 40 years after William Henry Perkins' discovery of synthetic mauveine, leading to the establishment of dye factories in England and Europe, Ludwig Rehn of Frankfurt-am-Main described three cases of bladder or "aniline" cancer in a group of 45 workers. Although later investigations incriminated 2-naphthylamine and benzidine rather than aniline, more recent epidemiological studies indicate that exposure of workers to simpler aromatic amines, especially *ortho*-toluidine and derivatives, increases the risk of bladder cancer (3,4). Bladder cancer was not produced by aromatic amines in experimental animals until 1938, but to duplicate the human effect in subhuman primates required only a few years of administration of 2-naphthylamine (5).

Similarly, with various substances, now recognized as human carcinogens, including arsenic, asbestos, 4-aminobiphenyl, benzene, chlornaphazine, and others, the effects were noted in exposed people before animal experiments showed a deleterious action. For example, although the leukemogenic action of benzene had long been described, many animal experiments failed in developing a neoplastic effect until the National Toxicology Program (NTP) bioassay of benzene yielded definitive positive results (6). On the other hand, some of the substances considered as carcinogens by various policymaking groups may be essential trace elements for one or the other form of life, as is the case for chromium, nickel, and possibly arsenic (7). Thus an informed, judicious approach to classifying carcinogens is needed.

In the remainder of the chapter we provide some current views on how chemical carcinogens act and what they affect in the exposed organism.

TYPES OF CARCINOGENS

It is considered that for carcinogens to be effective, they must interact with cellular constituents, including proteins, lipids, and most important, with the nucleic acids, the genetic material of the cell. Compounds that have structures permitting these types of reactions are direct acting; those that require metabolic activation are indirect acting. The nongenotoxic or epigenetic carcinogens have other mechanisms of action, as discussed later.

Direct Acting

Relatively few carcinogens are direct acting since the inate reactivity of such compounds also tends to make them unstable. Examples of such carcinogens are aziridine (ethyleneimine), β-propiolactone, bis(chloromethyl) ether, bis(2-chloroethyl)sulfide, diepoxybutane, ethylene oxide, methyl methane sulfonate, nitrogen mustard and derivatives, including cyclophosphamide, and propane sultone. These structures lead to alkylation of cellular macromolecules, often at the 7-position of guanine in nucleic acids, without the need for metabolic activation. Once in the organism, such molecules may be deactivated by reaction with water or by metabolism before reaching important cellular receptors. Conversely, metabolism may alter the characteristics of the molecule to make it more accessible to cellular receptors. Direct-acting carcinogens that are very reactive may not be potent because of all the intervening reactions before they reach a receptor. Often, compounds of intermediate reactivity are more potent in vivo than very reactive ones. Most direct-acting carcinogens do not represent an appreciable hazard to the general population. However, medical personnel involved in the treatment of patients with chemotherapeutic agents such as cyclophosphamide should be aware of the possible hazards from these drugs (8).

Indirect Acting

Indirect-acting carcinogens constitute those that are stable in the environment and thus are more likely to be contacted by the general population. Such agents, often called pro- or precarcinogens, require metabolic activation before they can interact with cellular macromolecules. In turn, metabolism is governed by many factors, including species, strain, sex, age, diet, enzyme inducers or inhibitors, immune status, plus other factors. Metabolic studies have identified species or strains that lack the enzyme systems necessary to metabolize certain procarcinogens to the activated form, exemplified by guinea pigs and steppe lemmings, which do not produce N-hydroxy derivatives of aromatic amines (9). Animals may lack a cellular receptor for the activated molecule, the case for some strains of mice that do not respond to polycyclic aromatic hydrocarbons (PAHs) because they lack the Ah receptor (10). Animals and humans who have low levels of the enzyme that acetylates aromatic amines, thus detoxifying them, are considered at somewhat greater risk of bladder cancer from exposure to aromatic amines (11,12).

Males and females may also differ in their responses to xenobiotics, including carcinogens; in some cases this difference correlated with higher levels of certain enzymes in males but did not hold in others (13). Newborn or very young animals are often quite sensitive to carcinogens because they generally have low levels of enzymes that detoxify xenobiotics. Diet plays a major role in determining the response to carcinogens. For example, diets high in fat increased the response to some carcinogens (14). The opposite, lowered response to carcinogens was noted in animals restricted to about 75% of the food eaten ad libitum (15). Diets high in certain constituents may protect against some types of carcinogens, while even deficient diets may alter the response to others. Enzyme inducers or inhibitors can alter, often quite dramatically, the response of animals to carcinogens. Traces of such substances are often present and may have considerable impact (16,17). The upshot is that there are several points in the metabolic pathway of an indirect-acting carcinogen where the process can be altered or influenced, either to enhance or suppress the action of the carcinogen.

Metabolic Aspects: P450 System

The initial metabolic reaction for most xenobiotics, including carcinogens, involves oxidation to either a detoxication product or to a form that is closer to the activated or ultimate carcinogen. The enzyme system responsible for many metabolic reactions is the P450 system; P450 is a hemoprotein distinguished by the wavelength of the carbon monoxide derivative of the reduced form, namely 450 nm. Previously, the over 100 forms of the system were named according to the method used to induce them. Currently, they have been classified according to a genetic evolutionary scheme (18), then on the protein name (19), and more recently a system based on chromosomal location has been suggested (20) (Table 1). Thus, depending on the time period, reports on metabolism of xenobiotics may employ various nomenclature systems for the P450 enzymes.

Genotoxic and Nongenotoxic or Epigenetic Carcinogens

Genotoxic carcinogens are those which either react as such with the genetic material of the cell, or are converted by metabolism to reactive intermediates that form

TABLE 1. Common P450 classifications of rats and mice and nomenclature according to various sytems

Trivial name	Protein name	Locus symbol
	Rats	
P450a1	P450IIA1	CYP2A1
P450a2	P450IIA2	CYP2A2
P450a3	P450IIA3	CYP2A3
P450b	P450IIB1	CYP2B1
P450c	P450IA1	CYP1A1
P450d	P450IA2	CYP1A2
P450e	P450IIB2	CYP2B2
P450f	P450IIC7	CYP2C7
P450g	P450IIC13	CYP2C13
P450h	P450IIC11	CYP2C11
P450i	P450IIC12	CYP2C12
P450j	P450IIE1	CYP2E1
	Mice	
P450P_1	P450IA1	Cyp1a-1
P450$_3$;P_2	P450IA2	Cyp1a-2
P450 15$_\alpha$oh-1	IIA3	Cyp2a-4
P450 15$_\alpha$oh-2		Cyp2a-5
P450pf26	P450IIB9	Cyp2b-9
P450pf 3/46	IIB10	Cyp2b-10
P450 16$_\alpha$	IID9	Cyp2d-9
P450cb	P450IID10	Cyp2d-10

Data from Nebert et al. (18–20).

adducts with the genetic material. The direct- and indirect-acting carcinogens discussed previously fall into this class. The nongenotoxic or epigenetic carcinogens do not appear to bind to the deoxyribonucleic acid (DNA) of the cell, although they may form adducts with other cellular constituents, and they have various mechanisms of action. A group of epigenetic carcinogens comprising hypolipidemic drugs, phthalate ester plasticizers, and trichloroacetic acid cause peroxisomal proliferation of the liver, eventually leading to liver tumors in mice and rats. Nevertheless, these agents did not damage DNA and were not mutagenic in the usual short-term test systems (21).

Some aliphatic hydrocarbons, unleaded gasoline, tetralin, limonene, and similar substances caused renal tumors in male rats, mediated through the presence of a male rat–specific protein, α_{2u}-globulin, in the kidney tubules. Upon combination with the xenobiotic or its metabolite, the protein was no longer metabolized normally; thus the complex remained in the kidney tubules, leading to hyaline droplet nephropathy, cell death, hyperplasia, and eventually tumors (22,23).

Several drugs previously used as sleeping aids led to liver tumors in rats, but intensive investigation has failed to show any appreciable interaction with liver DNA (24). Immunosuppressants, solid-state materials such as films and fibers of specific dimensions are also considered epigenetic carcinogens, as are hormones and substances that affect the function of an endocrine organ, as does ethylene thiourea (7). Physicochemical factors such as aberrant osmolarity or abnormal pH, induced by some unphysiological condition, may be involved, especially for the bladder (7,25). Compounds that led to formation of crystals and then calculi in the bladder, especially of male rats, often led to bladder tumors, particularly with administration of high levels over a lifetime; saccharin is in this category. Diverse types of compounds with equally varied mechanisms of action thus comprise the group of substances known as epigenetic carcinogens.

ORGANIC COMPOUNDS

The mechanisms of action for indirect-acting carcinogens which are organic chemicals are generally better understood than those for inorganic carcinogens. Metabolism is the first step along the activation pathway.

Aliphatic Compounds

Aliphatic compounds of great concern with respect to carcinogenicity are the short-chain halogenated aliphatics since these compounds have many uses. Sizable amounts are produced industrially for solvents, pesticides, and as intermediates in the manufacture of other materials. There also is some natural production, especially by marine organisms (26). A greater concern is that trihalomethanes and other compounds are by-products of water chlorination, presumably by reaction of humic acids in natural waters with chlorine (27).

One-Carbon Compounds

Halogenated one-carbon compounds, specifically dichloromethane (DCM) (methylene chloride), chloroform, and carbon tetrachloride, have shown carcinogenic effects in various animal systems. For these compounds, oxidation by P450 enzymes occurs to an appreciable extent (28). Although the specific human P450 responsible for oxidizing DCM has been delineated (29), this has not been done for all animal P450s. DCM is metabolized through two competing pathways (30); by oxidation the high-affinity saturable one goes through formyl chloride to carbon monoxide and to formaldehyde and formic acid, a urinary metabolite of DCM. The low-affinity pathway is glutathione dependent; formyl chloride may interact with glutathione to produce formic acid and carbon dioxide, or acylation of microsomal proteins or lipids may occur (30,31). Although DCM induced liver tumors in mice, it did not share the mitogenic properties of other mouse liver carcinogens (32).

A P450 inhibitor decreased the metabolic activation, toxicity, and binding of chloroform to protein in mice (33). Trichloromethanol, the primary oxidation product, degraded to phosgene, which in turn reacted with water, with protein, with cysteine (affording 2-oxothiazolidine 4-carboxylic acid), and possibly with glutathione.

The metabolism of carbon tetrachloride, also P450 mediated, proceeds through reductive dechlorination. One model includes a P450–Fe–CCl_3 complex that degrades to carbon monoxide, carbon dioxide, phosgene, formic acid, chloroform, and hexachloroethane, in addition to yielding protein- or lipid-bound complexes. The trichloromethyl radical $\cdot CCl_3$ was detected in the blood of rats given carbon tetrachloride (34), while a carbon dioxide $\cdot CO_2$ radical was derived from a glutathione-dependent reaction (35). Further work may differentiate the two pathways more clearly.

Two-Carbon Compounds

Unsaturated

Halogenated aliphatics with two-carbon and longer chains are metabolized by various paths, although P450 plays a major role. Vinyl chloride appears to be metabolized to a transient oxide (36). Because of the strained ring, this oxide reacts readily with nucleic acids. Besides alkylating the 7-position of guanine in DNA to yield 7-(2'-oxyethyl)guanine, vinyl chloride forms exocyclic products in the DNA which contain new rings, including N^2,3-ethenoguanine, 1, N^6-etheno-2'-deoxyadenosine, and 3,N^4-etheno-2'-deoxycytidine (37–39). It may be surmised that such structures would not readily be subject to the usual repair enzyme systems (40,41) and would interfere in normal cell replication.

The situation is more complex with trichloroethylene (TCE). Oxidation by P450, as for vinyl chloride, may produce a transient oxide (36), while another theory is that an intramolecular rearrangement occurs within an oxygenated TCE, leading to chloral without epoxide formation (42). The TCE oxide, if formed, was not an electrophile, for TCE was a weak mutagen and showed low levels of DNA binding (43). Whatever the intermediate, it rearranged to trichloroacetaldehyde, which was oxidized to trichloroacetic acid (TCA) or was reduced to trichlorethanol (44). TCA is a peroxisomal proliferator; it and dichloroacetic acid induced liver tumors in B6C3F1 mice (45,46). Various studies of TCE and TCA indicated that mice had higher body burdens of TCA after exposure to TCE than did rats (44,47), which may account for the relative lack of response of rats to TCE (48,49).

Tetrachloroethylene, also more effective in mice than in rats, underwent P450-mediated oxidation, yielding reactive metabolites in the liver and excretion of chlorinated compounds, especially TCA. Mice formed more of the toxic metabolites than did rats. A second metabolic route involved conjugation with glutathione to form S-1,2,2-trichlorovinyl-N-acetylcysteine, which was considered responsible for the nephrotoxicity of tetrachloroethylene (50,51).

Saturated

The saturated two-carbon halogenated compounds of interest as carcinogens are 1,2-dibromoethane (DBE) and 1,2-dichloroethane (DCE), both of which had had commercial use. DBE had been employed to fumigate grain and tropical and citrus fruits, and to scavenge lead in gasoline. DCE is an intermediate in production of vinyl chloride, in addition to lesser uses as a lead scavenger and grain fumigant. Both compounds were carcinogenic in rats and mice following oral administration, but DCE had lower toxicity and activity (52). By inhalation exposure, DBE was an active carcinogen (53), whereas DCE was not, even at levels manyfold those allowed in the industrial workplace (54). Administration of the enzyme inhibitor, disulfiram, together with DBE or DCE, potentiated the effect, probably by reducing the rate of elimination of the two compounds.

Both DDE and DCE were metabolized through two different paths; an oxidative route mediated through a P450 led to the haloalcohol, haloaldehyde, and haloacetic acid. The haloaldehydes reacted with cellular macromolecules (55). The second path involved coupling with glutathione to yield a hemisulfur mustard analog, followed by cyclization to an episulfonium ion that was an alkylating agent, leading to nucleic acid adducts (56,57). The binding of both DBE and DCE to cellular macromolecules in the respiratory epithelium of mice and rats could be detected, despite the difference in response to the compounds when given by inhalation (58).

Three-Carbon Compounds

The compound of interest in this group is 1,2-dibromo-3-chloropropane (DBCP), which was carcinogenic in mice and rats either after oral administration or by inhalation. Metabolism also proceeded through an oxidative route, affording oxides, alcohols, and aliphatic acids (59–61). In contrast to DBE and DCE, an episulfonium ion was not involved, but the potent mutagen 2-bromoacrolein was formed by microsomes (62). 2-Bromoacrolein readily formed various adducts with calf thymus DNA, yielding $1,N^2$-(6-hydroxy-7-bromo)propanodeoxyguanosine, $1,N^2$-(7-bromo-8-hydroxy)propanodeoxyguanosine, and 3-(bromooxypropyl)thymidine (63). What effect such exocyclic adducts would have on the function of the nucleic acids has not been reported.

The halogenated aliphatics thus constitute a class of compounds with a wide range of effects, from active only under certain conditions, exemplified by DCE, to fairly active under all conditions, as with DBE and DBCP. DBE and DBCP have genotoxic effects and form DNA adducts. Others such as carbon tetrachloride and TCE show minimal or no DNA binding. In addition, some members of this class, especially 1,1,1-trichloroethane, had minimal or no carcinogenic effects (64). Although glutathione conjugation is generally considered a detoxication reaction, with halogenated aliphatics this reaction often affords toxic metabolites (65).

Aromatic Compounds

Benzene

Benzene (BZ), the simplest aromatic compound, presents an intriguing puzzle, for BZ itself is toxic and carcinogenic (6,66), while most of its metabolites are

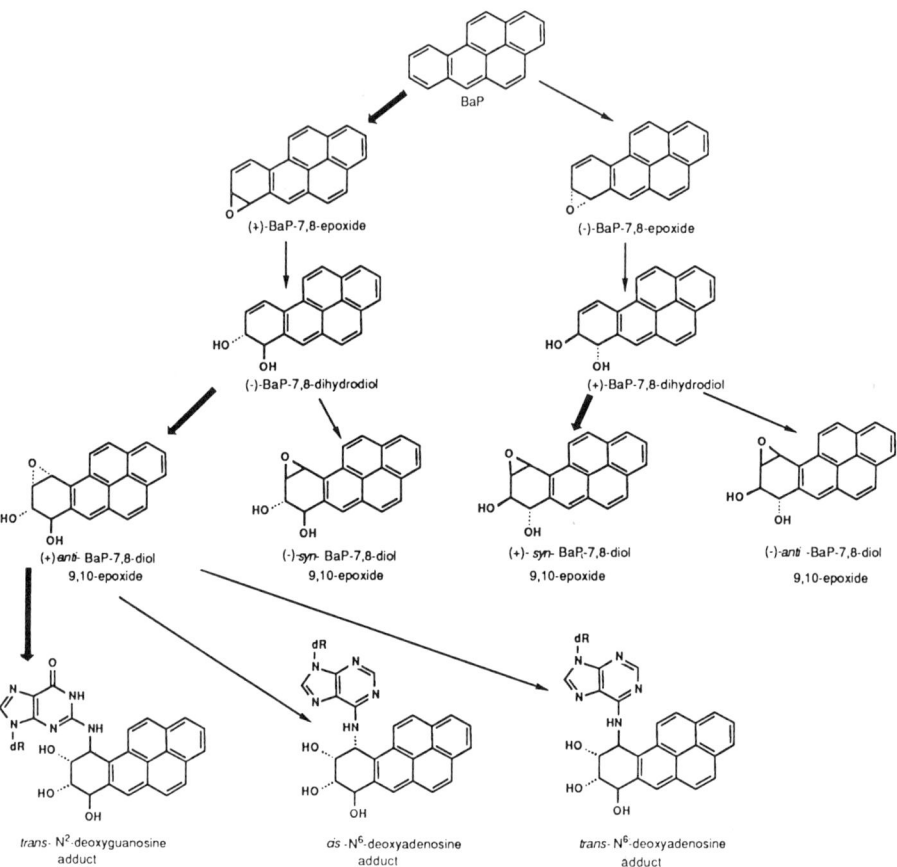

FIG. 1. Stereospecific metabolism and DNA binding of benzo[a]pyrene. [Reproduced with permission from Beland and Poirier (78).]

much less effective. BZ metabolism is generally mediated through P450IIE1 (67) to an epoxide that is a substrate for numerous other enzymes, affording various mono-, di-, and trihydroxylated derivatives, plus their glucuronide and sulfate conjugates. Phenylmercapturic acid, benzoquinone, muconaldehyde, and muconic acid were also detected (68,69).

The myelotoxicity of BZ was reproduced by coadministration of two metabolites, phenol and hydroquinone (70–72), but others concluded that this combination alone did not account entirely for the effects of BZ (73). Another hypothesis has been that oxygen radicals, generated through certain BZ metabolites, induce DNA damage (74). BZ bound to the nucleic acids and protein of rat liver, although not at a high level, but in a dose-related fashion (75). Below certain levels BZ binding could not be detected (76). However, the specific BZ adducts and their effects on the function of cellular macromolecules have not been delineated (77).

Polycyclic Aromatic Hydrocarbons

This subject has been reviewed numerous times, and a summary of both the metabolic activation of the prototype benzo[a]pyrene (BaP) and its adducts with DNA has appeared (78). Initial oxidation of BaP led to the formation of two enantiomers of a 7,8-epoxide that could be converted to phenols, be substrates for glutathione transferase leading to mercapturic acids, or be altered by epoxide hydrolase to dihydrodiols, which also existed as enantiomers. Further oxidation afforded diastereomeric diol epoxides which had different DNA binding and tumorigenic properties and were not formed in equal amounts. The major adduct is the $trans-N^2$-deoxyguanosine adduct, but cis- and $trans-N^6$-deoxyadenosine adducts have also been detected (Fig. 1). The significant feature of activation of polycyclic aromatic hydrocarbons was that the second epoxide group was located in an angular bay region of the hydrocarbon, leading to the *bay region hypothesis* as summarized by Jerina and Daly and their associates (79). Subsequent work has demonstrated the viability of the hypothesis with other hydrocarbons besides BaP (80).

The bay region hypothesis has not stifled investigation of other metabolic systems for activation of BaP and analogs. One-electron oxidation through peroxidases such as prostaglandin H synthase or by a peroxyl radical from fatty acid hydroperoxides has been proposed (81). In addition, further oxidation of 7,8-dihydroxy-7,8-dihydro BaP to an epoxide via a hydroperoxide-dependent mechanism, catalyzed by lipoxygenases in the presence of arachidonic acid or unsaturated fatty acids, has been investigated (82). Although the bay region diol epoxide of BaP, accomplished through different oxidation steps with different forms of P450, appears to dominate activation of BaP, other possible activation modes should not be overlooked.

Aromatic Amines and Aminoazo Dyes

When the carcinogenicity of aromatic amines and aminoazo dyes was established in animal experiments, they appeared somewhat unusual, since with a few exceptions, they were not active at the site of application. This led to the premise that metabolites were responsible for the effects.

The model compound for many such investigations was 2-acetylaminofluorene (2-AAF). Originally proposed for insecticidal use, it was never used as a pesticide after toxicity studies showed that it caused numerous types of tumors in rats and mice. However, 2-AAF became a model compound for research purposes, and it has been the subject of several reviews (9,83). Initial oxidation reactions of these amines or amides are largely mediated by the P450 mixed-function oxidases. Other oxidation systems are the flavine-dependent enzymes, and peroxidases, especially the prostaglandin H synthase system, for which benzidine and 2-aminofluorene are good substrates. The prostaglandin system was also effective for activation of the carcinogenic heterocyclic amine, 2-amino-3-methylimidazo[4,5f]quinoline and its methyl derivative, formed in very small amounts during cooking of protein-rich foods, to N-hydroxy derivatives (84).

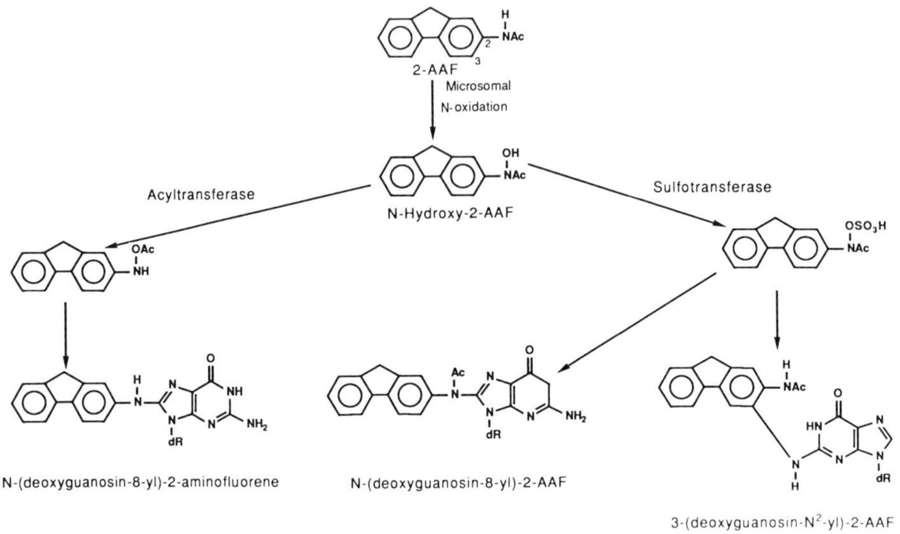

FIG. 2. Metabolic activation and DNA adducts of 2-acetylaminofluorene. [Reproduced with permission from Beland and Poirier (78).]

The ring-hydroxylated derivatives of 2-AAF were not carcinogenic, indicating that they were detoxication products. However, the N-hydroxy derivative was active, although further metabolic processes were necessary, including acylation or sulfation of the N-hydroxy group, through acyl- or sulfotransferase enzymes. The esters thus produced were highly reactive and readily formed DNA adducts, mainly at the C-8 of guanosine and to a lesser extent at other locations (Fig. 2) (8,78).

There are many complicating factors in these types of reactions, affording various minor products such as chloro derivatives of 2-AAF (85). Even the presence of albumin led to a decrease in guanosine binding and to formation of 1-, 3-, and 4-hydroxy derivatives of 2-AAF (86).

The detection of 4-aminobiphenyl (4-AB), a known bladder carcinogen, in tobacco smoke, has increased the efforts on the metabolic activation of 4-AB and related compounds. As with 2-AAF, N-oxidation, mediated through P450IA2, led to an oxidized product that formed an adduct with hemoglobin (87). Such adducts of 4-AB were readily detected in both smokers and nonsmokers, although levels were higher in smokers (88). The 4'-fluoro derivative of acetyl 4-AB was also activated by N-oxidation and sulfation (89), but an unusual product was formed with deoxyadenosine. Besides the expected 3-(deoxyadenosin-N^6-yl)-4'-fluoro-4-(acetylamino)biphenyl, a dearomatized adduct, 3-(deoxyadenosin-N^6yl)-4'-fluoro-4-(acetylimino)-3,4-dihydrobiphenyl, represented 3% to 6% of the total covalent binding (90). Similar products have not been reported from other aromatic amines.

Aminoazo dyes, exemplified by 4-dimethylaminoazobenzene, require an initial oxidative N-demethylation, accomplished by an amine oxidase of a flavine-dependent system, followed by N-hydroxylation and esterification as with aromatic amines. Concurrently, such dyes may be detoxified by ring hydroxylation, by glutathione conjugation, or by reductive splitting of the azo bond by the flavine-dependent enzyme, azo reductase. In mammals there is some azo reductase in the liver, but the intestinal bacteria are usually quite proficient at splitting azo dyes.

Historically, definitive binding of chemical carcinogens to cellular constituents, namely proteins, was first noted with aminoazo dyes (91). This finding eventually led to investigation of binding to the genetic material of the cell (92).

Nitrosamines

The dialkyl-N-nitrosamines are the most omnipotent of all carcinogens, for they have shown effects in more animal species than have other classes of carcinogens. P450 monooxygenases are involved in the activation of nitrosamines, and different forms may be effective with one nitrosamine but not another (93). Regardless of which P450 is involved, metabolic activation of nitrosamines proceeds through an unstable hydroxyalkylalkylnitrosamine that fragments spontaneously to an aldehyde and a nitrosoalkylamine. The latter intermediate rearranges to an alkyldiazonium hydroxide which dissociates to nitrogen and the activated alkyl carbocation which alkylates proteins and nucleic acids (8,78). The initial hydroxylation is the rate-limiting step in the process. Denitrosation and other competing reactions also occur to an appreciable extent (94).

Dialkylnitrosamines with longer carbon chains may be oxidized on other positions besides the one adjacent to the nitrosamine function. Dibutylnitrosamine (DBN) is converted to the 4-hydroxy derivative and then to a 4-carboxylic acid; both the compounds and the parent DBN are bladder carcinogens in rats. Additional oxidation reactions on intermediate carbons may yield various hydroxy and keto derivatives or shorten the carbon chain, analogous to fatty acid degradation. Nitrosamines derived from tobacco alkaloids have varied metabolic patterns since oxidation can occur on several positions, leading to many intermediate and end products. Some tobacco-derived nitrosamines are potent carcinogens (95).

Nitrosoureas do not require metabolism; at alkaline pH values they decompose spontaneously to afford the activated alkyl carbocation. In animals nitrosoureas have caused some unusual tumors. Some of these compounds are active transplacentally or affect organs or tissues not generally attacked by many other carcinogens.

Hydrazines, Azo and Azoxy Compounds, and Related Compounds

Hydrazine and its simpler derivatives are important industrial intermediates or rocket fuels, while the more complex hydrazines have been used medicinally or occur naturally in mushrooms. 1,2-Dimethylhydrazine (DHM) has long been used to induce intestinal tumors in rats and mice for various mechanistic studies. DMH is oxidized through microsomal oxidases to the carcinogen azomethane which on further oxidation affords azoxymethane, also an intestinal carcinogen. However, this is not the final stage; another oxidation step, mediated by P450IIE1 (96), leads to the relatively unstable methylazoxymethanol, which degrades to formaldehyde and methyldiazonium ion. The ion breaks down to nitrogen and an alkylating species, the methyl carbocation that forms nucleic acid adducts. Because of all the oxidation stages involved, selective inhibitors of these steps can be used to suppress tumor formation from DMH (97). Related to hydrazines are the carcinogenic dialkyltriazenes, which also appear to alkylate DNA via an alkyldiazonium ion (98).

Other Compounds

Under specific circumstances numerous other compounds may also be carcinogenic in animals. Urethane or ethyl carbamate causes lung tumors in mice and various types of tumors in infant rats. N-Hydroxylation is a metabolic reaction, but N-hydroxyurethane was not more active than urethane. However, a concept that urethane is dehydrogenated metabolically to vinyl carbamate, followed by epoxidation and attachment to DNA, has support in current experimental work (99).

Important industrial compounds that are carcinogenic in animals are acrylonitrile, acrylamide, and formaldehyde. Presumably, the first two are activated through epoxidation, yielding activated molecules that interact with DNA (100). Formaldehyde forms hydroxymethyl adducts on the exocyclic amino groups of deoxyguanosine, deoxycytidine, deoxyadenosine, and thymidine. In the affected area, the nasal mucosa, it formed DNA-protein cross-links (101). Model studies with monkeys suggested that the rate of formation of the complexes was lower than in rats, and that in humans the rate would be even less (102).

In the environment there are numerous naturally occurring carcinogens (103). The one with the most impact is aflatoxin B_1, a carcinogenic metabolite of the fungus *Aspergillus flavus*. Aflatoxin B_1 is also activated by epoxidation through a P450, across the double bond of its terminal furan ring. Although this epoxide has been prepared synthetically only within the past few years (104), previous investigation of the structures of the nucleic acid adducts and the hydrolysis products led to the premise that epoxidation was involved. The more readily available dichloride of aflatoxin B_1 has been used as a surrogate to study binding to nucleic acids (105), although the epoxide and dichloride have different properties chemically.

Safrole and estragole, which are structurally related, are natural products that have shown carcinogenic effects; both are hydroxylated on the propenyl side chain, followed by esterification with sulfate or acetate to yield reactive intermediates. These formed DNA adducts and appeared to account for the action of the parent compounds. Still other natural products, the pyrrolizidine alkaloids, occurring in plants such as comfrey, coltsfoot, and ragworts, are both toxic and carcinogenic to the liver. They are activated by dehydrogenation to reactive pyrrolic compounds that form carbonium-type electrophiles, capable of DNA reactions. The remainder of the alkaloid molecule was oxidized to reactive aldehydes which also formed adducts with deoxyguanosine. Another carcinogenic natural product is ptaquiloside, a norsesquiterpene glucoside from the bracken fern. Despite the carcinogenic effects of bracken demonstrated in both farm and laboratory animals, the fiddleheads of bracken are eaten as a spring vegetable in some countries (106). However, no mechanistic studies on ptaquiloside have appeared.

INORGANIC CARCINOGENS

Inorganic substances considered as carcinogens include arsenic and its compounds, asbestos and the related erionite, hexavalent chromium, and nickel. Although beryllium, cadmium, lead, and silica have also shown carcinogenic effects in animals, the evidence for such action in humans is less substantial (107).

Arsenic and Compounds

Arsenic occurs naturally, generally at low levels, but more significant levels are found in marine organisms as arsenorganic compounds. Occupational, extended medicinal use, or drinking water with high levels of arsenic have been the factors associated with increased risk of lung or skin cancer (108). Trivalent arsenic appears to be the toxic form and in this state does affect DNA synthesis and repair (109). In addition, arsenic caused amplification of the dihydrofolate reductase gene in mouse 3T6 cells, which may tie arsenic to protooncogene activation (110). Arsenic, in some form, is also considered an essential trace element (111). Consumption of seafood containing the organic forms of arsenic carries negligible risk (112).

Asbestos and Erionite

Asbestos and erionite are natural fibrous silicates. Commerically used forms of asbestos are chrysotile, anthophyllite, amosite, and crocidolite. Erionite occurs as a volcanic tuff in certain areas of Turkey, where it was used as building material, and it may also contaminate zeolite beds in other parts of the world. Long, thin fibers (>4 μm long; <0.25 μm in diameter) are much more active than thick fibers as inducers of bronchogenic carcinomas and mesotheliomas in exposed persons. The risk was multiplicative in asbestos workers who smoked (107).

Multiple mechanisms may be involved in the carcinogenicity of asbestos, for it induced chromosomal mutations in cells in culture but was inactive as a gene mutagen (113). Asbestos is a cocarcinogen and tumor promoter (114). There are data supporting a hypothesis that asbestos acts by generation of active oxygen species ($OH^.$ and O_2^-) which lead to lipid peroxidation and DNA strand breakage (115).

Chromium

On an epidemiological basis the carcinogenicity of chromium compounds is associated with the slightly soluble chromates (Cr^{6+}), while insoluble and very soluble salts of chromic acid or trivalent forms showed little or no carcinogenicity (107). When Cr^{6+} enters the cell several systems, such as P450, DT diaphorase, ascorbate, thiols, aldehyde oxidase, glutathione, and cysteine, all convert it to lower-valence states. The compounds thus formed caused DNA damage in the form of DNA interstrand cross-links, DNA-protein cross-links, and DNA strand breaks. These lesions led to changes in certain targeted genes (116). As is the situation with certain other elements, chromium is also an essential micronutrient in humans, being necessary for the metabolism of sugar and fats (117).

Nickel

Several epidemiological studies implicated nickel refining as a risk factor for cancers of the nasal cavity, lung, and possibly larynx (107). Further studies have pointed toward nickel subsulfide as an active material. However, by intramuscular injection, most forms of nickel produced local sarcomas in animals. The exact means by which nickel acts as a carcinogen have not been delineated, but it may act through lipid peroxidation, by inhibiting DNA replication and transcription, or by altering the conformational structure of DNA (118). Despite the carcinogenicity of certain forms of nickel, at low levels it is an essential micronutrient for both plants, where it is a component of the P450 system (119), and for mammals (118).

MODIFYING FACTORS

Current research in carcinogenesis has emphasized the processes by which carcinogens act, the stages in the process, the factors that enhance or suppress the effects of carcinogens, and how chemical carcinogenesis relates to biological factors in the target organism. The spotlight is not so much on the animal as on the molecular processes involved (120).

Initiation–Promotion–Progression

The phenomenon now known as initiation–promotion was discovered during experiments on mouse skin carcinogenesis with PAHs. A dose of PAH (initiator) so low that no tumors developed during the lifetime of the animal was applied; this initiation process was followed by regular periodic applications, usually twice weekly, of a solution of croton oil or resin (promoter), resulting in numerous tumors. Even a delay of one year before application of the promoter led to as many tumors as if the croton oil were applied a week or two after the initiator (121). Systematic investigation of these events led to the opinion that the initiator produces an irreversible and rapid but permanent change in the cell genome while the promoter affects gene expression and causes clonal expansion of the initiated cells, leading to hyperplasia. However, a promoter is essentially noncarcinogenic, does not bind to DNA, and is not mutagenic.

Many fractionation studies demonstrated that the active material in croton oil is tetradecanoylphorbol-13-acetate (TPA), but other natural products which are promoters are mezerein, okadaic acid, teleocidin, lyngbyatoxin, and others (122). Simpler compounds, such as phenol, dodecane, and anthralin, have also acted as promoters. In contrast to promoters, cocarcinogens are not active alone, but they enhance the action of a carcinogen when applied concurrently with the carcinogen; ethanol is an example, both experimentally (123) and in humans.

The phorbol esters act through specific receptors, specifically the calcium- and phospholipid-dependent protein kinase (protein kinase C) (124,125). Other substances with tumor-promoting activity (chlordane, kepone, heptachlor, lindane) also stimulated protein kinase C, with an effect comparable to that of TPA (126). The initiation–promotion concept has been applied to other organ systems, including liver, mammary gland, respiratory tract, colon, thyroid, and pancreas (121).

After initiation and the action of the promoter, the cell also undergoes progression, a stepwise process whereby the initiated cell evolves into a cancer (127–129). The actual mechanism by which the initiated cell converts to a neoplastic one is not known, but the loss of genes at specific chromosomal loci has been observed in several neoplasms. Although the three stages of initiation, promotion, and progression are well recognized, there have been hypotheses that many more stages are recognizable in the process of neoplastic development (130).

Inhibition–Prevention

Inhibition of carcinogenesis was noted during relatively early experiments in which sulfur mustard decreased the effect of tar on mouse skin (131). There was no continued systematic investigation of inhibition, although numerous reports showed such an effect under specific conditions. As examples, simpler structural analogs of PAHs (132), of 4-dimethylaminoazobenzene (133), or of 2-AAF (134) could decrease the effects of these carcinogens. Ablation of an endocrine organ, either surgically (135) or chemically (136), was also effective. Administration of toxic substances (copper salts) (137) or cytotoxic materials as actinomycin D (138) were investigated. Some of these results have been summarized in a review (139).

In retrospect, the inhibition of some carcinogens by simpler analogs may have been due to competition for receptor sites. Some of the toxic substances may have inhibited cell growth; endocrine ablation might have altered metabolic activation. More systematic examination of cancer inhibition has centered on the stage where the inhibitors act (17). Thus some prevent the formation of carcinogens from precursors, especially the nitrosamines; examples are ascorbic acid, propyl gallate, and tocopherols. Antioxidants may prevent the formation of toxic and carcinogenic substances, particularly from the fats in foodstuffs (140). Other inhibitors block the carcinogen from reaching the target site; many of these are relatively simple substances that occur in ordinary foods and beverages (17). Other substances may block the metabolic formation of the ultimate carcinogen by acting in specific steps of the pathway; others may induce enzymes involved in detoxication of the carcinogen, as do flavones and phenobarbital. Some inhibitors scavenge the activated forms of carcinogens. The variety of materials having such capabilities is large, with no single mechanism of action. For example, protease inhibitors, retinoids, selenium salts, citrus oils, tannic acid and its constituents, and allyl sulfides from garlic have shown activity against carcinogens of different structural classes (141–145). An isothiocyanate found in vegetables inhibited the potent nicotine-derived nitrosamine that occurs in tobacco smoke (146), as did citrus oils (143). There has been a great deal of experimental work on inhibition and prevention of cancer (147). The extrapolation to human use may be difficult.

Convergence of Chemical and Biological Carcinogenesis

Research on carcinogenesis has evolved from several aspects. The chemical related factor was involved in identifying carcinogens in the environment, in determining their effects in animal models, and in delineating the metabolic aspects of the process. From a biological viewpoint there was emphasis on the cellular processes controlling growth and related events. Some of this early research was on acute transforming or retroviruses which led rapidly to sarcomas in inoculated animals, especially chickens; the viruses contained additional genetic material which was originally derived from the host species and had become incorporated or transduced into the virus. This material was called an oncogene, and the normal cellular genetic material from which it was derived was considered a protooncogene (148). These genes occur in mammalian cells and function in regulatory mechanisms related to growth factors, to protein kinases, to regulatory proteins that bind phosphorylated guanosine, or to intranuclear or DNA-binding regulatory proteins (149).

The cellular protooncogenes may be activated to oncogenes by several mechanisms, including retroviral insertion, mutations, gene amplification, and chromosomal translocation (150). Point mutations, especially, and gene amplification may be induced by the action of chemical carcinogens, leading to activation of the cellular protooncogenes. Although the H- and K-*ras* (Harvey or Kirsten rat sarcoma) oncogenes were among the earliest to be identified (151), other oncogenes have been detected in rodent tumors, whether induced by chemical carcinogens (152–156) or of spontaneous origin (157).

The technological advances of recent years have facilitated delineation of the exact coding region where changes induced by chemical carcinogens, with subsequent activation of oncogenes, may occur (149). In addition to oncogenes, research has also stressed the presence of antioncogenes or tumor suppressor genes in the normal cell. These genes usually prevent the formation of tumors, but if they are mutated or otherwise altered, these genes are inactivated, allowing growth of the tumor (158,159). Thus chemical carcinogenesis may represent an intricate interplay between the genetic factors discussed and an activated moiety from the carcinogen.

REFERENCES

1. Shimkin MB. *Contrary to nature.* Washington, DC: US Department of Health, Education and Welfare; 1977.
2. Wagoner JK, Archer VE, Carroll BE, Holaday DA, Lawrence PA. Cancer mortality patterns among U.S. uranium miners and millers, 1950 through 1962. *J Natl Cancer Inst* 1964;32:787–801.
3. Stasik MJ. Carcinomas of the urinary bladder in a 4-chloro-*o*-toluidine cohort. *Int Arch Occup Environ Health* 1988;60:21–24.
4. Ward E, Carpenter A, Markowitz S, Roberts D, Halperin W. Excess number of bladder cancers in workers exposed to *ortho*-toluidine and aniline. *J Natl Cancer Inst* 1991;83:501–506.
5. Conzelman GM Jr, Moulton JE, Flanders LE III, Springer K, Crout DW. Induction of transitional cell carcinomas of the urinary bladder in monkeys fed 2-naphthylamine. *J Natl Cancer Inst* 1969; 42:825–836.
6. Huff JE, Haseman JK, DeMarini DM, et al. Multiple-site carcinogenicity of benzene in Fischer 344 rats and B6C3F1 mice. *Environ Health Perspect* 1989;82:125–163.
7. Weisburger EK. Mechanistic considerations in chemical carcinogenesis. *Regul Toxicol Pharmacol* 1990;12:41–52.
8. Weisburger EK. Chemical carcinogenesis in experimental animals and humans. In: Sirica AE, ed. *The pathobiology of neoplasia.* New York: Plenum Press; 1989:39–56.
9. Weisburger JH, Weisburger EK. Biochemical formation and pharmacological, toxicological, and pathological properties of hydroxylamines and hydroxamic acids. *Pharmacol Rev* 1973;25:1–66.
10. Thorgeirsson SS, Nebert DW. The Ah locus and the metabolism of chemical carcinogens and other foreign compounds. *Adv Cancer Res* 1977;25:149–193.
11. Glowinski IB, Weber WW. Genetic regulation of aromatic amine N-acetylation in inbred mice. *J Biol Chem* 1982;257:1424–1430.
12. Weber WW, Hein DW. N-Acetylation pharmacogenetics. *Pharmacol Rev* 1985;37:27–79.
13. Irving CC, Janss DH, Russell LT. Lack of *N*-hydroxy-2-acetylaminofluorene sulfotransferase activity in the mammary gland and Zymbal's gland of the rat. *Cancer Res* 1971;31:387–391.
14. Birt DF. The influence of dietary fat on carcinogenesis: lessons from experimental models. *Nutr Rev* 1990;48:1–5.
15. Cohen LA, Choi K, Wang C-X. Influence of dietary fat, caloric restriction, and voluntary exercise on *N*-nitrosomethylurea-induced mammary tumorigenesis in rats. *Cancer Res* 1988;48:4276–4283.
16. DiGiovanni J, Berry DL, Juchau MR, Slaga TJ. 2,3,7,8-Tetrachlorodibenzo-*p*-dioxin: potent anticarcinogenic activity in CD-1 mice. *Biochem Biophys Res Commun* 1979;86:577–584.
17. Wattenberg LW. Chemoprevention of cancer. *Cancer Res* 1985;45:1–8.
18. Nebert DW, Adesnik M, Coon MJ, et al. The P450 supergene family: recommended nomenclature. *DNA* 1987;6:1–11.
19. Nebert DW, Nelson DR, Adesnik M, et al. The P450 superfamily: updated listing of all genes and recommended nomenclature for the chromosomal loci. *DNA* 1989;8:1–13.
20. Nebert DW, Nelson DR, Coon MJ, et al. The P450 superfamily: update on new sequences, gene mapping and recommended nomenclature. *DNA Cell Biol* 1991;10:1–14.
21. Goel SK, Lalwani ND, Reddy JK. Peroxisome proliferation and lipid peroxidation in rat liver cancer. *Cancer Res* 1986;46:1324–1330.
22. Flamm WG, Lehman-McKeeman LD. The human relevance of the renal tumor-inducing potential of *d*-limonene in male rats: implications for risk assessment. *Regul Toxicol Pharmacol* 1991; 13:70–86.
23. Short BG, Burnett VL, Swenberg JA. Elevated proliferation of proximal tubule cells and localization of accumulated α_{2u}-globulin in F344 rats during chronic exposure to unleaded gasoline or 2,2,4-trimethylpentane. *Toxicol Appl Pharmacol* 1989;101:414–431.
24. Lijinsky W, Muschik GM. Distribution of the liver carcinogen methapyrilene in Fischer rats and its interaction with macromolecules. *J Cancer Res Clin Oncol* 1982;103:69–73.
25. Clayson DB. Bladder carcinogenesis in rats and mice: possibility of artifacts. *J Natl Cancer Inst* 1974;52:1685–1689.
26. Hoyt SD, Rasmussen RA. Determining trace gases in air and seawater. *Adv Chem Ser* 1985; 209:31–56.
27. Bull RJ, Meier JR, Robinson M, Ringhand HP, Laurie RD, Stober JA. Evaluation of mutagenic

and carcinogenic properties of brominated and chlorinated acetonitriles: by-products of chlorination. *Fundam Appl Toxicol* 1985;5:1065–1074.
28. Guengerich FP. Reactions and significance of cytochrome P-450 enzymes. *J Biol Chem* 1991; 226:10019–10022.
29. Guengerich FP, Kine D-H, Iwasaki MI. Role of human cytochrome P-450IIE1 in the oxidation of many low molecular weight cancer suspects. *Chem Res Toxicol* 1991;4:168–179.
30. Ottenwalder H, Jager R, Thier R, Bolt HM. Influence of P-450 inhibitors on the inhalative uptake of methyl chloride and methylene chloride in male B6C3F1 mice. *Arch Toxicol* [Suppl] 1989; 13:258–261.
31. Reitz RH, Mendrala AL, Guengerich FP. *In vitro* metabolism of methylene chloride in human and animal tissue: use in physiologically based pharmacokinetic models. *Toxicol Appl Pharmacol* 1989;97:230–246.
32. Lefevre PA, Ashby J. Evaluation of dichloromethane as an inducer of DNA synthesis in the $B_6C_3F_1$ mouse liver. *Carcinogenesis* 1989;10:1067–1072.
33. Letteron P, Degott C, Labbe G, Larrey D, Descatoire V, Tinel M, Pessayre D. Methoxsalen decreases the metabolic activation and prevents the hepatotoxicity and nephrotoxicity of chloroform in mice. *Toxicol Appl Pharmacol* 1987;91:266–273.
34. Reinke LA, Janzen EG. Detection of spin adducts in blood after administration of carbon tetrachloride to rats. *Chem Biol Interact* 1991;78:155–165.
35. Connor HD, La Cagnin CB, Knecht KT, Thurman RG, Mason RP. Reaction of glutathione with a free radical metabolite of carbon tetrachloride. *Mol Pharmacol* 1990;37:443–451.
36. Bartsch H, Mallaveille C, Barbin A, Planche G. Mutagenic and alkylating metabolites of haloethylenes, chlorobutadienes and dichlorobutenes produced by rodent or human liver tissues. Evidence for oxirane formation by P450-linked microsomal mono-oxygenases. *Arch Toxicol* 1979; 41:249–277.
37. Green T, Hathaway DE. Interactions of vinyl chloride with rat liver DNA *in vivo*. *Chem Biol Interact* 1978;22:211–224.
38. Fedtke N, Boucheron JA, Turner MJ Jr, Swenberg JA. Vinyl chloride-induced DNA adducts. I. Quantitative determination of N^2,3-ethenoguanine based on electrophore labeling. *Carcinogenesis* 1990;11:1279–1285.
39. Fedtke N, Boucheron JA, Walker VE, Swenberg JA. Vinyl chloride–induced DNA adducts. II. Formation and persistence of 7-(2′-oxyethyl)guanine and N^2,3-ethenoguanine in rat tissue DNA. *Carcinogenesis* 1990;11:1287–1292.
40. Lindahl T. DNA repair enzymes. *Annu Rev Biochem* 1982;51:61–87.
41. Dresler SL. DNA repair mechanisms and carcinogenesis. In: Sirica AE, ed. *The pathobiology of neoplasia*. New York: Plenum Press; 1989:173–197.
42. Miller R, Guengerich FP. Oxidation of TCE by liver microsomal cytochrome P-450: evidence of chlorine migration in a transient state not involving trichloroethylene oxide. *Biochemistry* 1982; 21:1090–1097.
43. Green T, Prout S. Species differences in response to trichloroethylene. II. Biotransformation in rats and mice. *Toxicol Appl Pharmacol* 1985;79:401–411.
44. Fisher, JW, Gargas ML, Allen BC, Andersen ME. Physiologically based pharmokinetic modeling with trichloroethylene and its metabolite, trichloroacetic acid, in the rat and mouse. *Toxicol Appl Pharmacol* 1991;109:183–195.
45. Nilsson R, Beije B, Preat V, Erixon K, Ramel C. On the mechanism of the hepatocarcinogenicity of peroxisome proliferators. *Chem Biol Interact* 1991;78:235–250.
46. Herren-Freund SL, Pereira M, Khoury MD, Olson G. The carcinogenicity of trichloroethylene and its metabolites, trichloroacetic acid and dichloroacetic acid, in mouse liver. *Toxicol Appl Pharmacol* 1987;90:183–189.
47. Bruckner JV, Davis DB, Blancato JN. Metabolism, toxicity, and carcinogenicity of trichloroethylene. *Crit Rev Toxicol* 1989;20:31–50.
48. NCI. *Carcinogenesis bioassay of trichloroethylene*. CAS 79-01-6, DHEW publication (NIH) 76-802. Bethesda, MD: National Cancer Institute; 1976.
49. NTP. *Carcinogenesis bioassay of trichloroethylene*.CAS 79-01-6, NIH publication 82-176. Research Triangle Park, NC: National Toxicology Program; 1982.
50. Dekant W, Metzler M, Henschler D. Identification of S-1,2,2-trichlorovinyl-N-acetylcysteine as a urinary metabolite of tetrachloroethylene: bioactivation through glutathione conjugation as a possible explanation of its nephrotoxicity. *J Biochem Toxicol* 1986;1:57–72.

51. Lock EA. Studies on the mechanisms of nephrotoxicity and nephrocarcinogenicity of halogenated alkenes. *Crit Rev Toxicol* 1988;19:23–43.
52. Weisburger EK. Carcinogenicity studies on halogenated hydrocarbons. *Environ Health Perspect* 1977;21:7–16.
53. NTP. *Carcinogenesis bioassay of 1,2-dibromoethane (CAS no 106-93-4) in F344 rats and B6C3F₁ mice (inhalation study)*. Technical Report Series 210; Research Triangle Park, NC: National Toxicology Program; 1982.
54. Cheever KL, Cholakis JM, El-Hawari AM, Kovatch RM, Weisburger EK. Ethylene dichloride: the influence of disulfiram or ethanol on oncogenicity, metabolism, and DNA covalent binding in rats. *Fundam Appl Toxicol* 1990;14:243–261.
55. Hill DL, Shih T-W, Johnston TP, Struck RF. Macromolecular binding and metabolism of the carcinogen 1,2-dibromoethane. *Cancer Res* 1978;38:2438–2442.
56. Koga N, Inskeep PB, Harris TM, Guengerich FP. S- [2-(N^7-Guanyl)ethyl]glutathione, the major DNA adduct formed from 1,2-dibromoethane. *Biochemistry* 1986;25:2192–2198.
57. Foureman GL, Reed DJ. Formation of S-[2-(N^7-guanyl)ethyl] adducts by the postulated S-(2-chloroethyl)cysteinyl and S-(2-chloroethyl)glutathionyl conjugates of 1,2-dichloroethane. *Biochemistry* 1987;26:2028–2033.
58. Brittebo EB, Kowalski B, Ghantous H, Brandt I. Epithelial binding of 1,2-dichloroethane in mice. *Toxicology* 1989;56:35–45.
59. Kluwe WM, Gupta BN, Lamb JC. The comparative effects of 1,2-dibromo-3-chloropropane (DBCP) and its metabolite, 3-chloro-1,2-propane oxide (epichlorohydrin), 3-chloro-1,2-propanediol (α-chlorohydrin), and oxalic acid, on the urogenital system of male rats. *Toxicol Appl Pharmacol* 1983;70:67–86.
60. Gingell R, Beatty PW, Mitschke HR, Mueller RL, Sawin VL, Page AC. Evidence that epichlorohydrin is not a toxic metabolite of 1,2-dibromo-3-chloropropane. *Xenobiotica* 1987;17:229–240.
61. Gingell R, Beatty PW, Mitschke HR, Page AC, Sawin VL, Putcha L, Kramer WG. Toxicokinetics of 1,2-dibromo-3-chloropropane (DBCP) in the rat. *Toxicol Appl Pharmacol* 1987;91:386–394.
62. Omichinski JG, Soderlund EJ, Dybing E, Pearson PG, Nelson SD. Detection and mechanism of the potent direct-acting mutagen 2-bromoacrolein from 1,2-dibromo-3-chloropropane. *Toxicol Appl Pharmacol* 1988;92:286–294.
63. Meerman JHN, Smith TR, Pearson PG, Meier GP, Nelson SD. Formation of cyclic 1,N^2-propanodeoxyguanosine and thymidine adducts in the reaction of the mutagen 2-bromoacrolein with calf thymus DNA. *Cancer Res* 1989;49:6174–6179.
64. Quast JF, Calhoun LL, Frauson LE. 1,1,1-Trichloroethane formulation: a chronic inhalation toxicity and oncogenicity study in Fischer 344 rats and B6C3F1 mice. *Fundam Appl Toxicol* 1989; 11:611–625.
65. Anders MW, Lash L, Dekant W, Elfarra AA, Dohn DR. Biosynthesis and biotransformation of glutathione S-conjugates to toxic metabolites. *Crit Rev Toxicol* 1988;18:299–309.
66. Maltoni C, Cilibert A, Cotti G, Conti B, Belpoggi F. Benzene, an experimental multipotential carcinogen: results of the long-term bioassays performed at the Bologna Institute of Oncology. *Environ Health Perspect* 1989;82:109–124.
67. Koop DR, Laethem CL, Schnier GG. Identification of ethanol-inducible P450 isozyme 3a (P450IIE1) as a benzene and phenol hydroxylase. *Toxicol Appl Pharmacol* 1989;98:278–288.
68. Sabourin PJ, Bechtold WE, Birnbaum LS, Lucier G, Henderson RF. Differences in the metabolism of inhaled ^{3}H-benzene by F344/N rats and B6C3F1 mice. *Toxicol Appl Pharmacol* 1988;94:128–140.
69. Travis CC, Quillen JL, Arms AD. Pharmacokinetics of benzene. *Toxicol Appl Pharmacol* 1990; 102:400–420.
70. Eastmond DA, Smith MT, Irons RD. An interaction of benzene metabolites reproduces the myelotoxicity observed with benzene exposure. *Toxicol Appl Pharmacol* 1987;91:85–95.
71. Smith MT, Yager JW, Steinmetz KL, Eastmond DA. Peroxidase-dependent metabolism of benzene's phenolic metabolites and its potential role in benzene toxicity and carcinogenicity. *Environ Health Perspect* 1989;82:23–29.
72. Snyder R, Dimitriadis E, Guy R, et al. Studies on the mechanism of benzene toxicity. *Environ Health Perspect* 1989;82:31–35.
73. Bois FY, Smith MT, Spear RC. Mechanisms of benzene carcinogenesis: application of a physiological model of benzene pharmacokinetics and metabolism. *Toxicol Lett* 1991;56:283–298.

74. Lewis JG, Stewart W, Adams DO. Role of oxygen radicals in induction of DNA damage by metabolites of benzene. *Cancer Res* 1988;48:4762–4765.
75. Lutz WK, Schlatter C. Mechanism of the carcinogenic action of benzene: irreversible binding to rat liver DNA. *Chem Biol Interact* 1977;18:241–245.
76. Mazzullo M, Bartoli S, Bonora B, et al. Benzene adducts with rat nucleic acids and proteins: dose-response relationships after treatment in vivo. *Environ Health Perspect* 1989;82:259–266.
77. Kalf GF. Recent advances in the metabolism and toxicity of benzene. *Crit Rev Toxicol* 1987; 18:141–159.
78. Beland FA, Poirier MC. DNA adducts and carcinogenesis. In: Sirica AE, ed. *The pathobiology of neoplasia*. New York: Plenum Press; 1989:57–80.
79. Wood AW, Chang RL, Levin W, et al. Mutagenicity and cytotoxicity of benz[a]anthracene diol epoxides and tetrahydro-epoxides: exceptional activity of the bay region 1,2-epoxide. *Proc Natl Acad Sci USA* 1977;74:2746–2750.
80. Dipple A, Moschel RC, Bigger CAH. Polynuclear aromatic carcinogens. In: Searle CE, ed. *Chemical carcinogens*. 2nd ed. Washington, DC: American Chemical Society; 1984:41–163.
81. Marnett LJ. Hydroperoxide-dependent oxygenation of polycyclic aromatic hydrocarbons and their metabolites. In: Harvey RG, ed. *Polycyclic hydrocarbons and carcinogenesis*. Washington, DC: American Chemical Society; 1985:307–326.
82. Hughes, MF, Chamulitrat W, Mason RP, Eling TE. Expoxidation of 7,8-dihydroxy-7,8-dihydrobenz[a]pyrene via a hydroperoxide-dependent mechanism catalyzed by lipoxygenases. *Carcinogenesis* 1989;10:2075–2080.
83. Weisburger EK. N-2-Fluorenylacetamide and derivatives. In: Sontag JM, ed. *Carcinogens in industry and the environment*. New York: Marcel Dekker; 1981:583–666.
84. Petry TW, Josephy PD, Pagano DA, Zeiger E, Knecht KT, Eling TE. Prostaglandin hydroperoxidase-dependent activation of heterocyclic aromatic amines. *Carcinogenesis* 1989;10:2201–2207.
85. Panda M, Novak M, Magonski J. Hydrolysis kinetics of the ultimate hepatocarcinogen N-(sulfonatooxy)-2-(acetylamino)fluorene: detection of long-lived hydrolysis intermediates. *J Am Chem Soc* 1989;111:4524–4525.
86. Kolanczyk RC, Rutko IR, Gutmann HR. The catalytic effect of bovine serum albumin on the ortho rearrangement of the potential ultimate carcinogen, N-(sulfooxy)-2-(acetylamino)fluorene, generated enzymatically from N-hydroxy-2-(acetylamino)fluorene and evidence for substrate specificity of the enzymatic sulfonation of arylhydroxamic acids. *Chem Res Toxicol* 1991;4:187–194.
87. Hammons GJ, Dooley KL, Kadlubar FF. 4-Aminobiphenyl-hemoglobin adduct formation as an index of in vivo N-oxidation by hepatic cytochrome P-450IA2. *Chem Res Toxicol* 1991;4:144–147.
88. Coghlin J, Gann PH, Hammond SK, Skipper PL, Taghizadeh K, Paul M, Tannenbaum SR. 4-Aminobiphenyl hemoglobin adducts in fetuses exposed to the tobacco smoke carcinogen in utero. *J Natl Cancer Inst* 1991;83:274–280.
89. van de Poll MLM, Tijdens RB, Vondracek P, Bruins AP, Meijer DKF, Meerman JHN. The role of sulfation in the metabolic activation of N-hydroxy-4'-fluoro-4-acetylaminobiphenyl. *Carcinogenesis* 1989;10:2285–2291.
90. van de Poll MLM, Venizelos V, Niessen WMA, Meerman JHN. An unusual dearomatized adduct formed by reaction of 4'-fluoro-4-(acetylamino)biphenyl N-sulfate with deoxyadenosine. *Chem Res Toxicol* 1991;4:318–323.
91. Miller EC, Miller JA. The presence and significance of bound aminoazo dyes in the livers of rats fed p-dimethylaminoazobenzene. *Cancer Res* 1947;7:468–480.
92. Miller EC, Miller JA. Mechanisms of chemical carcinogenesis. Nature of proximate carcinogens and interactions with macromolecules. *Pharmacol Rev* 1966;18:805–838.
93. Crespi CL, Penman BW, Leakey JAE, et al. Human cytochrome P450IIA3: cDNA sequence, role of the enzyme in the metabolic activation of promutagens, comparison to nitrosamine activation by human cytochrome P450IIE1. *Carcinogenesis* 1990;11:1293–1300.
94. Streeter AJ, Nims RW, Sheffels PR, et al. Metabolic denitrosation of N-nitrosodimethylamine in vivo in the rat. *Cancer Res* 1990;50:1144–1150.
95. Hoffmann D, Rivenson A, Chung F-L, Hecht SS. Nicotine derived N-nitrosamines (TSNA) and their relevance in tobacco carcinogenesis. *Crit Rev Toxicol* 1991;21:305–311.
96. Sohn OS, Ishizaki H, Yang CS, Fiala ES. Metabolism of azoxymethane, methylazoxymethanol and N-nitrosodimethylamine by cytochrome P450IIE1. *Carcinogenesis* 1991;12:127–131.
97. McLellan E, Bird RP. Effect of disulfiram on 1,2-dimethylhydrazine- and azoxymethane-induced aberrant crypt foci. *Carcinogenesis* 1991;12:969–972.

98. Kroeger-Koepke MB, Smith RH Jr, Goodnow EA, et al. 1,3-Dialkyltriazenes: reactive intermediates and DNA alkylation. *Chem Res Toxicol* 1991;4:334–340.
99. Leithauser MT, Liem A, Stewart BC, Miller EC, Miller JA. 1,N^6-Ethenoadenosine formation, mutagenicity and murine tumor induction as indicators of the generation of an electrophile epoxide metabolite of the closely related carcinogens ethyl carbamate (urethane) and vinyl carbamate. *Carcinogenesis* 1991;11:463–473, 1250.
100. Roberts AE, Kedderis GL, Turner MJ, Rickert DE, Swenberg JA. Species comparison of acrylonitrile epoxidation by microsomes from mice, rats and humans: relationship to epoxide concentrations in mouse and rat blood. *Carcinogenesis* 1991;12:401–404.
101. Heck Hd'A, Casanova M, Starr TB. Formaldehyde toxicity: new understanding. *Crit Rev Toxicol* 1990;20:397–426.
102. Casanova M, Morgan KT, Steinhagen WH, Everitt JI, Popp JA, Heck Hd'A. Covalent binding of inhaled formaldehyde to DNA in the respiratory tract of rhesus monkeys: pharmacokinetics, rat-to-monkey interspecies scaling, and extrapolation to man. *Fundam Appl Toxicol* 1991;17:409–428.
103. Weisburger EK. Carcinogenic natural products in the environment. In: Mehlman MA, ed. *Safety evaluation: toxicology, methods, concepts and risk assessment*. Princeton, NJ: Princeton Scientific; 1987: 243–266.
104. Baertsche SW, Raney KD, Stone MP, Harris TM. Preparation of the 8,9-epoxide of the mycotoxin aflatoxin B_1: the ultimate carcinogenic species. *J Am Chem Soc* 1988;110:7929–7931.
105. Lee F-L, Huang J-X, Bender W, Wu Z, Chang JCS. Evidence for the covalent binding of aflatoxin B_1-dichloride to cytosine in DNA. *Carcinogenesis* 1991;12:997–1002.
106. Hirono I. Carcinogenic principles isolated from bracken fern. *Crit Rev Toxicol* 1986;17:1–22.
107. IARC. *IARC monographs on the evaluation of carcinogenic risks to humans* [Suppl 7]. Lyon, France: International Agency for Research on Cancer; 1987.
108. IARC. *IARC monographs on the evaluation of the carcinogenic risk of chemicals to humans*. Vol 23. *Some metals and metallic compounds*. Lyon, France: International Agency for Research on Cancer; 1980.
109. Leonard A, Lauwerys RR. Carcinogenicity, teratogenicity and mutagenicity of arsenic. *Mutat Res* 1980;75:49–62.
110. Lee T-C, Tanaka N, Lamb PW, Gilmer TM, Barrett JC. Induction of gene amplification by arsenic. *Science* 1988;241:79–81.
111. Nielsen FH. Possible future implications of ultratrace elements in human health and disease. In: Prasad AS, ed. *Essential and toxic trace elements in human health and disease*, New York: Alan R Liss; 1988:277–292.
112. Sabbioni E, Fischbach M, Pozzi G, Pietra R, Gallorini M, Piette JL. Cellular retention, toxicity and carcinogenic potential of seafood arsenic. I. Lack of cytotoxicity and transforming potential of arsenobetaine in the BALB/3T3 cell line. *Carcinogenesis* 1991;12:1287–1291.
113. Barrett JC, Lamb PW, Wiseman RW. Multiple mechanisms for the carcinogenic effects of asbestos and other mineral fibers. *Environ Health Perspect* 1989;81:81–89.
114. Cameron G, Woodworth CD, Edmondson S, Mossman BT. Mechanisms of asbestos-induced squamous metaplasia in tracheobronchial epithelial cells. *Environ Health Perspect* 1989;80:101–108.
115. Mossman BT, Marsh JP. Evidence supporting a role for active oxygen species in asbestos-induced toxicity and lung disease. *Environ Health Perspect* 1989;81:91–94.
116. Wetterhahn KE, Hamilton JW. Molecular basis for hexavalent chromium carcinogenicity: effect on gene expression. *Sci Total Environ* 1989;86:113–129.
117. Anderson RA. Essentiality of chromium in humans. *Sci Total Environ* 1989;86:75–81.
118. Coogan TP, Latta DM, Snow ET, Costa M. Toxicity and carcinogenicity of nickel compounds. *Crit Rev Toxicol* 1989;19:341–384.
119. Eskew DL, Welch RM, Cary EE. Nickel: an essential micronutrient for legumes and possibly all higher plants. *Science* 1983;222:621–623.
120. Yuspa SH, Poirier MC. Chemical carcinogenesis: from animal models to molecular models in one decade. *Adv Cancer Res* 1988;50:25–70.
121. Peraino C, Jones CA. The multistage concept of carcinogenesis. In: Sirica AE, ed. *The pathobiology of neoplasia*. New York: Plenum Press; 1989:131–148.
122. Fujiki H, Sugimura T. New classes of tumor promoters: teleocidin, aplysiatoxin and palytoxin. *Adv Cancer Res* 1987;49:223–264.
123. Radike MJ, Stemmer KL, Brown PG, Larson E, Bingham E. Effect of ethanol and vinyl chloride on the induction of liver tumors: preliminary report. *Environ Health Perspect* 1977;21:153–155.

124. Blumberg PM. Protein kinase C as the receptor for the phorbol ester tumor promoter: sixth Rhoads Memorial Award Lecture. *Cancer Res* 1988;48:1–8.
125. Jeng AY, Blumberg PM. Biochemical mechanisms of action of the phorbol ester class of tumor promoter. In: Sirica AE, ed. *The pathobiology of neoplasia.* New York: Plenum Press; 1989:371–383.
126. Moser GJ, Smart RC. Hepatic tumor-promoting chlorinated hydrocarbons stimulate protein kinase C activity. *Carcinogenesis* 1989;10:851–856.
127. Sirica AE. Tumor progression and the clonal evolution of neoplasia. In: Sirica AE, ed. *The pathobiology of neoplasia.* New York: Plenum Press; 1989:217–229.
128. Cohen SM, Ellwein LB. Cell proliferation in carcinogenesis. *Science* 1990;249:1007–1011.
129. Pitot HC, Dragan YP. Facts and theories concerning the mechanisms of carcinogenesis. *FASEB J* 1991;5:2280–2286.
130. Fearon ER, Vogelstein B. A genetic model for colorectal tumorigenesis. *Cell* 1990;61:759–767.
131. Berenblum I. The modifying influence of dichloroethyl sulphide on the induction of tumours in mice by tar. *J Pathol Bacteriol* 1929;32:425–434.
132. Finzi C, Daudel P, Prodi G. Interference among polycyclic hydrocarbons in experimental skin carcinogenesis. *Eur J Cancer* 1968;3:497–501.
133. Crabtree HG. Retardation of azo-carcinogenesis by non-carcinogenic azo-compounds. *Br J Cancer* 1955;9:310–319.
134. Yamamoto RS, Glass RM, Frankel HH, Weisburger EK, Weisburger JH. Inhibition of the toxicity and carcinogenicity of N-2-fluorenyl-acetamide by acetanilide. *Toxicol Appl Pharmacol* 1968;13:108–117.
135. Huggins C, Briziarelli G, Sutton H Jr. Rapid induction of mammary carcinoma in the rat and the influence of hormones on the tumors. *J Exp Med* 1959;109:25–42.
136. Shay H, Gruenstein M, Shimkin MB. Inhibition of mammary cancer in rats by a dithiocarbamoylhydrazine (ICI-33,828). *Cancer Res* 1964;24:998–1001.
137. Fare G. The protective effects of beef and yeast extracts and copper acetate in the diet against rat liver carcinogenesis by 4-dimethylaminoazobenzene. *Br J Cancer* 1964;18:782–791.
138. Hennings H, Smith HC, Colburn NH, Boutwell RK. Inhibition by actinomycin D of DNA and RNA synthesis and of skin carcinogenesis initiated by 7,12-dimethylbenz[a]anthracene or β-propiolactone. *Cancer Res* 1968;28:543–552.
139. Wattenberg LW. Inhibitors of chemical carcinogenesis. *Adv Cancer Res* 1978;26:197–226.
140. Ito N, Hirose M. Antioxidants—carcinogenic and chemopreventive properties. *Adv Cancer Res* 1989;53:247–302.
141. Troll W, Wiesner R, Frenkel K. Anticarcinogenic action of protease inhibitors. *Adv Cancer Res* 1988;49:265–283.
142. Daniel EM, Stoner GD. The effects of ellagic acid and 13-*cis*-retinoic acid on N-nitrosobenzylmethylamine-induced esophageal tumorigenesis in rats. *Cancer Lett* 1991;56:117–124.
143. Wattenberg LW, Coccia JB. Inhibition of 4-(methylnitrosamino)-1-(3-pyridyl)-1-butanone carcinogenesis in mice by D-limonene and citrus fruit oils. *Carcinogenesis* 1991;12:115–117.
144. Muktar H, Das M, Khan WA, Wang ZY, Bik DP, Bickers DR. Exceptional activity of tannic acid among naturally occurring plant phenols in protecting against 7,12-dimethylbenz(a)anthracene-, benzo(a)pyrene-, 3-methylcholanthrene-, and N-methyl-N-nitrosourea-induced skin tumorigenesis in mice. *Cancer Res* 1988;48:2361–2365.
145. Hu P-J, Wargovich MJ. Effect of diallyl sulfide on MNNG-induced nuclear aberrations and ornithine decarboxylase activity in the glandular stomach mucosa of the Wistar rat. *Cancer Lett* 1989;47:153–158.
146. Morse MA, Eklind KT, Hecht SS, et al. Structure–activity relationships for inhibition of 4-(methylnitrosamino)-1-(3-pyridyl)-1-butanone lung tumorigenesis by arylalkyl isothiocyanates in A/J mice. *Cancer Res* 1991;51:1846–1850.
147. Jacobs MM, ed. *Vitamins and minerals in the prevention and treatment of cancer.* Boca Raton, FL: CRC Press; 1991.
148. Westin EH. Oncogenes. In: Sirica AE, ed. *The pathobiology of neoplasia.* New York: Plenum Press; 1989:275–290.
149. Diwan BA, Rice JM. Organ and species specificity in chemical carcinogenesis and tumor promotion. In: Sirica AE, ed. *The pathobiology of neoplasia.* New York: Plenum Press; 1989:149–171.
150. Anderson MW, Reynolds SH. Activation of oncogenes by chemical carcinogens. In: Sirica AE, ed. *The pathobiology of neoplasia.* New York: Plenum Press; 1989:291–304.

151. Barbacid M. *ras* Genes. *Annu Rev Biochem* 1987;56:779–829.
152. Balmain A, Brown K. Oncogene activation in chemical carcinogenesis. *Adv Cancer Res* 1988; 51:147–182.
153. Burns PA, Bremmer R, Balmain A. Genetic changes during mouse skin tumorigenesis. *Environ Health Perspect* 1991;93:41–44.
154. Cooper CS. The role of non-*ras* transforming genes in chemical carcinogenesis. *Environ Health Perspect* 1991;93:33–40.
155. Vogt PK, Bos TJ. *jun*: Oncogene and transcription factor. *Adv Cancer Res* 1990;55:1–35.
156. Spencer CA, Groudine M. Control of c-*myc* regulation in normal and neoplastic cells. *Adv Cancer Res* 1991;56:1–48.
157. Fox TR, Watanabe PG. Detection of a cellular oncogene in spontaneous liver tumors of B6C3F1 mice. *Science* 1985;228:596–597.
158. Sager R. Tumor suppressor genes: the puzzle and the promise. *Science* 1990;246:1406–1412.
159. Weinberg RA. Oncogenes, antioncogenes, and the molecular basis of multistep carcinogenesis. *Cancer Res* 1989;49:3713–3721.

2

Chemicals Causally Associated with Cancers in Humans and in Laboratory Animals

A Perfect Concordance

James Huff

Environmental Carcinogenesis Program, National Institute of Environmental Health Sciences, Research Triangle Park, North Carolina 27709

Cancer—a multidisease phenomenon—remains as much a mystery nowadays as it was when first described as *karkinos* (meaning "new growth," from the Greek word for "crab"). We have learned much about this disease in the last century; yet as a collection of maladies "contrary to nature" (1), not nearly enough is understood to stem the devastating tide that has begun to consume more and more lives around the globe as population life spans lengthen. Known causes of cancer include both external factors (chemicals, radiation, viruses) and internal factors (hormones, immune conditions, inherited genes) as well as aging. Diet seems to be targeted as a major causative, but the growing volume of information is often contradictory.

In any event, in the United States alone, estimates of the number of new cancer cases for the year 1993 indicate that 1,170,000 humans will be diagnosed with cancer (2). This figure does not include carcinoma in situ or basal and squamous cell cancers of the skin, which will afflict more than 700,000 people annually. Most of the latter cancers, together with *all* those induced by alcoholic beverages (17,000) and tobacco smoking (160,000), are preventable—nearly 900,000.

Unfortunately, even though we do know certain causes of cancer, for the most part we do not know the causes of the overwhelming majority of cancers (3,4). In the decade of the 1980s, for instance, there were more than 4,500,000 cancer deaths, 9,000,000 new cancer cases, and 12,000,000 people under medical care for cancer. The numbers keep rising (5–7), and predictions (albeit perhaps conservative) indicate that 1 in 3, about 85,000,000 Americans now living, will eventually develop cancer (2). One consensus influencing factor associated with cancer causation centers on our modern industrialized and chemically based society. While making our lives longer and better in every sense, we now equally know that this revolution has not been without adverse health impact. We are devoting considerable effort to identifying and then overcoming or changing unhealthy practices and habits that lead to or exacerbate diseases.

Chemicals are typically reactive—reactive for a designed purpose. Most if not all chemicals interact with biological components. Some (e.g., pesticides, bactericides, warfare agents; antibiotics) are structured specifically to kill organisms. Others are designed to overcome disease and illness (e.g., drugs). Most are probably made for other purposes, yet still "react" with biologic constituents, tissues, organs, and systems. Thus, not surprisingly, chemicals do cause toxic effects, including cancer. Fortunately, not all chemicals are considered potentially carcinogenic either to humans (8–10) or to animals (11–15), and the proportion of chemicals eventually identified to cause cancer in experimental animals or humans is predicted to be relatively low (16,17). However, given the long latency period for developing cancer, and awareness that the chemical industry has comparatively recently reduced exposures to hazardous chemicals, occupationally associated cancers in humans will continue to be discovered (18,19).

Those chemicals identified as being causally associated with cancers in humans—that have been adequately evaluated experimentally—have all been shown to cause cancer in laboratory animals; in each instance at least one organ or tissue site of cancer was common to both mammalian species (20–24) (see the chapter, "Chemically Associated Respiratory Carcinogenesis in Rodents and in Humans," by Huff). This knowledge, together with patent similarities in biologic mechanisms of carcinogenesis across species (25–32), confirms the scientific and public health logic that chemicals shown clearly to be carcinogenic in animals should be considered as being likely and anticipated to present cancer risks to humans (8–10). So far, 100 to 150 "agents" or "exposure circumstances" have been identified (10).

PURPOSE

This chapter includes a list of the "known" and generally accepted chemicals, mixtures of chemicals, exposure circumstances, lifestyles and personal or cultural habits, occupations, viruses, living conditions, and physical agents that have been causally associated with cancers in humans. The collection is not fully complete, and may contain agents that might or might not be fully endorsed as consensus human carcinogens. People interested in suggesting additions to or deletions from this compilation are urged to write to me, with appropriate rationale or supporting evidence. Primarily, these major sources of information were used: (a) International Agency for Research on Cancer (IARC) monographs on carcinogenic risks to humans (12), (b) U.S. Public Health Service's annual reports on carcinogens (as prepared and coordinated by the National Toxicology Program) (8), (c) series of carcinogenesis bioassay reports by the National Cancer Institute and the NTP (13,14),

(4) PHS's survey of compounds tested for carcinogenicity (33) and IARC directories of agents being tested for carcinogenicity (34), and (5) other available scientific literature (e.g., refs. 21,23) (see the chapter, "Chemically Associated Respiratory Carcinogenesis in Rodents and in Humans," by Huff).

In particular, comparisons are made between those agents (re: chemical, mixture of chemicals, exposure circumstance) causing or strongly associated with cancer in humans and the same agents that have been studied in experimental animals. Answers to two specific questions were sought: Did the agent causing cancer in humans also cause cancer in laboratory animals, and was a carcinogenic response seen in the same organ or tissue as discovered in humans exposed to the same agent? In a companion review (see the chapter, "Chemically Associated Respiratory Carcinogenesis in Rodents and in Humans," Huff) we evaluated the evidence of chemically associated carcinogenesis for those chemicals and exposure circumstances identified as causing lung/respiratory tract cancers in humans, and compared these findings with those from experimental animals exposed to the same agents. Concordances for carcinogenesis and for organ site (lung) were exceptional.

BACKGROUND AND PERSPECTIVE

Since 1971 the International Agency for Research on Cancer (IARC), an autonomously functioning agency within the World Health Organization, has been evaluating available epidemiological and experimental evidence for carcinogenicity of chemicals, mixtures of chemicals, industrial processes, occupations, lifestyle and cultural habits, and exposure circumstances ("agents") (9,10,12,21). A few more than 110 are now recognized as being, or strongly implicated as being, carcinogenic to humans (10,35). Of the fewer than 1,000 agents that have been evaluated adequately for carcinogenicity in laboratory animals, a varying spectrum of data from studies on humans is available for only about 20% to 25%. So far (as of May 1993), 60 agents are linked unequivocally to cancer in humans, and another 51 are considered as strongly suspected of being carcinogenic to humans (10) (Table 1). Importantly, another 206 agents or groups of agents are considered by IARC to be "possibly carcinogenic to humans." Other agents have been declared by additional organizations or in the literature as being carcinogenic to humans with which IARC Working Groups have not fully agreed or for which the IARC has not yet evaluated (or in some cases reevaluated) the available data.

For 450 additional agents, IARC has decided that these are "unclassifiable as to carcinogenicity to humans." So far, only one chemical has been placed into group 4: "probably not carcinogenic to humans": caprolactam (36). This category was agreed upon in the absence of any case reports or epidemiological studies of carcinogenicity to humans (9,37). Thus IARC has evaluated or reevaluated the epidemiological and experimental data on 768 "entities" as divided into 702 agents and groups of agents, 40 mixtures, and 26 exposure circumstances.

TABLE 1. *Distribution of IARC evaluations of carcinogenicity classified according to carcinogenic risk to humans*

IARC grouping and categories		Number of agents
Group 1:	Carcinogenic to humans	60
	Agents and groups of agents	36
	Mixtures	11
	Exposure circumstances	13
Group 2A:	Probably carcinogenic to humans	51
	Agents and groups of agents	42
	Mixtures	5
	Exposure circumstances	4
Group 2B:	Possibly carcinogenic to humans	206
	Agents and groups of agents	191
	Mixtures	13
	Exposure circumstances	2
Group 3:	Cannot be classified as to carcinogenicity to humans	450
	Agents and groups of agents	432
	Mixtures	11
	Exposure circumstances	7
Group 4:	Probably not carcinogenic to humans	1
Total		768
	Agents and groups of agents	702
	Mixtures	40
	Exposure circumstances	26

Data from IARC (10) and Vanio, Coleman, and Wilbourn (22). Contains numerical listings data from *IARC Monographs*, Volumes 1–58.

HUMAN AND ANIMAL CONCORDANCE

Not all of these 111 agents in groups 1 and 2A have been or can be evaluated in animals because some are industrial processes or "occupations," some are environmental and cultural risk factors, and some are unknown or uncharacterized mixtures of agents [e.g., "contents" of Boston Harbor "causes" liver tumors in flounder (45)]. Moreover, Tomatis et al. (21) have identified other environmental risk factors as causally associated with human cancers: hepatitis B virus, human T-cell leukemia virus, ionizing radiation, and ultraviolet radiation, and another five risk factors for which an association with the occurrence of human cancer has been observed yet a causal relation has not been fully established: *Clonorchis sinensis, Schistosomia haematobium, Opisthorchis vivarrini*, Epstein–Barr virus, and papilloma virus.

Table 2 contains a list of those group 1 and group 2A agents (and group 2B or others where appropriate) that have been evaluated in humans and in animals, target organs are listed for humans, the species corresponding with the same organ response is given, and other species (and sexes) showing carcinogenicity for that agent having additional or different target sites. For the 206 agents in group 2B, the evidence has been considered less than what is considered necessary for inclusion in groups 1 and 2A, and these have been placed into the grouping considered "possibly carcinogenic to humans." Some confusion and differences of opinion may exist in

TABLE 2. Shared organ and tissue sites of chemically caused cancers in humans and in animals[a]

		Common organ or tissue sites of cancer	
	Chemical or agent	Human	Animal[b]
•	Acrylonitrile	Lung	R [+]
		Prostate	
		Brain, GIT [+3]	
+•	Aflatoxins	Liver	R, H, M, P, Du, F
		Lung	M [+]
+	Alcoholic beverages	Oral cavity, pharynx, larynx, esophagus, liver, [breast]	[I; R?, +?]
+•	4-Aminobiphenyl	Urinary bladder	Ra, M [R]
+•	Analgesics and phenacetin	Renal	R, M [+]
		Urinary bladder	R
	Androgenic steroids (oxy-metholone; testosterone)	Liver	
		Liver?	[ND]
		Prostate, [liver?]	R [M, +]
+	Arsenic and As compounds	Lung [+5], skin	M, H
+•	Asbestos	Lung, pleura, peritoneum	R, M, H
		GIT, larynx	R
+	Azathioprine	Lymphoma [+3]	R [+], M
+	Benzene	Leukemia [+3]	R [+], M [+]
+	Benzidine	Urinary bladder	D [M, R, H] [+]
•	Beryllium and Be compounds	Lung	Mo, R [+], [Ra]
	Bischloroethyl nitrosourea (BCNU)	Leukemia	[R, +]
+•	Bis(chloromethyl) ether and chloromethylmethyl ether	Lung	R [+], M [+], H
•	1,3-Butadiene	Leukemia	M, [+]
		Lymphatic cancers	M, [+], [R] [+]
•	Cadmium and Cd compounds	Lung	R [+], [M, +]
		Prostate	R, M
		[Renal]	
+	Chlorambucil	Leukemia	R, M [+]
	Chloramphenicol	Leukemia	[I]
+•	Chlorination and by-products	Urinary bladder	R [+], [M]
		Colon and rectum	
+	Chlornaphazine [bis(2-chloroethyl)-2-naphthylamine]	Urinary bladder	[R, M] [−]
	Chlorophenols	Lymphoma [+]	R [+], [M +]
	Chlorophenoxy herbicides	Lymphoma [+]	R [+], [M +]
	p-Chloro-o-toluidine	Urinary bladder	[R, M]
+	Chromium(VI) compounds	Lung [+1]	R [M]
+	Ciclosporin	Lymphoma [+]	Mo, M
+	Coal tars	Skin	Ra, M
		Lung [+1]	R, M
+	Coal-tar pitches	Skin [+]	M
	Creosotes	Skin [+]	M [+]
		Scrotum	
+	Cyclophosphamide	Urinary bladder	R
		Leukemia	R, M
	2,4-D	Lymphoma	D, [R]
•	DDT and related compounds	Pancreas	[R+]
		Lymphoma	M [+]
		Lung	M [+]
		Breast	

TABLE 2. (Continued.)

	Chemical or agent	Common organ or tissue sites of cancer Human	Animal[b]
•	Dibromoethane (EDB)	Lymphoma	[R [+], M [+]]
	Dichloromethane	[Liver]	M [+]
		[Pancreas]	R [+]
	Diesel engine exhaust	Lung	R, M
		Urinary bladder	
+•	Diethylstilbestrol (DES)	Cervix/vagina	H [+], M [+]
		Breast	R [+], M [+]
		Endometrium	H [+], Mo
		Testes	
	Dimethylformamide	Testes	[I]
+	Erionite	Pleura, peritoneum	R, M
+	Estrogen (replacement)	Endometrium	[H]
		Breast	
+	Estrogens, nonsteroidal	(see Diethylstilbestrol)	(see DES)
+	Estrogens, steroidal	Endometrium	M, GP, M, R [H]
		Breast	
•	Ethyl acrylate	Colon	[R, M]
		Rectum	
•	Ethylene oxide	Leukemia	R [+], M [+]
		[Stomach]	R
•	Formaldehyde	Nasopharynx	R
		Nasal cavity	
		[Lung]	
•	Gasoline, aviation	Kidney	R, [M]
		[Leukemia]	
	Hair dyes	Leukemia	R [+], M [+]
		Urinary bladder	R [+], M [+]
	Ionizing radiation	Leukemia	Species?
		Skin	Species?
		Other organs	Species?
•	Lead and compounds	[Lung]	M [+]
		[Stomach and GIT]	
		[Renal]	R [+], M [+]
	Maté, hot "tea"	Upper GIT	[ND]
+•	Melphalan	Leukemia	M [R]
+•	8-Methoxypsoralen + UV	Skin	M
+	Methyl-CCNU [1-(2-chloro-ethyl)-3-(4-methylcyclo-hexyl)-1-nitrosourea]	Leukemia	[R]
•	4,4'-Methylene bis-(2-chloro-aniline) (MOCA)	[Urinary bladder]	D, [R [+], M]
•	4,4'-Methylene dianiline diHCl (MDA)	"Infante"	R [+], M [+]
+	Mineral oils (untreated)	Skin	Mo, Ra, M
+	MOPP (M or P evaluated)	Leukemia	R [+], M [+]
+•	Mustard gas (sulfur mustard)	Lung	M [+]
		Larynx/pharynx	
+	Myleran (1,4-butanediol dimethanesulfonate)	Leukemia	M
+	2-Naphthylamine	Urinary bladder	R, H, D, P, [M]
		[Liver]	M
+	Nickel compounds	Lung	R, M, H, Ra
		Nasal sinus	
		[Larynx]	

TABLE 2. (Continued.)

	Chemical or agent	Common organ or tissue sites of cancer Human	Animal[b]
	Nitrogen mustard		
•	Ochratoxin A		
+	Oral contraceptives (combined)	Liver	
+	Oral contraceptives (sequential)	Endometrium	
•	Phenacetin	Kidney	
	Polychlorinated biphenyls		
+•	Radon and decay products	Lung	R, D
•	Reserpine	[Breast]	M, [R+, M+]
•	Rockwool/slagwool	Lung	R [+]
+	Shale oils	Skin, scrotum [Colon]	Ra, M [+], [R]
•	Silica, crystalline	Lung	R [+]
+	Solar radiation	Skin	[ND] ?
+	Soots	Skin, scrotum Lung [Esophagus]	M R
	Sulfuric acid mist and other strong inorganic acid mists	Lung Larynx	[ND]
	Talc	Uterus	[R, +]
+	Talc with asbestiform fibers	Lung [+1] [Mesothelium]	[I]
•	2,3,7,8-TCDD	Lung Skin (soft tissue sarcoma) [Thyroid gland]	R [+], M [+] M [+], H R [+], M [+]
	Tamoxifen	Uterus Endometrium Liver	R
+	Thiotepa	Leukemia	R [+], M [+]
+	Tobacco smokeless products	Oral cavity [Pharynx, esophagus]	[I]
	o-Toluidine	Urinary bladder	R [+], Ra?, GP?, [M]
+	Tobacco smoke	Respiratory tract [+10]	R, H
+	Treosulfan	Leukemia	[ND]
+•	Vinyl chloride	Liver Lung GIT [+5]	R [+], M [+], H [+] M [+], Ra [+] H [+]

[a]Chemicals and exposure circumstances listed are those having evidence of carcinogenesis in humans *and* (for most cases) in laboratory animals as well (e.g., Treosulfan has not been studied in animals). Abbreviations: + (preceding chemical name), agents evaluated as group 1 human carcinogens by IARC; • (preceding name), evidence of carcinogenicity first observed in experimental animals and subsequently in humans; [organ/system], site possibly related to exposure; [+], one or more additional sites of carcinogenesis; [initials], species with induced cancers at sites *other than those* observed specifically in humans; [I], inadequate studies; [ND], no experimental data available; GIT, gastrointestinal tract.

[b]D, dogs; Du, ducks; F, fish; GP, guinea pigs; H, hamster; M, mice; Mo, monkeys; P, primates; R, rats; Ra, rabbits.

distinguishing between those agents in IARC group 2A and those in IARC group 2B: for group 2A the agents typically (but not always) have "limited evidence of carcinogenicity in humans" and "sufficient evidence of carcinogenicity in experimental animals," as contrasted to agents in group 2B that may exhibit "limited evidence of carcinogenicity in humans" and less than "sufficient evidence of carcinogenicity in experimental animals" or have no data in humans and "sufficient evidence in experimental animals." Obviously, placement of an agent in one or the other category entails scientific judgment of the particular IARC Working Group, in addition to the totality of the weight of the evidence, including mechanisms of carcinogenic activity as well as other relevant information (15,28,30,31,39–41). Thus one needs to study and examine the actual IARC Monograph (and the original papers leading to the decisions) to best understand the placement of an agent into a particular category of evidence. Methods and guidelines for developing and assigning levels of evidence of carcinogenicity from experiments in animals have been reported (42,43).

Additionally, I have included certain chemicals in Table 2 that have either not been evaluated by IARC, and that have relatively recent reports of evidence of carcinogenicity in humans. Some may be listed because they "would be" carcinogenic to humans: for example, benzidine-based congener dyes, which etiologically are difficult to separate from benzidine exposures and in most cases are "more carcinogenic" than the parent compound in experimental animals. One might consider vinyl bromide (group 2A) as a group 1 chemical based on the closeness of the physicochemical properties to vinyl chloride and more so on the remarkable and unique similarities in carcinogenic responses in animals (e.g., both induced angiosarcomas of the liver and tumors of Zymbal's gland).

As mentioned, the primary collective sources of this information come from the IARC Monographs Series (12) the NCI/NTP Technical Report Series (14), the DHHS Reports on Carcinogens (8), the IARC Supplement 7 (9), the U.S. Public Health Service series on chemicals tested for carcinogenicity (33), Tomatis et al., (21) Huff and Rall (23), Huff (15,44,45), Vainio et al. (22), Vainio and Wilbourn (24,35), and the chemical bioassay and carcinogenesis literature. In a few instances where the evidence from humans has not yet been evaluated by independent groups (e.g., DHHS or IARC), I have taken the opportunity to interpret the available findings on reported associations between exposure and human cancers (15,23), and appropriate references are given in ref. 46 and in the foregoing sources to allow others to judge the levels of evidence (e.g., refs. 15,42) (see the chapter, "Chemically Associated Respiratory Carcinogenesis in Rodents and in Humans," by Huff).

Obviously, the agents listed in Table 1 should not be considered complete, and others will surely be added in the future. For some, the evidence of carcinogenicity came first from experimental carcinogenesis (see refs. 15,47), however, the possibility exists that the evidence of agent-associated carcinogenesis in humans may in fact predate the experimental evidence, and I would appreciate learning about any such errors in awareness, together with appropriate reference citations. For some, the levels of evidence of carcinogenesis in humans may be reflected in case reports (recall vinyl chloride) or in bits of evidence cumulated over time (e.g., refs. 48–51). In any event these are my opinions, and those readers who wish to suggest additions, deletions, or modifications to this list are encouraged to do so.

Because epidemiological data are often absent, or/and past exposure data are unavailable, public health decisions must continue to be based largely on animal data. Historically, this logical concept has served the public well as preventive medicine. Thus while we hope that subsequent epidemiologic studies on the recognized animal chemical carcinogens do not identify additional causal associations with human cancer, these chemical carcinogenesis results in laboratory animals frequently, if not almost always, constitute the primary basis for identifying and predicting potential human health hazards (25,52–59). Several chemicals identified first as causing cancer in laboratory animals have subsequently been shown to be associated with human cancers.

In 1979, Tomatis reported seven chemicals that initially were found to cause cancer in experimental carcinogenesis studies, and at some later time evidence of carcinogenicity in humans came forth (47). The possibility exists that perhaps clinical or epidemiological investigations were stimulated by these data (45). This collection of chemicals has been expanded since the early disclosure (12,21,45,57) and now includes upward of 30 chemicals that are causally or probably associated with cancer in humans whereby the first implication of carcinogenesis was discovered in experimental animals (46). These are preceded by bullets in Table 2.

Certain chemicals with convincing experimental findings in laboratory animals, and with varying levels of human evidence, would seem to be candidates for further follow-up evaluation and confirmation as human carcinogens; several have been included in Table 2. For other chemicals exhibiting clear evidence in laboratory animals, with no available studies in humans, exposure cohorts should be identified and evaluated for possible carcinogenicity (45). That is, using our limited data set, one could begin to identify exposure cohorts for 45 of the 326 chemicals (14%) causing cancer in each of the four sex-species experiments and 26 of the 326 chemicals (8%) causing cancer in 3-of-4 experiments (11,15). Obviously, these could be further divided into priority classes by the strength of evidence of carcinogenicity. A few have already been acted on. Once these are investigated, chemicals causing cancer in fewer experiments could be pursued.

As stated by Doll (18,19), and unfortunately, the final number of proven occupational (and I might add, environmental) carcinogens may eventually be quite large—quite large in the numerical sense, but as a percentage of chemicals currently in commerce eventually estimated to be potentially carcinogenic to animals or humans, we believe the final figure will be quite low, perhaps 10% or less (16,17). Thus we must continue in our scientific and public health efforts to identify potential carcinogenic hazards to humans, and those agents considered to inflict undue harm should no longer be permitted unregulated exposures.

Regarding identified etiologies of cancer in humans, Doll and Peto (3) argue that the causes of 97% of human cancers can be explainable, with a large proportion

(10% to 70%; best estimate, 35%) being due to or strongly associated with diet. Using the most relevant and common sites of human cancer, Schmahl et al. (4) estimate that only one-third of the cancers (in the Federal Republic of Germany) can be assigned etiologically to exogenous carcinogenic agents or lifestyle. These authors stress that indirect primary prevention, based on the probable summation of subcarcinogenic effects of single carcinogens identified from animal experiments, may lead to a reduction in carcinogen-induced cancers, even if the effects of a particular carcinogenic compound cannot be determined precisely. Regarding the influence of diet on the incidence and mortality of cancer, Schmahl et al. (4) agree with Byers and Graham (60), who indicate that the relationship between dietary factors and cancer rises has not revealed a single unequivocal conclusion of causality. Much work is being devoted to this issue and perhaps more strenuous answers will be forthcoming.

The decades-old question remains: How convinced should we be that consensus experimental carcinogens will with reasonable confidence predict cancers in populations exposed to the same chemical or similar exposure circumstance? History, biology, and the theme of this chapter support the concept of extrapolating carcinogenesis findings from animals to humans. Even more basic, will chemicals shown conclusively to cause cancers in laboratory animals also eventually be found to cause cancer in humans? Ignoring for the moment the important and controversial issue of exposure, the answer is yes. The scientific correctness and public health prudency of this acknowledgment come not only from the cross-mammalian consistency but from the clearness of knowing that nearly one-third of those agents considered carcinogenic to humans were discovered first in animals.

SUMMARY

Certain chemicals, mixtures of chemicals, exposure circumstances, lifestyles and personal or cultural habits, occupations, viruses, living conditions, and physical agents have been causally associated with cancers in humans. Fortunately, not all of these possibilities are considered potentially carcinogenic to humans or to animals, and the proportion of agents eventually identified as causally associated with cancer in humans or experimental animals is predicted to be relatively low. Focusing on chemicals, those so far identified as causing cancers in humans have all been shown to cause cancer in laboratory animals; in every instance at least one site of cancer was common to both mammalian species. For a sizable number, the initial awareness of carcinogenic activity came from laboratory experiments. This knowledge, together with clear similarities in mechanisms of carcinogenesis across mammalian species, led to the scientific logic and the international public health strategy that chemicals (or other agents or exposure circumstances) shown clearly to be carcinogenic in animals should be considered as being likely and anticipated to present cancer risks to humans. To date, 150 to 200 agents or exposures have been identified, with more expected.

Data reported elsewhere show that nearly 25% to 30% of the agents, substances, or chemicals that have been causally or strongly associated with cancer in humans were first identified as being carcinogenic in experimental animals (46). If more attention would have been given to these findings, perhaps some unnecessary suffering and death could have been avoided. Similarly, for those chemicals shown unequivocally to cause cancer in laboratory animals that have not as yet had any epidemiological investigations, one should reduce or eliminate all avoidable exposures. Meanwhile, cohorts being exposed to these agents should be identified and evaluated. Finally, to continue to ignore or debate experimental data for reasons of uncertainty or until mechanisms of carcinogenicity are clarified should not be tolerated or condoned. Public health and human life must continue to take preference.

ACKNOWLEDGMENTS

The author thanks Dr. Michael Waalkes and Dr. Jerrold Ward, National Cancer Institute, for asking him to write a chapter on evidence of carcinogenicity in humans and animals, and for offering significant comments regarding orientation and contents. Dr. Richard Griesemer, National Institute of Environmental Health Sciences, and Dr. J. Ward, NCI, reviewed the manuscript and made valuable suggestions. Donna Mayer was most helpful with administrative efforts and reference coordination.

REFERENCES

1. Shimkin MB. *Contrary to nature.* DHEW publication (NIH) 76–720. Washington, DC: US Department of Health and Human Services; 1977. 498 pp.
2. ACS. *Cancer facts and figures—1993.* Atlanta, GA: American Cancer Society; 1993. 30 pp.
3. Doll R, Peto R. The causes of cancer. *J Natl Cancer Inst* 1981;66:1191–1308. Also, *The causes of cancer.* Oxford: Oxford Medical Publications, Oxford University Press; 1981:1191–1312.
4. Schmahl D, Preussmann R, Berger MR. Causes of cancer: an alternative view to Doll and Peto. *Klin Wochenschr* 1989;67:1169–1173.
5. Bailer JC III, Smith EM. Progress against cancer. *N Engl J Med* 1986;314:1226–1232.
6. Davis DL, Hoel DG. Trends in cancer mortality in industrial countries. *Ann NY Acad Sci* 1990;609:1–347.
7. Miller BA, Ries LAG, Hankey BF, Kosary CL, Edwards BK, eds. *Cancer statistics review: 1973–1989.* Bethesda, MD: National Cancer Institute; 1992.
8. DHHS/NTP. *Annual reports on carcinogens.* Research Triangle Park, NC: National Toxicology Program, US Department of Health and Human Services; 1978–1993; seventh report.
9. IARC. *IARC monographs on the evaluation of carcinogenic risks to humans: overall evaluations of carcinogenicity: an updating of IARC monographs volumes 1 to 42* [Suppl 7]. Lyon, France: International Agency for Research on Cancer; 1987. 440 pp.
10. IARC. Lists of IARC evaluations. *IARC monographs on the evaluation of carcinogenic risks to humans.* Lyon, France: International Agency for Research on Cancer; May 1993. 35pp.
11. Huff JE, Haseman JK. Long-term chemical carcinogenesis experiments for identifying potential human cancer hazards. Collective data base of the National Cancer Institute and National Toxicology Program (1976–1991). *Environ Health Perspect* 1991;96:23–31.
12. IARC. *IARC monographs on the evaluation of carcinogenic risks to humans.* Vols 1–58. Lyon, France: International Agency for Research on Cancer; 1972–1993.
13. NCI. *NCI bioassay of "chemical" for possible carcinogenicity.* Carcinogenesis technical report series 2–100, 202–205. Bethesda, MD: National Cancer Institute; 1976–1980.

14. NTP. *NTP toxicology and carcinogenesis studies of "chemical" ("CAS no") in F344/N rats and B6C3F1 mice ("exposure route")*. Technical report series 201, 206–443. Research Triangle Park, NC: National Toxicology Program; 1980–1993.
15. Huff JE. Issues and controversies surrounding qualitative strategies for identifying and forecasting cancer causing agents in the human environment. *Pharmacol Toxicol* 1993;72[Suppl 1]:12–27.
16. Huff JE, Hoel DG. Perspective and overview of the concepts and value of hazard identification as the initial phase of risk assessment for cancer and human health. *Scand J Work Environ Health* 1992; 18[Suppl 1]:83–89.
17. Fung V, Huff JE, Weisburger E, Hoel DG. Predictive strategies for selecting 379 NCI/NTP chemicals evaluated for carcinogenic potential: scientific and public health impact. *Fundam Appl Toxicol* 1993;20:413–436.
18. Doll R. Occupational cancer: problems in interpreting human evidence. *Ann Occup Hyg* 1984; 28:291–305.
19. Doll R. Occupational cancer: a hazard for epidemiologists. *Int J Epidemiol* 1985;14:22–31.
20. Wilbourn J, Haroun L, Heseltine E, Kaldor J, Partensky C, Vainio H. Response of experimental animals to human carcinogens: an analysis based upon the IARC monographs programme. *Carcinogenesis* 1986;7:1853–1863.
21. Tomatis L, Aitio A, Wilbourn J, Shuker L. Human carcinogens so far identified. *Jpn J Cancer Res* 1989;80:795–807.
22. Vainio H, Coleman M, Wilbourn J. Carcinogenicity evaluations and ongoing studies: the IARC databases. *Environ Health Perspect* 1991;96:5–9.
23. Huff JE, Rall DP. Relevance to humans of carcinogenesis results from laboratory animal toxicology studies. In: Last JM, Wallace RB eds. *Maxcy–Rosenau–Last's public health and preventive medicine*. 13th ed. Norwalk, CT: Appleton & Lange; 1992:433–440, 453–457, 1257 pp.
24. Vainio H, Wilbourn J. Identification of carcinogens within the IARC monograph program. *Scand J Environ Health* 1992;18[Suppl 1]:64–73.
25. Bertram JS, Kolonel LN, Meyskens FL Jr. Rationale and strategies for chemoprevention of cancer in humans. *Cancer Res* 1987;47:3012–3031.
26. Boyd JA, Barrett JC. Genetic and cellular basis of multistep carcinogenesis. *Pharmacol Ther* 1990; 46:469–486.
27. Vainio H, Cardis E. Estimating human cancer risk from the results of animal experiments: relationship between mechanism and dose-rate and dose. *Am J Ind Med* 1992;21:5–14.
28. Vainio H, Heseltine E, McGregor D, Tomatis L, Wilbourn J. Working group on mechanisms of carcinogenesis and the evaluation of carcinogenic risks (meeting report). *Cancer Res* 1992;52:2357–2361.
29. Barrett JC. [1992]. Mechanism of action of known human carcinogens. In: Vainio H, Magee P, McGregor D, McMichael A, eds. *Mechanisms of carcinogenesis in risk identification*. IARC scientific publication 116. Lyon, France: International Agency for Research on Cancer; 1992:115–134. 615pp.
30. Barrett JC. Mechanisms of multistep carcinogenesis and carcinogen risk assessment. *Environ Health Perspect* 1993;100:9–20.
31. Huff JE. Mechanisms, chemical carcinogenesis, and risk assessment. *Ramazzini Newsl* 1993;3:47–50.
32. Lijinsky W. Species differences in carcinogenesis. *In Vivo* 1993;7:65–72.
33. PHS. *Survey of compounds which have been tested for carcinogenic activity*. Bethesda, MD: National Cancer Institute; 1951–1993.
34. IARC. *IARC directory of agents being tested for carcinogenicity*. Nos 1–15. Lyon, France: International Agency for Research on Cancer; 1973–1992.
35. Vainio H, Wilbourn J. Cancer etiology: agents causally associated with human cancer. *Pharmacol Toxicol* 1993;72[Suppl 1]:4–11.
36. Huff JE, Ward JM. Caprolactam: no evidence of carcinogenicity in F344/N rats and B6C3F1 mice. In: *An industry approach to chemical risk assessment, caprolactam and related compounds as a case study*. Pittsburgh, PA: Industrial Health Foundation; 1984:115–119.
37. IARC. Caprolactam. In: *IARC monographs on the evaluation of the carcinogenic risks of chemicals to humans*. Vol 39. Lyon, France: International Agency for Research on Cancer; 1986:247–276. 403pp.
38. Huff JE, Bucher JR, Yang RSH. Carcinogenesis studies in rodents for evaluating risks associated with chemical carcinogens in aquatic food animals. *Environ Health Perspect* 1991;90:127–132.

39. IARC. *Mechanisms of carcinogenesis in risk identification. A consensus report of an IARC monographs working group.* IARC internal technical report 91/002. Lyon, France: International Agency for Research on Cancer; 1991. 60 pp.
40. Vainio H, Magee P, McGregor D, McMichael AJ, eds. *Mechanisms of carcinogenesis in risk identification.* IARC scientific publication 116. Lyon, France: International Agency for Research on Cancer; 1992:1–615.
41. Barrett JC, Wiseman RW. Molecular carcinogenesis in humans and rodents. In: Klein-Szanto A, Anderson M, Barrett JC, Slaga TJ, eds. *Comparative molecular carcinogenesis.* vol 376. New York: Wiley, 1992:1–30.
42. Huff JE. A historical perspective of the classification developed and used for chemical carcinogens by the National Toxicology Program during 1983–1992. *Scand J Work Environ Health* 1992;18 [Suppl 1]:74–82.
43. IARC. Preamble. In: *IARC monographs on the evaluation of carcinogenic risks to humans.* Vol 58. *Beryllium, cadmium, mercury, and exposures in the glass manufacturing industry.* Lyon, France: International Agency for Research on Cancer; 1993.
44. Huff JE, McConnell EE, Haseman JK, Boorman GA, Eustis SL, Schwetz BA, Rao GN, Jameson CW, Hart LG, Rall DP. Carcinogenesis studies: results from 398 experiments on 104 chemicals from the U.S. National Toxicology Program. *Ann NY Acad Sci* 1988;534:1–30.
45. Huff JE, Haseman JK, Rall DP. Scientific concepts, value, and significance of chemical carcinogenesis studies. *Annu Rev Pharmacol Toxicol* 1991;31:621–652.
46. Huff JE. Chemicals and cancer in humans: first evidence in experimental animals. *Environ Health Perspect* 1993;100:201–210.
47. Tomatis L. The predictive value of rodent carcinogenicity tests in the evaluation of human risks. *Annu Rev Pharmacol Toxicol* 1979;19:511–530.
48. Zeise L, Huff JE, Salmon AG, Hooper NK. Human risks from 2,3,7,8-tetrachlorodibenzo-p-dioxin and hexachlorodibenzo-p-dioxins. *Adv Mod Environ Toxicol* 1990;17:293–342.
49. Huff JE, Salmon A, Hooper K, Zeise L. Long-term carcinogenesis studies on 2,3,7,8-tetrachlorodibenzo-pp-dioxin and hexachlorodibenzo-p-dioxins. *Cell Biol Toxicol* 1991;7:67–94.
50. Huff JE. 2,3,7,8-TCDD: a potent and complete carcinogen in experimental animals. *Chemosphere* 1992;25:173–176.
51. Lucier GW, Clark GC, Tritscher AM, Sewall CH, Heuvel JP, Huff JE. Mechanistic-based reasoning for assessing carcinogenic risk of TCDD. *Annu Rev Pharmacol Toxicol* [in press].
52. Montesano R, Bartsch H, Vaino H, Wilbourn J, Yamasaki H. *Long-term and short-term assays for carcinogens. A critical appraisal.* IARC scientific publication 83. Lyon, France: International Agency for Research on Cancer; 1986. 564 pp.
53. Staff Group on Chemical Carcinogenesis. Office of Science and Technology, Executive Office of the President. Chemical carcinogens: a review of the science and its associated principles. *Fed Reg* 1985;50:10371–10442. Also, *Environ. Health Perspect,* 1986;67:201–282.
54. OTA. *Assessment of technologies for determining cancer risks from the environment.* Washington, DC: Office of Technology Assessment, Congress of the United States; 1981. 240pp.
55. OTA. *Identifying and regulating carcinogens.* Washington, DC: Office of Technology Assessment, Congress of the United States; 1987. 215pp.
56. OTA. *Research on health risk assessment.* Washington, DC: Office of Technology Assessment, Congress of the United States [*in press*].
57. Rall DP, Hogan MD, Huff JE, Schwetz BA, Tennant TW. Alternatives to using human experience in assessing health risks. *Annu Rev Public Health* 1987;8:355–385.
58. Tomatis L, Aitio A, Day NE, Heseltine E, Kaldor J, Miller AB, Parkin DM, Riboli E. *Cancer: causes, occurrence and control.* IARC scientific publication 100. Lyon, France: International Agency for Research on Cancer; 1990. 352 pp.
59. Huff JE. Design strategies, results, and evaluations of long-term chemical carcinogenesis studies. *Scand J Work Environ Health* 1992;18[Suppl 1]:31–37.
60. Byers T, Graham S. The epidemiology of diet and cancer. *Adv Cancer Res* 1984;41:1–61.

3

Hepatocarcinogenesis in the Rat

Ryohei Hasegawa and Nobuyuki Ito

First Department of Pathology, Nagoya City University Medical School, Nagoya, 467 Japan

Analysis of experimental liver carcinogenesis is an old research theme dating back to early successful attempts to induce hepatocellular carcinomas with a variety of chemicals in rats (1). Subsequent studies revealed that focal populations with an aberrant phenotypic expression may be preneoplastic in character, and several trials have been performed to classify preneoplastic and neoplastic lesions. The morphological sequence of events in liver cancer pathogenesis may be similar in all animal species studied. However, specific differences in the histogenesis and morphology of tumors between strains of a given species and between species have been found. A discussion of the terminology and diagnosis of hepatoproliferative lesions should therefore also be prefaced by an explanation of the diagnostic process. In this chapter we review histopathologic typing of proliferating lesions of the rat liver, their characteristics, and their usefulness in risk assessment.

TYPING OF PROLIFERATIVE LESIONS IN THE RAT LIVER

The liver is composed of two types of epithelial cells—hepatocytes and bile duct cells—as well as sinusoidal lining cells of several types and other stromal supporting cells. Although all of these cell types can be associated with proliferative lesions, many classification schemes focus only on lesions of the epithelial components of the liver. Several authors have classified the various tumor types and associated lesions using terms that reflect their own concepts or prejudices regarding histogenesis (2–7). Although it is obvious that such exercises do not alter the histologic appearance of the lesions as viewed through the microscope, the general understanding of the biological nature of the lesions has changed and the terminology applied has also undergone review within recent years. The most recent suggestion for classification is replacement of the term *hyperplastic* or *neoplastic nodule* with *hepatocellular adenoma* (5–7).

Hepatocellular Proliferative Lesions

The significance of experimentally induced proliferative liver changes in rats for determining carcinogenic risk to humans is limited almost entirely to epithelial lesions. A variety of types of hepatocellular proliferative lesions have been proposed, the differences between them being due primarily to variation in understanding of early proliferative changes. Most progress has been made in the identification and characterization of preneoplastic liver lesions, in particular foci of cellular alteration and of more advanced nodular lesions, which may be used as endpoints in carcinogenicity studies (8–14). It has recently become widely accepted that hepatocellular focal lesions can be classified into three major categories, separate from other diffuse proliferative or regenerative lesions: (a) foci of cellular alteration, (b) neoplastic or hyperplastic nodules (hepatocellular adenomas), and (c) hepatocellular carcinomas.

Foci of Cellular Alteration

Small altered lesions of hepatic parenchymal cells without compression of the surrounding liver tissue are termed *foci* or *areas* when large. The architectural pattern within the lesion is usually little altered from the normal, but solid lesions with unclear sinusoidal patterns and plates of the hepatocytes are also observed. Foci may merge imperceptively into the surrounding parenchyma, but generally, a demarcation line is apparent. Cellular atypia are generally absent. The lesions are now further classified into several subtypes, based on different cytoplasmic staining patterns.

Diffusely basophilic cell foci are made up of a more or less homogeneous populations of basophilic cells that may be arranged in somewhat irregular plates. The foci are composed of enlarged cells that contain increased free ribosomes but are poor in glycogen. The activity of glycogen synthetase and phosphorylase is drastically reduced: the glucose-6-phosphate dehydrogenase (G6PD) and glyceraldehyde-3-phosphate dehydrogenase activities are considerably increased. Basophilic cell foci are considered to be a prestage of hepatocellular carcinomas (7,15). *Tigroid basophilic cell foci* consist of cells that may be the same size or smaller than normal hepatocytes. Their hepatic cords may be slightly tortuous, and the cellular density of the foci may be increased compared with the surrounding liver parenchyma. Instead of homogeneous basophilia, clumps of basophilic material representing cisternae of rough endoplasmic reticulum are distributed in a clear or eosinophilic background. The activity of glucose-6-phosphatase (G6Pase) or adenosine triphosphatase (ATPase) is variable, while γ-glutamyltranspeptidase (GGT) and placental glutathione S-transferase (GST-P) activities are almost always absent.

Eosinophilic (acidophilic) foci are composed of cells with similar or more acidophilic staining of the cytoplasm than normal liver cells. The characteristic ground-glass appearance of the cell cytoplasm is due to a proliferation of the smooth endoplasmic reticulum. The cells usually store excess glycogen, and since the cytoplasm is usually increased in amount, are consequently enlarged. Clear cells may also be present in small numbers in eosinophilic foci. Many authors reported decreased activity of G6Pase, ATPase, glycogen phosphorylase, adenylate cyclase, and acid or alkaline nuclease, and increased activity of GGT, G6PD, epoxide hydrase, uridine diphosphate-glucuronyl transferase (UDP-GT), cytochrome P450, and GST-P within these lesions (10). The enzyme histochemical pattern of small foci, however, may be rather heterogeneous.

Clear cell foci are composed of clear pale cells distinct from the surrounding liver tissue because of their storage of more glycogen than normal hepatocytes. The cell size may be unaltered or slightly enlarged. Both eosinophilic and clear cell foci have been referred to as glycogen storage foci (16). *Amphophilic cell foci* have been described only recently (17). The foci are composed of enlarged cells whose cytoplasm stains diffusely eosinophilic with a definite basophilic tint, resulting in an amphophilic appearance. The cells have a decreased glycogen content and an increased activity of the mitochondrial enzyme succinate dehydrogenase and the peroxisomal enzyme catalase as well as G6PD and acid phosphatase. Both GGT and GST-P are totally lacking, as in tigroid cell foci. Amphophilic foci have also been referred to as atypical eosinophilic foci (18). *Mixed cell foci* may exhibit mixtures of any of the two or three types described above.

Neoplastic or Hyperplastic Nodules (Hepatocellular Adenomas)

The histology and cytology of neoplastic or hyperplastic nodules in the rat have been described in detail (5–7,10,19–21). The most striking features are sharp demarcation at the periphery or at least a portion of it, and apparent compression of the surrounding liver tissue. The lesions are further characterized by a loss of the normal lobular architecture of the liver parenchyma. The neoplastic or hyperplastic nodule is a manifestation of the process of hepatocarcinogenesis, earlier stages of which are represented by the foci and areas of cellular alteration described above and some are reversible (22,23). Some nodules are associated with apparent gland formation and can be subclassified into two types—solid and trabecular—based on their architectural patterns. Subtypes similar to those for foci of cellular alteration are also observable in terms of constituent, basophilic, eosinophilic, clear, and mixed cell types.

The term *hepatocellular adenoma* has been reintroduced by Brooks and Roe (21) to separate this entity clearly from hepatocellular hyperplasia, which is not neoplastic but may be regenerative change (6), and the term *hyperplastic* or *neoplastic nodule* is no longer recommended by some authors (5,6). Although there is still no clear-cut criterion for a separation of hepatocellular hyperplasia from neoplastic changes (24), there is a strong possibility that hyperplastic (neoplastic) nodules and hepatocellular adenomas can be distinguished from hepatocellular hyperplasias by positivity for GGT, GST-P, or other marker enzyme staining within the lesions as discussed later (Fig. 1)

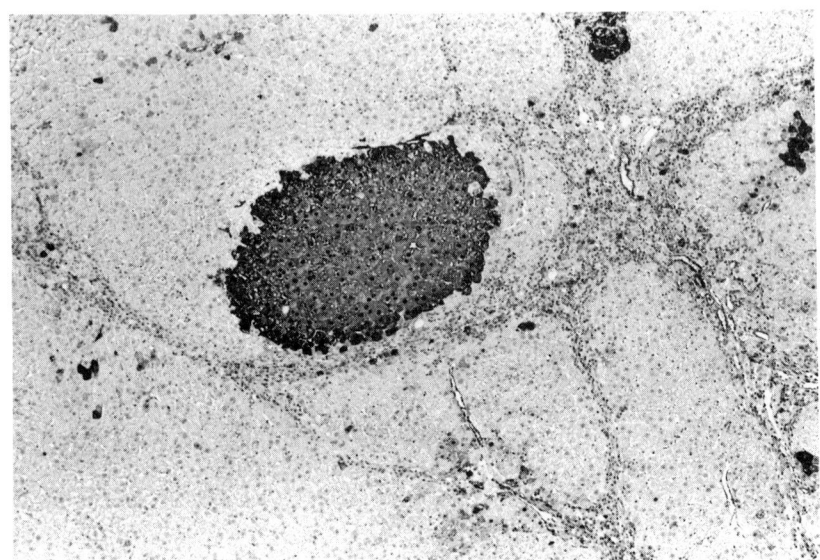

FIG. 1. GST-P-positive hyperplastic nodule observed among regenerative hyperplasias.

Hepatocellular Carcinomas

Hepatocellular carcinomas (HCCs) are distinguishable from hyperplastic nodules or hepatocellular adenoma by nuclear or cellular atypism, architectural pattern, and cellularity. There are three histological types of rat hepatocellular carcinoma based on the architectural patterns of hepaticlike cell arrangement: trabecular, adenoid (pseudoglandular), and solid types (3,7,25,26). A pseudocapsule may be found along the edge of some lesions. Each subtype can be further divided into well, moderately, and poorly differentiated carcinomas, based on degree of architectural and cellular atypia. Well-differentiated trabecular hepatocellular carcinomas are most commonly found in the rat. Bile duct–like formations are sometimes observed within the lesion as mentioned below.

Intrahepatic Cholangiocellular Lesions

A large proportion of bile duct proliferative lesions are reflections of aging, infections, or chemically derived liver toxicity (3,7). Except in frank cholangiocellular carcinomas, it is rather difficult to identify neoplastic characteristics. *Bile duct hyperplasia* consists of clusters and chains of bile ducts occurring most commonly within or adjacent to portal triads. The duct structure is associated with only limited amounts of collagenous stroma. The lesion commonly appears in old rats and may not be related to neoplasia. *Biliary cysts* are cystic dilatations of bile ducts. They

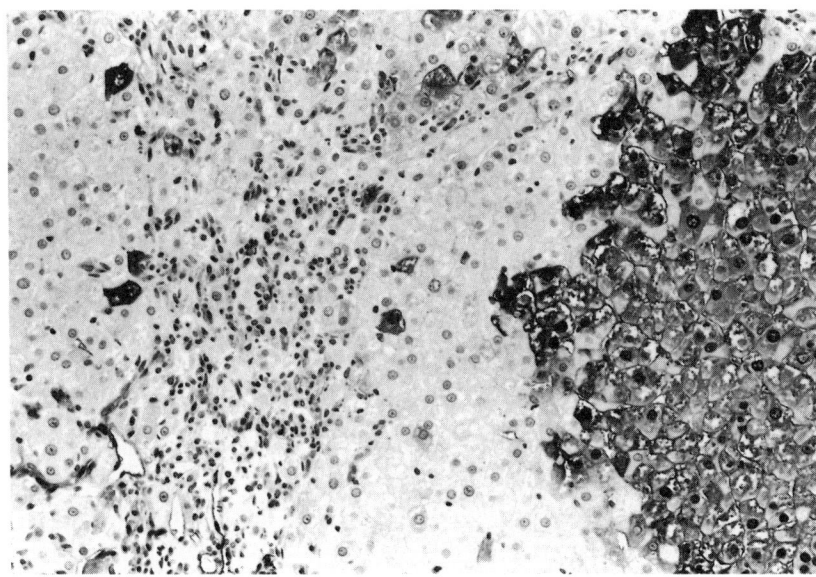

FIG. 2. Oval cells are weakly positive to GST-P staining as well as several single hepatocytes.

occur as single or multiple, simple or multilobular forms. The conglomerate cystic area gives the impression that the lumen of each individual cyst represents a greatly dilated canalicule. Neoplastic characteristics are not evident.

Oval cell hyperplasia is a proliferation of small cells with scanty cytoplasm and an oval pale nucleus. The lesion is usually associated with atrophic hepatic cell cords and develops first in the portal region and may be confined to this area or may extend into the center of the lobule. Several lines of evidence suggest that the origin of these cells is the epithelium of the canals of Hering (bile ductules), but transition from hepatocytes has also been reported (7). Glandular patterns, partly associated with cells of gastrointestinal type, are observed occasionally (27). It is usually seen in association with other evidence of hepatic toxicity or in hepatocellular tumors. Oval cells and duct epithelial cells are usually positive for GST-P staining (Figs. 2 and 3). *Cholangiofibrosis* is composed of bile duct–like glands and large amounts of collagen-rich connective tissue, and shows nodular growth. The epithelial cells are usually intensely basophilic, and typical intestinal cell metaplasia is occasionally observed. Architectural and cellular atypia is often marked, and it is sometimes difficult to distinguish the lesion from cholangiocellular carcinoma.

Neoplastic lesions of bile duct origin could be classified into cholangiocellular adenomas and carcinomas (7). *Cholangiocellular adenomas* (cholangiomas) are composed of uniform, well-differentiated glands morphologically similar to biliary ductules. Scant fibrous tissues are present between the ductules. Nodular growth is apparent and the adjacent liver parenchyma is often compressed due to marked expansion of the tumors. The lining of cuboidal or columnar epithelial cells is

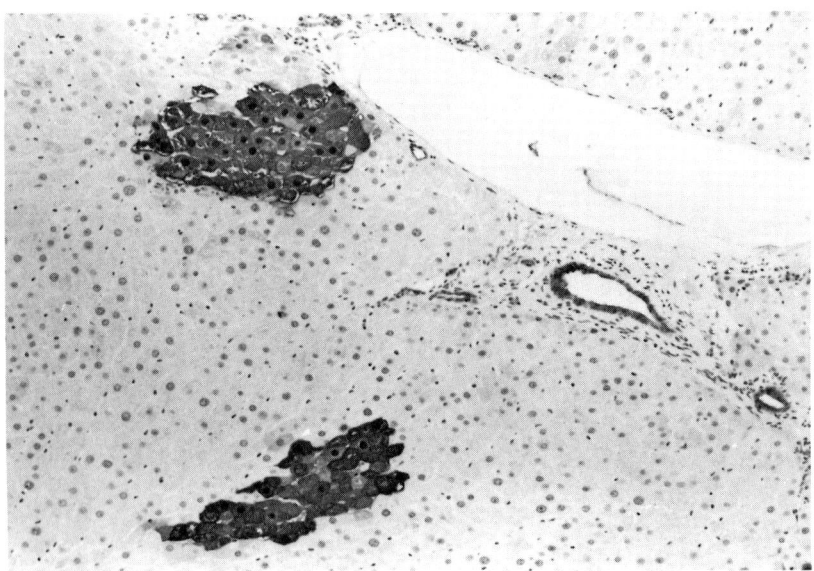

FIG. 3. Epithelial cells of the bile ducts are positive to GST-P staining. Two hepatic positive foci are also clearly observable as contrasted with normal hepatocytes.

slightly atypical and mitotic figures are rare. *Cholangiocellular carcinomas* consist of ductural structure lined by atypical single or stratified cuboidal or columnar cells. Glandular, solid, or papillary patterns are observed. There is often a high mitotic index. The tumors typically contain abundant scirrhous stroma. In contrast to cholangiocellular adenomas, they undergo clear-cut invasive growth.

Rarely observed in rodents are *mixed hepatocholangiocellular adenomas and carcinomas*. The adenomas are morphologically similar to hepatocellular adenomas, but also contain areas of neoplastic bile duct epithelium. Hepatocholangiocellular carcinomas similarly involve elements of both hepatocellular carcinoma and cholangiocellular carcinoma within the same lesion (Figs. 4 to 6). Transitions between the two architectural elements are observed. Commonly, hepatocellular carcinomas have partly associated with cholangiocellular carcinomas, and the presence of bile ducts within an hepatocellular carcinoma is in itself not sufficient to warrant this diagnosis. As a rule, it is important to confirm the production or storage of both bile and mucous substances in the cholangiocellular carcinoma portion. McConnell et al. (28) recommended not combining hepatocellular carcinomas and cholangiocarcinomas in data evaluation.

Hepatoblastoma

Hepatoblastoma is a primitive type of neoplasm rarely observed in rats. It consists of immature hepatic cells, which are normally observed in the liver of the

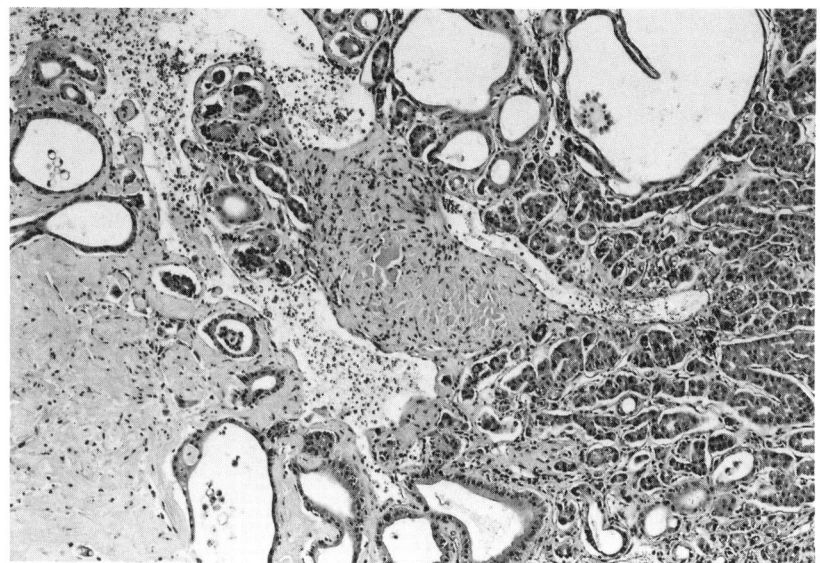

FIG. 4. Mixed hepatocholangiocellular carcinoma induced by 3'-Me-DAB.

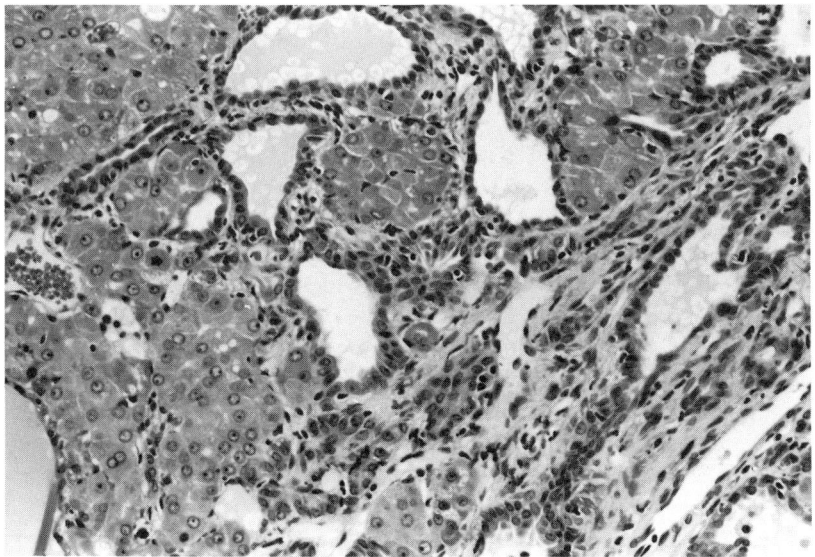

FIG. 5. Higher magnification of the tumor shown in Fig. 4.

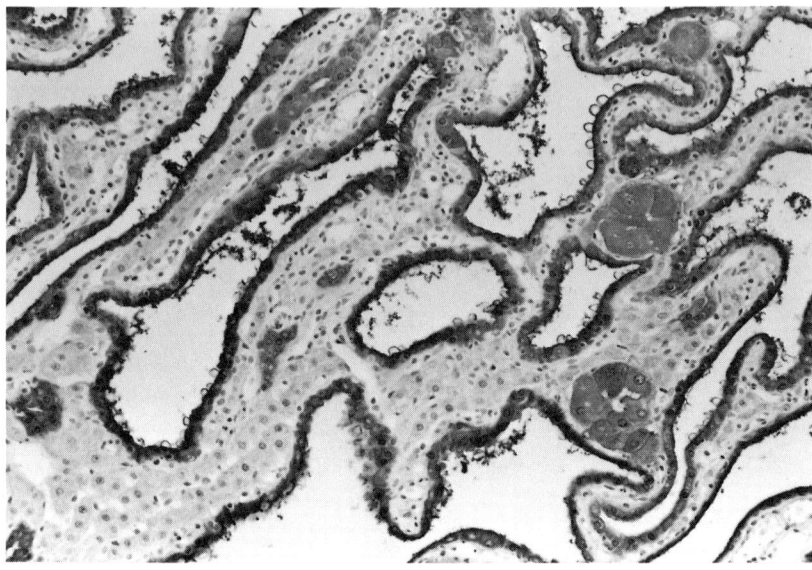

FIG. 6. GST-P immunohistochemistry of a different portion of the tumor shown in Fig. 4.

fetus, and other neoplastic epithelial and mesenchymal elements. A characteristic feature of some tumors is the presence of peculiar "organoids" formed by vascular channels surrounded by tumor cells. The cells in the outer portion of the organoid structures tend to form rosettes. In such cases it is difficult to distinguish the lesion from tumors of hemangioendothelial cell origin.

CHARACTERISTICS OF PRENEOPLASTIC LIVER CELL LESIONS

Significance of Preneoplastic Lesions in Hepatocarcinogenesis

As noted above, histopathologic changes evident in altered cell foci have been analyzed extensively by many authors (3,5–8,10,29). Foci of cellular alteration occur spontaneously in aging rats (30) and regularly precede the development of hepatocellular tumors. Their incidence, size, and multiplicity are usually increased, and the time taken for their development is usually decreased by the administration of hepatocarcinogens or hepatopromoters. In our early study (11,22), the sequential development of hepatocellular carcinomas from foci of cellular alterations, mostly eosinophilic and clear cell foci but also basophilic foci, was followed up to 50 weeks after a single injection of diethylnitrosamine (DEN) and 6 weeks' subsequent administration of 2-acetylaminofluorene (2-AAF) or α-hexachlorocyclohexane (α-HCH). The reliability of hyperplastic foci or nodules (foci of cellular alteration or hepatocellular adenomas) as indicator populations of carcinogenicity was confirmed. Hyperplastic (neoplastic) nodules were increased first and then gradually decreased as degenerative areas in nodules increased. Hepatocellular carcinomas therafter appeared. Precise quantitative analysis indicated that about 2% of hyperplastic nodules develop into hepatocellular carcinomas. Based on these observations, we prefer not to use the term *hepatocellular adenoma* for the lesion.

It has been well recognized that different morphological features may reflect different biological potential. Thus studies have indicated that while foci represent an early stage in neoplastic development and that at least some foci have the capacity to progress to tumors, not all may be related to carcinogenesis (18,22). It was reported in a review of F344 rat liver from several carcinogenicity tests that hepatocarcinogenesis was associated with an increase in the diffusely basophilic or amphophilic cell foci and also with an increase in clear cell foci, but common spontaneous eosinophilic or tigroid basophilic foci were not so clearly associated with exposure to hepatocarcinogens (18). In our observation, however, eosinophilic foci as well as clear cell foci are well correlated with GST-P positivity rather than basophilic foci. It is well known that quantitative analysis of GST-P-positive foci is a reliable method to predict the carcinogenic potential of chemicals (11,31–33).

Thus it is now generally accepted that hyperplastic foci and nodules, both eosinophilic and basophilic, are preneoplastic. Therefore, the lesions have attracted interest as possible endpoints for carcinogenicity testings by a number of authors and therefore applied as indicators of liver carcinogenesis (8–14,34). Focal fatty changes without a specific lobular distribution have also been referred to as *vacuolated* or *fat-storing* cell foci of cellular alteration. However, the lesion is commonly seen under a variety of circumstances and is considered degenerative rather than proliferative in character.

The term *hepatocellular adenoma* was reintroduced by Brooks and Roe (21) to separate this entity clearly from hepatocellular hyperplasia. There are, however, two points for discussion. First, the term *adenoma* itself implies irreversibility. The fact that not all nodules precede tumorigenic course but some might be reversible in nature (22,23) leads us to use the term *hyperplastic nodule* instead of *adenoma* for possible reversible lesions. The term *adenoma* may be used for those that are apparently progressive and relatively large ones, although it is practically difficult to separate them. Another point is a practical approach to distinguish neoplastic focal lesions from regenerative hyperplastic changes. Hepatocellular hyperplasia is defined as a focal or multifocal regenerative or compensatory proliferation of hepatocytes (5,6) and is not necessarily related to hepatic neoplasia. Two salient characteristics are essential for diagnosis for hepatocellular hyperplasia: lack of cytologic or histologic features of neoplasia and evidence of prior or ongoing hepatocyte damage within the liver parenchyma (5,6). Hepatocellular hyperplasia therefore essentially represents regeneration associated with hepatocyte damage, increased mitosis, chronic inflammation, or bile duct hyperplasia. Morphologically, this pattern resembles cirrhosis in other species, and under these conditions lesions should not be assumed automatically to be important hepatocellular changes in the course

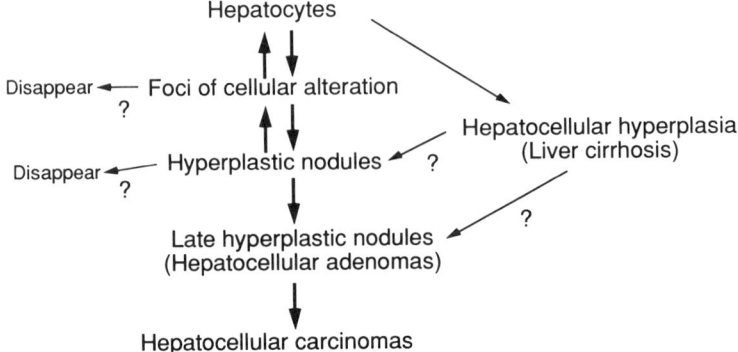

FIG. 7. Possible histogenesis of hepatocellular neoplasias.

of hepatocarcinogenesis in the rat. They are possibly distinguishable from preneoplastic lesions by GST-P staining as mentioned above (Fig. 1).

Possible histogenesis of hepatic tumors is shown in Fig. 7. Hepatocellular hyperplasia is not thought to be a neoplastic lesion but rather a regenerative lesion associated with liver cirrhosis. However, the neoplastic cells generated in the lesions as in human liver cirrhosis are a main source of carcinoma development. Foci and nodules may be reduced in number by remodeling or apoptosis if the carcinogenic stimuli are withdrawn. Hepatocellular adenoma may correspond to late or persistent hyperplastic nodules we have studied (22).

Phenotypic Alterations in Preneoplastic Lesions

Landmarks in studying early stages of hepatocarcinogenesis were the findings of foci characterized by excessive storage of glycogen (16,35) and a reduction in the activity of the microsomal enzyme G6Pase (36,37). A sequence of cellular alterations has been inferred which leads from clear and eosinophilic hepatocytes storing glycogen in excess to basophilic hepatoma cells poor in glycogen. The failure of such foci, as well as hyperplastic and neoplastic nodules, to accumulate iron in the siderotic liver has also been reported (38). A number of histochemically or immunohistochemically demonstrable alterations in enzyme parameters, both negative and positive, have been examined for their usefulness as early indicators of neoplasia (10,39–43), which are observable as negative and positive lesions (Fig. 8).

Thus foci frequently show decreased activities of G6Pase and ATPase (36), glucokinase (36), acid and alkaline nucleases (44,45), glycogen phosphorylase (46,47), adenyl cyclase (48), and L-pyruvate kinase (36). Elevation in activity or amounts of enzyme protein has been found for GGT (49), G6PD (47,50), epoxide hydrolase (51,52), UDP-GT (53), hexokinase (36), and GST-P (42,43,54). Various isozymes of cytochrome P450 (55–59) and α-fetoprotein (60,61) are variable in expression patterns. Although GGT was earlier regarded as a most useful enzyme for detection

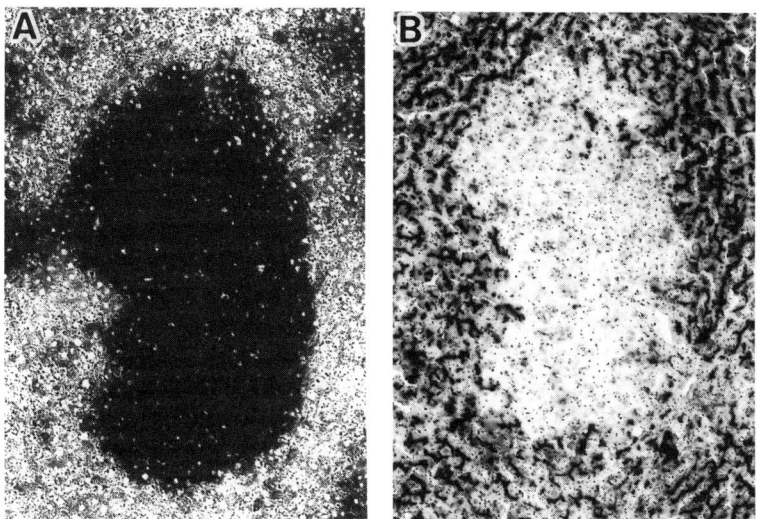

FIG. 8. Serial sections of an eosinophilic focus. **A:** positive for G6PD histochemistry; **B:** negative for ATPase histochemistry.

of foci (8,39,48), investigations have demonstrated a marked advantage for GST-P as a positive immunohistochemical marker (Fig. 9) (42,54).

Foci and tumors induced by hepatocarcinogenic peroxisome proliferators such as clofibrate are unusual in not being detected by the same altered enzyme expression as typical carcinogen-induced lesions (Fig. 10) (62,63). Examination of the effects

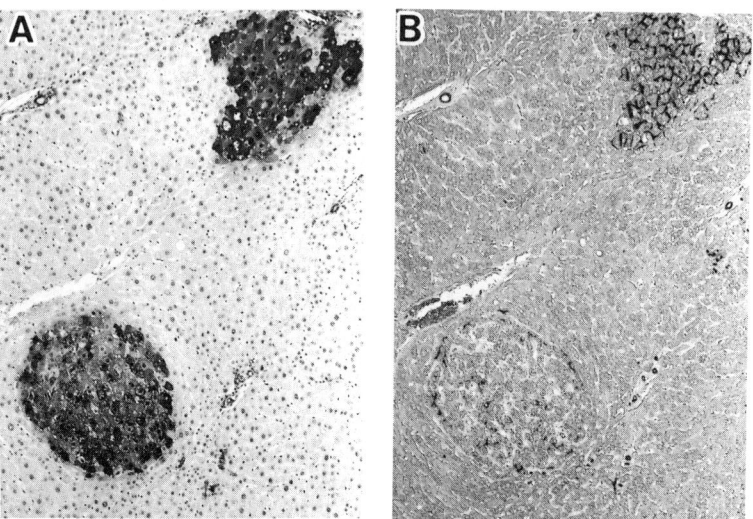

FIG. 9. Some GST-P-positive foci are only weakly stained or unstained for GGT on acetone-fixed formalin-embedded sections. **A:** GST-P immunohistochemistry; **B:** GGT histochemistry.

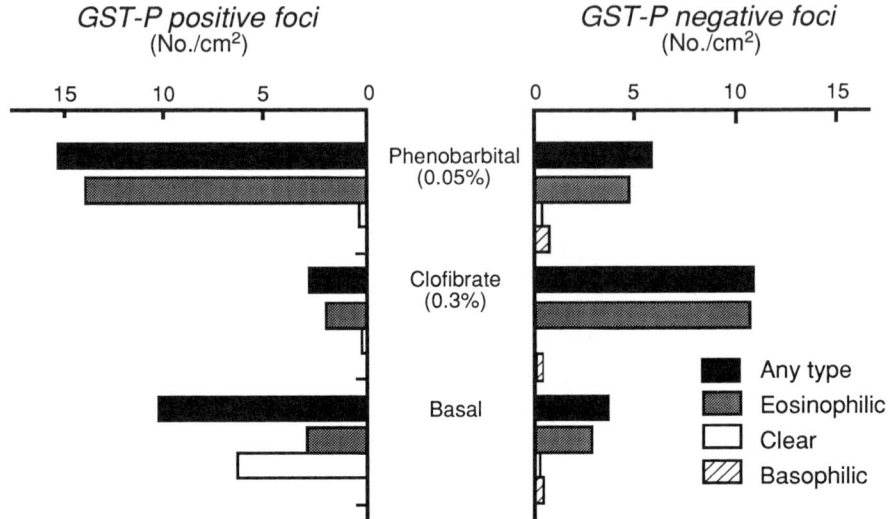

FIG. 10. Number of foci of different types based on GST-P positivity in a rat liver treated with clofibrate for 6 weeks after DEN initiation. (Protocol shown in Fig. 16.)

of prolonged administration of clofibrate at a dose of 0.3% in the diet on neoplastic lesion development after DEN injection (200 mg/kg, i.p.) resulted in a large number of HCC, about a half of these being GST-P negative, and DEN alone induced a few HCC, all of which were GST-P positive (64). Similar findings were obtained for foci and nodules; the proportion of GST-P-negative lesions increased with time, and carcinogenicity could not be predicted by evaluation of GST-P positive foci at any point during the experiment. Clofibrate alone did not induce carcinomas. None of the peroxisome proliferators examined—clofibrate, di(2-ethylhexyl)phthalate (DEHP), di(2-ethylhexyl)adipate (DEHA), and trichloroacetic acid (TCA)—increased lesions characterized by changes in marker enzymes such as GGT, G6PD, ATPase, G6Pase, and catalase on histochemical examination of frozen samples (Fig. 11). Immunohistochemistry of acetone-fixed sections using antibodies against enoyl CoA hydratase (ECH), a hepatic peroxisomal enzyme (65), carbonic anhydrase III (CA III) (66), and manganese superoxide dismutase (Mn-SOD) (67) showed negative expression in foci; the majority of lesions were less clear than with GST-P staining (64). ECH-negative foci were not observable in DEN alone and DEN–phenobarbital groups since in this case background hepatocytes also did not bind the antibody (68).

3,2′-Dimethyl-4-aminobiphenyl (DMAB)–DNA adducts were not formed within foci, as evidenced by immunohistochemical analysis after DMAB, a wide-spectrum genotoxic carcinogen, was injected to rats 24 h before sacrifice (Fig. 12) (64). The findings mean the resistance of foci for exogenous toxic agents are presumably related to lowered P450 levels and glutathione S-transferase induction.

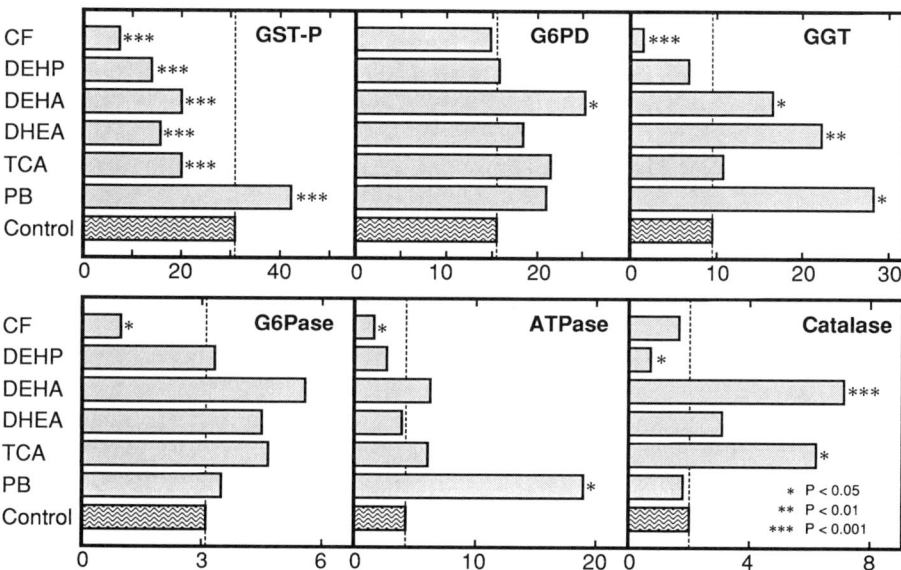

FIG. 11. Number of foci in rat liver treated with peroxisome proliferator after DEN initiation. (Protocol shown in Fig. 16.)

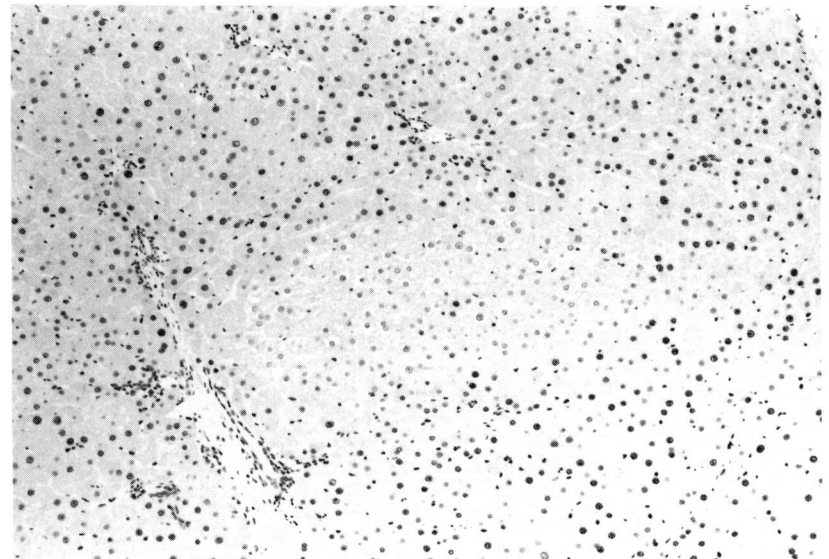

FIG. 12. Immunohistochemistry for DNA–DMAB adducts on the liver of a rat injected with DMAB 1 h prior to sacrifice. Adduct formation observable as a dark stain in nuclei are almost not demonstrated in cells within a focus.

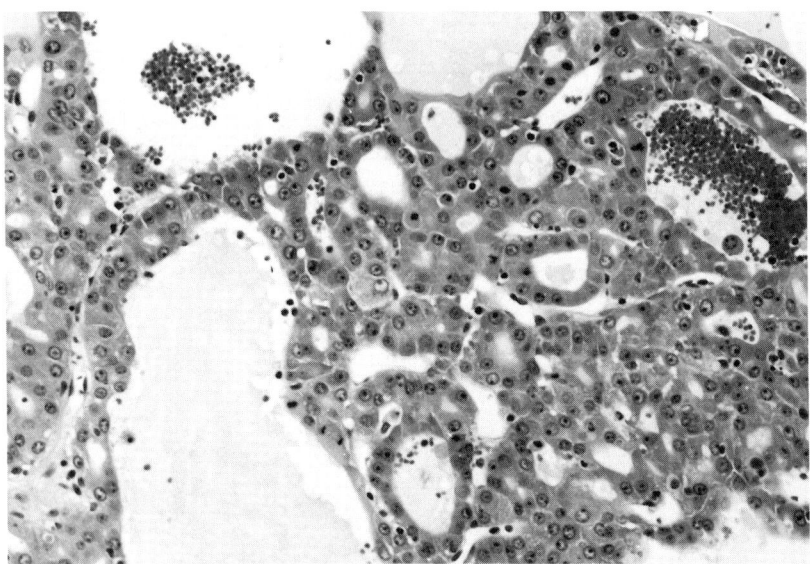

FIG. 13. Pseudoglandular pattern in a hepatocellular carcinoma.

In purely practical terms, GST-P has particular advantages for detection and quantitation work because the ease of immunohistochemical staining enables rapid processing of large numbers of specimens, and the clear contrast recognition allows the use of a semiautomatic image analysis system.

Some Biological Aspects in Hepatic Lesions

The putative preneoplastic lesions show characteristic alterations of key enzymes of carbohydrate metabolism, indicating a switching from glycogen-dependent glucose homeostasis to utilization via the pentose phosphate pathway and glycolysis (69). This has the advantage of providing increased response for anabolic reaction.

In the liver, GGT and GST-P are normally expressed only in the epithelial cells lining the bile ducts (Fig. 3). Early preneoplastic lesions are usually homogeneously stained for both enzymes, although marked heterogeneity is sometimes observed in late nodules or HCC. Since hepatic cells are developmentally derived from bile ducts, these enzymatic changes can be regarded as a functional dedifferentiation of hepatocytes to ductal cells. Similar phenotypic expression of ductal cell characteristics by hepatocytes can also be demonstrated in glandular elements frequently observed within hepatocellular carcinomas (Fig. 13) and in rarely observed combined hepatocholangiocellular tumors (Figs. 4 and 5). GST-P immunostaining demonstrates a clear contrast in positivity between different histologic elements of hepatocholangiocellular tumor (Fig. 6). Based on the foregoing opinion that hepatocytes mimic bile duct characteristics during carcinogenesis, recent findings, such as an increased level of *p*-glycoprotein staining within preneoplastic hepatic foci (70), appear to provide evidence of a directed shift to a mere "selfish" phenotype. It is thus possible to hypothesize that preneoplastic lesions in the liver show biological dedifferentiation, with the alterations acting to endow resistance of preneoplastic foci to hepatotoxic agents, as well as enhanced growth potential.

MULTISTAGE CARCINOGENESIS IN THE RAT LIVER

The original concept of the multistage nature of neoplastic development evolved from experiments conducted on epidermal carcinogenesis in the mouse skin and demonstrated thereafter in other organs. In experimental liver carcinogenesis, Peraino et al. (71) first reported a two-stage model using 2-AAF as an initiator and phenobarbital as a promoter, and this feature of hepatic tumor induction was later confirmed by many authors, including our group (11,72–74). An additional stage of progression has been recognized increasingly as the process whereby characteristics of malignant neoplasia evolve and a higher degree of autonomy and invasion is achieved (75–77). Several authors have applied the multistage hypothesis to liver carcinogenesis.

Initiation

The stage of initiation that occurs first in the natural history of neoplastic development is generally agreed to reflect permanent and irreversible changes in the initiated cell (78). A plausible assumption is that it is related to genetic alteration, fixed during cellular replicative DNA synthesis and cell division (79). Mutagenic agents causing direct DNA damage *in vitro* also often possess tumor-initiating potency, but the correlation is very much less than perfect. Thus mutations cannot in all circumstances be equated with initiation. A number of workers have adapted a pragmatic approach and recognize initiation in terms of quantitatively evaluated numbers of preneoplastic focal lesions (80). Single GST-P-positive cells (Fig. 14) have also been termed *initiated hepatic cells* by some authors (81). However, since many enzyme-altered cells and foci demonstrate a reversible phenotype, the present authors do not agree with using the term *initiated cells*, preferring *phenotypically altered cells* for such populations.

Using male F344 rats in a Solt–Farber protocol (72), we have compared the tumor-initiating potential of five potent hepatocarcinogens—DEN, aflatoxin B_1, 2-AAF, 3′-methyl-4-dimethylaminoazobenzene (3′-Me-DAB), and dimethylnitrosamine—at different doses (82). The results indicated that DEN injected at a necrogenic dose was most effective for reliable induction of hyperplastic nodules. In a separate experiment (83), DEN was once again revealed to be strongest in terms of foci development among three carcinogens—DEN, *N*-hydroxyacetylaminofluorene, and aflatoxin B_1—in an 8-week experiment involving promotion by phenobarbital or 3′-Me-DAB for 6 weeks after a single injection and partial hepatectomy (PH) per-

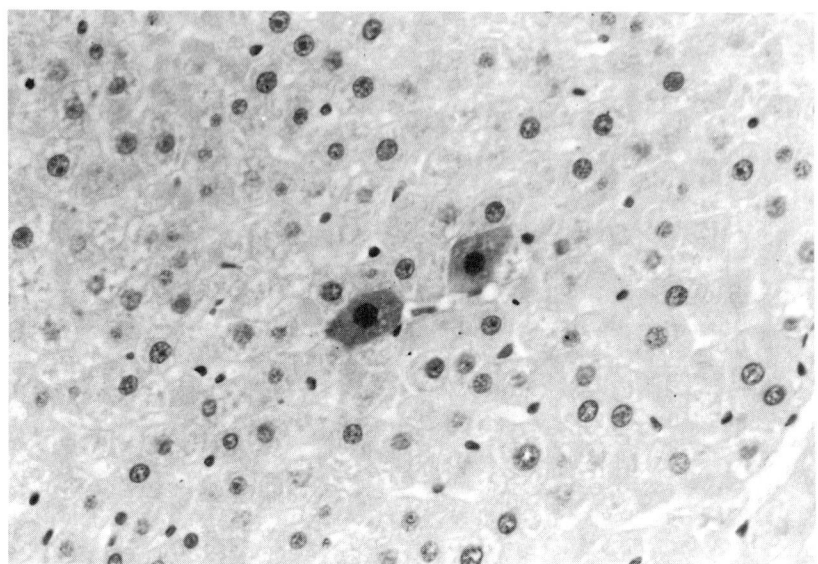

FIG. 14. Two single positive cells for GST-P immunohistochemistry.

formed at the end of week 3. In these experiments, results for quantitative analyses of preneoplastic foci were dependent on the dose of carcinogens used in the initiation step. Although the values for foci differed between the carcinogens, attention should be drawn to the fact that the promoting agents used effectively increased numbers and areas of enzyme-altered foci irrespective of the initiating agents.

Promotion

Promotion means the selection and clonal proliferation of initiated cells by a chemical compound or other factors (9). The principal characteristic of promotion that distinguishes it from the stages of initiation and progression is its operational reversibility (9,22,34). Theoretically, genetic alteration is not required for this stage, but continuous increased proliferation and/or selective toxicity to normal hepatocytes might be important for manifestation of promoting activity (62). Thus promoting agents may increase the risk of cancer development by increasing the proliferation rate and enhancing the likelihood of propagating a genetic error. As hepatopromoting agents in the rat, microsomal enzyme inducers, hypolipidemic agents, steroid hormones, dietary factors, and miscellaneous exogenous factors are included (9,31,32,62).

Complete carcinogens are considered to possess both initiation and promotion activities (34,62). In fact, the organotropism of carcinogenicity might be determined primarily by promoting activity. Based on these concepts we have established a medium-term bioassay for carcinogens, as introduced below.

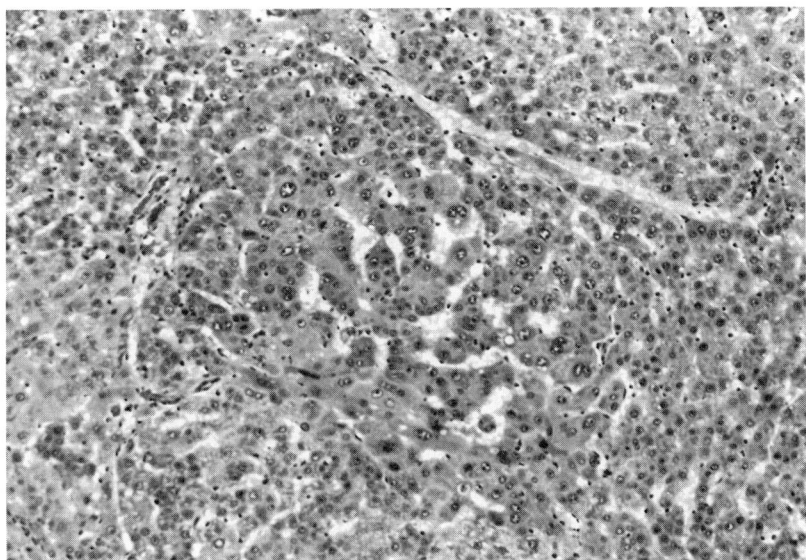

FIG. 15. Small focus of malignant transformation within a hyperplastic nodule (focus in focus/nodule).

Progression

The stage of progression is characterized primarily by the evolution of karyotypic instability and the development of irreversibly aneuploid, malignant neoplasms (76,84,85). The malignancy is related directly to increased growth rate, invasiveness, metastatic capability, and biochemical changes in the malignant cell. Agents that act only during progression, or at least advance a cell from the promotion to progression stages, have not yet been definitely characterized in most systems. However, the initiation–promotion–initiation format proposed by Potter (86) and Pitot et al. (87) resulted in a rapid high incidence of carcinomas when the usual initiation–promotion format was followed by application of a direct-acting mutagen, such as an alkylating agent, as a second genetic insult. A similar regimen has been used to induce foci within foci in experimental multistage hepatocarcinogenesis (88). We also demonstrated an accelerated malignant transformation from neoplastic nodules to hepatocellular carcinomas by the second hit protocol with DEN expanded from our initiation (DEN)–promotion (phenobarbital) protocol and observed carcinomas developing in hyperplastic nodules (unpublished data) and observed malignant transformation in hyperplastic nodules (Fig. 15). Nevertheless, the normal occurrence of foci within foci in standard initiation–promotion protocols is infrequent for rat liver.

Cell Proliferation and Liver Carcinogenesis

As reported elsewhere (89–91), rapid cell proliferation is a prerequisite for effective initiation by a single carcinogen treatment. Our own and other workers' results have further shown an enhancing effect during the promotion phase (9,11,92). The development of foci is clearly related to differences in levels of DNA synthesis and cell turnover between cells within foci and in the surrounding tissue (93). Such differences are most obvious after partial hepatectomy when rats are administered 2-acetylaminofluorene, a hepatotoxic carcinogenic agent that blocks normal cell division (92).

Development of hepatocellular tumors in LEC rats, mutant animals derived from the Long–Evans strain (94), has been reported to be lowered by therapy of copper metabolism or reduced intake of copper, suggesting that the normally extensive liver injury is related to hepatocellular carcinoma development (95). Similar histopathological changes associated with increased hepatocellular damage and cell replication are observable in cases of liver tumors induced in rats maintained on a choline-deficient diet (96,97) or in some types of transgenic animals in which the promoter region of *trans* genes was replaced by albumin or metallothionein promoter (98–100). According to the hypothesis proposed by Cohen and Ellwein (101), development of liver cell tumors in these cases could be explained simply by the increased cell replication, although genetic changes could also be involved.

Genetic Factors and Oncogenes

In an earlier publication (102), increased expression of c-Ha-*ras* and c-*myc* was reported to occur in some, but not all, hepatocellular carcinomas. Moreover, increased expression of these protooncogenes was noted in cells of foci during the stage of promotion (102,103). Other workers have demonstrated increased expression of the c-Ha-*raf* and c-*myc* genes in primary hepatomas induced by 3′-Me-DAB (104,105). However, in multistage hepatocarcinogenesis of the rat, transcriptional activation of proto- and cellular oncogenes has not been identified consistently. For example, the increase in c-Ha-*ras* gene expression in altered hepatic foci after a necrogenic dose of DEN was reported by Galand and associates (106), but mutational activation of the gene could not be demonstrated by Sakai and Ogawa (107) and Li et al. (108).

Sequential protooncogene expression has been demonstrated during rat liver regeneration. When growth is stimulated in the normally quiescent adult rat liver by partial hepatectomy, steady-state levels of messenger RNAs for c-*fos*, c-*myc*, and p53 are increased in sequence during the prereplicative phase which precedes DNA synthesis, and *ras* p21 protein increases much later at the time of DNA replication and cell division (109). Other authors reported sequential and transient expression of c-*fos*, c-*jun*, c-*myc*, c-Ha-*ras*, and c-Ki-*ras* protooncogene RNA transcripts in virtually all hepatocytes of adult rat liver by *in situ* hybridization after a single dose of carbon tetrachloride (110). Protooncogene products thus represent valuable markers of cellular activation preceding and accompanying various aspects of tissue repair reactions. In our observations, increased expression of c-*jun* and c-*fos* in the rat liver was most strongly associated with cell proliferation induced by DEN toxicity and partial hepatectomy (64). In hepatitis B virus transgenic mice, Pasquinelli et al. (111) found that multiple oncogenes and tumor suppressor genes are structurally and functionally intact during hepatocarcinogenesis. Noninsertional activation or inactivation of cellular growth control genes is also not common (112,113), and incidences of *ras* gene mutations are very variable between tumor types in humans (114). It is therefore time to reevaluate the role of alterations in oncogene expression or structure in the hepatocarcinogenic process as well as the role of tumor suppressor genes (115).

PRENEOPLASTIC LESIONS AND RISK ASSESSMENT

The existence of discrepancies between short-term mutagenicity and conventional long-term carcinogenicity testings dictates the necessity of a suitable *in vivo* assay system which could bridge the gap between the short- and long-term tests (116), and several models have been introduced (12–14,72,73). Therefore, a medium-term liver bioassay has been established in our laboratory for rapid detection of carcinogenic agents utilizing preneoplastic GST-P-positive foci of rat liver as endpoint marker lesions. The liver is an obvious choice as the best organ with which to assess carcinogenicity in bioassay systems since the process of liver carcinogenesis has been well studied, and furthermore, more than half of known carcinogens show carcinogenicity in this organ (117–119).

A number of protocols for rapid induction of preneoplastic hepatic foci have been proposed using rat liver (73,120), but most of them have not been tested for general use in risk assessment. Using immunohistochemically demonstrated GST-P-positive foci as endpoint marker lesions, we have established a liver medium-term bioassay model of 8 weeks' duration based on the two-stage hypothesis of carcinogenesis (11,33). In our early studies, hyperplastic nodules (121) and then GGT-positive foci (122) were used as preneoplastic marker lesions. However, after Sato and his colleagues raised an antibody against GST-P (43,123), we have shifted to immunohistochemical demonstration of GST-P-positive foci as endpoint lesions (42,54). Use of immunohistochemically demonstrated GST-P has practical advantages because the ease of immunohistochemical staining enables rapid processing of large numbers of specimens and the clear contrast recognition allows the use of a semiautomatic image analysis system.

Figure 16 shows the protocol now employed in our laboratory for medium-term bioassays. Male F344 rats are given a single intraperitoneal injection of DEN (200 mg/kg) to initiate hepatocarcinogenesis, and beginning 2 weeks later, are given test compound for 6 weeks. Animals are subjected to PH at week 3. Liver slices fixed in ice-cold acetone are immunohistochemically stained for quantitative analysis of

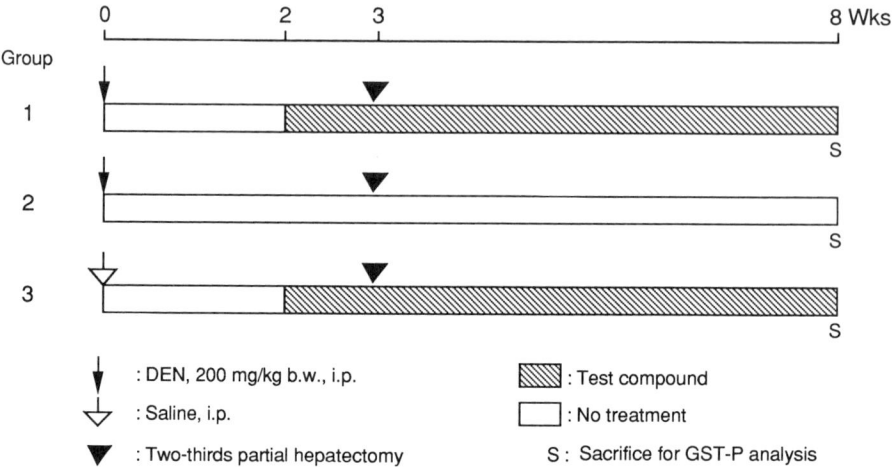

FIG. 16. Protocol of the medium-term liver bioassay for carcinogens. Six-week-old male F344 rats are used (15 rats per group). [Data from Ito et al. (11,31–33).]

GST-P-positive foci more than 0.2 mm in diameter. The results in numbers and areas of foci per unit area of liver section are assessed.

A total of 237 compounds have so far been tested in this system and the results compared with reported *Salmonella*/microsome and long-term carcinogenicity test findings (31,32). Of the 237 compounds (Table 1), 96 exerted positive effects on GST-P-positive foci development, most of them being liver carcinogens (51 chemicals). The positive rate is extremely high (97%, 28 of 29 compounds) for genotoxic hepatocarcinogens and satisfactory (86%, 23 of 27 chemicals) for nongenotoxic hepatocarcinogens (Table 2). The positive rate for carcinogens targeting organs other than the liver, however, is relatively low (24%).

In addition to four well-known hepatocarcinogenic peroxisome proliferators—clofibrate, DEHP, DEHA, and TCA—the bile duct proliferator, 4,4'-diaminodiphenylmethane (124), and dehydroepiandrosterone (125) were negative, although

TABLE 1. *Results of 237 chemicals examined in the liver medium-term bioassay (%)*

Carcinogenicity	Mutagenicity (Ames test)			Total
	+	−	?	
Hepatocarcinogens	28/29 (97)[a]	23/27 (86)[b]	0/1 (0)[c]	51/57 (89)
Nonhepatocarcinogens	7/25 (28)	3/14 (21)	0/2 (0)	10/41 (24)
Noncarcinogens	0/6 (0)	2/32 (6)[d]	0/2 (0)	2/40 (5)
Unknown	3/13 (23)	22/60 (37)	8/26 (31)	33/99 (33)
Total	38/73 (52)	50/133 (38)	8/31 (26)	96/237 (41)

[a] 4,4'-Diaminodiphenylmethane (DDPM) was negative.
[b] Clofibrate, di(2-ethylhexyl)adipate, di(2-ethylhexyl)phthalate, and trichloroacetic acid were negative.
[c] Dehydroepiandrosterone was negative.
[d] Malathion and vinclozolin were positive.

TABLE 2. Results for nongenotoxic hepatocarcinogens in the medium-term liver bioassay

Increased	Aldrin[a]
	Auramine O
	Barbital[a]
	Chlordane[a]
	Chlorendic acid
	Chlorobenzilate[a]
	p,p'-DDT
	Dieldrin[a]
	Ethenzamide[a]
	17α-Ethinyl estradiol
	DL-Ethionine
	Hexachlorobenzene
	α-Hexachlorocyclohexane
	Phenobarbital
	Prochloraz[a]
	Propiconazole[a]
	Safrole
	Sulpyrin[a]
	Tannic acid
	Thioacetamide
	Triadimefon[a]
	Trifluralin[a]
	Urethane
No change	Di(2-ethylhexyl)adipate[a,b]
	Trichloroacetic acid [a,b]
Decreased	Clofibrate[b]
	Di(2-ethylhexyl)phthalate[b]

[a] Carcinogenicity in the mouse liver.
[b] Peroxisome proliferator.

these are all categorized as liver carcinogens (so called false negatives). Dehydroepiandrosterone is known to cause peroxisome proliferation. With regard to the carcinogenicity of peroxisome proliferators, it is important to remember that they depress GST-P expression, and the lesions associated with their hepatocarcinogenicity are not positive for this marker enzyme (62,63).

Of 41 nongenotoxic carcinogens examined, 26 compounds proved positive in this system. Many are chlorinated compounds showing carcinogenicity in the liver (118) and antioxidants (126), which are usually negative in the Ames test. Liver carcinogens reported to be carcinogenic only in mice were also detected at a high rate (11 chemicals). Among 15 nongenotoxic carcinogens that did not exert positive effects in the present system, 11 compounds are nonhepatocarcinogens. Four nongenotoxic hepatocarcinogens are peroxisome proliferators, as mentioned above.

There are several chemicals testing positive in our liver foci system that were reported not to be hepatocarcinogenic in long-term carcinogenicity tests in rats. However, it may be possible that these chemicals are indeed weak hepatocarcinogens or hepatopromoters (32). Our results for hepatocarcinogens indicate that preneoplastic lesions detected by GST-P expression are meaningful precursors for hepatocellular carcinomas, and their quantitative analysis can accurately predict hepatocarcinogenic potential. The validity of this system as a practical tool for rapid detection of carcinogenic and chemopreventive agents of hepatocarcinogenesis has been discussed in detail elsewhere (11,31–33).

CONCLUSIONS

Since the rat liver is the most common target organ of carcinogenic agents, appropriate classification and evaluation of neoplastic and preneoplastic lesions is urgently required. Recent developments in molecular biology have provided pathologists with valuable techniques such as immunohistochemistry and blotting approaches which are providing a deeper understanding of carcinogenesis. Every effort should be made to support and facilitate this process so that liver cancer can be controlled in the future.

REFERENCES

1. Sasaki T, Yoshida T. Experimental induction of hepatocarcinoma by feeding with o-aminoazotoluene. *Virchows Arch* 1935;295:175–200.
2. Squire RA, Levitt MH. Report of a workshop on classification of specific hepatocellular lesions in rats. *Cancer Res* 1975;35:3214–3223.
3. Stewart HL, Williams G, Keysser CH, Lombard LS, Montali RJ. Histologic typing of liver tumors of the rat. *J Natl Cancer Inst* 1980;64:179–206.
4. Hayashi Y. Histologic typing of liver tumors in rats, mice and hamsters. A workshop report. *Exp Pathol* 1985;28:140–141.
5. Maronpot RR, Montgomery CA Jr, Boorman GA, McConnell EE. National Toxicology Program nomenclature for hepatoproliferative lesions of rats. *Toxicol Pathol* 1986;14:263–273.
6. Rinde E, Chiu A, Hill R, Haberman B. *Proliferative hepatocellular lesions of the rat. Review and future use in risk assessment*. Washington DC: US Environmental Protection Agency; 1986:1–22.
7. Bannasch P, Zerban H. Tumours of the liver. In: Turusov V, Mohr U, eds. *Pathology of tumours in laboratory animals*. Vol 1. *Tumours of the rat*. 2nd ed. Lyon, France: IARC Scientific Publications; 1990:199–240.
8. Williams GM. Phenotypic properties of preneoplastic rat liver lesions and applications to detection of carcinogens and tumor promoters. *Toxicol Pathol* 1982;10:3–10.
9. Schulte-Hermann R. Tumor promotion in the liver. *Arch Toxicol* 1985;57:147–158.
10. Bannasch P. Preneoplastic lesions as end points in carcinogenicity testing. I. Hepatic neoplasia. *Carcinogenesis* 1986;7:689–695.
11. Ito N, Imaida K, Hasegawa R, Tsuda H. Rapid bioassay methods for carcinogens and modifiers of hepatocarcinogenesis. *CRC Crit Rev Toxicol* 1989;19:385–415.
12. Oesterle D, Deml E. Detection of chemical carcinogens by means of the "rat liver foci bioassay." *Exp Pathol* 1990;39:197–206.
13. Dragan YP, Rizvi T, Xu YH, Hully JR, Bawa N, Campbell HA, Maronpot RR, Pitot HC. An initiation–promotion assay in rat liver as a potential complement to the 2-year carcinogenesis bioassay. *Fundam Appl Toxicol* 1991;16:525–547.
14. Williams GM. Phenotypic properties of preneoplastic rat liver lesions and applications to detection of carcinogens and tumor promoters. *Toxicol Pathol* 1982;10:3–10.
15. Bannasch P, Zerban H, Hacker HJ. Foci of altered hepatocytes, rat. In: Jones TC, Mohr U, Hunt RD, eds. *Digestive system*. Monographs on pathology of laboratory animals. Berlin: Springer-Verlag; 1985:10–30.
16. Bannasch P. The cytoplasm of hepatocytes during carcinogenesis. Light and electron microscopic investigations of the nitrosomorpholine-intoxicated rat liver. *Recent Results Cancer Res* 1968;19:1–100.
17. Weber E, Moore MA, Bannasch P. Enzyme histochemical and morphological phenotype of am-

phophilic cell and amphophilic/tigroid cell neoplastic nodules in rat liver after combined treatment with dehydroepiandrosterone and N-nitrosomorpholine. *Carcinogenesis* 1988;9:1049–1054.
18. Harada T, Maronpot RR, Morris RW, Boorman GA. Observations on altered hepatocellular foci in National Toxicology Program two-year carcinogenicity studies in rats. *Toxicol Pathol* 1989;17: 690–706.
19. Farber E. Hyperplastic liver nodules. *Methods Cancer Res* 1973;7:345–375.
20. Bannasch P. Cytology and cytogenesis of neoplastic (hyperplastic) hepatic nodules. *Cancer Res* 1976;36:2555–2562.
21. Brooks PN, Roe FJC. Hepatocellular adenoma, liver, rat. In: Jones TC, Mohr U, Hunt RD, eds. *Digestive system*. Monographs on pathology of laboratory animals. Berlin: Springer-Verlag; 1985: 47–52.
22. Tatematsu M, Takano T, Hasegawa R, Imaida K, Nakanowatari J, Ito N. A sequential quantitative study of the reversibility or irreversibility of liver hyperplastic nodules in rats exposed to hepatocarcinogens. *Gann* 1980;71:843–855.
23. Ito N, Hananouchi M, Sugihara S, Shirai T, Tsuda H, Fukushima S, Nagasaki H. Reversibility and irreversibility of liver tumors in mice induced by the α isomer of 1,2,3,4,5,6-hexachlorocyclohexane. *Cancer Res* 1976;36:2227–2234.
24. Bannasch P, Zerban H. Modulation of hepatocellular phenotype and proliferation in liver cirrhosis. In: Boyer JL, Bianochi L, eds. *Liver cirrhosis*. Lancaster, PA: MTP Press; 1987:27–38.
25. Schauer A, Kunze E. Liver tumours of the rat. In: Turusov VS, ed. *Pathology of tumours in laboratory animals*. Vol 1. *Tumours of the rat*. Pt 2. Lyon, France: IARC Scientific Publications; 1976:41–72.
26. Popp JA, Scortichini BH, Carvey LK. Quantitative evaluation of hepatic foci of alteration occurring spontaneously in Fischer 344 rats. *Fundam Appl Toxicol* 1985;5:314–319.
27. Tatematsu M, Ho RH, Kaku T, Ekem JK, Farber E. Studies on the proliferation and fate of oval cells in the liver of rats treated with 2-acetylaminofluorene and partial hepatectomy. *Am J Pathol* 1984;114:418–430.
28. McConnell EE, Solleveld HA, Swenberg JA, Boorman GA. Guideline for combining neoplasms for evaluation of rodent carcinogenesis studies. *J Natl Cancer Inst* 1986;76:283–289.
29. Emmelot P, Scherer E. The first relevant cell stage in rat liver carcinogenesis. A quantitative approach. *Biochem Biophys Acta* 1980;605:247–304.
30. Ward JM, Henneman JR. Naturally-occurring age-dependent glutathione S-transferase π immunoreactive hepatocytes in aging female F344 rat liver as potential promotable targets for nongenotoxic carcinogens. *Cancer Lett* 1990;52:187–195.
31. Ito N, Tsuda H, Tatematsu M, Inoue T, Tagawa Y, Aoki T, Uwagawa S, Kagawa M, Ogiso T, Masui T, Imaida K, Fukushima S, Asamoto M. Enhancing effect of various hepatocarcinogens on induction of preneoplastic glutathione S-transferase placental form positive foci in rats: an approach for a new medium-term bioassay system. *Carcinogenesis* 1988;9:387–394.
32. Hasegawa R, Ito N. Liver medium-term bioassay in rats for screening of carcinogens and modifying factors in hepatocarcinogenesis. *Food Chem Toxicol* 1992;30:979–992.
33. Ito N, Shirai T, Hasegawa R. Medium-term bioassay for carcinogens. In: Vainio H, Magee PN, McGregor DB, McMichael AJ, eds. *Mechanisms of carcinogenesis in risk assessment*. Lyon, France: IARC Scientific Publications, 1992:353–388.
34. Pitot HC, Dragan YP. Facts and theories concerning the mechanisms of carcinogenesis. *FASEB J* 1991;5:2280–2286.
35. Bannasch P, Müller HA. Lichtmikroskopische Untersuchungen über die Wirking von N-Nitrosomorpholin auf die Leber von Ratte und Mause. *Arzneim Forsch* 1964;14:805–814.
36. Fischer G, Ruschenburg I, Eighnbrodt E, Katz N. Decrease in glucokinase and glucose-6-phosphatase and increase in hexokinase in putative preneoplastic lesions of rat liver. *J Cancer Res Clin Oncol* 1987;113:430–436.
37. Gössner W, Friedrich-Freksa H. Histochemische Untersuchungen über die Glucose-6-Phosphatase in der Rattenleber während der Cancerisierung durch Nitrosamine. *Z Naturforsch* 1964;19b:862–864.
38. Williams G, Klaiber M, Parker SE, Farber E. Nature of early appearing, carcinogen-induced liver lesions resistant to iron accumulation. *J Natl Cancer Inst* 1976;57:157–165.
39. Hanigan MH, Pitot HC. γ-Glutamyl transpeptidase, its role in hepatocarcinogenesis. *Carcinogenesis* 1985;6:165–172.
40. Hendrich S, Pitot HC. Enzymes of glutathione metabolism as biochemical markers during hepatocarcinogenesis. *Cancer Metastasis Rev* 1987;6:155–178.

41. Tsuda H, Ozaki K, Uwagawa S, Takahashi S, Hakoi K, Kato T, Fukushima S, Sato K, Ito N. Analysis of the effects of modifying agents on proliferation and enzyme phenotype in focal preneoplastic and neoplastic liver lesions in rats. In: Columbano A, et al, eds. *Chemical carcinogenesis*. Vol 2. New York: Plenum Press; 1991:219–229.
42. Tatematsu M, Mera Y, Ito N, Satoh K, Sato K. Relative merits of immunohistochemical demonstration of placental A, B and C forms of glutathione S-transferase and histochemical demonstration of γ-glutamyltransferase as markers of altered foci during liver carcinogenesis in rats. *Carcinogenesis* 1985;6:1621–1626.
43. Sato K, Kitahara A, Satoh K, Ichikawa T, Tatematsu M, Ito N. The placental form of glutathione S-transferase as a new marker protein for preneoplasia in rat chemical carcinogenesis. *Gann* 1984; 75:199–202.
44. Taper HS, Fort L, Brucher JM. Histochemical activity of alkaline and acid nucleases in the rat liver parenchyma during N-nitrosomorpholine carcinogenesis. *Cancer Res* 1971;31:913–916.
45. Taper HS, Lans M, de Garlache J, Fort L, Roberfroid M. Morphological alterations and DNase deficiency in phenobarbital promotion of N-nitrosomorpholine initiated rat hepatocarcinogenesis. *Carcinogenesis* 1983;4:231–234.
46. Scherer E, Emmelot P. Kinetics of induction and growth of enzyme-deficient islands involved in hepatocarcinogenesis. *Cancer Res* 1976;36:2544–2554.
47. Hacker HJ, Moore MA, Mayer D, Bannasch P. Correlative histochemistry of some enzymes of carbohydrate metabolism in preneoplastic and neoplastic lesions in the rat liver. *Carcinogenesis* 1982;3:1265–1272.
48. Ehemann V, Mayer D, Hacker HJ, Bannasch P. Loss of adenyl cyclase activity in preneoplastic and neoplastic lesions induced in rat liver by N-nitrosomorpholine. *Carcinogenesis* 1986;7:567–573.
49. Ogawa K, Solt DB, Farber E. Phenotypic diversity as an early property of putative preneoplastic populations in liver carcinogenesis. *Cancer Res* 1980;40:725–733.
50. Klimek F, Mayer D, Bannasch P. Biochemical microanalysis of glycogen content and glucose-6-phosphate dehydrogenase activity in focal lesions of rat liver induced by N-nitrosomorpholine. *Carcinogenesis* 1984;5:265–268.
51. Enomoto K, Ying TS, Griffin MJ, Farber E. Immunohistochemical study of epoxide hydrolase during experimental liver carcinogenesis. *Cancer Res* 1981;41:3281–3287.
52. Kuhlmann WD, Krichan R, Kunz W, Guenthner TM, Oesch F. Focal elevation of liver microsomal epoxide hydrolase in early preneoplastic stages and its behavior in the further course of hepatocarcinogenesis. *Biochem Biophys Res Commun* 1981;98:417–423.
53. Fischer G, Ullrich D, Katz N, Bock WK, Schauer A. Immunohistochemical and biochemical detection of uridine-diphosphate-glucuronyltransferase (UDP-GT) activity in putative preneoplastic liver foci. *Virchows Arch B Cell Pathol* 1983;42:193–200.
54. Tatematsu M, Mera Y, Inoue T, Satoh K, Sato K, Ito N. Stable phenotypic expression of glutathione S-transferase placental type and unstable phenotypic expression of γ-glutamyltransferase in rat liver preneoplastic and neoplastic lesions. *Carcinogenesis* 1988;9:215–220.
55. Schulte-Hermann R, Roome N, Timmermann-Trosiener I, Schuppler J. Immunohistochemical demonstration of a phenobarbital-inducible cytochrome P450 in putative preneoplastic foci of rat liver. *Carcinogenesis* 1984;5:143–153.
56. Buchmann A, Kuhlmann WD, Schwarz M, Kunz HW, Wolf CR, Moll E, Friedberg T, Oesch F. Regulation and expression of four cytochrome P450 isozymes, NADPH-cytochrome P450 reductase, the glutathione transferase B and C and microsomal epoxide hydrolase in preneoplastic and neoplastic lesions in rat liver. *Carcinogenesis* 1985;6:513–521.
57. Tsuda H, Moore MA, Asamoto M, Inoue T, Ito N, Satoh K, Ichihara A, Nakamura T, Amelizad Z, Oesch F. Effect of modifying agents on the phenotypic expression of cytochrome P-450, glutathione S-transferase molecular forms, microsomal epoxide hydrolase, glucose-6-phosphate dehydrogenase and γ-glutamyltranspeptidase in rat liver preneoplastic lesions. *Carcinogenesis* 1988; 9:547–554.
58. Degawa M, Miura S, Hashimoto Y. Expression and induction of cytochrome P450 isozymes in hyperplastic nodules of rat liver. *Carcinogenesis* 1991;12:2151–2156.
59. Buchmann A, Schwarz M, Schmitt R, Wolf CR, Oesch F, Kunz W. Development of cytochrome P-450-altered preneoplastic and neoplastic lesions during nitrosamine-induced hepatocarcinogenesis in the rat. *Cancer Res* 1987;47:2911–2918.
60. Tamaoki T, Fausto N. Expression of the α-fetoprotein gene during development, regeneration, and

carcinogenesis. In: Stein GS, Stein JL, eds, *Recombinant DNA and cell proliferation*. New York: Academic Press; 1984:145–168.
61. Lemire JM, Fausto N. Multiple α-fetoprotein RNAs in adult rat liver: Cell type-specific expression and differential regulation. *Cancer Res* 1991;51:4656–4664.
62. Moore MA, Kitagawa T. Hepatocarcinogenesis in the rat: the effect of promoters and carcinogens *in vivo* and *in vitro*. *Int Rev Cytol* 1986;101:125–173.
63. Rao MS, Reddy JK. Peroxisome proliferation and hepatocarcinogenesis. *Carcinogenesis* 1987; 8:631–636.
64. Ito N, Hasagawa R, Imaida K, Masui T, Takahashi S, Shirai T. Pathological markers for nongenotoxic agent-associated carcinogenesis. *Toxicol Lett* 1992;64/65:613–620.
65. Yokoyama Y, Tsuchida S, Hatayama I, Satoh K, Narita T, Rao MS, Reddy JK, Yamada J, Suga T, Sato K. Loss of peroxisomal enzyme expression in preneoplastic lesions induced by peroxisome proliferators in rat liver. *Carcinogenesis* 1992;13:265–269.
66. Nagase T, Sugiyama T, Kuwata S, Tarui S, Deutsch HF, Taniguchi N. Analysis of polypeptides in the liver of a novel mutant (LEC rats) to hereditary hepatitis and hepatoma by two-dimensional gel electrophoresis: identification of P92/6.8 as carbonic anhydrase III and triosephosphate isomerase. *Comp Biochem Physiol* 1991;99:193–201.
67. Kawaguchi T, Noji S, Uda T, Nakashima Y, Takeyasu A, Kawai Y, Takagi H, Tohyama M, Taniguchi N. A monoclonal antibody against COOH-terminal peptide of human liver manganese superoxide dismutase. *J Biol Chem* 1989;264:5762–5767.
68. Yokoyama Y, Tsuchida S, Hatayama I, Sato K. Lack of peroxisomal enzyme inducibility in rat hepatic preneoplastic lesions induced by mutagenic carcinogens: contrasted expression of glutathione S-transferase P form and enoyl CoA hydratase. *Carcinogenesis* 1993;14:393–398.
69. Bannasch P, Hacker HJ, Klimek F, Mayer D. Hepatocellular glycogenesis and related pattern of enzymatic changes during hepatocarcinogenesis. *Adv Enzyme Regul* 1984;22:97–121.
70. Bradley G, Sharma R, Rajalakshmi S, Ling V. P-Glycoprotein expression during tumor progression in the rat liver. *Cancer Res* 1992;52:5154–5161.
71. Peraino C, Fry RJM, Staffeldt E. Reduction and enhancement by phenobarbital of hepatocarcinogenesis induced in the rat by 2-acetylaminofluorene. *Cancer Res* 1971;31:1506–1512.
72. Solt D, Farber E. New principle for the analysis of chemical carcinogenesis. *Nature* 1976;263: 701–703.
73. Goldsworthy TL, Hanigan M, Pitot HC. Models of hepatocarcinogenesis in the rat: contrasts and comparisons. *CRC Crit Rev Toxicol* 1986;17:61–89.
74. de Gerlache J, Lans M, Preat V, Taper H, Roberfroid M. Comparison of different models of rat liver carcinogenesis: conclusions from a systemic analysis. *Toxicol Pathol* 1984;12:374–382.
75. Foulds L. The experimental study of tumor progression: a review. *Cancer Res* 1954;14:327–339.
76. Pitot HC. Progression: the terminal stage of carcinogenesis. *Jpn J Cancer Res* 1989;80:599–607.
77. Nowell PC. Mechanisms of tumor progression. *Cancer Res* 86;46:2203–2207.
78. Boutwell RK. Some biological aspects of skin carcinogenesis. *Prog Exp Tumor Res* 1954;4:207–250.
79. Ishikawa T, Takayama S, Kitagawa T. Correlation between time of partial hepatectomy after a single treatment with diethylnitrosamine and induction of adenosine triphosphatase-deficient islands in rat liver. *Cancer Res* 1980;40:4261–4264.
80. Pitot HC. Altered hepatic foci: their role in murine hepatocarcinogenesis. *Annu Rev Pharmacol Toxicol* 1990;30:465–500.
81. Moore MA, Nakagawa K, Satoh K, Ishikawa T, Sato K. Single GST-P positive liver cells: putative initiated hepatocytes. *Carcinogenesis* 1987;8:483–486.
82. Imaida K, Shirai T, Tatematsu M, Takano T, Ito N. Dose responses of five hepatocarcinogens for the initiation of rat hepatocarcinogenesis. *Cancer Lett* 1981;14:279–283.
83. Shirai T, Imaida K, Ohshima M, Fukushima S, Lee MS, King MC, Ito N. Different responses to phenobarbital promotion in the development of γ-glutamyl transpeptidase positive foci in the liver of rats initiated with diethylnitrosamine, 2-hydroxy-2-acetylaminofluorene or aflatoxin B_1. *Jpn J Cancer Res (Gann)* 1985;76:16–19.
84. Sargent L, Xu YH, Sattler GL, Pitot HC. Ploidy and karyotype of hepatocytes isolated from enzyme-altered foci in two different protocols of multistage hepatocarcinogenesis in the rat. *Carcinogenesis* 1989;10:387–391.
85. Schere E. Neoplastic progression in experimental hepatocarcinogenesis. *Biochem Biophys Acta* 1984;738:219–236.

86. Potter VR. A new protocol and its rationale for the study of initiation and promotion of carcinogenesis in rat liver. *Carcinogenesis* 1981;2:1375–1379.
87. Pitot HC, Barsness L, Goldsworthy T, Kitagawa T. Biochemical characterization of stages of hepatocarcinogenesis after a single dose of diethylnitrosamine. *Nature* 1978;271:456–457.
88. Scherer E, Feringa AW, Emmelot P. Initiation–promotion–initiation: induction of neoplastic foci within islands of precancerous liver cells in the rat. *Models Mech Etiol Tumor Promot* 1984;56:57.
89. Cayama E, Tsuda H, Sarma DSR, Farber E. Initiation of chemical carcinogenesis requires cell proliferation. *Nature* 1978;275:60–62.
90. Craddock VM. Cell proliferation and experimental liver cancer. In: Cameron HM, Linsell DA, Warwick GP, eds. *Liver cell cancer*. Amsterdam: Elsevier; 1976:153–201.
91. Scherer E, Emmelot P. Kinetics of induction and growth of precancerous liver-cell foci, and liver tumor formation by diethylnitrosamine. *Eur J Cancer* 1975;11:689–696.
92. Hasegawa R, Tsuda H, Shirai T, Kurata Y, Masuda A, Ito N. Effect of timing of partial hepatectomy on the induction of preneoplastic liver foci in rats given hepatocarcinogens. *Cancer Lett* 1986;32:15–23.
93. Tatematsu M, Aoki T, Kagawa M, Mera Y, Ito N. Reciprocal relationship between development of glutathione S-transferase positive liver foci and proliferation of surrounding hepatocytes in rats. *Carcinogenesis* 1988;9:221–225.
94. Sasaki M, Yoshida MC, Kagami K, Takeichi N, Kobayashi H, Dempo K, Mori M. Spontaneous hepatitis in an inbred strain of Long–Evans rats. *Rat News Lett* 1985;14:4–6.
95. Kang JH, Togashi Y, Li Y, Miki T, Takeichi N, Enomoto K, Mori M, Hosokawa M. Inhibition of spontaneous development of hepatocellular carcinoma in LEC rats by administration with D-penicillamine. *Proceedings of the Japanese Cancer Association 51st annual meeting*; 1992, no 21.
96. Shinozuka H, Katyal SL, Perera MIR. Choline deficiency and chemical carcinogenesis. *Adv Exp Med Biol* 1986;206:253–267.
97. Nakae D, Yoshiji H, Mizumoto Y, Horiguchi K, Shiraiwa K, Tamura K, Denda A, Konishi Y. High incidence of hepatocellular carcinomas induced by a choline deficient L-amino acid defined diet in rats. *Cancer Res* 1992;52:5042–5045.
98. Dunsford HA, Sell S, Chisari FV. Hepatocarcinogenesis due to chronic liver cell injury in hepatitis B virus transgenic mice. *Cancer Res* 1990;50:3400–3407.
99. Orian JM, Tamakoshi K, Mackay IR, Brandon MR. New murine model for hepatocellular carcinoma: transgenic mice expressing metallothionein-ovine growth hormone fusion gene. *J Natl Cancer Inst* 1990;82:393–398.
100. Sepulveda AR, Finegold MJ, Smith B, Slagle BL, DeMayo JL, Shen RF, Woo SLC, Butel JS. Development of a transgenic mouse system for the analysis of stages in liver carcinogenesis using tissue-specific expression of SV40 large T-antigen controlled by regulatory elements of the human α-1-antitrypsin gene. *Cancer Res* 1989;49:6108–6117.
101. Cohen SM, Ellwein LB. Cell proliferation in carcinogenesis. *Science* 1990;249:1007–1011.
102. Beer DG, Schwarz M, Sawada N, Pitot HC. Expression of H-*ras* and c-*myc* protooncogenes in isolated γ-glutamyltranspeptidase-positive hepatocytes and hepatocellular carcinomas induced by diethylnitrosamine. *Cancer Res* 1986;46:2435–2439.
103. Embleton MJ, Butler PC. Reactivity of monoclonal antibodies to oncoproteins with normal rat liver, carcinogen-induced tumors, and premalignant liver lesions. *Br J Cancer* 1988;57:48–52.
104. Makino R Hayashi K, Sato S, Sugimura T. Expressions of the c-Ha-*ras* and c-*myc* genes in the rat liver tumors. *Biochem Biophys Res Commun* 1984;119:1096–1101.
105. Cote GJ, Lastra BA, Cook JR, Huang DP, Chiu JF. Oncogene expression in rat hepatoma and during hepatocarcinogenesis. *Cancer Lett* 1985;26:121–126.
106. Galand P, Jacobovitz D, Alexandre K. Immunohistochemical detection of c-Ha-*ras* oncogene p21 product in pre-neoplastic and neoplastic lesions during hepatocarcinogenesis in rats. *Int J Cancer* 1988;41:155–161.
107. Sakai H, Ogawa K. Mutational activation of Ha-*ras* and K-*ras* genes is absent in *N*-nitroso-*N*-methylurea-induced liver tumors in rats. *Jpn J Cancer Res* 1990;81:437–439.
108. Li H, Lee GH, Nomura K, Ohtake K, Kitagawa T. Low frequency of *ras* activation in 2-acetylaminofluorene- and 3′-methyl-4-(dimethylamino)azobenzene-induced rat hepatocellular carcinomas. *Cancer Lett* 1991;56:17–24.
109. Thompson NL, Mead JE, Braun L, Goyette M, Shank PR, Fausto N. Sequential protooncogene expression during rat liver regeneration. *Cancer Res* 1986;46:3111–3117.
110. Herbst H, Milani S, Schuppan D, Stein H. Temporal and special patterns of proto-oncogene expression at early stages of toxic liver injury in the rat. *Lab Invest* 1991;65:324–333.

111. Pasquinelli C, Bhavani K, Chisari FV. Multiple oncogenes and tumor suppressor genes are structurally and functionally intact during hepatocarcinogenesis in hepatitis B virus transgenic mice. *Cancer Res* 1992;52:2823–2829.
112. Ganem D, Varmus HE. The molecular biology of the hepatitis B viruses. *Annu Rev Biochem* 1987; 56:651–693.
113. Ganem D. Oncogenic viruses of marmots and men. *Nature (London)* 1990;347:230–232.
114. Bos JL. *Ras* oncogenes in human cancer: a review. *Cancer Res* 1989;49:4682–4689.
115. Smith ML, Yeleswarapu L, Scalamogna P, Locker J, Lombardi B. p53 mutations in hepatocellular carcinomas induced by a choline-devoid diet in male Fischer 344 rats. *Carcinogenesis* 1993;14: 503–510.
116. Ward JM, Ito N. Development of new medium-term bioassays for carcinogens. *Cancer Res* 1988; 48:5051–5054.
117. IARC. *IARC monographs on the evaluation of carcinogenic risks to humans. Overall evaluations of carcinogenicity: an updating of IARC monographs volumes 1 to 42* [Suppl 7]. Lyon, France: IARC Scientific Publications; 1987.
118. Zeiger E. Carcinogenicity of mutagens: predictive capability of the *Salmonella* mutagenesis assay for rodent carcinogenicity. *Cancer Res* 1987;47:1287–1296.
119. Ashby J, Tennant RW. Definitive relationship among chemical structure, carcinogenicity and mutagenicity for 301 chemicals tested by the U.S. NTP. *Mutat Res* 1991;25:229–306.
120. Diwan BA, Ward JM, Rice JM. Modification of liver tumor development in rodents. In: Ito N, Sugano H, eds. *Modification of tumor development in rodents*. Vol 33. Basel: S Karger; 1991: 76–107.
121. Ito N, Tatematsu M, Nakanishi K, Hasegawa R, Takano T, Imaida K, Ogiso T. The effects of various chemicals on the development of hyperplastic liver nodules in hepatectomized rats treated with *N*-nitrosodiethylamine or *N*-2-fluorenylacetamide. *Gann* 1980;71:832–842.
122. Tsuda H, Hasegawa R, Imaida K, Masui T, Moore MA, Ito N. Modifying potential of thirty-one chemicals on the short-term development of γ-glutamyl transpeptidase-positive foci in diethylnitrosamine-initiated rat liver. *Gann* 1984;75:876–883.
123. Satoh K, Kitahara A, Soma Y, Inaba Y, Hatayama I, Sato K. Purification, induction, and distribution of placental glutathione transferase: a new marker enzyme for preneoplastic cells in the rat chemical carcinogenesis. *Proc Natl Acad Sci USA* 1985;82:3964–3968.
124. Lamb JC, Huff JE, Haseman JK, Murthy ASK, Lilga H. Carcinogenesis studies of 4,4'-methylenedianiline dihydrochloride given in drinking water to F344/N rats and B6C3F$_1$ mice. *J Toxicol Environ Health* 1986;18:325–337.
125. Rao MS, Subbarao V, Kumar S, Yeldandi AV, Reddy JK. Phenotypic properties of liver tumors induced by dehydroepiandrosterone in F344 rats. *Jpn J Cancer Res* 1992;83:1179–1183.
126. Ito N, Hirose M. Antioxidants: carcinogenic and chemopreventive properties. *Adv Cancer Res* 1989;53:247–302.

Carcinogenesis, edited by
M.P. Waalkes and J.M. Ward.
Raven Press, Ltd., New York © 1994.

4
Susceptibility Factors of Gastrointestinal Tract Carcinogenesis

Kosaku Sakamoto, *Huimian Xu, and †Abulkalam M. Shamsuddin

*Department of Surgery, Maki Hospital, Takasaki, Gunma, T370 Japan; *Department of Oncology, First Affiliated Hospital, China Medical University, Shenyang, China 110001; †Department of Pathology, University of Maryland School of Medicine, Baltimore, Maryland 21201*

EPIDEMIOLOGY OF GASTROINTESTINAL CANCER

Cancers of the digestive system are the second-most-common cause of deaths (next to that of respiratory system) from malignant neoplasms in the United States (1). The number of estimated new cancer cases for the major gastrointestinal organs (esophagus, stomach, colon, and rectum) will be larger than that of lung cancer in 1993 (1). Since the best means of reducing mortality from the disease and improving the posttherapeutic life quality at present consists of detection of a pathologically early stage and prevention, a clear understanding of the mechanism of carcinogenesis and its susceptibility factors is vital.

Epidemiological study is a fundamental process in elucidating the etiology of a particular disease. A large number of studies have suggested a variety of environmental and hereditary causative factors for gastrointestinal cancers (GICs). In contrast to lung cancer, where smoking is clearly identified as the major risk factor, the etiological factors for GICs are not without controversy. However, it has generally been recognized that there is a wide variation in the incidence of GICs throughout the world (2), which points strongly to environmental factors. For instance, the incidence of large intestinal cancer (LIC) in Denmark is higher (about double) than that in Finland. Other instances are: (a) the incidence of LIC of black people in the United States is higher than that of Nigerian people, despite the fact that they share a similar hereditary background; (b) the incidence of gastric cancer (GC) among Japanese immigrants in Hawaii is lower than that of native Japanese in Japan, whereas their LIC incidence is higher than that of the latter (3,4); (c) GCs are particularly frequent in Japan, Chile, Iceland, Finland, and part of the south central region of the former Soviet Union; and (d) the prevalence of esophageal cancer in Durban in Africa, Puerto Rico, and part of south central Russia is extremely high.

Numerous studies have suggested that dietary factors are the most important environmental risk factors for GICs. Humans consume a variety of foodstuffs and cooked food that contain various types of natural mutagens and carcinogens, as well as many natural antimutagens and anticarcinogens. Consumption of different proportions of these synergistic or mutually antagonistic substances could explain, at least in part, the differences in incidence in various parts of the world.

Risk Factors for Gastrointestinal Cancer

Risk factors of GICs could be considered from three major points of view: environmental, genetic, and immunological. Among them, the environmental factors are considered to play a major role in the GI carcinogenesis. Numerous epidemiological and laboratory studies have suggested possible involvement of various substances present in the GI tract as carcinogenic agents, which include nitrosamines and nitroso compounds formed from nitrate and nitrite in the diet (5), mold carcinogens (sterigmatocystin and aflatoxin), fatty acid, bile acids, fecal steroids, protein metabolites, bacterial flora, and their products having mutagenic or promoting activity, such as fecapentaenes and diacylglycerol. Other carcinogens, such as benzo[*a*]pyrene and other polycyclic aromatic hydrocarbons, may affect the GI mucosa via hematogenic route. These agents are degraded into terminal metabolites, may form adducts with DNA, RNA, or other cellular macromolecules, or may act as initiator and/or promoter through the generation of oxygen radicals. It is postulated that several carcinogens are generated *in vivo* through iron-catalyzed lipid peroxidation. Inflammatory reactions also involve the generation of superoxide anion free radicals by phagocytes. This reaction includes a process of hydroxyl free radical ($\cdot OH$) production from superoxide anion free radicals ($^-O_2$) combined with H_2O_2.

$$\cdot O_2^- + Fe^{3+} \rightarrow Fe^{2+} + O_2$$
$$H_2O_2 + Fe^{2+} \rightarrow Fe^{3+} + OH + \cdot OH^-$$

These processes are believed to be responsible for enhanced tumor formation in various tissues. Thus the superoxide anion free radicals act as DNA-damaging initiating agents as well as important promoters. Interestingly enough, there is evidence that superoxides generated by human neutrophils induced neoplastic transformation of immortalized C3H10T 1/2 fibroblasts both *in vivo* and *in vitro* (6). Furthermore, free radical generation by human neutrophils is enhanced when they are cocultured with human colon adenocarcinoma cells. Neutrophils are also observed during the very early stage of histogenesis of colorectal cancer in both experimental models and humans.

As regards genetic risk factors, a large number of studies have unveiled a plethora of oncogenes that appear to be involved in promotion, proliferation, transformation, and tumor suppressor activities. Recently, the importance of tumor suppressor genes in carcinogenesis has gained popularity. Numerous studies have revealed frequent mutation or allelic loss of p53 gene in human cancer cells from various organs as well as in experimental tumor cell lines transformed by oncogene.

A study by Sugimura (7) has pointed out that there is a high incidence of second or third primary cancers in other organs following complete cure of primaries. Thus cancer is a multifactorial disease, among which genetically defined factor(s) may play a crucial role in developing malignancies.

While most of the potent chemical carcinogens are metabolized into ultimate carcinogenic forms that couple with DNA and macromolecules, various experimental observations suggest that there are interindividual variations in the ability to metabolize the carcinogens. These variations have been attributed to the differences in enzyme activities involved in metabolic conversion of procarcinogens. Recent epidemiological study also suggests possible involvement of acromegaly as risk factor for GICs (8). Increased secretion of growth hormone is considered to be at play.

Negative Risk Factors of Gastrointestinal Cancer

It is apparent that humans consume not only carcinogenic substances, but also anticarcinogens, which have protective activity for cancer development. Most anticarcinogens are categorized as antioxidants which mitigate or circumvent the action of oxygen radicals (9). Endogenous oxygen radicals are generated from hydrogen peroxide and superoxide mainly through lipid peroxidation and inflammation reaction in tissue. Various enzymes have antioxidant activities, which include superoxide dismutase, glutathione peroxidase, DT-diaphorase, and glutathione transferases. Also known to have antioxidant activity are some of the small molecular substances in the edible stuffs: vitamin E, β-carotene, selenium, glutathione, ascorbic acid, and others (9). Uric acid, generated in humans from nucleic acid metabolites and dietary purines, is also known to be a potent antioxidant. Inositol hexaphosphate ($InsP_6$, phytic acid), which is rich in the cereals and legumes, is recognized to be an anticarcinogen, its mechanism(s) of action notwithstanding (10). Since Finnish people apparently consume more $InsP_6$ in the diet than do the Danes, the anticarcinogenic activity of $InsP_6$ contributing to the difference in large intestinal cancer incidence between Denmark and Finland could be explained at least in part (11,12).

Another negative risk factor for cancer is immune defense mechanism or surveillance. A major part of the surveillance mechanism for neoplastic cells is considered to be mediated by natural killer (NK) cells and macrophages. Although mixed-lymphocyte tumor cell culture and many other experimental evidence shows that cancer patients retain an immune response against their own neoplastic cells, the specific T-cell-mediated immune reactions appear to be less important in carcinogenesis surveillance. One explanation to support this contention is the evidence that athymic nude mice, who are devoid of matured T cells and incidentally, harbor intact NK cell activity, do not have a high incidence of spontaneous malignant tumor development. In humans, patients with Chediak–Higashi syndrome, which accompanies an impairment of NK activity, have a high incidence of malignant tumors.

SUSCEPTIBILITY FACTORS OF GASTROINTESTINAL CANCER

Environmental Factors

The term *susceptibility* in conjunction with a particular disorder implies a host's character. The concept contrasting to *susceptibility factor* is *risk factor*. Therefore, an environmental factor itself can participate with host susceptibility only indirectly. The former affects the latter through modifying the host's otherwise normal resistance to develop malignancy.

Nonspecific injury and chronic inflammatory lesions may fall into this category. Examples of these lesions are leukoplakia in the esophagus, chronic gastritis (intestinal metaplasia), nodular hyperplasia in the liver, chronic cholecystitis, chronic pancreatitis, and inflammatory bowel disease (ulcerative colitis and Crohn's disease). In these inflammatory lesions, there is an increase in the mitotic activity of epithelial cells. In addition, a variety of inflammatory cells of mesenchymal origin, including neutrophils and macrophages, are accumulated. They are well known to be a potent generator of mutagens (by way of free radicals).

Genetic Factors

The strongest evidence supporting the involvement of genetic factors for carcinogenesis susceptibility is the presence of cancer family syndrome and development of colorectal cancers in familial polyposis coli. Numerous studies have attempted to elucidate the responsible mechanism of carcinogenesis in high-risk individuals, which include defective DNA repair or the impaired defense mechanism against DNA injury by carcinogenic agents, interindividual differences in enzyme activities of carcinogen metabolism, and defective immune response.

It is well known that experimental animals show various strain/species differences in susceptibility to chemical carcinogens (13–16). In the rat carcinogenesis model using N-methyl-N'-nitro-N-nitrosoguanidine (MNNG), ACI strain rat is susceptible for gastric carcinoma development, while Baffalo strain is resistant (17). F_1 rats by reciprocal cross mating of resistant and susceptible strains showed that the resistance was inherited by autosomal dominant mode. In the mouse model of 1,2-dimethylhydrazine (DHM)-induced colorectal carcinogenesis, ICR/Ha strain is susceptible and C57BL/Ha is relatively resistant (14,15). Study by Deschner et al. (16) suggested the presence of gene(s) repressing metabolism of DMH to methylazoxymethanol (MAM), the more proximate carcinogen. Moreover, the repressor genes responsible for DMH resistance appear to be associated with maternal X chromosome.

Another evidence that susceptibility factors to carcinogenesis are controlled by the person's ability to metabolize procarcinogens has been brought by various experimental studies in humans (18). It is well known that most of the environmental (chemical) carcinogens are inert by themselves and need to be metabolized by cytochrome P450-dependent monooxygenases before they exert mitogenic activity. It is the dogma that the ultimate metabolites form adducts with DNA, having escaped from the usual DNA repair processes along with oncogene expression and suppressor gene inactivation to bring about the transformation. The metabolic activation of the procarcinogen to the ultimate carcinogen is regulated by cytochrome P450 genes. Since the expression of P450 genes are regulated at various steps (transcription and posttranscription), susceptibility to chemical carcinogens may be influenced by those substances (hormones and enzymes) that affect each of the steps of gene expression (19). A marker enzyme of these activities is aryl hydrocarbon hydroxylase (AHH).

Immunological Factors

Immunological factors also contribute to susceptibility to cancer development. In the long line of sequential events in multistep carcinogenesis (from initiation to established tumor formation), the nonspecific immune system may take part in a surveillance step normally protecting the host. Impaired natural killer (NK) cell and/or macrophage-mediated defense mechanism is considered to be responsible for increased incidence of malignant tumor development in humans and experimental animals. Impairment of NK cell function results from various drugs and chemicals, including carcinogens (12).

Although the function of suppressor T cells is demonstrated by using transplantable tumor cell lines in animals, it is speculative whether T cells play a particular role in allowing transformed cells to sneak through the immune surveillance mechanism. A more realistic explanation for the sneak-through phenomenon is that the host does not recognize the transformed cells as "nonself," through several putative mechanisms: (a) the fact that transformed cells do not express alien antigenicity, and (b) antigenic modulation.

ORGAN-ORIENTED SUSCEPTIBILITY FACTORS

Esophagus Cancer

Of the different cancers in various regions of the gastrointestinal tract, that of the esophagus is the most deadly, with a mere 6% five-year survival rate. Worldwide, it is the sixth most common cancer, fourth in the subset of developing countries (20). Host susceptibility to esophageal cancer appears to be mostly a function of the environment (physical, cultural, even political); inherent (or genetic) susceptibility plays a very minor role, if at all. The strongest argument in favor of environmental factors, often highly localized, as the most important determinants of its susceptibility comes from the geographic epidemiology of esophageal cancer. Cancer of the esophagus shows a 500-fold difference in prevalence between the high- and low-incidence areas, that being a close second only to cancer of the liver, which shows a nearly 700-fold difference (21,22).

A literal geographic belt can be drawn across the high-incidence areas in Asia: on the west, beginning from the southern shore of the Caspian Sea, through Iran, Soviet Central Asia, Afghanistan, Siberia, and Mongolia to northwest China on the east (22). In addition, there are pockets, albeit small, of areas in India, Singapore, and Japan that also have a high incidence. The fact that in China the high incidence of esophageal cancer in humans is paralleled by a similarly high incidence in domestic fowl and that up to 44% of the poultry developing the cancer belonged either to the patients or to their neighbors points strongly to the susceptibility factors in food common to the diet of the birds and their human masters (23,24). On the one hand, these include the presence of such carcinogens as nitrosamines and fungal toxins, and the deficiency of vitamins (e.g., vitamin C), minerals (molybdenum, selenium, etc.) and miscellaneous nutrients, on the other (25). Similar observations made in other parts of the world incriminate general items of habitual use, such as alcohol, tobacco, and opium as the vehicle, if not the causative agents, for esophageal cancer. Listed below [Sales and Levin (22)] are various categories of susceptibility factors for esophageal carcinoma.

1. Physical
    a. Extreme temperature: hot food and drinks
    b. Caustic burns resulting in strictures (lye strictures)
    c. Achalasia, irradiation, diverticula
2. Chemical carcinogens
    a. Nitrosamines
    b. Alcohol
    c. Tobacco
    d. Opiates
    e. Fungal toxins
3. Nutritional deficiencies
    a. Plummer–Vinson syndrome
    b. Vitamins and minerals
4. Predisposing conditions and diseases
    a. Precancerous lesions of the esophagus
    b. Gastroesophageal reflux
    c. Chronic infections (fungal, viral, etc.)
    d. Celiac sprue, idiopathic steatorrhea
    e. Tylosis plantaris et palmaris

Physical Factors

That physical insult to the esophagus may play an important role in carcinogenesis has been speculated on the basis of the observations in high-incidence areas: for instance, tea-gruel drinking in Japan, high-temperature food and drink ingestion in Singapore and Iran. Consumption of coarse food and poorly milled grains has also been implicated, but associated deficiency of important nutrients in these areas cannot be totally ruled out (22). From a total of 2,414 patients with caustic burns following lye ingestion, Appleqvist and Salmo (26) reported 63 patients (2.6%) with carcinoma of the esophagus (lye stricture always being the site where carcinoma developed) after an average of 41 years.

Achalasia is a rather uncommon disorder of motility of esophagus which literally means "failure of relaxation" perhaps due to a loss of myenteric ganglion cells in the wall of the esophagus, which in turn is usually idiopathic except in Chaga's disease, which is caused by *Trypanosoma cruzi*, in which the parasite destroys the ganglion cell. Esophageal cancer appears to arise in achalasia in 1% to 7% of cases, which is perhaps due to chronic inflammation secondary to retention of food, which in turn is due to failure of relaxation of the esophagus (24). Similar mechanisms are likely to be at play in congenital or acquired diverticula of the esophagus, where the stagnation of food gives rise to chronic irritation and inflammation and a high risk of cancer.

Chemical Carcinogens

Nitrosamines are the most suspected of all carcinogens for cancers of the esophagus and stomach, and produce cancer in the experimental models. A variety of amines and peptides could be nitrosated, and nitrosamines can form in the mammalian stomach from percursor nitrites under acidic conditions. Low levels of nitrosamines are present in nitrite-cured meat and fish in the industrialized West, which enjoys a relatively low incidence of esophageal cancer. However the levels of nitrosamines, nitrates, and nitrate are quite high in the food and drinking water of high-incidence areas in China. But extensive studies in Iran have failed to show such a correlation. In any event, nitrosamines can alkylate DNA and produce o-alkylated purines, resulting in mispair and transition mutations (27).

Although numerous epidemiological studies, particularly those from France, Puerto Rico, and other areas in the United States, have implicated alcohol as a causative agent for esophageal cancer, alcohol *per se* is not carcinogenic (27). It may, however, increase the risk of carcinogenesis or enhance the process by increasing the permeability of the cell membranes, by increasing the metabolism of carcinogenesis, by acting as a tumor promoter, or by suppressing cellular immunity, notwithstanding the fact that studies of the effect of alcohol on models of chemical carcinogenesis have yielded contradictory results (27).

A synergistic relationship between alcohol and tobacco appears to exist as regards increasing the risk for esophageal cancer. Alcohol causes a persistence of O^6-methylguanine (the putative lesion in the DNA responsible for dimethylnitrosamine-induced carcinogenesis), and depression of the DNA repair enzyme O^6-methylguanine transferase; thus carcinogens in tobacco could provide the initiating stimulus, and owing to alcohol, the induced DNA damage is allowed to persist (27). Besides alcohol, a variety of other euphoria-inducing substances, such as opium and marijuana, have been implicated in enhancing the susceptibility toward esophageal cancer; however, the laboratory data regarding these are limited at the time and the readers are referred to a comprehensive review on this subject by Mufti et al. (27).

In China, pickled vegetables, a popular food item in high-incidence areas, are prepared by fermenting the vegetables under water in ceramic containers until they are covered with mold (22): thus the search for fungal mycotoxins, particularly since it is known that a variety of fungal species produce potent mycotoxins, some of which are known carcinogens, such as aflatoxins. Indeed, a positive correlation was found between the rate of esophageal cancer mortality and the consumption of pickled vegetables (28). As it turns out, the popular pickled vegetables in high-incidence areas are contaminated most commonly with the fungus *Geotrichum candidum*. Extracts of these moldy food items are mutagenic and induce *in vitro* transformation (29). *Fusarium* species also are common contaminants not only in the Linxian area of China but also in the Transkei in South Africa. The *Fusarium* species produce a large amount of T-2 toxin (a trichothecene), which is a potent carcinogen in experimental models (30).

Nutritional Deficiencies

With the exception of the high-incidence areas in France, it is suspected that deficiency of a variety of nutritional substances may, either alone or in addition, play an important role in enhancing susceptibility to esophageal cancer. Deficiencies of trace metals such as selenium, molybdenum, and zinc have been reported from high-incidence areas of esophageal cancer as well as in patients with esophageal carcinomas (27,31–33). Besides being a constituent of a number of metalloenzymes (including those involved in the synthesis of DNA and RNA), zinc appears to play an important role in the initiation and promotion of carcinogenesis as well as in immunocompetence of the host. Notwithstanding the exact mechanism(s) by which zinc deficiency enhances the susceptibility of esophageal cancer, Gabrial et al. (34) demonstrated a reduction in experimental esophageal carcinomas by zinc. Similarly, selenium, a constituent of glutathione peroxidase, appears to act during both the initiation and promotion stages of carcinogenesis, and supplementation by selenium exerts a chemopreventive effect in other models as well (35).

Patients with Plummer–Vinson syndrome (also known as Kelly–Patterson syndrome, iron-deficiency anemia, esophageal web, and dysphagia in middle-aged women) have an increased susceptibility to esophageal carcinoma. It is not exactly known how iron deficiency increases the susceptibility of esophageal cancer, but improved nutrition has virtually eliminated Plummer–Vinson syndrome from once-endemic areas of Sweden (27).

Ascorbic acid (vitamin C) is known to inhibit nitrosation both *in vitro* and *in vivo* and reduces the mutagenic activity of gastric juice following oral ingestion (36). Gastric juice collected at various intervals following oral administration of 1 g of ascorbic acid showed an interindividual variation of response in nitrite content (37). However, if the basal level of *N*-nitroso compound was high, ascorbic acid administration reduced the nitrites significantly (37). Thus ascorbic acid may play an important role in inhibition of nitrosation and hence in carcinogenesis of the stomach and esophagus.

Predisposing Conditions and Diseases

A few conditions of the esophagus in addition to those noted under physical factors and those related to nutritional deficiencies render enhanced susceptibility of the organ to cancer. These can be lumped under the term *precancerous lesions of the esophagus* and include Barrett's esophagus, chronic esophagitis (due to chronic infections by fungal or viral agents), and dysplasia of the esophagus (38–40). Gastroesophageal reflux is one condition that is quite common and predispose to chronic inflammation of the esophagus and hence increases the susceptibility to cancer. The risk of esophageal cancer originating from severe dysplasia is 140 times higher than that of the normal population, and Anani et al. have demonstrated the existence of the sequence healthy mucosa→dysplasia→*in situ* carcinoma→invasive carcinoma during its pathogenesis (40). Interestingly, as in other organs, there also seems to be a field defect as regards the presence of precancerous changes in the esophagus (40), whereby multifocal changes of different degrees of dysplasias and microscopic carcinomas are seen throughout the esophagus as if the entire field of the esophagus is affected by carcinogenic stimuli. However, only a few of these foci appear to progress to invasive cancer (40). There is a striking analogy with that of the large intestine as regards these field effects (discussed later in the section on the large intestine).

At this point it may be beneficial to recall that the normal epithelium of the esophagus is composed of nonkeratinizing squamous epithelium and DNA synthesis, and mitosis in the normal is seen only in the deep basal layer of cells (38). Barrett's esophagus is an abnormal condition where the normal squamous epithelium of the distal esophagus (above the gastroesophageal junction) is replaced by columnar epithelium and renders the area highly susceptible to cancer, in this special situation, usually adenocarcinomas. Rubio and Aberg (39) have shown that Barrett's esophagus may also be in association (without a cause–effect relationship) with squamous carcinomas at sites distant from the Barrett's. Barrett's esophagus is caused by the persistent (chronic) reflux of gastric juice into the lower esophagus, resulting in chronic inflammation leading to metaplastic changes with increased cell proliferation (38). That fungal infection may play an important role in susceptibility to esophageal cancer by way of various carcinogenic mycotoxins has already been alluded to. Viral infections have also been incriminated; the most serious candidates have been the human papilloma virus (HPV). However, pilot studies to detect the presence of HPV genome in esophageal papillomas (benign neoplasms) have been unrewarding (41). A few diseases that do not directly affect the esophagus, such as celiac sprue, idiopathic steatorrhea, and tylosis plantaris et palmaris, carry an increased risk for esophageal carcinomas (22).

Finally, recent interest in the genetic control of cell proliferation, differentiation, and cancer has resulted in studies of the p53 gene, which encodes 53-kDa cellular protein. Alteration of the gene (inactivation by point mutation, loss of heterozygosity at or near the p53 gene locus) may be responsible for rendering the organism susceptible to cancer—cancer of the esophagus by no means excluded (42,43).

In summary, owing to extensive and ongoing epidemiological studies, a variety of factors (besides the physical deformities of the esophagus) have been identified that make the organ susceptible to cancer. These studies have revealed factors that may be candidates for initiating agents and conditions that promote carcinogenesis (such as chronic inflammation) by enhancing cell proliferation; the roles of others are yet to fit into the dogma of the initiation–promotion model.

Experimental Carcinogenesis in Rodents

A multitude of animal models are exploited to increase our insight into tumor development in humans, to assess risk factors in the human environment, and to evaluate antineoplastic substances (44). Carcinogenesis models that have a high organ specificity to esophagus were reported long ago by Druckrey (45). He demonstrated that almost all nonsymmetrical dialkylnitrosamines were specific carcinogens to esophagus in rats. Among them, methylalkylnitrosamines have the highest efficiency and organ specificity. Irrespective of the route of administration, methylalkylnitrosamines induced esophageal carcinomas of both exophytic and sessile forms. Subsequently, Stinson demonstrated N-methyl-N-benzylnitrosamine (MBZN) to be a more potent inducer of esophageal neoplasms in F344 rats (46). Papillomas are the most predominant tumor in these animal models, and this is a major discrepancy with the human disease, where papillomas are a rarity. It is postulated that MBZN is activated by cytochrome P450 and causes methylation of the DNA, thus forming O^6-methylguanine adducts in the esophageal epithelium (47–49). O^6-methylguanine is a mutagenic adduct and induced guanine-to-adenine point mutations in DNA (50–52). Recently, Barch et al. demonstrated H-*ras* oncogene point mutations (GGA to GAA in the codon 12) in 67% of the DNA of papillomas induced by MBZN in SD rats (53). This point mutation codes for glycine, substituted by glutamate, at the twelfth amino acid of the *ras* P^{21} protein. Using a monoclonal antibody raised against mutant *ras* P^{21} protein, Barch et al. observed the expression of H-*ras* mutation in 20% of squamous papillomas, 13.6% of hyperplastic lesions, and 10% of dysplastic lesions, concluding the fact that activation of *ras* oncogene may be an early event in the neoplastic transformation of this animal model.

Animal models are utilized for the study of modifying factors of esophageal carcinogenesis. Lin et al. demonstrated that dietary zinc deficiency at the initiation phase of MBZN carcinogenesis significantly enhanced the esophageal neoplasia, while supplementation of zinc suppressed the tumor development (54). Zinc deficiency is associated with alcohol treatment in rats and alcohol drinking in humans. According to Barch et al., dietary zinc deficiency increased the MBZN-induced formation of O^6-methylguanine in the esophageal DNA in rats (55). In contrast to the zinc deficiency, supplementation of ellagic acid in the diet reduced the incidence of MBZN-induced esophageal carcinoma (56) and selectively reduced the MBZN-induced formation of O^6-methylguanine adducts without reducing total methylation of esophageal DNA (57).

Gastric Cancer

Gastric cancer has been the commonest cancer and a leading cause of cancer death worldwide until 1988. Although its incidence has steadily decreased over the last five decades in the United States and western Europe, it is very common in eastern Asia, South America, and eastern Europe (58–61). The evaluation of risk and carcinogenesis has been based on data from three principal sources:

1. *Epidemiologic studies related to genetic, dietary, and environmental factors.* Worldwide studies on the epidemiology of gastric cancer help us to understand the correlation between possible cause and risk factors and the development of gastric cancer. One remarkable finding involves the different incidence in various countries and continents, which is inversely related to socioeconomic status and is associated with poor nutrition, especially eating habits, and other environmental influences.

2. *Histogenesis and pathological changes associated with carcinoma.* There is a strong association of gastric cancer with precursor conditions and lesions such as chronic atrophic gastritis, intestinal metaplasia, gastric epithelial dysplasia, and gastric postresection stump. Based on the classification of Lauren (62), there are two major histological types of gastric cancer: the diffuse and intestinal types. The incidence of the diffuse type is relatively even in all populations; geographical variations in incidence are due primarily to variation in intestinal type. As mentioned above, all of the precursor lesions lead to gastric cancer of the intestinal type (63).

3. *Molecular genetic mechanisms.* Progress in molecular genetics research has revealed a consistent set of genetic alterations in various human cancers, possibly corresponding to multistep tumor development. Gastric cancer is no exception, and multiple genetics alterations, including oncogene mutation, rearrangement, amplification, and chromosomal loss of heterozygosity by carcinogenic activation, have been observed (64,65). Environmental factors related to initiation, promotion, and progression play an essential role in gastric carcinogenesis.

In this review we consider the information that we have on the epidemiology of gastric cancer. A description of how this has been used to develop a hypothesis of the mechanism of carcinogenesis in this disease follows. Finally, we discuss the evidence in support of that hypothesis.

TABLE 1. Food and food components suggested to be associated with high or low risk of GC

High risk	Low risk
Added salt	High fat
Salted food (fish, bacon)	Milk
Smoked food (meat, fish)	High intake of fresh fruits and vegetables
Fish (fresh, dried, salted)	Vitamin C
Animal and cooked fat	Vitamin E
Fried foods	Selenium
Rice and rice cakes	
Potatoes	
Cooked cereals	
Canned fruits	
Fava beans	
Alcohol	
Cabbage	
Beef	
Chocolate	
Hot tea	

Adapted from Geboers et al. (67).

Epidemiological Investigation of Gastric Carcinogenesis

Naturally occurring carcinogens in diets have been shown to be one of the important factors in the etiology of various cancers, including that of the stomach (66). Recent reviews have summarized the evidence for involvement of dietary factors in gastric carcinogenesis (67,68) and show that food or food components have a positive or negative association with gastric cancer risk (Tables 1 and 2).

Geboers et al. (67) have looked at the evidence of the role of salt in gastric carcinogenesis; the significant positive relations between salt as measured by 24-h urinary sodium and gastric cancer from three countries with different gastric cancer incidence are in support of the salt hypothesis; levels of sodium excretion were lowest in the United States, intermediate in Chile, and highest in Japan, parallel with the incidence of gastric carcinoma. A subsequent study demonstrated that salt in hypertonic solution in the stomach (a) induced a dose-response increased DNA synthesis and ornithine decarboxylase activity in a manner similar to nitrosocar-

TABLE 2. Characteristics of diets consumed by populations with high risk of GC

1. Low intake of animal fats and protein
2. High intake of starches and carbohydrates, mainly grains
3. High salt intakes
4. High dietary nitrate intake (from water and/or foodstuffs)
5. Low intake of fresh fruits
6. Low intake of raw vegetables and salads

Adapted from Geboers et al. (67).

cinogens (69); (b) enhanced the carcinogenic action of nitrosamines, such as MNNG, thereby acting as a cocarcinogen, and (c) had a significant promoting activity for stomach cancer when given after administration of a carcinogen (70).

The hypothetical etiology of stomach cancer can be summarized as follows: a hypertonic salt solution in the stomach delays emptying of the stomach by the pylorus following the activation of duodenal osmoreceptors and damages the stomach mucosa, first causing hypertrophic gastritis, then atrophic gastritis, and finally, intestinal metaplasia (71). The pH of the stomach rises with atrophy of the stomach mucosa and enhances the conversion of nitrates to nitrites by bacterial overgrowth; at this stage, nitrates in the food may increase the risk of stomach cancer. Therefore, it may be extrapolated that a high salt content in the stomach may exert cocarcinogenic and promotional activity (72).

Smoked foods such as smoked fish and meat have been demonstrated to contain a significant level of benzopyrene, a known carcinogen (73), and have also been demonstrated to have the capability of inducing cancers in laboratory animals (74). Retrospective studies of diets of stomach cancer patients and controls have offered some support to the smoked meat and stomach cancer hypothesis. A twofold increase in stomach cancer risk associated with more frequently reported consumption of smoked meats and a similar level of risk elevation for consumption of smoked fish has been reported from a study in Canada (75). In a prospective study in Japan, consumption of broiled fish was found to be associated with a 70% increase in the relative risk for gastric cancer (76).

Given the large number of investigations of diet and stomach cancer, it is inevitable that many different food items will show some association with the risk of gastric cancer, for example, in a retrospective study consumption of chocolate was found to be reported more often by stomach cancer patients than by controls (75). The consumption of popular soybean paste soup was associated with a reduced risk, whereas consumption of fava beans was found more common in high-risk regions in Colombia (77). Hoey et al. (78) compared the diet histories of French stomach cancer patients and controls; they observed increased relative risks for alcohol consumption, particularly red wine. Hirayama (79) has shown an association between cigarette use and stomach cancer risk in Japan. More recently, Carner et al. (80) compared smokers and nonsmokers with gastric cancer. ^{32}P-Postlabeling of human gastric biopsy DNA showed smokers to have higher adduct levels than those of nonsmokers ($p<0.01$: mean smoker$=15.4$ adduct/10^8, nonsmoker$=5.5$ adduct/10^8) and suggested that smoking may play a role in gastric cancer induction. As regards the inhibitors of carcinogens in the diet, it is very possible that some of the reduction in incidence is related to the changes in diet and lifestyle that accompany increased socioeconomic status, resulting in increased intake of animal proteins or a variety of vitamins (81). Alternatively, there may be decreased intake of smoked and salt food as access to refrigeration improves. The beneficial effects of cold storage are said to be due to its mold-inhibiting properties and to the inhibition of nitrite formation in preserved food (82). Laboratory data have shown that dietary vitamin A is capable of inhibiting experimentally induced cancer. Vitamin A deficiency has been shown to lead to hyperplasia and papillomatosis in the forestomach of rats and mice (83). Experimental data suggest that ascorbic acid acts as an inhibitor of nitrite-mediated intragastric nitrosation (36,37,84). The urinary excretion of noncarcinogenic nitrosamines has been shown to be particularly inhibited by dietary supplementation with vitamin C. It should be noted that other substances are capable of inhibiting *in vivo* nitrosation, including vitamin E, tannins, and polyphenols (84). Vegetable consumption may play a protective role by mechanisms other than the inhibition of nitrosation. Cruciferous vegetables contain indoles and isothiocyanates, which affect polycyclic aromatic hydrocarbon metabolism; therefore, it has been linked to risk reduction at other gastrointestinal sites in humans and to the inhibition of chemical carcinogenesis in laboratory animals (85).

Recently, the effect of subcutaneous administration of deoxycorticosterone acetate (DOCA) plus p.o. treatment with NaCl solution on gastric carcinogenesis induced by MNNG and the effect of p.o. potassium supplementation on the enhanced induction of gastric carcinogenesis in DOCA–NaCl-hypersensitive rats were investigated using Wistar rats (86). It was found that administration of DOCA and NaCl increased the norepinephrine concentration in the gastric wall and promoted gastric carcinogenesis, and that potassium supplementation decreased the norepinephrine concentration in the gastric wall and suppressed gastric carcinogenesis in DOCA–NaCl-hypertensive rats. Inasmuch as the norepinephrine concentration has been used as a marker of sympathetic nervous system activity, these findings suggest that the sympathetic nervous system plays an important role in gastric carcinogenesis, probably associated with cell proliferation of antral epithelial cells (86). Benjamin et al. (87) show that Japanese-style fermented soy sauce (Shoyu) by itself (without nitrite) exhibited a pronounced anticarcinogenic effect on benzo[*a*]pyrene-induced mouse forestomach neoplasia. Soy sauce produced a significant dose-dependent reduction in forestomach neoplasms, which appeared to be maximal when soy sauce constituted 20% of the diet. Moreover, the anticarcinogenic effect was neither enhanced nor diminished by nitrite. Soy sauce was found to contain antioxidant activity which may be related to the observed anticarcinogenic effect.

In modern times, the family histories of gastric cancer patients have been examined extensively to ascertain the frequency of gastric cancer. No simple inherited form of stomach cancer has been identified. An estimated 10% of gastric cancers will exhibit some degree of familial aggregation; related to the possible influence of genetics in gastric cancer etiology is the association of the ABO blood group with risk (88). Stomach cancer patients are more likely to be of blood group A than is the general population. Analysis of data pooled from multiple studies indicate that persons of blood group A have approximately a 20% increase in the relative risk for stomach cancer compared to all other groups (89). Haenszel et al. (90) have reported that the increased risk associated with blood group A was characteristic only of patients with cancer of diffuse histological type, which may suggest a greater genetic component in etiology of this type of stomach cancer than for the intestinal type.

Most cancers were demonstrated to have an association with social class; this association is particularly strong for stomach cancer. The rate in lower socioeconomic groups is two to three times higher than in more affluent classes (91). The epidemiology of gastric cancer has been reviewed periodically and different surveys of the field have focused on different factors. In the earliest assessments greater importance tended to be attached to the role of individual susceptibility. More recently, the focus has shifted toward environmental sources of risk. The other major development has been the much greater attention to the role of diet in recent studies. The linkages between laboratory and population studies are best reflected perhaps in development and refinement of a hypothesis regarding ingestion of nitrates and the *in vivo* formation or inhibition of carcinogenic nitrosamines.

N-Nitroso Compounds and Chemogastric Carcinogenesis

Since *N*-nitroso compounds and gastric carcinogenesis were demonstrated by Magee and Barnes in 1956 (92), the carcinogenic potential of over 200 *N*-nitroso compounds (NNC) has been established in 40 animal species so far tested (93,94). *N*-Nitroso compounds have been identified in various environmental situations. Exposure to humans may be through ingestion, inhalation, dermal contact, and *in vivo* formation, the latter primarily in the gastrointestinal tract and probably representing the main source of human exposure. The site most commonly regarded to be at risk from endogenous NNC synthesis *in vivo* is the stomach. It has been demonstrated in the stomach of both animals and human. Trace amounts of *N*-nitrosopiperidine have been detected in the gastric juice after ingestion of nitrite-containing homogenized food (95). Certain *N*-nitrosamines such as *N*-nitrosoproline (N-PRO) are excreted in the urine and feces virtually unchanged (96). Stillwell et al. demonstrated increased urinary excretion of nitrate and *N*-nitrosoproline in individuals with precancerous lesions of the stomach, such as intestinal metaplasia and dysplasia of the stomach, and in populations at high risk for gastric cancer (97).

The endogenous formation of *N*-nitroso compounds in the human stomach has also been demonstrated following introduction of the *N*-nitrosoproline test (98). The major source of gastric juice nitrite is the bacterial reduction of nitrate, which occurs primarily in the oral cavity but also in the stomach. Gastric juice nitrite concentration has been shown to correlate with the severity of dysplasia. Correa et al. (99,100) proposed a postulated etiopathology of intestinal-type gastric cancer via a multistage sequence of events. Initiation of this sequence is due to the loss of gastric acid and to the development of gastric atrophy. Under these conditions, a resident flora of nitrate-reducing bacteria is established whose metabolic products (nitroso compounds) induce atrophic gastritis followed by intestinal metaplasia with increasing severity of epithelial dysplasia and eventually, cancer (Fig. 1). Experimental animals fed with secondary amines and a high nitrite concentration show tumor induction typical of the corresponding *N*-nitroso compounds. Bile reflux has been associated with an increased incidence of gastric cancer observed in the stump following certain types of partial gastrectomy. Comparisons between precursors to

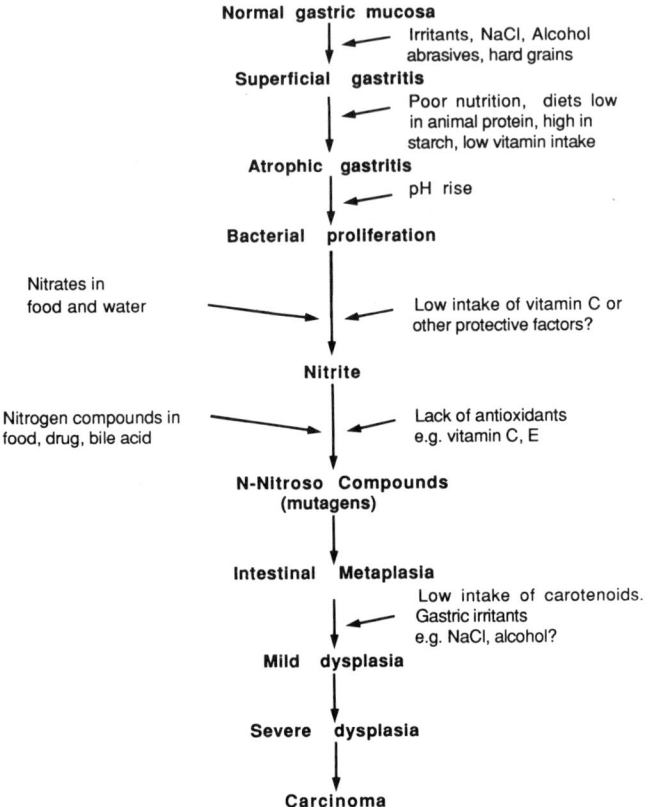

FIG. 1. Model for gastric carcinogenesis. [Adapted from Correa (100).]

N-nitroso compounds in bulked samples of pentagastrin-stimulated (A) and bile-contaminated gastric juice (B) are available. Overall, type B has been found to contain over four times as much precursors to N-nitrosodimethylamine (NDMA) and N-nitropyrrolidine (NPyr) as compared with the very low yield from type A; thus bile salt or other constituents of duodenal juice could play a role in gastric carcinogenesis. Coupled with gastric carcinogenesis are series of premalignant histological changes, including atrophic gastritis, intestinal metaplasia, and dysplasia. In addition, evidence has been provided in a number of studies that bacteria can promote formation of the nitroso compounds, and several possible mechanisms have been proposed (101). First, the action of the bacteria may involve merely the reduction of nitrate to nitrite coupled with acidification of milieu by the products of bacterial metabolism; both of these processes promote the acid-catalyzed reactions of nitrite. Second, N-nitrosation could be stimulated by the products of bacterial metabolism. Finally, the bacterial enzymes themselves could catalyze the N-nitrosation process. It has been demonstrated that denitrifying bacteria can catalyze N-nitrosation reactions, the rate of reaction being several orders of magnitude greater than those observed with nondenitrifiers (102). Leach et al. (101) have calculated from their own studies that considerably greater concentration of *N*-nitrosomorpholine would be formed by bacterial catalysis under conditions relevant to the achlorhydric stomach than would be produced by chemical nitrosation as in acidic stomach. In this relation, a specific type of bacteria, *Campylobacter (Helicobacter) pylori*, recently identified in human stomach mucosa as a possible etiological agent of gastritis, may also contribute to gastric carcinogenesis by inducing chronic irritation or inflammation. The role of chronic tissue injury has also been implicated in a later stage of carcinogenesis, possibly through continuous generation of reactive oxygen species such as a superoxide anion and hydroxy radicals known to produce oxidative DNA base damage. Parsonnet et al. (103) demonstrated a direct association between *Helicobacter pylori* infection and gastric cancer; the 89.2% prevalence of infection in patients with intestinal gastric cancer greatly exceeded the rate of infection in patients with diffuse gastric cancer. This finding suggests that *H. pylori* may be a cofactor in the development of intestinal gastric cancer. Several areas of high gastric cancer risk in the United States and abroad have been found to have a high prevalence of *H. pylori* infection and chronic atrophic gastritis (104,105). There are several mechanisms by which a bacterial infection might induce carcinogenesis. First, infection may result in rapid cell turnover, which in turn increases the risk for mutagenesis. Cells in mitosis with exposed single-stranded DNA are at substantially higher risk of mutation than are cells at rest; inflammation also causes production of damaging agents that can cause mutation. Prolonged inflammation might also overcome the body's natural ability to repair the DNA damage caused by either inflammation-induced mutagens or exogenous mutagens (106,107). *H. pylori* itself might also produce mutagens that act directly at the site of infection (103). To determine simultaneously the relevance of several gastric juice factors to gastric carcinogenesis, 56 patients with unoperated stomachs undergoing endoscopy for dysplasia had gastric juice aspirated and analyzed for pH, ascorbic acid, total bile acids, nitrite, nitrate, and total NNCs. The results showed that patients with chronic atrophic gastritis had higher pH values and a higher incidence of *H. pylori* infection than did normal subjects, whereas patients with chronic gastritis and intestinal metaplasia had higher gastric juice pH values and total bile acid concentrations and lower gastric ascorbic acid concentrations than those with chronic gastritis and no intestinal metaplasia, but both those with gastritis and those with intestinal metaplasia had no significant elevation in nitrite or total NNCs in fasting gastric juice (108).

Since stomach is the first resting place of all food and drinks, it is therefore more likely that gastric cancer may have a multifactorial etiology. There is a large body of evidence relating gastric luminal factors, particularly gastric bacterial flora and nitrite concentration, to the progression from atrophic gastritis through intestinal metaplasia, increasing severe dysplasia to gastric cancer.

Analysis of Carcinogens: Macromolecular Adducts

The progression in technology development has produced a number of highly promising laboratory methods which are available to monitor humans and animals with carcinogens accurately by analysis of carcinogen macromolecular adducts in tissues and body fluid. These methods have been applied to two different approaches to monitoring the macromolecular adducts: one involves the quantitation of adduct in DNA or the protein of particular tissues to provide useful information on the internal dose of carcinogens. Using a highly sensitive radioimmunoassay to detect O^6-methyldeoxyguanosine (O^6-MEDG) in DNA from human esophageal and stomach cancer; 27 of 30 tissue samples showed high levels of O^6-MEDG (up to 160 fmol/mg DNA) (109,110). The ^{32}P-postlabeling method, which detects carcinogen-modified DNA nucleotides that are postlabeled enzymatically with ^{32}P, has also been applied to several human tissues. This method is extremely sensitive and can detect as few as one adduct per 10^9 unmodified nucleotides in a small quantity of DNA (80). Another promising approach is to quantitate excised DNA adducts excreted in urine by an immunoassay and also by photon-counting synchronous fluorescence spectroscopy (111). Urinary excretion of alkylated DNA bases (e.g., 3-methyladenine and 7-carboxylmethylguanine) has been quantitated in the urine of animals fed NNCs such as nitrosodimethylamine and *N*-nitrosoglycocholic acid, a gastric carcinogen derived from nitrosated bile acid conjugate. Low levels of 3-methyladenine have also been detected in human urine (112).

Protooncogene Activation and Expression

Protooncogenes are cellular genes with a fundamental role in cell growth, development, and differentiation. They can be activated by carcinogens through a variety of molecular mechanisms resulting in qualitative and quantitative changes of their products. These mechanisms include point mutation, rearrangement, amplification, and chromosomal loss of heterozygosity (113). Although stomach cancer is a common malignancy in humans, little is known about the oncogenes that may be associated with the origin or development of tumors. Until recently, findings of amplified and single base mutation of several oncogenes have been reported in gastric tissues, with most studies focusing on *ras* and *myc* genes, but the incidence of these alterations is low compared to those in colorectal cancer, another major cancer of the gastrointestinal tract (114–120).

Oncoprotein Expression in Gastric Cancer

Ras-activated mutated N-*ras* and K-*ras* genes have been detected by transfection assay using DNA prepared directly from gastric carcinomas (116,118,121). Fujita et al. (122) extracted DNA from seven patients with advanced gastric cancer and transferred it into NIH/3T3 cells without demonstrable transformation and failed to demonstrate the presence of point mutations. An immunohistochemical analysis of *ras* P^{21} expression in 11 gastric tumors using monoclonal antibody RAP-5 showed more reactivity in the cancer than in adjacent normal mucosa (123). Immunohistochemically, P^{21} was detected in 11% of early cancers and in 43.8% of advanced cancers, in which the immunoreactivity correlated with the depth of tumor invasion and was stronger in metastatic tumor than in primary ones. c-Ha-*ras* P^{21}-positive tumors were associated with significantly worse prognosis than were negative tumors in patients followed up to 3 years after gastrectomy. Ohuchi et al. (124) demonstrated an elevated level of c-Ha-*ras* P^{21} expression in advanced gastric cancers, with generally decreased expression in an early stage of gastric cancer, dysplasia, and nonneoplastic lesions adjacent to cancer; but it is overexpressed in early gastric cancer of diffuse and intestinal types compared to the normal mucosa. Ranzani et al. (125) analyzed c-Ha-*ras* 1 locus polymorphisms in an Italian population with a high risk of developing gastric carcinoma. Thirteen different alleles were detected, but there was no evidence that the inheritance of any allele predisposes to gastric malignancy.

Studies of the expression of TGF-α and c-Ha-*ras* P^{21} in 174 gastric carcinomas comprising 27 early gastric cancer and 147 advanced ones showed the presence of TGF-α immunoreactivity in 25.9% of early cancers and 78.4% of advanced lesions (126). Of the 67 cases positive for P^{21}, 88.1% showed synchronous expression of TGF-α. Expression of both markers correlated with depth of tumor invasion, presence of metastasis, and prognosis. Shibuya et al. (114) found that 3 of 16 human gastric cancers maintained as solid tumors in nude mice carried amplified c-*myc* genes. c-*myc* RNA was obviously elevated in rapidly growing and poorly differentiated tumors, whereas it was only slightly elevated in slower growing better-differentiated tumor. Others have noted the presence of amplified c-*myc* genes in 2% to 7% of gastric cancer (127,128). Variable expression of c-*myc* genes occurs in about 50% of gastric cancers (129); however, Allum et al. (130) evaluated the presence of P62-c-*myc* in a series of archival specimens of gastric cancer and found no relations with the degree of tumor cell differentiation, but there was a tendency for intestinal tumors to stain more frequently than diffuse type in nonneoplastic mucosa. Staining occurs more commonly in patients with gastritis than in patients with normal mucosa, and was especially marked in atrophic gastric mucosa, showing intestinal metaplasia type IIb. Others also found low levels of expression in normal gastric mucosa, and increased expression was found in inflamed metaplastic and dysplastic mucosa (131). Restriction fragment length polymorphism (RFLP) of the L-*myc* gene, related to the progression of human gastric carcinoma, has also been demonstrated (132). Sakamoto et al. (119) analyzed DNA from 21 primary human gastric carcinomas, 16 metastatic cancers in lymph nodes, and 21 apparently normal examples of gastric mucosa for their ability to induce neoplastic transformation of NIH/3T3 cells. Three samples were shown to have transforming activity, the transformants were tumorigenic in nude mice, and their DNA can induce secondary transformants. The transforming gene was cloned since it did not share homology with transforming sequences; it was termed *hst* for "human stomach tumor." The ability of nonneoplastic mucosa to transform the NIH/3T3 cells could be explained in one of several ways. The first possibility is that the transforming genes were activated in nonneoplastic gastric mucosa, but other genetic changes were required to develop tumors. It is well established that carcinogenesis occurs through a series of multiple steps and that at least two cooperating oncogenes are required to convert a normal cell to a malignant cell (133). Another possibility is that sequence change resulted from the transfection process. Finally, a transformation sequence may be a regulatory sequence that enhances the expression of transforming gene in NIH/3T3 cells (119). A systematic study on 50 cases of gastric carcinoma characterized by different clinical parameter has been carried out in which DNA from neoplastic and control tissue sample was hybridized by the Southern blotting technique with probes homologous to seven different protooncogenes: c-*myc*, c-*erb* B2, c-Ki-*ras*, c-H2-*ras*, c-N-*ras*, *hst*, and c-*mos*. The authors found amplification of c-*myc*, c-*erb* B2, c-Ki-*ras*, and *hst* oncogene, and also demonstrated a statistically significant association between amplification and both tumor progression and presence of metastasis (64). Therefore, amplification represents a late event in the temporal development of gastric cancer. Current interest is concentrated on tumor suppressor genes in malignant tumors such as p^{53} gene, whose mutation may play an important role in the development of many common human malignancies (134). In gastric cancer, however, p^{53} gene mutations have not been detected in the primary site or been detected at low levels, but have been demonstrated mostly in metastases and cell lines (65,135). Tamura et al. (136) studied mutation of the p^{53} gene after tumor cell enrichment by cell sorting based on difference in DNA content and PCR single-strand conformation polymorphism analysis in 24 surgical specimens of primary gastric cancer. p^{53} mutations were detected in exons 4 to 8 in 64% (9 of 14) of aneuploid tumors but in none of the 10 diploid tumors examined. Four of five tumors containing two or three aneuploid subpopulations showed the presence of p^{53} gene mutations. No correlation was found between the presence of p^{53} mutation and the degree of histological differentiation of tumor. These findings suggest that p^{53} gene mutations are related to DNA ploidy alterations as relatively late events of carcinogenesis in gastric cancer. In addition, loss or inactivation of genes at specific chromosomal loci has been considered to be one of the important mechanisms during the development of human tumors. Allele loss on chromosome 17_p is a common event in gastric carcinoma, regardless of histological type, and allele loss on chromosome 5_q may play a role in the carcinogenesis of well-differentiated adenocarcinoma (137). Additionally, allele losses on chromosomes 1_q and 7_p may be involved in the progression of well-differentiated adenocarcinoma (137).

Oncogene Expression in Precancerous Lesion

A few studies have shown that foci of intestinal metaplasia (IM) of gastric mucosa express oncogene products (138). Ciclitira et al. (131) reported increased expression of the P62 product of c-*myc* oncogene in inflammatory, metaplastic, and dysplastic gastric mucosa. Some expression was also found in the epithelial cells of the mucus neck region. *Ras* gene expression may be associated with cellular transformation, while the product of *myc* gene may reflect excessive replication. Studies of the growth factor expression in gastric cancer and normal gastric tissue using reverse transcriptase polymerase chain reaction (RT-PCR) indicate that there are qualitative differences between them (139). The induction of expression of FGF, bFGT, FGFS, *hst*, and PDGFB may be important in malignant transformation of normal gastric cells to gastric cancer. Rearranged TPR-MET oncogene expression in several gastric cancer cell lines may indicate that TPR-MET oncogene may be associated with gastric tumorigenesis process (140). Expression of this gene at the early stage of superficial gastritis suggests a functional role of this oncogene during the initial stage of gastric carcinogenesis.

Histogenesis and Precursors of Human Gastric Cancer

Histopathologically, the development of gastric cancer can be looked at whether or not it is through dysplastic changes in the mucosa. Precancerous changes of stomach can be defined as broad or narrow. The term *broad* reflects the result of epidemiological, pathological, and clinical studies which imply that the altered mucosa has a higher probability of developing into cancer than does the normal mucosa, which includes atrophic gastritis, intestinal metaplasia, chronic peptic ulcer scar, and long-standing postoperative gastric remnants. The *narrow* definition encompasses those changes that are associated with malignancy from the aspects of histological similarities of the lesion to carcinoma *in situ* but may not fulfill all the histological criteria of invasive malignancy (141). As has been done for other organs, the term *precancerous* with regard to the stomach should be subdivided into two separate categories: *precancerous conditions* and *precancerous lesions*. The former term is a clinically defined state that involves an elevated risk of cancer compared with the normal population, including chronic atrophic gastritis, chronic peptic ulcer, polyps, anemia, Ménétrièr disease, and postoperation. By contrast, precancerous lesions are defined as a group of histopathological abnormalities in which cancer is more likely to occur than is its apparently normal counterpart. The intestinal metaplasia and epithelial dysplasia of the stomach are the histological substrates of precancerous lesions (142,143). A number of studies elucidated either precancerous conditions or precancerous lesions essentially related only to the intestinal type, and no conclusive finding could be found about diffuse carcinoma.

Intestinal Metaplasia and Histogenesis

In the classification of intestinal metaplasia (IM) based on morphology and mucin secretion, three main IM phenotypes have been identified (144): type 1, also termed mature, complete, or small intestinal type; type II, or incomplete type; and type III, also called immature, incomplete, or colonic type. Other variants of intestinal metaplasia have been described, based on the staining patterns of goblet cell mucous secretion, particularly its content in O-acylated sialomucins (145). Despite different classifications of IM and the terminology used, there has been general agreement that sulfomucin-positive incomplete-colonic-type III variants are significantly associated with gastric cancer of the intestinal type, whereas types I and II are not. Filipe et al. show a 20% to 30% incidence of IM in a large number of gastric biopsies which is prevalent in gastric carcinoma (65%). Type I IM is the most common (approximately 70%) and prevalent type in all conditions. The nonsulfated incomplete type shows approximately an even prevalence (20% to 25%) in chronic gastritis, gastric ulcer, and carcinoma. In contrast, type III IM was found in approximately 10% of IM-positive biopsies. Thus the nonsulfated phenotypes I and II are common to both benign conditions (approximately 95%) and carcinoma (64%), and type III is more selective for carcinoma and its high prevalence (77% to 80%) in mucosa adjacent to early gastric cancer and microcarcinoma has been well documented in gastrectomy specimen by Japanese authors (146,147). It is important to note that IM is more common in the intestinal than in the diffuse type of gastric cancer.

Dysplasia with Early Gastric Carcinoma

For histological expression of precancerous changes, the term *dysplasia* has been used by many authors. According to the grades of cellular atypia and structural abnormality, dysplastic changes of gastric mucosa can be classified into three grades: mild, moderate, and severe, which corresponds to the changes in group classification: namely, group I (benign lesion with slight atypia), group II (borderline lesion between benign and malignant), and group III (probable carcinoma or quite suspicious of carcinoma but not fulfilling the histological criteria of malignancy) (148). From a theoretical viewpoint, severe dysplasia and early change of carcinoma have to be clearly separated, but in reality the changes do overlap. Zhang et al. (143,149) classified the dysplasia into three pathological types which are able to reflect the histopathological characteristics associated with early gastric cancer. The cryptous type, which is most common and is frequently associated with intestinal metaplasia, originates at the bottom of the IM crypt. The adenomatous type (flat adenoma, atypical epithelial lesion, or IIa subtype), which histopathologically shows obvious proliferation of epithelia and distorted or dilated crypts, called *borderline lesions*, is seen most often in broad-based mucosal elevation. This lesion is irreversible and maintains the same microscopic and histological features for a fairly long time; early gastric cancer may fall into this group. The regenerative type, which occurs simultaneously with chronic ulcerative and erosive lesions of gastric mucosa, is less frequently associated with gastric carcinoma (150).

In summary, the histogenesis of gastric cancer cannot be determined exactly from the results of the present endoscopic follow-up study with biopsy. However it is presumed that gastric cancer not developing through dysplasia is far more frequent than that which develops through changes of moderate or severe dysplasia in cancer of diffuse type, the reverse situation being seen in intestinal cancer.

Experimental Carcinogenesis in Rodents

Animal models of gastric cancer have contributed enormously to extending the insight into mechanisms of chemical carcinogenesis and to identifying susceptibility factors. Rodents have forestomach, which is not present in primates, including humans. Therefore, it should be taken into account that some of the experimental data describing forestomach lesions may not simulate the human situation.

Since Sugimura and Fujimura succeeded in inducing adenocarcinoma in the glandular stomach of rats by oral administration of N-methyl-N'-nitro-N-nitrosoguanidine (MNNG) (151), many subsequent investigators have confirmed MNNG to be one of the most potent and reproducible carcinogens for gastric neoplasia. Other compounds that induced glandular neoplasia in rats include 3-methylcholanthrene (152), 12-dimethylbenz[a]anthracene (DMBA) (153), 2,7-bis(acetylamino)fluorenylene (2,7-FAA) (154), alcoholic solution of 4-hydroxyaminoquinoline 1-oxide (155), and aflatoxin-containing diet (156).

The African rodent *Praomys* (*Mastomys*) *natalensis* is known to develop spontaneous tumors in glandular stomach: carcinoids and adenocarcinoma (157). The spontaneous carcinoids of *Mastomys* are histologically analogous to those in humans. Recently, experimental gastric carcinoids have been induced in rats treated either with omeprazole (158), a proton pump inhibitor that blocks acid secretion, or with a long-acting H_2 blocker, loxtidine (159). Hypergastrinemia induced by an abrogation of acid feedback mechanism is postulated to cause the enterochromaphin-like cell hyperplasia associated with carcinoids.

Numerous investigations have identified a variety of modifying factors that enhanced or inhibited chemical carcinogen–induced gastric neoplasia in rodents. These factors included genetic susceptibility factors (17), surfactants (160), chronic proliferative conditions (161–165), sodium chloride (166,167), potassium chloride (168), ethanol (169), change in gastric acidity (170–172), specific reconstruction after gastrectomy (173), bile reflux (174,175), bile salts (176), norepinephrine (177), low-protein diet (178), epidermal growth factor (179), somatostatin (165), monoamine oxidase inhibitor (180), vasoacting amines (181), and spontaneous and chemically induced hypertension (86,182) (these are enhancing factors); and tetragastrin (183), phenolic antioxidants (184), phenylalanine (185), γ-amino-n-butyric acid (186), and 6-hydroxydopamine (183) (these are suppressing factors).

Inbred strains of rodents that differ in susceptibility to chemical carcinogens provide a useful model for identifying particular genetic loci relevant to carcinogenesis. Morino et al. demonstrated that in the rat carcinogenesis model by MNNG, the gene controlling resistance to carcinoma development was inherited in an autosomal dominant mode (17).

Various surfactants may facilitate the absorption of chemical carcinogens. Fukushima et al. reported that combined administration of various surfactants with MNNG enhanced the development of histologically poorly differentiated adenocarcinomas (160).

The association of chronic proliferative conditions with increased susceptibility to chemical carcinogens is also widely accepted in gastric carcinogenesis. Proliferative conditions induced by various agents have been attributed to one of the risk factors, which include iodoacetamide (162), aspirin (187), norepinephrine concentrations in the gastric wall (177), and prostaglandin deficiency (188).

The tissue level of norepinephrine is increased by various agents. According to Tatsuta et al. (182), spontaneously hypertensive rats contained significantly higher levels of norepinephrine in fundic and antral gastric wall than those in control Wistar rats. Concomitantly, the labeling indices in the fundic and antral mucosa were significantly higher in the former than in the latter. In parallel with these findings, spontaneously hypertensive rats developed a significantly higher incidence and number of gastric glandular carcinomas per rat than did the control Wistar rats in the MNNG carcinogenesis model. Similar results were confirmed by experimental hypertensive rat model, which was induced by deoxycorticosterone acetate–NaCl (86). In this animal model, supplementation of potassium chloride reduced the blood pressure, the incidence of gastric cancers, and the number of tumors per animal. The tissue level of norepinephrine and labeling indices were also significantly suppressed by oral potassium chloride. Additional studies further confirmed the role of tissue norepinephrine in gastric carcinogenesis by MNNG. Increase in tissue norepinephrine concentration was induced by a low-protein diet, which correlated with gastric cancer incidence (178). Tyrosine methyl ester significantly increased the tumor incidence, labeling index, and tissue norepinephrine level (180). Along those lines, cysteamine reduced the incidence of MNNG-induced gastric carcinomas in rats, while the monoamine oxidase inhibitor furazolidone attenuated the effect of cysteamine and increased the tissue level of norepinephrine (180). Administration of L-phenylalanine reduced the incidence and number of glandular adenocarcinomas by MNNG, increased the basal serum gastrin level, and decreased the norepinephrine concentration in the antral gastric wall as well as the labeling index in antral mucosa (185).

Prostaglandin E2 liberated in the gastric juice was reduced by MNNG (188) but increased during the period when the animals became tumor bearers (189), suggesting a positive association of prostaglandins in gastric carcinogenesis. γ-Amino-n-butyric acid (GABA) decreased the proliferation of antral mucosa and suppressed the incidence and number of gastric cancers in rats by MNNG (186).

Induction of ornithine decarboxylase (ODC) activity and DNA synthesis *in vitro* are used as markers for screening gastric cancer promoters (190,191). Using these markers, Furihata et al. suggested the potential promoter activity of glyoxal and methylglyoxal (192,193); these findings were later confirmed by Takahashi et al. using a rat–MNNG initiation model (194). Glyoxal treatment enhanced the incidence of adenocarcinoma in the pylorus of the glandular stomach, while methyl glyoxal increased hyperplasia in the pyloric mucosa.

Sodium chloride has a strong promoter activity in the MNNG-induced carcinogenesis model, in addition to its coinitiating activity. The incidence of adenocarcinomas was elevated when the rats were given NaCl following initiation by combined MNNG and NaCl (166,167) Enhanced tumor induction by NaCl is attributed to diffuse proliferative changes in the surface epithelium of the glandular stomach.

It is to be noted here that in a low-dose model of MNNG carcinogenesis of rat stomach, adenocarcinomas were composed mainly of tumor cells of gastric type (pyloric gland cell type and surface mucous cell type) and that the area of intestinal metaplasia in pyloric mucosa was less than 1% (195). In addition, adenomatous hyperplasia without intestinal-type cells (intestinal-absorptive cell type and goblet cell type) appeared sequentially first, whereas those with intestinal cells arose later, indicating that intestinal metaplasia may not be a preneoplastic change in this carcinogenesis model.

Bile and bile salts are also considered to be promoters for gastric carcinogenesis. Association of bile flux into the stomach with promotion of gastric carcinoma has been demonstrated (173). Bile reflux may cause disruption of gastric mucosal barrier and induce chronic epithelial cell injury, in addition to enhancing absorption of potential carcinogens. Some of the bile salts (taurocholic acid and sodium taurocholate) mixed in the diet have been demonstrated to act as promoters in MNNG-induced gastric carcinogenesis (176,189). Partial gastrectomy in rats combined with MNNG reduced the carcinoma induction period by more than 10 weeks compared to those without gastrectomy (174). In this model, duodenal reflux (including bile) into the remnant of stomach increased the number of tumors.

Intestinal Cancer

Small Intestine

The small intestine (jejunum and ileum) is an organ where carcinomas are extremely low in contrast to other sites in the gastrointestinal tract (197). Several reasons for this low incidence are speculated: (a) the mucosal epithelial turnover rate is so rapid that neoplastic cells, if they have emerged, cannot settle and remain in the mucosa; (b) the movement of small intestinal content is too fast to allow carcinogenic interaction with the cells; and (c) bacterial flora in the small intestine is quantitatively and qualitatively different from that in the large intestine.

According to Miles et al. (198), malignant tumors in the small intestine comprised carcinoids (39%), adenocarcinomas (20%), lymphomas (19%), leiomyosarcomas (13%), undifferentiated carcinomas (8%), and others. From the small number of reports on carcinoma developing in the small intestine, we might be able to extrapolate several susceptibility factors for carcinogenesis. They include genetically defined predisposition to cancer, long-standing Crohn's disease, chronic repeated inflammatory stimulation to aberrant tissue, and celiac disease.

Inherited Predisposition to Cancer

Patients with Peutz–Jeghers syndrome are reported to develop small intestinal carcinomas (199–206). Peutz–Jeghers syndrome (PJS) (207) is inherited as an autosomal dominant trait and characterized by mucocutaneous pigmentation and gastrointestinal hamartomas, which are not generally regarded as potentially premalignant. Based on 72 cases with PJS complicating malignant tumors, Spigelman et al. (199) speculated the presence of gene(s) regulating the growth and differentiation of gastrointestinal tract and they proposed the hamartoma–carcinoma sequence in the PJS (199); the hamartoma consists of relatively normal mucosal cells and abnormal amounts and arrangement of smooth muscle cells.

Crohn's Disease

Cancers complicated by Crohn's disease are found predominantly in the right side of the colon (208). However, association of increased risk of small intestinal cancers and Crohn's disease has been supported by numerous reports (209–212). On the basis of literature throughout the world, Collier et al. (210) reported 78 patients with Crohn-related adenocarcinoma of the small intestine. In contrast to the *de novo* cancer, of which approximately 76% occur in the duodenum and jejunum and 24% in the ileum (209), Crohn-associated adenocarcinomas of the small intestine appear to be in parallel with the disease distribution: jejunum 24% to 30% and ileum 67% to 76% (208,210). Although numerous studies have identified a diversity of pathophysiologic mechanisms of inflammatory bowel disease (211), susceptibility factors responsible for its malignant complication are yet to be clearly understood. However, prolonged chronic stimuli secondary to the inflammatory reaction is considered to be a reasonable explanation for the factors. At the site of inflammation is a variety of pathophysiological alterations, including (a) migration of immune competent cells (macrophage, T-cell populations, B-cell populations, and particularly, elevated level of cytotoxic Leu7$^+$ cells), (b) increased production of IgG, (c) deposition of complement component in the mucosa, (d) increased expression of histocompatibility complex class II antigens, (e) demonstration of cell-mediated and humoral immunity directed against epitopes common to enterobacterial antigens and enterocytes surface determinants, (f) increased activity of interleukin-1 and interleukin-6 as well as altered expression of interleukin-2 and its receptor, and (g) enhanced production of diverse mediators of the inflammatory response, such as several eicosanoid products of arachidonic acid metabolism (prostaglandin, thromboxane products, and thromboxane synthetase) and 5-lipoxygenase products (leukotrien B$_4$). These cytokines, eiconsanoids, and oxygen free radicals cause sustained damage of tissue and modification of immune surveillance mechanism. A common feature of Crohn's disease is formation of strictures and fistulas, which commonly causes partial bowel obstruction. The stagnant flow of intestinal content may contribute to the interaction of carcinogens and cells. Hawker et al. (208) reported that 29.5% of adenocarcinoma of the small intestine in Crohn's disease occurred in bypassed loops. While Hoffman et al. (212) and Collier et al. (210) report that a bypass operation delays the detection of complicating tumors, the possibility cannot be excluded that it may contribute to alteration of the bacterial flora.

Epithelial dysplasia is considered to play an important role in carcinogenesis (208,213). Interestingly enough, Simpson et al. (214) reported dysplasia and carcinoma *in situ* adjacent to and distant (10 cm) from foci of adenocarcinoma of the small intestine complicated by Crohn's disease. Their observation lends support to the field effect theory of carcinogenesis.

Cancers Originating from Aberrant Tissue

Heterotopic tissues localized in the small intestine are rare. They are usually found incidentally at abdominal laparatomy. Clinical manifestations are uncommon. A rare carcinoma was reported which developed in the jejunal aberrant pancreatic tissue (215). In their review Barbosa et al. stated that pancreatic tissue in the aberrant site is more prone to malignant transformation than is that of the pancreas proper (216).

Celiac Disease

National Registry Study of celiac disease in the United Kingdom demonstrated an extremely high incidence of malignant neoplasms, particularly lymphomas (217). Of 259 histologically confirmed malignancies in 235 patients with celiac disease, 51.4% were malignant lymphomas, the predominant histological type being malignant histiocytosis, and the commonest site of this lesion, the small intestine. Of 116 invasive nonlymphomatous malignancies, 16.4% were adenocarcinoma of the small intestine followed by 8.6% of squamous carcinoma of the esophagus. Celiac disease is a metabolic intolerance for dietary gluten. The jejunal biopsy findings of celiac disease consist of subtotal or severe partial villous atrophy and crypt hyperplasia accompanied by an unusually increased number of plasma cells and lymphocytes infiltration in the lamina propria. A gluten-free diet improves both clinical symptoms and signs and histopathological findings of the follow-up biopsies. A reasonable explanation for the increased incidence of small intestinal malignancies in the celiac disease is lacking. Swinson et al. (217) postulated several mechanisms: increased permeability of the small intestine for environmental carcinogens, vitamin A deficiency, and increased susceptibility to an as-yet-unidentified oncovirus due to immunological disturbances.

Large Intestine

Carcinoma of the large intestine (colon and rectum) is a major cancer of the gastrointestinal (GI) tract in the United States and other industrialized Western countries (1). It is ranked among the leading causes of cancer death. We review risk factors of the large intestinal cancers, precursors of carcinomas, inherited and acquired predisposing conditions/diseases, and finally, a method of screening susceptible, high-risk individuals.

TABLE 3. Diet and large intestinal cancer[a]

Dietary factors	Draser and Irving (1973)	Armstrong and Doll (1975)	Howell (1975)	Wynder and Hirayama (1977)	Liu et al. (1979)	IARC (1977)	Jensen et al. (1982)
Cereals		−	−				−
Wheat							0
Rice			−				
Legumes			−				
Sugars			+				
Meat		+	+	+		+	0
Milk			+	+		−	0
Fat and oil			+	+			0
Animal protein	+	+					
Animal fat	+						
Total fat	+	+			+	−	0
Saturated fatty acid					+		−
Unsaturated fatty acid					+		0
Fiber	0	−			−	−	−

Modified from Zaridze (218).
[a] +, Positive correlation; −, negative correlation; 0, no correlation.

Colorectal Cancer Risk Factors

Numerous epidemiological and laboratory studies have revealed a possible relationship between colorectal cancer and various dietary factors (Table 3) (218). These studies suggest that various substances present in the large intestinal lumen may act directly or indirectly as carcinogenic agents; these include fatty acid, catalytic ferrous ion, bile acids, fecal steroids, protein metabolites, and bacterial flora and their products having mutagenic/promoting activity, such as fecapentaenes (219) and diacylglycerol (220). Recently, Ito et al. (221) reported that 2-amino-1-methyl-6- phenylimidazo[4,5,b]pyridine (PhIP) produced during cooking induces a high incidence of mammary and colonic carcinoma in F344 rats. It is postulated that several carcinogens are generated *in vivo* through iron-catalyzed lipid peroxidation (222). The ultimate products are hydroxyl free radicals ($\cdot$OH), which, in conjunction with superoxide anions ($^-O_2$), act as DNA-damaging initiator and/or promoter.

Some of the experimental tumor promoters are known to be activators of protein kinase C (PKC), a key enzyme in the intracellular signal transduction and growth control (223). When extracellular signal is transferred to membrane-bound receptor complex, the agonist-stimulated receptor complex activates the phospholipase C in the membrane to hydrolyze phosphatidylinositol 4,5-bisphosphate (PIP_2), generating the second messengers inositol triphosphate ($InsP_3$) and diacylglycerol (DAG). While $InsP_3$ mobilizes intracellular calcium ($[Ca^{2+}]_i$) from multiple calcium compartments, DAG in collaboration with $[Ca^{2+}]_i$ activates PKC (223–225).

Morotomi et al. (220) demonstrated that DAG is produced *in vitro* by normal human intestinal microflora combined with certain bile acids. This evidence points to possible correlation between a high-fat meat diet, increased bile acid secretion, intestinal bacterial flora, and colon cancer risk.

DAG in the feces also acts as an endogenous promoter, which increases the Na^+/H^+ exchange at the plasma membrane, leading to a rise in cytoplasmic pH (226). One of the earliest events in growth stimulation generated by growth factors (platelet-derived growth factor, epidermal growth factor) is an increase in sodium influx into quiescent cells, and this process is coupled with hydrogen efflux. By using two mouse strains that are either DMH sensitive (CF_1) or DMH resistant (DBA/2), Davis et al. (227) observed an increase in the influx of sodium in the distal colon of CF_1, while DMH treatment had no effect on sodium transport in the distal colon of DBA/2. Thus Na^+/H^+ exchange, resulting in intracellular alkalinization, may have an important role in the initial event of colon carcinogenesis. However, other investigators (228), using rodent lymphocytes stimulated by 12-*O*-tetradecanoylphorbol 13-acetate and ionomycin, observed that an increased level of c-*fos* mRNA, an early response to mitogens, was unaffected by inhibition of the Na^+/H^+ antiport or even in the absence of Na^+ when alkalinization was prevented by means of nigericin. They observed similar results using human T-lymphocytes stimulated by phytohemagglutinin. It appears that further investigation is necessary to have a clearer concept on the proliferation and intracellular alkalinization signal coupling hypothesis.

$[Ca^{2+}]_i$-regulating PKC activity plays another important role in carcinogenesis. In the regulation of cell functions, initiation of gene transcription is essentially a very important step. This step is controlled by an RNA polymerase, which is a substrate of various protein kinases (229). The second messengers, such as cAMP, DAG, $[Ca^{2+}]_i$, $InsP_3$ and $InsP_4$ (230), regulate the activity of relevant kinases, which include protein kinase A, PKC, and calcium/calmodulin-dependent protein kinase (CaM-KII). These kinases activate specific gene expression. Some of the membrane-associated oncogene products, such as *src* and *ras* protein, have inositol lipid kinase activity (231–233), which converts phosphatidylinositol to phosphatidylinositol 4,5-bisphosphate. The activated *ras* gene may result in uncontrolled phosphodiesteric cleavage to produce $InsP_3$. On the other hand, point mutation of *ras* oncogene at codon 12 has been shown to be devoid of intrinsic GTPase activity. While GTPase activity of normal *ras* gene products autoregulates its function, deregulation of GTPase activity in mutant could result in uncontrolled production of $InsP_3$ and DAG (234,235). Various reports demonstrated a prevalence of point mutation of K-*ras* gene codon 12 in sporadic colorectal cancers (236,238). Similar point mutation in codon 12 of K-*ras* 2 protooncogene was also reported in adenomas (236–239), in some of the adenocarcinomas (240,241), and less frequently in polyposis (241,242).

Although environmental factors play a major role in colorectal carcinogenesis, genetically defined factors play an important role. This includes inherited predisposition to cancer (familial polyposis coli syndromes, and hereditary nonpolyposis colorectal cancers, which are known as Lynch syndrome I and II) (243–254) and most recently an inherited mutation of the p53 suppressor gene (255–257). It is a current dogma that irrespective of various hereditary factors or specific environmental factors, the development of colorectal cancers may share common molecular mechanisms, where multiple mutational activations of oncogenes take place and are coupled with mutational inactivation or deletion of tumor suppressor genes or abrogation of suppressor gene products function.

Another aspect of colon cancer risk factors is association with host's immune defense mechanism. It is well recognized that various diseases that accompany impairment of immune defense mechanism eventually develop cancers in various organs, including colon and rectum. Areas of crypt atypia adjacent to the lymphoid aggregates are not uncommon (258), and there is experimental evidence that some early cancers may appear in those areas (258–260). More specifically, experimental evidence also indicates (12) that *in vivo* treatment by (DMH) suppressed mouse natural killer (NK) cell activity by 38.1%. By contrast, augmentation of NK cell activity, brought about by additional treatment with inositol hexaphosphate, correlated well with suppressed colon carcinogenesis. It is well known that intestinal mucosa harbors particularly enriched distribution of large granular lymphocytes (LGL) that show a high level of NK cell activity (261). These data indicate that NK cells in the normal intestine play a major role in surveillance mechanism.

Precursors of Carcinomas

A large number of experimental and clinicopathological studies indicate that a variety of histological abnormalities can be precursors of colorectal carcinomas. They include hyperplastic polyps, adenomatous polyps, villous adenomas, flat adenomas, and dysplastic mucosa that appear in a long-standing chronic state of ulcerative colitis and Crohn's disease. Historically, there were two major hypotheses regarding the histogenesis, each being mutually exclusive (262,263). One was the polyp–cancer hypothesis and the other was the so-called *de novo* cancer hypothesis. It has become necessary to change the interpretation of the facts in the light of new evidence, making the hypothesis a theory and the theory a fact (264). Shamsuddin et al. (265–267) and others (268) observed microscopic carcinomas affecting single or several crypts. They were in the flat nonpolypoid mucosa of the colon, which might be difficult to determine by conventional diagnostic maneuvers. From these observations they documented the notion that large intestinal carcinomas can and do arise directly from the flat mucosa as well as arising from polyps in humans (258,259,269). Shamsuddin proposed a unified concept that large intestinal carcinomas may arise directly from the nonpolypoid mucosa as well as through a polyp–cancer sequence. This hypothesis allows a reasonable explanation for the evidence that most carcinomas in the right hemicolon are fungating exfoliating growth, which might arise from polyps, while most of those in the left hemicolon are sessile infiltrating growth, probably from the flat nonpolypoid mucosa. Ando et al. reported that the frequency of point mutations in the c-K-*ras* oncogene in human colorectal adenomas with severe atypia was higher than that in carcinomas, suggesting that many colorectal carcinomas may not be induced through adenomas with severe atypia (239). (For a more detailed discussion of these issues, see ref. 269.)

Inherited Predisposition to Colorectal Cancer

Inherited predisposition to colorectal cancer is divided into two categories: hereditary discrete colorectal polyp–cancer syndrome [familial adenomatous polyposis (FAP)] and hereditary nonpolyposis colorectal cancer (HNPCC; Lynch syndrome).

Familial Adenomatous Polyposis and Gardner's Syndrome. Familial adenomatous polyposis (FAP) is inherited as an autosomal dominant trait with nearly 100% penetrance characterized by the presence of numerous adenomas (at least 100) in the large intestine, most of which develop in childhood and increase in number with age. Gardner's syndrome (GS) is a phenotypic variant of FAP characterized by multiple adenomatous polyps throughout the entire GI tract. Patients with FAP or GS left untreated will inevitably develop colorectal cancer at a relatively young age and comprises about 1% of all colorectal cancer deaths (270). In addition, FAP and GS demonstrate a diversity of accompanying neoplastic lesions other than those in the gastrointestinal tract. These include tumors of ecto-, meso-, and endodermal tissues. The incidence of carcinomas is higher in the distal colon and rectum than in the proximal colon. Carcinomas of the large intestine in FAP seem to be induced from numerous preceding polyps; hence they are multicentric. As a clinical marker for FAP, *congenital hypertrophy of the retinal pigment epithelium* (CHRPE) has been evaluated (271,272). However, the definitive diagnosis for FAP, based on genetic/molecular markers, is yet to be developed.

FAP gene has been detected on chromosome 5q (273–277). Others have identified allelic losses in colon cancers developed in FAP patients on chromosome 17, 18, and 22 and less frequently on chromosomes 6 and 12 (278–281). It has been demonstrated that the DNA of a colon carcinoma–derived cell line from a FAP patient had transforming activity for NIH/3T3 cells, whereas skin fibroblast DNA from the same patient did not (240,282). The transforming gene is a human activated c-K-*ras* 2 oncogene with a point mutation in codon 12. K-*ras* 2 point mutation at codon 12 has also been demonstrated in adenomas (239,283). More recently, FAP locus genes were identified in chromosome 5q21 (284,285). These genes on 5q21 are considered to be important not only for the inheritance of FAP and GS, but also for development of the noninherited form of colorectal cancer. The MCC gene on 5q21 has been shown to be somatically altered in tumors from sporadic colorectal cancer patients. APC gene on 5q21 was found to have point mutations in germ line cells from FAP and GS patients. These genes are characterized as suppressor genes.

Peutz–Jeghers Syndrome. Although the incidence of colorectal cancers associated with Peutz–Jeghers syndrome (PJS) is low, rare cases are reported that are complicated with adenomas and adenocarcinomas in the colon (199,286,287). In the PJS, polyps [the majority of which are histologically hamartomas (287)] in the upper GI tract are usually more frequent in number than those in the colon and rectum. Reflecting these distribution pattern of polyps, the number of colon cancers reported by Spigelman et al. (199) is smaller than those of the small intestine and stomach.

Juvenile Polyposis. The average age of diagnosis of juvenile polyposis (JP) is 6 years (288). Polyps are small in number or sometimes solitary, and are seen more often in colon and rectum. The accompanying symptoms are blood in the stool and severe anemia. Although polyps in JP are usually nonneoplastic, some cases with adenomatous tumors have been reported (289). Family members of the JP have a high incidence of colon carcinomas (288,290).

Turcot Syndrome. Turcot's syndrome is believed to be a variant of FAP that represents one manifestation of the pleiotropic gene mutation responsible for the association between colorectal polyposis and neural gliomas (including medulloblastomas), both of which predispose highly to malignancy (291). Interestingly enough, an unusual sensitivity to DNA alkylating agents and radiation has been demonstrated both in fibroblasts from a patient with Turcot's syndrome (292,293) and skin fibroblasts from a family with Gardner's syndrome (294). Based on these observations, Rutz et al. (291) speculate a possible association between increased sensitivity and heterozygosity of a functional growth suppressor gene on chromosome 5 that is related with FAP.

Hereditary Nonpolyposis Colorectal Cancer. Hereditary nonpolyposis colorectal cancer is classified arbitrarily into two subtypes: HNPCC type a or Lynch syndrome I (site-specific nonpolyposis colorectal cancer) and HNPCC type b or Lynch syndrome II (cancer family syndrome) (245–252,295). Lynch syndrome I is characterized by (a) an autosomal dominant trait of inherited susceptibility to colorectal cancer, which has no relationship with polyps; (b) an earlier age onset than sporadic colorectal cancer, which does not fall into this syndrome; (c) right-sided (proximal) colon predilection for cancer development; and (d) synchronous or metachronous multicentricity of the cancer emergence (295–297).

Lynch syndrome II (cancer family syndrome, CFS) is featured by all the criteria described above (Lynch syndrome I) plus additional association with extracolonic cancers, particularly endometrial carcinoma (245,298). Other sites harboring cancers associated with Lynch syndrome II are ovary, stomach, small intestine, pancreas, urinary tract, and larynx (247,249,253,254).

In HNPCC, the diagnosis is not easy to establish in individual patients because of the requirement of extensive pedigree study over a period of several years. In addition, neither genetic nor molecular markers specific for HNPCC are available. However, several biochemical and cytopathological abnormalities would help us to understand the predisposition to cancer. Tetraploidy of cultured skin fibroblasts is often increased in individuals affected by heritable colon cancer, while that in the normal person is not demonstrable (299). Colonic epithelial proliferation, as measured by a labeling index using [^{3}H]thymidine or bromodeoxyuridine incorporation, has been shown to be of value for estimating increased risk of colon cancer in HNPCC (300).

Acquired Predisposition to Colorectal Cancer

Ulcerative Colitis. That ulcerative colitis complicates colorectal cancer is supported by numerous reports (211,301–304). The risk of colorectal cancer complication is increased significantly in persons with ulcerative colitis (UC) affecting the entire colon (305–308), and with left-sided hemicolon (309). It is particularly high among those patients who develop UC in young age, and having a long history (10 years or more) of the disease with remission and exacerbation (310). According to Sugita et al. (304), the interval between the onset of the disease and the development of cancer is virtually the same in patients with extensive colitis and those with left-sided colitis (about 21 years).

Pseudopolyp and epithelial dysplasia have been pointed out as precancerous changes in the mucosa (262,303,308,311). In view of the observation that c-Ki-*ras* mutations in codon 12 are infrequent (3.6%) in ulcerative colitis–associated carcinoma or dysplasia while those in sporadic colon carcinomas were 52%, Burmer et al. speculate distinct genetic pathways in the carcinogenesis mechanism between them (236). Prophylactic total colectomy may be recommended when severe dysplasia and pseudopolyps are established during long-term surveillance by colonoscopy (302,312–314).

Crohn's Disease. Crohn's disease is one of the inflammatory bowel diseases that have increased incidence of colorectal cancer (267,302,315–319). According to Ekbom et al. (320), the relative risk of cancer in Crohn's disease is 1.0 when the disease is confined within the terminal ileum, 3.2 when the terminal ileum and part of the colon are involved, and 5.6 when only colon is affected. Moreover, the relative risk is particularly high (20.9) for patients in whom Crohn's disease with colonic involvement is diagnosed before age 30. Because of the nature of Crohn's disease, which involves full thickness of the affected intestine and develops fistulas between intestine and surrounding tissue, the clinical manifestations associated with Crohn's disease–complicated large intestinal carcinoma are not simple. However, epithelial dysplasia in Crohn's disease, which may play a role in carcinogenesis, is analogous to that in ulcerative colitis (318).

Radiation Therapy. Large intestinal cancer is a late complication that may develop following pelvic radiation therapy. Since Slaughter and Southwick (321) first reported a case of radiation-induced carcinomas of the large intestine, several cases have been published (266,322). Most of the cases developed cancer 20 to 30 years after the irradiation therapy. In general, the radiation-affected segment shows severe narrowing due to fibrosis. The mucosa is featured by a variety of dysplastic crypts with mesenchymal cell infiltration. Radiation-induced carcinoma of the large intestine is another example where cancers emerge without going through a benign polyp–cancer sequence.

Ureterosigmoidostomy. Ureterosigmoidostomy, which is usually performed as pediatric surgery for congenital malformation, is considered to be a high risk factor for developing large intestinal cancer (323–327). The experimental study by Crissey et al. suggested that carcinogens in both the urine and feces were cooperatively responsible for development of carcinoma (328). Kalble et al. reported an increased urinary nitrite and N-nitrosamine excretion in patients who developed carcinoma at the ureterocolonic junction (326).

Rectovaginal Fistula. Rectovaginal fistula is a complication of delivery (329) or of Crohn's disease (330,331). Left untreated, it can be a risk factor over the long run for developing rectal or anal carcinoma due to a mechanism similar to that in ureterosigmoidostomy.

Schistosomiasis. Association of helminthic infection with colon cancer has been reported from a province in China (332) and from Tanzania (333), where intestinal schistosomiasis is endemic. Although Cheevers did not find sufficient evidence for positive correlation between schistosomiasis and colon cancer (334), Ming-Chai et al., based on studies with 454 colorectal cancers, observed several analogies between schistosomiasis- and ulcerative colitis–related cancers (335,336). Other investigators found mild to severe dysplasia in 36 (60%) of 60 cases of surgical specimen from schistosomiasis (337).

Barrett's Esophagus. Barrett's esophagus is defined as an abnormality in the lower esophageal epithelium, where the normal squamous epithelial cells are replaced with columnar cells because of repeated peptic esophagitis. The complication of colon carcinoma with Barrett's esophagus has been reported by several investigators (338–340). Pero et al. (341) attributed the susceptibility of carcinomas in both colon and columnar epithelial-lined esophagus to the defective DNA repair mechanism; however, there is no definitive evidence that will reasonably explain the association of Barrett's esophagus with large intestinal carcinoma. Meltzer et al. (43) observed site-specific expression of c-Ha-*ras* protooncogene in ulcerative colitis and Barrett's esophagus, in which the expression was greater in proximal colon than in distal colon and undetectable in Barrett's esophagus.

Identification of Susceptible, High-Risk Individuals

Identification by screening of asymptomatic, normal-appearing individuals, who are at high risk of developing CR cancer is the most important strategy for effective prevention and mortality improvement. For this purpose, markers associated with CR cancer and precancerous lesion, which include mucopolysaccharides, blood group antigen–related glycoconjugates, carcinoembryonic antigen, cytoskeletal proteins, and mucus component antigens, have been studied widely (269). Before discussing a method for detection of susceptible individuals for CR cancer and precancer, we provide a brief review of the background for the rationale of this approach.

Morphogenesis of Colorectal Carcinomas. The morphological changes during experimental and human carcinogenesis in their very early phases should provide us some insight into the mechanism. Studies of azoxymethane-induced early lesions in

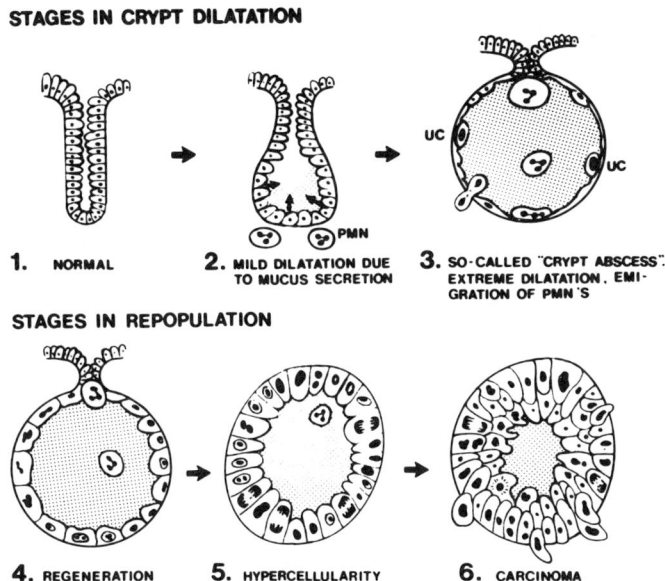

FIG. 2. Morphogenesis of colon carcinoma. In the very early (primary) stage, mucus secretion is increased, resulting in moderately dilated crypts (2). In the intermediate stage, the crypt is further dilated (enormously) and epithelial cells become flattened; migrating polymorphonuclear leukocytes are commonly observed in the lumen (3). In the later stage, the distended crypts are repopulated by epithelial cells with an increased N/C ratio, bizarre nuclei, and nucleoli. [From Shamsuddin et al. (349), with permission.]

rat colon epithelium revealed that prior to definitive malignant transformation, there is marked dilatation and distortion of the crypts (342,343) followed by atypical and dysplastic crypts. Figure 2 is a schematic representation of the various changes early in colon carcinogenesis.

Very early (primary) stage. There is an increase in mucus secretion as well as the exhausted appearance of mucous cells in the crypt (mild crypt dilatation). The regulation of mucus secretion from intestinal goblet cells is site-specific (344–346). The surface goblet cells secrete mucin in response to surface-active chemical irritants (such as mustard oil, alcohol, hypertonic saline, bile salts, and bacterial enterotoxins), while crypt goblet cells secrete mucin in response to cholinergic agonists (acetylcholine, pilocarpine, carbachol), vasoactive histamine, and electrical field stimulation. It is speculated that electrolyte/fluid and mucin secretory processes are regulated independently in the intestine and the calcium–calmodulin systems may be involved in stimulus–secretion coupling in goblet cells. However, it is not clear what kind of stimuli are responsible for the crypt dilatation connected with precarcinogenic change.

Intermediate stage. Following the very early stage, there is an enormous dilatation of crypt lumen with extremely low flattened epithelial cells. The hyperdistended lumen is filled with mucin, mostly sialomucin, and characterized by polymorphonuclear cells' infiltration. Changes of mucin properties in the carcinogen affected mucosa are abnormalities associated with malignant transformation, which precede overt morphological transformation (347). Of particular interest and importance is the role of polymorphonuclear leukocytes as a generator of mutagen (6), which is evidenced by the *in vitro* demonstration that there is an enhancement of free-radical production by human neutrophils when they are cocultured with human colon adenocarcinoma cells (348).

Crypt repopulation stage. In the later stage, the hyperdistended crypts are repopulated by epithelial cells showing an increased nuclear/cytoplasmic ratio and bizarre nuclei and nucleoli. Mitotic figures are commonly observed. These cells may be regenerated from surviving undifferentiated stem cells, which perhaps became dysplastic through the various mechanisms involved during transformation.

The changes in experimental models described above have their counterpart in human diseases; virtually identical changes are seen in human precancerous lesions, such as polyps, ulcerative colitis, and Crohn's disease (349,350). The fact that these changes are also seen to a variable degree in an otherwise normal mucosa remote from cancer has led to the concept of the field effect, discussed below.

Field Effect Theory of Colorectal Carcinogenesis. Extensive experimental and histopathological study on animals and humans by Shamsuddin et al. showed that normal-appearing mucosa of the surgically resected colon that is remote from carcinoma sites is morphologically and histochemically similar to the pre-neoplastic and neoplastic changes observed in experimental models (both *in vivo* and *in vitro*) of carcinogenesis (351–353). The interpretation of these observations is that carcinogens cause simultaneous changes throughout the entire colon which are responsible for the multifocal occurrence of abnormalities in mucosa remote from an obvious cancer. There may be quantitative and qualitative differences by sites in the degree of neoplastic changes, depending on the influence of carcinogenic agents and on the site-specific susceptibility (15). These changes may be expressed as morphological changes (atypia or dysplasia) or biochemical changes (altered antigenicity, new enzyme, protein, hormone synthesis, altered receptor expression, oncogene product, and altered mucin production (347). Burmer and Loeb (236) demonstrated mutations of codon 12 in K-*ras* 2 oncogene not only in the carcinomas and less frequently in adenomas but also in regions of histologically benign mucosa adjacent to the carcinoma in some cases. Other investigators (354) observed abnormal findings of DNA ploidy and proliferative pattern (as determined by S-phase fraction) in superficial colonic epithelium adjacent to and distant from foci of colorectal cancer. These and other evidence support the field effect theory of large intestinal carcinogenesis.

Such a concept would allow us to examine an accessible part of the large intestine (i.e., the rectum) and to predict the condition of the rest of the organ by virtue of the field effect. Exploration of this concept and development of a marker has resulted in just that. People who have colonic cancer or precancerous lesions or those who are at a high risk can now be identified by using the marker β-D-Gal-(1→3)-D-GalNAc in rectal mucin by a simple enzymatic test (355). Early results show that this approach may be quite useful in screening susceptible persons (356,357). For a more detailed discussion, see ref. 269.

Experimental Carcinogenesis in Rodents

Animal models have made a great contribution toward understanding the mechanism of colon carcinogenesis. Since Lorenz and Stewart first reported the chemical carcinogen–induced intestinal tumors in mice (358), numerous studies have identified the carcinogenic activity of various substances, including 7,12-dimethylbenz-[*a*]anthracene (359), methylcholanthrene (358), 4-aminodiphenyl, 3,2-dimethyl-4-aminodiphenyl (360), 3,2'-dimethyl-4-aminobiphenyl (361), methylazoxymethanol (MAM) (362), 1,2-dimethylhydrazine (DMH) (363), azoxymethane (AOM) (364), methylnitrosourea (365), N-methyl-N'-nitro-N-nitrosoguanidine (366), and fecapentaene-12 (367). Some of the carcinogens were found in foodstuffs. These include products of cycad gymnosperms, cycasin (methylazoxymethanol β-D-glucoside), MAM, other azoxy-containing compounds, and mushroom-derived hydrazine derivatives. These carcinogenic substances, in combination with various rodent strains, served to investigate the factors that modify the susceptibility of colon carcinogenesis.

Numerous factors have been identified as enhancers or suppressors of colon carcinogenesis. These include genetic predisposition (368), chronic inflammation (369,370), dietary fat (371–374), bacterial flora (375), bile (366,376), vitamin A deficiency (377,378), dietary fiber (379–381), inositol compounds (10), dopamine antagonist (382), selenium (383), oltipraz (384), neurotensin (385), calorie restriction (386), spontaneous hypertension (387), tissue norepinephrine level (388), glucarate (389), magnesium hydroxide (390), body activity stress, or voluntary exercise (391,392).

Colon crypt is a unit structure where epithelial cell proliferation and turnover takes place. Factors or substances that enhance the cell proliferation in the crypt are considered to be associated with carcinogenic promoter. Various endogenous substances have been reported to enhance cell proliferation. Attention has been focused on the noradrenergic and cholinergic fibers near the basal region of crypts. Tutton and Barkla (393) demonstrated that chemical sympathectomy decreased the mitotic rate, suggesting that norepinephrine locally liberated from sympathetic nerves might stimulate cell proliferation. This hypothesis was confirmed by spontaneously hypertensive rats (387), in which tissue norepinephrine concentration and labeling index in the distal colon mucosa were significantly higher than those of normotensive control rats, which was in parallel with colon tumor incidence induced by AOM. Moreover, cysteamine inhibited the AOM-induced colon tumor incidence by suppressing the norepinephrine level in colon tissue and labeling indices of colon mucosa (388).

Chronic inflammation of the colon increases the susceptibility of carcinogenesis. Chronic colitis model in mice was reported by Okayasu et al. (370). Administration of 5% dextran sulfate sodium in drinking water produced a pathological feature morphologically and symptomatically similar to the chronic ulcerative colitis in humans.

According to Deschner and Raicht, bile has a strong trophic action on colon epithelial cells (394,395). When bile flow to the intestine was eliminated, a number of mitotic figures and DNA synthesis in the large intestine were decreased, migration of cells to the luminal surface was retarded, and generation time (cell cycle) was prolonged. In addition, cholic acid, supplemented in the diet, induced a marked increase in cell proliferation and in cell migration rate in the colon epithelium (396). Narisawa et al. demonstrated that lithocholic or taurocholic acid, which was intrarectally instilled with carcinogens, increased the number of adenomatous polyp development in the large intestine (366). However, according to Cameron et al., suppression of crypt cell proliferation by parenteral feeding (associated with decreased bile secretion) during and shortly after the initiation stage of carcinogenesis did not reduce the incidence of colon tumor, suggesting that other factors in addition to enhanced cell proliferation may possibly be involved in the promotion of colon carcinogenesis (380).

Burkitt advocated that dietary fiber had a protective role in the development of large intestinal cancer (397). However, a number of subsequent investigations resulted in controversy. Neither fecal bulk nor fecal transit time, both being influenced by the dietary fiber, had an association with colonic tumor formation. Depending on the types of dietary fiber, colon carcinogenesis is either protected or enhanced (380). Barnes et al. observed that wheat bran was protective on DMH-induced colon carcinogenesis, while corn bran was associated with increased tumor development (398). They neglected the fact that wheat bran was rich in inositol hexaphosphate ($InsP_6$, phytic acid), while corn bran does not contain $InsP_6$. Shamsuddin and Sakamoto (10) describe that when administered to animals in drinking water, $InsP_6$ is antineoplastic in rodent carcinogenesis models. This activity is augmented further when $InsP_6$ is combined with inositol. Concomitantly, cell proliferation in the crypts is suppressed by inositol compounds (10).

Vitamin A deficiency causes enhancement in DMH-induced tumor development (399). The mechanism is attributed to its antioxidant and cellular differentiation activity, the latter being investigated most extensively using respiratory epithelium and urothelium.

Selenium is shown to protect AOM-induced colon carcinogenesis. Dietary benzylselenocyanate, a novel organoselenium compound, increases liver cytochrome P450 and induces hydroxylation of AOM and oxidation of MAM in the rat liver, thus resulting in decreased delivery of MAM to the colon epithelium via a hematogenic route (383).

Arachidonic acid metabolites have a complex biological activity, some of which have a counteracting effect on each other on the same target organ. For example, prostaglandins, which are produced locally in the colon epithelium via the cyclooxygenase pathway, inhibited colon epithelial cell proliferation (400), while in the MNNG-induced colon carcinogenesis model, the intrinsic PGE2 level in the cancerous lesion was significantly higher than that of normal-appearing mucosa (401). The intrinsic PGE2 level in the colon was also more elevated in the MNNG-treated group than in the control normal group, suggesting the role of PGE2 as a promoter in the development and proliferation of carcinoma. This conflicting evidence should make us consider other factors, such as the biological activities of intermediate metabolites (endoperoxides, prostaglandins, thromboxanes, and prostacyclin) on inflammatory cells, endocrine cells, and neurogenic cells.

SUMMARY AND CONCLUSIONS

Development of GI tract carcinoma is a function of multiple factors, among which environmental carcinogens play a major role, while genetic and immunological factors also contribute, often interacting with each other. Susceptibility factors of GI tract carcinogenesis could be governed by a variety of genes controlling the normal cellular physiology and protooncogenes, including their mutational alterations as well as environmental risk factors. With the increase in detailed knowledge of the mechanism in each step of the carcinogenesis process, we can gradually make steady progress toward a clearer understanding of carcinogenesis. Hopefully, this will lead to clues for identifying susceptible persons at an early stage, resulting in prevention of this dreadful disease.

ACKNOWLEDGMENTS

The authors wish to thank Millie Michalisko and Sabrina Mercer of the publication staff for preparing the manuscript. This chapter is contribution No. 3160 from the Pathobiology Laboratory.

REFERENCES

1. Boring CC, Squires TS, Tong T. Cancer statistics, 1993. *CA* 1993;43:7–26.
2. Doll R. The geographical distribution of cancer. *Br J Cancer* 1969;23:1–8.
3. Haenszel W, Berg JW, Segi M, Kurihara M, Locke FB. Large bowel cancer in Hawaiian Japanese. *J Natl Cancer Inst* 1973;51:1765–1779.
4. Wynder EL, Kajitani T, Ishikawa S. Environmental factors of cancer of the colon and rectum. *Cancer* 1969;23:1210–1220.
5. Bartsch H, Ohshima H, Pignatelli B. Inhibitors of endogenous nitrosation. Mechanism and implications in human cancer prevention. *Mutat Res* 1988;202:307–324.
6. Weitzman SA, Weitberg AB, Clark EP, Stossel TP. Phagocytes as carcinogens: malignant transformation induced by human neutrophils. *Science* 1985;227:1231–1233.
7. Sugimura T. Multiple primary cancers: biology and its significance on cancer control program. *Proc Am Assoc Cancer Res* 1991;32:457–458.
8. Ron E, Gridley G, Hrubec Z, Page W, Arora S, Fraumeni JF Jr. Acromegaly and gastrointestinal cancer. *Cancer* 1991;68:1673–1677.
9. Ames BN. Dietary carcinogens and anticarcinogens. Oxygen radicals and degenerative diseases. *Science* 1983;221:1256–1264.
10. Shamsuddin AM, Sakamoto K. Antineoplastic action of inositol compounds. In: Wattenberg L, Lipkin M, Boone CW, Kelloff G, eds. *Cancer chemopreventive agents.* Boca Raton, FL: CRC Press; 1992;285–308.

11. Shamsuddin AM, Elsayed AM, Ullah A. Suppression of large intestinal cancer in F344 rats by inositol hexaphosphate. *Carcinogenesis* 1988;10:577–588.
12. Baten A, Ullah A, Tomazic VJ, Shamsuddin AM. Inositol-phosphate-induced enhancement of natural killer cell activity correlates with tumor suppression. *Carcinogenesis* 1989;10:1595–1598.
13. Bralow SP, Gruenstein M, Meranze DR. Host resistance to gastric adenocarcinomatosis in three strains of rats ingesting N-methyl-N'-nitro-N-nitrosoguanidine. *Oncology* 1973;27:168–180.
14. Evans JT, Shows TB, Sproul EE, Paolini NS, Mittelman A, Hauschka TS. Genetics of colon carcinogenesis in mice treated with 1,2-dimethylhydrazine. *Cancer Res* 1977;37:134–136.
15. James JT, Shamsuddin AM, Trump BF. Comparative study of the morphologic, histochemical, and proliferative changes induced in the large intestine of ICR/Ha and C57BL/Ha mice by 1,2-dimethylhydrazine. *J Natl Cancer Inst* 1983;71:955–964.
16. Deschner EE, Hakissian M, Long FC. Genetic factors controlling inheritance of susceptibility to 1,2-dimethylhydrazine. *J Cancer Res Clin Oncol* 1989;115:335–339.
17. Morino K, Ohgaki H, Matsukura N, Kawachi T, Sugimura T. Genetic study of host factors in gastrocarcinogenesis in rats. In: Bartsch H, Armstrong B, eds. *Host factors in human carcinogenesis*. Lyon, France: International Agency for Research on Cancer; 1982:153–156.
18. Autrup H, Harris CC. Metabolism of chemical carcinogens by human tissues. In: Harris CC, Autrup HN, eds. *Human carcinogenesis*. New York: Academic Press; 1983:169–194.
19. Nebert DW. P450 genes: structure, evolution, and regulation. *Annu Rev Biochem* 1987;56:945–993.
20. Perkin DM, Laara E, Muir CS. Estimates of the world-wide frequency of sixteen major cancers in 1980. *Int J Cancer* 1988;41:184–197.
21. Burkitt D. Epidemiological feature of gastrointestinal cancer. *Front Gastrointest Res* 1979;4:86–95.
22. Sales D, Levin B. Incidence, epidemiology and predisposing factors. In: DeMeester TR, Levin B, eds. *Cancer of the esophagus*. Orlando, FL: Grune & Stratton; 1985:1–19.
23. Priester WA. Esophageal cancer in North China: high rates in human and poultry populations in the same areas. *Avian Dis* 1975;19:213–215.
24. Duranceau A. Epidemiological trends and etiologic factors of esophageal carcinoma. In: Delarue NC, Wilkins EW Jr, Wong J, eds. *International trends in general thoracic surgery*. Vol 4. *Esophageal cancer*. St. Louis, MO: CV Mosby; 1988:3–10.
25. Munoz N, Crespi M, Wahrendorf J, Bang LJ. An intervention trial on precursor lesions for esophageal cancer in a high incidence area of China. In: Jacobs MM, ed. *Vitamins and minerals in the prevention and treatment of cancer*. Boca Raton, FL: CRC Press; 1991:61–68.
26. Appleqvist P, Salmo M. Lye corrosion carcinoma of the esophagus: a review of 63 cases. *Cancer* 1980;45:2655–2658.
27. Mufti SI, Garewal HS, Watson RR. Role of environment, drugs of abuse, and nutritional factors in the etiology and prevention of cancers of oral cavity and esophagus. In: Watson RR, ed. *Biochemistry and physiology of substance abuse*. Vol 2. Boca Raton, FL: CRC Press; 1990:1–23.
28. Yang CS. Research on esophageal cancer in China: a review. *Cancer Res* 1980;40:2633–2644.
29. Cheng SJ, Sala M, Li MH, et al. Mutagenic, transforming, and promoting effect of pickled vegetables from Linxian county, China. *Carcinogenesis* 1980;1:685–692.
30. Schoental R, Joffe AZ, Yagen B. Cardiovascular lesions and various tumors in rats given T-2 toxin a trichothecene metabolite of *Fusarium*. *Cancer Res* 1979;39:2179–2189.
31. Burrell RJW, Roach WA, Shadwell A. Esophageal cancer of the Bantu of the Transkei associated with mineral deficiency in garden plants. *J Natl Cancer Inst* 1966;36:201–209.
32. Moberhan S, Dowlatshahi K, Diba YY. Hair zinc levels from a normal population of north east Iran with a high incidence of esophageal carcinoma. *Clin Res* 1980;28:598A.
33. Mellow MH, Layne EA, Lipman TO, Kaushik M, Hostetler C, Smith JC. Plasma zinc and vitamin A in human squamous carcinoma of the esophagus. *Cancer* 1983;51:1615–1620.
34. Gabrial GN, Shrager TF, Newberne PM. Zinc deficiency, alcohol and a retinoid: Association with esophageal cancer in rats. *J Natl Cancer Inst* 1982;68:785–789.
35. Milner JA. Rationale and possible mechanisms by which selenium inhibits mammary cancer. In: Jacobs MM, ed. *Vitamins and minerals in the prevention and treatment of cancer*. Boca Raton, FL: CRC Press; 1991:95–111.
36. O'Connor HJ, Habibzedah N, Schorah CJ, Axon ATR, Riley SE, Garner RC. Effect of increased intake of vitamin C on the mutagenic activity of gastric juice and intragastric concentrations of ascorbic acid. *Carcinogenesis* 1985;6:1675–1676.

37. Kyrtopoulos SA, Pignatelli B, Karkanias G, Golematis B, Esteve J. Studies in gastric carcinogenesis V. The effects of ascorbic acid on N-nitroso compound formation in human gastric juice *in vivo* and *in vitro*. *Carcinogenesis* 1991;12:1371–1376.
38. Mufti SI, Zirvi KA, Garewal HS. Precancerous lesions and biologic markers in esophageal cancer. *Cancer Detect Prev* 1991;15:291–301.
39. Rubio CA, Aberg B. Barrett's mucosa in conjunction with squamous carcinoma of the esophagus. *Cancer* 1991;68:583–586.
40. Anani PA, Gardiol D, Savary M, Monnier P. An extensive morphological and comparative study of clinically early and obvious squamous cell carcinoma of the esophagus. *Pathol Res Pract* 1991; 187:214–219.
41. Chang F, Janatuinen E, Pikkarainen P, Syrjanen S, Syrjanen K. Esophageal squamous cell papillomas. Failure to detect human papillomavirus DNA by *in situ* hybridization and polymerase chain reaction. *Scan J Gastroenterol* 1991;26:535–543.
42. Hollstein M, Sidransky D, Vogelstein B, Harris CC. p53 Mutations in human cancer. *Science* 1991;253:49–53.
43. Meltzer SJ, Yin J, Huang Y, et al. Reduction to homozygosity involving p53 in esophageal cancers demonstrated by the polymerase chain reaction. *Proc Natl Acad Sci USA* 1991;88:4976–4980.
44. Takahashi M, Imaida K. Modification of tumor development in the gastrointestinal tract. In: Ito N, Sugano H, eds. *Progress in experimental tumor research*. Vol 33. *Modification of tumor development in rodents*. Basel: S Karger; 1991:58–75.
45. Druckrey H. Organospecific carcinogenesis in the digestive tract. In: Nakahara W, Takayama S, Sugimura T, eds. *Topics in chemical carcinogenesis*. Baltimore: University Park Press; 1972:73–103.
46. Stinson SF. Animal model: esophageal carcinoma in the rat induced with methyl-alkyl-nitrosamines. *Am J Pathol* 1979;96:871–874.
47. Fong LYY, Lin HJ, Lee CLH. Methylation of DNA in target and non-target organs of the rat with methylbenzylnitrosamine and dimethylnitrosamine. *Int J Cancer* 1979;23:679–682.
48. Hodgson RM, Wiessler M, Kleihues P. Preferential methylation of target organ DNA by the esophageal carcinogen N-nitrosomethylbenzylamine. *Carcinogenesis* 1980;1:861–866.
49. Umbenhauer D, Wild CP, Montesano R, et al. O^6-Methyl-deoxyguanosine in oesophageal DNA among individuals at high risk of oesophageal cancer. *Int J Cancer* 1985;36:661–665.
50. Saffhill R. The competitive miscoding of O^6-ethylguanine and O^6-ethylguanine and the possible importance of cellular deoxynucleoside 5'-triphosphate pool sizes in mutagenesis and carcinogenesis. *Biochim Biophys Acta* 1986;866:53–60.
51. Abbott PJ, Saffhill R. DNA synthesis with methylated poly(dC-dG) templates. Evidence for a competitive nature to miscoding by O^6-methylguanine. *Biochim Biophys Acta* 1979;562:51–61.
52. Hill-Perkins M, Jones MD, Karran P. Site-specific mutagenesis in vivo by single methylated or deaminated purine bases. *Mutat Res* 1986;162:153–163.
53. Barch DH, Jacoby RF, Brasitus TA, Radosevich JA, Carney WP, Iannaccone PM. Incidence of Harvey *ras* oncogene poit mutations and their expression in methylbenzylnitrosamine-induced esophageal tumorigenesis. *Carcinogenesis* 1991;21:2373–2377.
54. Lin HJ, Cahn WC, Fong LYY, et al. Zinc levels in serum, hair and cancer tumors from patients with esophageal cancer. *Nutr Rep Int* 1977;15:632–635.
55. Barch DH, Fox CC. Dietary zinc deficiency increases the methylbenzylnitrosamine-induced formation of O^6-methylguanine in the esophageal DNA of the rat. *Carcinogenesis* 1987;8:1461–1464.
56. Mandal S, Stoner GD. Inhibition of N-nitrosobenzylmethylamine-induced esophageal tumorigenesis in rats by ellagic acid. *Carcinogenesis* 1990;11:55–61.
57. Barch DH, Fox CC. Selective inhibition of methylbenzylnitrosamine-induced esophageal tumorigenesis in rats by ellagic acid. *Cancer Res* 1988;48:7088–7092.
58. Muir C, Waterhouse J, Mack T, Powell J, Whelan S. *Cancer incidence in five continents*. Vol 5, no 88. Lyon, France: IARC Scientific Publications; 1987.
59. Parkin DM. *Cancer occurrence in developing countries*. No. 75. Lyon, France: IARC Scientific Publications; 1986.
60. Waterhouse J, Muir C, Shanmugaratnamk ET. *Cancer incidence in five continents*. No 42. Lyon, France: IARC Scientific Publications; 1986.
61. Whelan SL, Parkin DM, Masuyer E. *Patterns of cancer in five continents*. No 102. Lyon, France: IARC Scientific Publications; 1990.

62. Lauren P. The two main histological types of gastric carcinoma: diffuse and so-call intestinal type. *Acta Pathol Microbiol Scand* 1965;64:31–39.
63. Hill MJ. *Epidemiology and mechanism of gastric carcinogenesis: new trends in gastric cancer.* Norwell, MA: Kluwer; 1990:3–12.
64. Ranzani GN, Pellegata NS, Previdere C, et al. Heterogeneous protooncogene amplification with tumor progression and presence of metastases in gastric cancer patients. *Cancer Res* 1990;50:7811–7814.
65. Kim J-H, Takahashi T, Chiba I, et al. Occurrence of p53 gene abnormalities in gastric carcinoma tumors and cell lines. *J Natl Cancer Inst* 1991;83:938–943.
66. Ames BN. Identifying environmental chemicals causing mutation and cancer. *Science* 1979;204:587–593.
67. Geboers J, Johossens JV, Kesteloot H. *Diet and human carcinogenesis.* New York: Excerpta Medica; 1985:81–95.
68. Graham S, Schotz W, Martino P. Alimentary factors in the epidemiology of gastric cancer. *Cancer* 1972;30:927–938.
69. Furihata C, Sato Y, Hosaka M, Matsushima T, Furukawa F, Takahashi M. NaCl induce ornithine decarboxylase and DNA synthesis in rat stomach mucosa. *Biochem Biophys Res Commun* 1984;121:1027–1032.
70. Takahashi M, Hasegawa R. *Nutrition and cancer.* Tokyo: Japan Scientific Societies Press; 1986:1–18.
71. Correa P. In: Sherlock P, Morson BC, eds. *Precancerous lesions of gastrointestinal tract.* New York: Raven Press; 1983:145–153.
72. Garland B, Ibrahim M, Grimson R. In cancer epidemiology: assessment of past diet. *Am J Epidemiol* 1982;116:577(abst).
73. Thorsteinsson T. Polyciclic hydrocarbons in commercially- and home-smoked foods in Iceland. *Cancer* 1969;23:457.
74. Dungal N. The special problem of stomach cancer in Iceland with particular reference to dietary factors. *JAMA* 1961;178:789–798.
75. Risch HA, Jain M, Choi NW, et al. Dietary factors and the incidence of cancer of the stomach. *Am J Epidemiol* 1985;122:947–959.
76. Ikeda M, Yoshimoto K, Yoshimura T. A cohort study on the possible association between broiled fish intake and cancer. *GaNN* 1983;74:640–648.
77. Correa P, Cuello C, Fajardo LF, Haenszel W, Bolanos O, deRamirez B. Diet and gastric cancer: nutrition survey in a high-risk area. *J Natl Cancer Inst* 1983;70:673–678.
78. Hoey J, Montvernay C, Lambert R. Wine and tobacco: risk factors for gastric cancer in France. *Am J Epidemiol* 1981;113:668–674.
79. Hirayama T. Epidemiology of stomach cancer in Japan. *Jpn J Clin Oncol* 1984;14:159–168.
80. Garner RC, Craven JL, Hall R, Dyke GW. P^{32} postlabelling of human gastric biopsy DNA. *Proc Am Assoc Cancer Res* 1991;32:233(abst).
81. Jedrychowski WA, Popiela T. Gastric cancer in Poland: a decreased malignancy due to changing nutritional habits of the population. *Neoplasma* 1986;33:97–106.
82. Weisberger JH, Raineri R. Dietary factors and the etiology of gastric cancer. *Cancer Res* 1975;35:3469–3474.
83. Saffiotti U, Montesano R, Sellakumar A, Borg SA. Experimental cancer of the lung: inhibition by vitamin A of the induction of tracheobronchial squamous metaplasia and squamous cell tumors. *Cancer* 1967;20:857–864.
84. Stehr P, Gloninger NF, Kuller L, Marsh GM, Radford EP, Weinberg GB. Dietary vitamin A deficiencies and stomach cancer. *Am J Epidemiol* 1985;121:65–70.
85. Wattenberg LW. Inhibitors of chemical carcinogenesis. *Adv Cancer Res* 1977;26:197–226.
86. Tatsuta M, Iishi H, Baba M, Taniguchi H. Enhanced induction of gastric carcinogenesis by N-methyl-N'-nitro-N-nitrosoguanidine in deoxycorticosterone acetate–NaCl hypertensive rats and its inhibition by potassium chloride. *Cancer Res* 1991;51:2863–2866.
87. Benjamin H, Storkson J, Nagahara A, Pariza MW. Inhibition of Benzo(a)pyrene-induced mouse forestomach neoplasia by dietary soy sauce. *Cancer Res* 1991;51:2940–2942.
88. Dodd GD. Genetics and cancer of the gastrointestinal system. *Radiology* 1977;123:263–275.
89. Roberts JAF. Some associations between blood groups and disease. *Br Med Bull* 1959;15:129–133.
90. Haenszel W, Kurihara M, Locke FB, Shimuza K, Segi M. Stomach cancer in Japan. *J Natl Cancer Inst* 1976;56:265–278.
91. Teppo L, Pukkala E, Hakama M, Hakulinen T, Herva A, Saxen E. Way of life and cancer incidence in Finland. *Scand J Soc Med* 1980[suppl];19:1–84.

92. Magee PN, Barnes JM. The production of malignant primary hepatic tumors in the rat by feeding dimethyl-nitrosamine. *Br J Cancer* 1956;10:114–122.
93. Bogovski P, Bogovski S. Animal species in which *N*-nitroso compounds induce cancer. Special report. *Int J Cancer* 1981;27:471–474.
94. Schmaal D, Scherf HR. Carcinogenic activity of *N*-nitroso-diethylamine in snakes. In: O'Neill IK, et al, eds. *N-nitroso compounds: occurrence, biological effects and relevance to human cancer.* No 57. Lyon, France: IARC Scientific Publications; 1984:677–682.
95. Walters CL, Carr FPA, Dyke CS. Nitrite sources and nitrosamine formation *in vitro* and *in vivo*. *Food Chem Toxicol* 1979;17:473–479.
96. Ohshima H, Bartsch H. Quantitative estimation of endogenous nitrosation in human by monitoring *N*-nitroproline excreted in the urine. *Cancer Res* 1981;41:3658–3662.
97. Stillwell WG, Glogowski J, Xu H-X, et al. Urinary excretion of *N*-nitrosoproline, 3-methyladenine, and 7-methylguanine in a Colombian population at high risk for stomach cancer. *Cancer Res* 1991;51:190–194.
98. Ohgaki H, Matsukura N, Morino K, Kawachi T, Sugimura T, Takayama S. Carcinogenicity in mice of mutagenic compounds from glutamic acid and soybean globulin pyrolysates. *Carcinogenesis* 1984;5:815–819.
99. Correa P, Haenszel W, Cuello C, Tannenbaum S, Archer M. A model for gastric cancer epidemiology. *Lancet* 1975;2:58–60.
100. Correa P. A human model of gastric carcinogenesis. *Cancer Res* 1988;48:3554–3560.
101. Leach SA, Thompson M, Hill M. Bacterially catalysed N-nitrosation reaction and their relative importance in the human stomach. *Carcinogenesis* 1987;8:1907–1912.
102. Leach SA, Cook AR, Challis BC. Exposures and mechanisms. In: Bartsch H, et al, eds. *The relevance of N-nitroso compounds to human cancer.* No 84. Lyon France: IARC Scientific Publications; 1987:396–399.
103. Parsonnet J, Vandersteen D, Goates J, Sibley RK, Pritikin J, Chang Y. *Helicobacter pylori* infection in intestinal and diffuse type gastric adenocarcinomas. *J Natl Cancer Inst* 1991;83:640–643.
104. Fox JG, Correa P, Taylor NS, et al. *Campylobacter pylori*-associated gastritis and immune response in a population at increased risk of gastric carcinoma. *Am J Gastroenterol* 1989;84:775–781.
105. Jaskiewicz K, Louwrens HD, Woodroof CW, et al. The association of *Campylobacter pylori* with mucosal pathological changes in a population at risk for gastric cancer. *S Afr Med J* 1989;75:417–419.
106. Ames BN, Gold LS. Chemical carcinogenesis: too many rodent carcinogens. *Proc Natl Acad Sci USA* 1990;87:7772–7776.
107. Ames BN, Gold LS. Too many rodent carcinogens: mitogenesis increases mutagenesis. *Science* 1990;249:970–997.
108. Sobala GM, Pignatelli B, Schorah CJ, et al. Level of nitrite, nitrate, *N*-nitroso compounds, ascorbic acid and total bile acid in gastric juice of patients with and without precancerous conditions of stomach. *Carcinogenesis* 1991;12(2):193–198.
109. Lu SH, Ohshima H, Fu H-M, et al. Urinary excretion of *N*-nitrosamino acids and nitrate by inhabitants of high- and low-risk areas for esophageal cancer in northern China: endogenous formation of nitrosoproline and its inhibition by vitamin C. *Cancer Res* 1986;46:1485–1491.
110. Lu SH, Yang WX, Guo LP, et al. In: Bartsch H, et al, eds. *The relevance of N-nitroso compounds to human cancer, exposures and mechanisms.* No 84. Lyon, France: IARC Scientific Publications; 1987:538–543.
111. Autrup H, Bradley KA, Shamsuddin AKM, Wakhisi J, Wasunna A. Detection of putative adduct with fluorescence characteristics identical to 2,3-edihydro-2-(7'-guanyl)-3-hydroxyaflatoxin B1 in human urine collected in Muranga district. *Carcinogenesis* 1983;4:1193–1195.
112. Shuker DEG, Bailey E, Farmer PB. In: Bartsch H, et al, eds. *The relevance of N-nitroso compounds to human cancer, exposures and mechanisms.* No 84. Lyon, France: IARC Scientific Publications; 1987:407–441.
113. Ranzani GN, Pellegata NS, Previdere C. Heterogeneous protooncogene amplification correlates with tumor progression and presence of metastasis in gastric cancer patients. *Cancer Res* 1990;50:7811–7814.
114. Shibuya M, Yokota J, Ueyama Y. Amplification and expression of a cellular oncogene (c-*myc*) in human gastric adenocarcinoma cells. *Mol Cell Biol* 1985;5:414–418.
115. Yokota J, Yamamoto T, Toyoshima K, et al. Amplification of c-*erb*B-2 oncogene in human adenocarcinoma *in vivo*. *Lancet* 1986;1:765–766.

116. Bos JL, Vries MV, Marshall CJ, Veeneman GH, van Boom JH, Van der Eb AJ. A human gastric carcinoma contains a single mutated and an amplified normal allele of the Ki-*ras* oncogene. *Nucleic Acids Res* 1986;14:1209–1217.
117. Deng G, Lu Y, Chen S, et al. Activated c-Ha-*ras* oncogene with a guanine to thymine transversion at the twelfth codon in a human stomach cancer cell line. *Cancer Res* 1987;47:3195–3198.
118. O'Hara BM, Tainsky MA, Blair DG. Mechanism of activation of human *ras* genes cloned from a gastric adenocarcinoma and a pancreatic carcinoma cell line. *Cancer Res* 1986;46:4695–4700.
119. Sakamoto H, Mori M, Taira M, et al. Transforming gene from human stomach cancer and a noncancerous portion of stomach mucosa. *Proc Natl Acad Sci USA* 1986;83:3997–4001.
120. Shimizu K, Nakatsu Y, Sekiguchi M, et al. Molecular cloning of an activated human oncogene, homologous to v-*raf*, from primary stomach cancer. *Proc Natl Acad Sci USA* 1985;82:5641–5645.
121. Yasui W, Sumiyoshi H, Yamomoto T, et al. Expression of Ha-*ras* oncogene product in *ras* gastrointestinal carcinomas induced by chemical carcinogens. *Arch Pathol Jpn* 1987;37:1731–1741.
122. Fujita J, Ohuchi N, Yao T, et al. Frequent overexpression, but not activation by point mutation, of *ras* genes in primary human gastric cancers. *Gastroenterology* 1987;93:1339–1345.
123. Tahara E, Yasui W, Tantyama K, et al. Ha-*ras* oncogene product in human gastric carcinoma: correlation with invasiveness, metastasis or prognosis. *Jpn J Cancer Res* 1986;77:517–522.
124. Ohuchi N, Horan Hand P, Merlo G, et al. Enhanced expression of c-Ha-*ras* P21 in human stomach adenocarcinoma defined by immunoassays using monoclonal antibody and *in situ* hybridization. *Cancer Res* 1987;47:1413–1420.
125. Ranzani GN, Salerno-Mele P, Maltoni M, Talarico D, Della Valle G, Amadori D. Study on c-Ha-*ras*-1 locus polymorphism in an Italian population with high incidence of gastric cancer. *Mol Biol Med* 1988;5:145–153.
126. Yamomoto T, Hattori T, Tahara E. Interaction between transformed TGF growth factor-alpha and c-Ha-*ras* P21 in progression of human gastric carcinoma. *Pathol Res Pract* 1988;183:663–669.
127. Koda T, Matsushima S, Sasaki A, Danjo Y, Kakinuma M. c-*myc* gene amplification in primary stomach cancer. *Jpn J Cancer Res* 1985;76:551–554.
128. Nomura N, Yamomoto T, Toyoshima K, et al. DNA amplification of c-*myc* and c-*erb*B-i genes in a human stomach cancer. *Jpn J Cancer Res* 1986;77:1188–1192.
129. Tsuboi K, Hirayoshi K, Takeuchi K, et al. Expression of the c-*myc* gene in human gastrointestinal malignancies. *Biochem Biophys Res Commun* 1987;146:699–704.
130. Allum WH, Newbold KM, Macdonald F, Russell B, Stokes H. Evaluation of P62 c-*myc* in benign and malignant gastric epithelia. *Br J Cancer* 1987;56:785–786.
131. Ciclitira PJ, Macartney JC, Evan G. Expression of c-*myc* in non-malignant and per-malignant gastrointestinal disorders. *J Pathol* 1987;151:293–296.
132. Kawashima K, Imoto K, Izawa M. Restriction fragment length polymorphism (RFLP) of L-*myc* is related to the progression of human colon and stomach cancers. *Proc Jpn Acad* 1987;63:300–303.
133. Land H, Parada LF, Weinberg RA. Tumorigenic conversion of primary embryo fibroblasts requires at least two cooperating oncogenes. *Nature* 1983;304:596–602.
134. Nigro JM, Baker SJ, Preisinger AC, et al. Mutations in p[53] gene occur in diverse human tumor types. *Nature* 1989;342:705–708.
135. Yamada Y, Yoshida T, Hayashi K, Sekiya T, Yokota J, Hirohashi S, Nakatani K, Nakano H, Sugimura T, Terada M. p[53] Gene mutations in gastric cancer metastases and in gastric cancer cell lines derived from metastases. *Cancer Res* 1991;51:5800–5805.
136. Tamura G, Kihana T, Nomura K, Terada M, Sugimura T, Hirohashi S. Detection of frequent p[53] gene mutations in primary gastric cancer by cell aborting and polymerase chain reaction single-strand conformation polymorphism analysis. *Cancer Res* 1991;51:3056–3058.
137. Sano T, Tsujino T, Yoshida K, et al. Frequent loss of heterozygosity on chromosome 1_q, 5_q and 17_p in human gastric carcinomas. *Cancer Res* 1991;51:2926–2931.
138. Noguchi M, Hirohashi S, Shimosato Y. Histologic demonstration of antigens reactive with anti-P21-*ras* monoclonal antibody (RAP-5) in human stomach cancers. *J Natl Cancer Inst* 1980;77:379–385.
139. Schwartz GK, Davis BM, Altorki N, Nanus DM, Kelsen DP, Albino AP. Growth factor RNA transcript expression in gastric cancer using reverse transcriptase polymerase chain reaction (RT-PCR). *Proc AACR* 1991;32:46(abst).
140. Soman NR, Correa P, Ruiz BA, Wagon GN. Molecular genetic model for gastric tumorigenesis. *Proc AACR* 1991;32:138(abst).
141. Nagayo T. Histogenesis and precursors of human gastric cancer. In: Reed PI, et al, eds. *New trends in gastric cancer*. Norwell, MA: Kluwer; 1990;13.
142. Jass JR. A classification of gastric dysplasia. *Histopathology* 1983;7:181–193.

143. Zhang YC. Epithelial dysplasia of stomach and its relationship with gastric cancer. In: Ming S-C, ed. *Precursors of gastric cancer*. New York: Praeger; 1984:41–52.
144. Fillipe MI, Jass JR. Intestinal metaplasia subtype and cancer risk. In: Fillipe MI, Jass JR, eds. *Gastric carcinoma*. New York: Churchill Livingstone; 1986:87–115.
145. Segura DI, Montero C. Histochemical characterization of different types of intestinal metaplasia in gastric mucosa. *Cancer* 1983;52:498–505.
146. Hirota T, Okada T, Itabashi M, et al. In: Ming S-C, ed. *Precursors of gastric cancer*. New York: Praeger; 1984:179–193.
147. Matsukura N, Zuzuki K, Kawachi T, et al. Distribution of marker enzymes and mucin in intestinal metaplasia in human stomach and relation of complete and incomplete types of intestinal metaplasia to minute gastric carcinoma. *J Natl Cancer Inst* 1980;65:231–240.
148. Morson BC, Sobin LH, Grundmann E, Johansen A, Nagoyo T, Serck-Hanssen A. Precancerous condition and epithelial dysplasia. *J Clin Pathol* 1980;33:711–721.
149. Zhang YC, Zhang PF, Wang MX, et al. Epithelial dysplasia of stomach and its relationship with gastric cancer. *Proceedings of the 6th Asia Pacific cancer conference*, Sendai, Japan; 1983:33.
150. Ming S-C. Pathological features and significance of gastric dysplasia. In: Ming S-C, ed. *Precursors of gastric cancer*. New York: Praeger; 1984:9–27.
151. Sugimura T, Fujimura S. Tumor production in glandular stomach of rats by N-methyl-N'-nitro-N-nitrosoguanidine. *Nature* 1967;216:943–944.
152. Hare WV, Stewart HL, Bennett JG, et al. Tumor of the glandular stomach induced in rats by intramural injection of 20-methylcholanthrene. *J Natl Cancer Inst* 1952;12:1019–1025.
153. Grant R. Cancer induction in the glandular stomach of rats at sites of implanted 7,12-dimethylbenz[*a*]anthracene. *J Natl Cancer Inst* 1966;37:353–364.
154. Morris HP, Wagner BP, Ray FE, et al. Comparative carcinogenic effects of N,N'-2,7-fluorenylene-bisacetamide by intraperitoneal and oral routes of administration to rats, with particular reference to gastric carcinoma. *J Natl Cancer Inst* 1962;29:977–1011.
155. Mori K, Ohta A, Murakami T, et al. Carcinomas of the glandular stomach and other organs of rats induced by 4-hydroxyaminoquinoline 1-oxide hydrochloride. *Gann* 1969;60:627–630.
156. Butler WH, Barnes JM. Carcinoma of the glandular stomach in rats given diets containing aflatoxin. *Nature* 1966;209:90.
157. Randeria JD. Animal model: carcinoids and adenocarcinoma of the glandular stomach of *Praomys (Mastomys) natalensis*. *Am J Pathol* 1979;96:359–362.
158. Ekman L, Hansson E, Havu N, et al. Toxicological studies on omeprazole. *Scand J Gastroenterol* 1985;108:53–69.
159. Poynter D, Pick CR, Harcourt RA, et al. Association of long-lasting unsurmountable histamine H_2 blockade and gastric carcinoid tumors in the rats. *Gut* 1985;26:1284–1295.
160. Fukushima S, Tatematsu M, Takahashi M. Combined effect of various surfactants on gastric carcinogenesis in rats treated with N-methyl-N'-nitro-N-nitrosoguanidine. *Gann* 1974;65:371–376.
161. Nagai T, Pfeiffer CJ, Fujimura M, Hattori T, Tobe T. Susceptibility of healed gastric ulcers to chemical carcinogenesis in rats and implications of cellular kinetic changes. *Cancer Res* 1984;44:5828–5835.
162. Takahashi M, Shirai T, Fukushima S, Hahanouchi M, Hirose M, Ito N. Effect of fundic ulcers induced by iodoacetamide on development of gastric tumors in rats treated with N-methyl-N'-nitro-N-nitrosoguanidine. *Gann* 1976;67:47–54.
163. Takahashi M, Shirai T, Fukushima S, et al. Ulcer formation and associated tumor production in multiple sites within the stomach and duodenum of rats treated with N-methyl-N'-nitro-N-nitrosoguanidine. *J Natl Cancer Inst* 1981;67:473–479.
164. Tatsuta M, Iishi M, Baba M, Yamamura H, Taniguchi H. Enhancement by prolonged administration of caerulein of experimental carcinogenesis induced by N-methyl-N'-nitro-N-nitrosoguanidine in rat stomach. *Cancer Res* 1988;48:6332–6335.
165. Tatsuta M, Iishi H, Baba M, Taniguchi H. Enhancement by somatostatin of experimental gastric carcinogenesis induced by N-methyl-N'-nitro-N-nitrosoguanidine in Wistar rats. *Cancer Res* 1989;49:5534–5536.
166. Takahashi M, Kokubo T, Furukawa F, Kurokawa Y. Effects of sodium chloride, saccharin, phenobarbital and aspirin on gastric carcinogenesis in rats after initiation with N-methyl-N'-nitro-N-nitrosoguanidine. *Gann* 1984;75:494–501.
167. Takahashi M, Kokubo T, Furukawa F, Kurokawa Y, Tatemastu M, Hayashi Y. Effect of high salt diet on rat gastric carcinogenesis induced by N-methyl-N'-nitro-N-nitrosoguanidine. *Gann* 1983;74:28–34.

168. Tatsuta M, Iishi H, Baba M, et al. Protective effect by potassium chloride against gastric carcinogenesis induced by N-methyl-N'-nitro-N-nitrosoguanidine. *Jpn J Cancer Res* 1991;82:280–285.
169. Iishi H, Tatsuta M, Baba M, Taniguchi H. Promotion by ethanol of gastric carcinogenesis induced by N-methyl-N'-nitro-N-nitrosoguanidine in Wistar rats. *Br J Cancer* 1989;59:719–721.
170. Tahara E, Shimosato F, Taniyama K, Ito N, Kosako Y, Sumiyoshi H. Enhanced effect of gastrin on rat stomach carcinogenesis induced by N-methyl-N'-nitro-N-nitrosoguanidine. *Cancer Res* 1982;42:1781–1787.
171. Tatsuta M, Itoh T, Okuda S, Taniguchi H, Tamura H. Effect of prolonged administration of gastrin on experimental carcinogenesis in rat stomach induced by N-methyl-N'-nitro-N-nitrosoguanidine. *Cancer Res* 1977;37:1808–1810.
172. Tatsuta M, Iishi H, Baba M, Mikuni T, Taniguchi H. Effect of propranolol and cimetidine on cysteamine inhibition of gastric carcinogenesis induced in Wistar rats by N-methyl-N'-nitro-N-nitrosoguanidine. *Int J Cancer* 1989;43:464–467.
173. Longhaus P, Hegar RA, Hohenstein J, Bunte H. Operation-sequel carcinoma: an experimental study. *Hepatogastroenterology* 1981;28:34–40.
174. Dahm K, Werner B, Eichen R, Mitschke H. Experimental cancer of the gastric stump. In: Herfarth Ch, Schlag P, eds. *Gastric cancer*. Berlin: Springer-Verlag; 1979:44–59.
175. Sherensheva NI, Patjutko Jul, Klimenkov AA, Turusov VS. Experimental carcinoma of the stomach in rats with chronic ulcers and following gastric surgery. *Arch Geschwulstforsch* 1987;57:91–98.
176. Kobori O, Watanabe J, Schimizu T, Shoji M, Morioka Y. Enhancing effect of taurocholate on N-methyl-N'-nitro-N-nitrosoguanidine-induced stomach tumorigenesis in rats. *Gann* 1984;75:651–654.
177. Tatsuta M, Iishi H, Baba M, Taniguchi H. Enhancement by tyrosine methyl ester of gastric carcinogenesis induced by N-methyl-N'-nitro-N-nitrosoguanidine in Wistar rats. *Int J Cancer* 1991;48:785–788.
178. Tatsuta M, Iishi H, Baba M, Uehara H, Nakaizumi A, Taniguchi H. Enhanced induction of gastric carcinogenesis by N-methyl-N'-nitro-N-nitrosoguanidine in Wistar rats fed a low-protein diet. *Cancer Res* 1991;51:3493–3496.
179. Yasui W, Takekura N, Kameda T, Oda N, Ito M, Tahara E. Effect of epidermal growth factor on rat stomach carcinogenesis induced by N-methyl-N'-nitro-N-nitrosoguanidine. *Acta Pathol Jpn* 1990;40:165–171.
180. Tatsuta M, Iishi H, Baba M, Taniguchi H. Attenuating effect of the monoamine oxidase inhibitor furazolidone on the anti-carcinogenetic effect of cysteamine on gastric carcinogenesis induced by N-methyl-N'-nitro-N-nitrosoguanidine in Wistar rats. *Int J Cancer* 1991;48:605–608.
181. Tatsuta M, Iishi H, Baba M. Inhibition by neostigmine and isoproterenol and promotion by atropine of experimental carcinogenesis in rat stomach by N-methyl-N'-nitro-N-nitrosoguanidine. *Int J Cancer* 1989;44:188–189.
182. Tatsuta M, Iishi H, Baba M, Taniguchi H. Enhancement of experimental gastric carcinogenesis in spontaneously hypertensive rats by N-methyl-N'-nitro-N-nitrosoguanidine. *Cancer Res* 1989;49:794–798.
183. Tatsuta M, Iishi H, Baba M, Taniguchi H. Effect of 6-hydroxydopamine on gastric carcinogenesis and tetragastrin inhibition of gastric carcinogenesis induced by N-methyl-N'-nitro-N-nitrosoguanidine in Wistar rats. *Cancer Res* 1989;49:4199–4203.
184. Hirose M, Mutai M, Takahashi S, Yamada M, Fukushima S, Ito N. Effect of phenolic antioxidants in low dose combination on forestomach carcinogenesis in rats pretreated with N-methyl-N'-nitro-N-nitrosoguanidine. *Cancer Res* 1991;51:824–827.
185. Iishi H, Tatsuta M, Baba M, Okuda S, Taniguchi H. Protection by oral phenylalanine against gastric carcinogenesis induced by N-methyl-N'-nitro-N-nitrosoguanidine in Wistar rats. *Br J Cancer* 1990;62:173–176.
186. Tatsuta M, Iishi H, Baba M, Nakaizumi A, Ichii M, Taniguchi H. Inhibition by γ-amino-n-butyric acid and baclofen of gastric carcinogenesis induced by N-methyl-N'-nitro-N-nitrosoguanidine in Wistar rats. *Cancer Res* 1990;50:4931–4934.
187. Tsung-Hsien C, Yu-Chung L, Kwang-Yung L, Cheng-Hsien S, Yee-Ping C. Cocarcinogenic action of aspirin on gastric tumors induced by N-nitroso-N-methylnitroguanidine in rats. *J Natl Cancer Inst* 1983;70:1067–1075.
188. Materia A, Selecchia G, Spaziani E, et al. Role of prostaglandins in the early phases of experimental gastric carcinogenesis in the rat. *J Cancer Res Clin Oncol* 1989;115:253–258.
189. Silecchia G, Materia A, Spaziani E, et al. Sequential evaluation of gastric intraluminal prostaglan-

din E2 release, acid secretion and DNA-flow cytometry in N-methyl-N'-nitro-N-nitrosoguanidine gastric carcinogenesis in the rat. *Cancer Lett* 1990;49:73–80.
190. Furihata C, Sato Y, Yamakoshi A, Takimoto M, Matsushima T. Inductions of ornithine decarboxylase and DNA synthesis in rat stomach mucosa by 1-nitrosoindole-3-acetonitrile. *Jpn J Cancer Res* 1987;78:432–435.
191. Furihata C, Yamakoshi A, Matsushima T. Inductions of ornithine decarboxylase and DNA synthesis in rat stomach mucosa by formaldehyde. *Jpn J Cancer Res* 1988;79:917–920.
192. Furihata C, Yoshida D, Matsushima T. Potential initiating and promoting activities of diacetyl and glyoxal in rat stomach mucosa. *Jpn J Cancer Res* 1985;76:809–814.
193. Furihata C, Sato Y, Matsushima T. Inductions of ornithine decarboxylase and DNA synthesis in rat stomach mucosa by methylglyoxal. *Carcinogenesis* 1985;6:91–94.
194. Takahashi M, Okamiya H, Furukawa F, et al. Effects of glyoxal and methylglyoxal administration on gastric carcinogenesis in Wistar rats after initiation with N-methyl-N'-nitro-N-nitrosoguanidine. *Carcinogenesis* 1989;10:1925–1927.
195. Tatematsu M, Furihata C, Katsuyama T, et al. Independent induction of intestinal metaplasia and gastric cancer in rats treated with N-methyl-N'-nitro-N-nitrosoguanidine. *Cancer Res* 1983;43:1335–1341.
196. Salmon RJ, Laurent M, Thierry JP. Effect of taurocholic acid feeding on methyl-nitro-N-nitrosoguanidine induced gastric tumors. *Cancer Lett* 1984;22:315–320.
197. Robey-Cafferty SS, Silva EG, Cleary KR. Anaplastic and sarcomatoid carcinoma of the small intestine: a clinicopathological study. *Hum Pathol* 1989;20:858–863.
198. Miles RM, Crawford D, Duras S. The small bowel tumor problem. An assessment based on a 20 year experience with 116 cases. *Ann Surg* 1979;189:732–740.
199. Spigelman AD, Murday V, Phillips RKS. Cancer in the Peutz–Jeghers syndrome. *Gut* 1989;30:1588–1590.
200. Aneiros J, Matamala M, Garcia del Moral R, Lopez JJ, Aguilar D, Camara M. Hamartomatous solitary polyp with malignant progression in the jejunum. A histochemical and immunohistochemical study by light and electron microscopy. *Acta Pathol Jpn* 1988;38:1031–1040.
201. Reid JD. Intestinal carcinoma in the Peutz–Jeghers syndrome. *JAMA* 1974;229:833–834.
202. Utsunomiya J, Gocho H, Miyanaga T, et al. Peutz–Jeghers syndrome: its natural course and management. *Johns Hopkins Med J* 1975;136:71–82.
203. Bussey HJR, Veale AMO, Morson BC. Genetics of gastrointestinal polyposis. *Gastroenterology* 1978;74:1325–1330.
204. Perzin KH, Bridge MF. Adenomatous and carcinomatous changes in hamartomatous polyps of the small intestine (Peutz–Jeghers syndrome): report of a case and review of the literature. *Cancer* 1982;49:971–983.
205. Trau H, Schewach-Millet M, Fisher BK, Tsur H. Peutz–Jeghers syndrome and bilateral breast carcinoma. *Cancer* 1982;50:788–792.
206. Giardiello FM, Welsh SB, Hamilton SR, et al. Increased risk of cancer in Peutz–Jeghers syndrome. *N Engl J Med* 1987;316:1511–1514.
207. Jeghers H, McKusick VA, Katz KH. Generalized intestinal polyposis and melanin spots of the oral mucosa, lips and digits. *N Engl J Med* 1949;241:993–1005.
208. Hawker PC, Gyde SN, Thompson H, Allan RN. Adenocarcinoma of the small intestine complicating Crohn's disease. *Gut* 1982;23:188–193.
209. McPeak CJ. Malignant tumors of the small intestine. *Am J Surg* 1967;114:402–411.
210. Collier PE, Turowski P, Diamond DL. Small intestinal adenocarcinoma complicating regional enteritis. *Cancer* 1985;55:516–521.
211. Podolsky DK. Inflammatory bowel disease. *N Engl J Med* 1991;325:928–937, 1008–1016.
212. Hoffman JP, Taft DA, Wheelis RF, Walker JH. Adenocarcinoma in regional enteritis of the small intestine. *Arch Surg* 1977;112:606–611.
213. Binder V. Incidence of colonic cancer in inflammatory bowel disease. *Scand J Gastroenterol* 1989 [Supp.]; 170:78–82.
214. Simpson S, Traube J, Riddel RH. The histologic appearance of dysplasia (precarcinomatous change) in Crohn's disease of the small and large intestine. *Gastroenterology* 1981;81:492–501.
215. Persson GE, Boiesen PT. Cancer of aberrant pancreas in jejunum. *Acta Chir Scand* 1988;154:599–601.
216. Barbosa JC, Dockerty MB, Waugh JM. Pancreatic heterotopia. Review of the literature and report of 41 authenticated surgical cases, of which 25 were clinically significant. *Surg Gynecol Obstet* 1946;82:527–542.

217. Swinson CM, Slavin G, Coles EC, Booth CC. Coeliac disease and malignancy. *Lancet* 1983;1: 111–115.
218. Zaridze, DG. Environmental etiology of large-bowel cancer. *J Natl Cancer Inst* 1983;70:389–400.
219. Shamsuddin AM, Ullah A, Baten AM, Hale E. Stability of fecapentaene-12 and its carcinogenicity in F-344 rats. *Carcinogenesis* 1991;12:601–607.
220. Morotomi M, Guillem JG, LoGerfo P, Weinstein IB. Production of diacylglycerol, an activator of protein kinase C, by human intestinal microflora. *Cancer Res* 1990;50:3595–3599.
221. Ito N, Hasegawa R, Sano M, Tamano S, Esumi H, Takayama S, Sugimura T. A new colon and mammary carcinogen in cooked food, 2-amino-1-methyl-6-phenylimidazo[4,5-*b*]pyridine (PhIP). *Carcinogenesis* 1991;12:1503–1506.
222. Graf E, Mahoney JR, Bryant RG, Eaton JW. Iron-catalyzed hydroxyl radical formation. Stringent requirement for free iron coordination site. *J Biol Chem* 1984;259:3620–3624.
223. Nishizuka Y. The role of proteinkinase C in cell surface signal transduction and tumor promotion. *Nature (London)* 1984;308:693–698.
224. Nishizuka Y. The molecular heterogeneity of proteinkinase C and its implications for cellular regulation. *Nature (London)* 1988;344:661–665.
225. Berridge MJ, Irvine RF. Inositol phosphates and cell signalling. *Nature* 1989;341:197–205.
226. Moolenaar WH, Tsien RY, van der Saag PT, de Laat SW. Na^+/H^+ exchange and cytoplasmic pH in the action of growth factors in human fibroblasts. *Nature* 1983;304:645–648.
227. Davis RJ, Weidema WF, Sandle GI, Palmer L, Deschner EE, DeCosse JJ. Sodium transport in a mouse model of colonic carcinogenesis. *Cancer Res* 1987;47:4646–4650.
228. Grinstein S, Smith JD, Onizuka R, Cheung RK, Gelfand EW, Benedict S. Activation of Na^+/H^+ exchange and the expression of cellular protooncogenes in mitogen- and phorbol ester-treated lymphocytes. *J Biol Chem* 1988;263:8658–8665.
229. Sawadogo M, Sentenae A. RNA Polymerase B(II) and general transcription factors. *Annu Rev Biochem* 1990;59:711–754.
230. Mitchell RH. A second messenger function for inositol tetrakisphosphate. *Nature* 1986;324:613.
231. Cartwright CA, Kamps MP, Meisler AI, Pipas JM, Eckhart W. $pp60^{c-src}$ Activation in human colon carcinoma. *J Clin Invest* 1989;83:2025–2033.
232. Macara I, Marinetti GV, Balduzzi PC. Transforming protein of avian sarcoma virus, VR2 is associated with phosphatidylinositol kinase activity: possible role in tumorigenesis. *Proc Natl Acad Sci USA* 1983;81:2728–2732.
233. Sugimoto Y, Whitman M, Cantley LC, Erikson RL. Evidence that the Rous sarcoma virus transforming gene product phosphorylates phosphatidylinositol and diacylglycerol. *Proc Natl Acad Sci USA* 1984;81:2117–2121.
234. McGrath JP, Capon DJ, Goeddel DV, Levinson AD. Comparative biochemical properties of normal and activated human *ras* 21 protein. *Nature* 1984;310:644–649.
235. Sweet RW, Yokoyama S, Kamata T, Feramisco J, Rosenberg M, Gross M. The product of *ras* is a GTPase and the T24 oncogenic mutant is deficient in this activity. *Nature* 1984;311:273–275.
236. Burmer GC, Loeb LA. Mutations in the K-*ras* 2 oncogene during progressive stages of human colon carcinoma. *Proc Natl Acad Sci USA* 1989;86:2403–2407.
237. Bos JL, Fearon ER, Hamilton SR, Verlaan de Vries M, van Boom JH, van der Eb AJ, Vogelstein B. Prevalence of *ras* gene mutations in human colorectal cancers. *Nature* 1987;327:293–297.
238. Forrester K, Almoquera C, Han K, Grizzle WE, Pepucho M. Detection of high incidence of K-*ras* oncogenes during human colon tumorigenesis. *Nature (London)* 1987;327:298–303.
239. Ando M, Maruyama M, Oto M, Takemura K, Endo M, Yuasa Y. Higher frequency of point mutations in the c-K-*ras* 2 gene in human colorectal adenomas with severe atypia than in carcinomas. *Jpn J Cancer Res* 1991;82:245–249.
240. Yuasa Y, Oto M, Sato C, et al. Colon carcinoma K-*ras* 2 oncogene of a familial polyposis coli patient. *Jpn J Cancer Res* 1986;77:901–907.
241. Sasaki M, Okamoto M, Sato C, et al. Loss of heterozygosity in colon tumors from patients with FAP non-FPC. *Cancer Res* 1989;49:4402–4406.
242. Farr CJ, Marshall CJ, Easty DJ, Wright NA, Powell SC, Paraskeva C. A study of *ras* gene mutations in colonic adenomas from familial polyposis coli patients. *Oncogene* 1988;3:673–678.
243. Harnden DG. Genetic predisposition to colorectal cancer. In: Seitz HK, Simanowski UA, Wright NA, eds. *Colorectal cancer*. Berlin: Springer-Verlag; 1989:24–43.
244. Alm T. Hereditary adenomatosis of the colon and rectum. In: Lynch PM, Lynch HT, eds. *Colon cancer genetics*. New York: Van Nostrand Reinhold; 1985:30–51.

245. Lynch HT, Kimberling WJ, Alban WA, et al. Hereditary nonpolyposis colorectal cancer (Lynch syndromes I and II), Part I and II. *Cancer* 1985;56:934–951.
246. Lynch PM, Lynch HT, Lynch JF. Hereditary nonpolyposis colon cancer: epidemiologic and clinical–genetic features. In: Lynch PM, Lynch HT, eds. *Colon cancer genetics*. New York: Van Nostrand Reinhold; 1985:52–98.
247. Lynch HT, Voorhees GJ, Lanspa SJ, McGreevy PS, Lynch JF. Pancreatic carcinoma and hereditary nonpolyposis colorectal cancer: a family study. *Br J Cancer* 1985;52:271–273.
248. Lynch HT. Frequency of hereditary nonpolyposis colorectal cancer. *Gastroenterology* 1986;90:486–492.
249. Lynch HT, Kriegler M, Christiansen TA, Smyrk T, Lynch JF, Watson P. Laryngeal carcinoma in a Lynch syndrome II kindred. *Cancer* 1988;62:1007–1013.
250. Lynch HT, Watson P, Lanspa SJ, et al. Natural history of colorectal cancer in hereditary nonpolyposis colorectal cancer (Lynch syndromes I and II). *Dis Colon Rectum* 1988;31:439–444.
251. Lynch HT, Watson P, Kriegler M, et al. Differential diagnosis of hereditary nonpolyposis colorectal cancer (Lynch syndromes I and II). *Dis Colon Rectum* 1988;31:372–377.
252. Lynch HT, Lanspa SJ, Smyrk TC, et al. Historical and natural cancer history facets of the Lynch syndromes. In: Utsunomiya J, Lynch HT, eds. *Hereditary colorectal cancer*. Tokyo: Springer-Verlag; 1990:17–25.
253. Lynch HT, Smyrk TC, Lynch PM, et al. Adenocarcinoma of the small bowel in Lynch syndrome II. *Cancer* 1989;64:2178–2183.
254. Lynch HT, Ens JA, Lynch JF. Lynch syndrome II and urological malignancies. *J Urol* 1990;143:24–28.
255. Vogelstein B, Fearon ER, Hamilton SR, et al. Genetic alterations during colorectal-tumor development. *N Engl J Med* 1988;319:525–532.
256. Baker SJ, Preisinger AC, Jessup JM, et al. p^{53} Gene mutations occur in combination with 17p allelic deletions as late events in colorectal tumorigenesis. *Cancer Res* 1990;50:7717–7722.
257. Purdie CA, O'Grady J, Piris J, Wyllie AH, Bird CC. p53 Expression in colorectal tumors. *Am J Pathol* 1991;138:807–813.
258. Shamsuddin AKM, Phelps PC, Trump BF. Human large intestinal epithelium. Light microscopy, histochemistry and ultrastructure. *Hum Pathol* 1982;13:790–803.
259. Shamsuddin AM, Hogan ML. Large intestinal carcinogenesis. II. Histogenesis and unusual features of low dose azoxymethane induced carcinomas in Fischer 344 rats. *J Natl Cancer Inst* 1984;73:1297–1305.
260. Hillon P, Martin MS, Piard F, Jacquot JF. Relation between adenomas and colorectal-associated lymphoid tissue in familial polyposis coli. *Dig Dis Sci* 1990;35:1307–1308.
261. Luini W, Boraschi D, Alberti S, Aleotti A, Tagliabue A. Morphological characterization of a cell population responsible for natural killer activity. *Immunology* 1981;43:663–668.
262. Morson BC, Dawson IMP, Day DW, Jass JM, Price AB, Williams GT. Benign epithelial tumors and polyps. In: Morson BC, Dawson IMP, et al, eds. *Gastrointestinal pathology*. Oxford: Blackwell; 1990:563–596.
263. Spjut HJ. Pathology of neoplasms. In: Spratt JS, ed. *Neoplasms of the colon, rectum, and anus*. Philadelphia: WB Saunders; 1984:159–204.
264. Burkit DP. Large bowel carcinogenesis: an epidemiological jigsaw puzzle. *J Natl Cancer Inst* 1975;54:3–6.
265. Shamsuddin AKM, Bell HB, Petrucci JV, Trump BF. Carcinoma *in situ* and "microinvasive" adenocarcinoma of colon. *Pathol Res Pract* 1980;167:374–379.
266. Shamsuddin AKM, Elias EG. Rectal mucosa: malignant and premalignant changes after radiation therapy. *Arch Pathol Lab Med* 1981;105:150–151.
267. Shamsuddin AM, Kato Y, Kunishima N, Sugano H, Trump BF. Carcinoma *in situ* in flat mucosa of large intestine: report of a case with significance in strategies for early detection. *Cancer* 1985;56:2849–2854.
268. Kuramoto S, Oohara T. Flat early cancers of the large intestine. *Cancer* 1989;64:950–955.
269. Shamsuddin AM. *Diagnostic assays for colon cancer*. Boca Raton, FL: CRC Press; 1991.
270. Bussey HJR. *Familial polyposis coli: family studies, histopathology, differential diagnosis, and results of treatment*. Baltimore: Johns Hopkins University Press; 1975.
271. Baba S, Tsuchiya M, Machida H, Yamada M. Retinal pigmentations in familial adenomatous polyposis, and linkage study on gene probes on chromosome 5q. In: Utsunomiya J, Lynch HT, eds. *Hereditary colorectal cancer*. Tokyo: Springer-Verlag; 1990:91–96.

272. Blair NP, Trempe CL. Hypertrophy of the retinal pigment epithelium associated with Gardner's syndrome. *Am J Ophthalmol* 1980;90:661–667.
273. Bodmer W, Bailey C, Bodmer J, et al. Localization of the gene for familial adenomatous polyposis on chromosome 5. *Nature* 1987;328:614–616.
274. Leppart M, Dobbs M, Scambler P, et al. The gene for familial polyposis coli maps to the long arm of chromosome 5. *Science* 1987;238:1411–1413.
275. Solomon E, Voss R, Hall V, et al. Chromosome 5 allele loss in human colorectal carcinomas. *Nature* 1987;328:616–619.
276. Nakamura Y, Lathrop M, Leppert M, et al. Localization of the genetic defect in familial adenomatous polyposis within a small region of chromosome 5. *Am J Hum Genet* 1988;43:638–644.
277. Rees M, Leigh SEA, Delhanty JDA, Jass JR. Chromosome 5 allele loss in familial and sporadic colorectal adenomas. *Br J Cancer* 1989;59:361–365.
278. Baker SJ, Fearon ER, Nigro JM, et al. Chromosome 17 deletions and p53 gene mutations in colorectal carcinomas. *Science* 1989;244:217–221.
279. Boman BM, Wildrick DM, Alfaro SR. Chromosome 18 allele loss at the D18S6 locus in human colorectal carcinomas. *Biochem Biophys Res Commun* 1988;155:463–469.
280. Miyaki M, Seki M, Okamoto M, et al. Allele loss and K ras mutation involved in the development of colorectal tumors in patients with familial adenomatous polyposis. In: Utsunomiya J, Lynch HT, eds. *Hereditary colorectal cancer*. Tokyo: Springer-Verlag; 1990:445–452.
281. Okamoto M, Sasaki M, Sugio K, et al. Loss of constitutional heterozygosity in colon carcinoma from patients with FPC. *Nature* 1988;331:273–277.
282. Needleman SW, Yuasa Y, Srivastava S, Aaronson SA. Normal cells of patients with high cancer risk syndromes lack transforming activity in the NIH/3T3 transfection assay. *Science* 1983;222:173–175.
283. Sasaki M, Sugio K, Sasazuki T. K-*ras* activation in colorectal tumors from patients with familial polyposis coli. *Cancer Res* 1990;50:2576–2579.
284. Kinzler KW, Nilbert MC, Su L-K, et al. Identification of FAP locus genes from chromosome 5q21. *Science* 1991;253:661–665.
285. Nishisho I, Nakamura Y, Miyoshi Y, et al. Mutations of chromosome 5q21 genes in FAP and colorectal cancer patients. *Science* 1991;253:665–669.
286. Narita T, Eto T, Ito T. Peutz–Jeghers syndrome with adenomas and adenocarcinomas in colonic polyps. *Am J Surg Pathol* 1987;11:76–81.
287. McAllister AJ, Richards KF. Peutz–Jeghers syndrome: experience with twenty patients in five generations. *Am J Surg* 1977;134:717–720.
288. Lipkin M. Identification of populations with increased susceptibility to cancer of the large intestine. In: Lynch PM, Lynch HT, eds. *Colon cancer genetics*. New York: Van Nostrand Reinhold; 1985:128–156.
289. Rozen P, Baratz P. Familial juvenile colonic polyposis with associated colon cancer. *Cancer* 1982;49:1500–1503.
290. Smilow PC Pryor CA Jr, Swinton NW. Juvenile polyposis coli: a report of three patients in three generations of one family. *Dis Colon Rectum* 1966;9:248–254.
291. Rutz HP, de Tribolet N, Calmes JM, Chapius G. Long-time survival of a patient with glioblastoma and Turcot's syndrome. *J Neurosurg* 1991;74:813–815.
292. Barfknecht TR, Little JB. Abnormal sensitivity of skin fibroblasts from familial polyposis patients to DNA alkylating agents. *Cancer Res* 1982;42:1249–1254.
293. Li FP, Little JB, Bech-Hansen NT, et al. Acute leukemia after radiotherapy in a patient with Turcot's syndrome. *Am J Med* 1983;74:343–348.
294. Little JB, Nove J, Weichselbaum RR. Abnormal sensitivity of diploid skin fibroblasts from a family with Gardner's syndrome to the lethal effects of x-irradiation, ultra-violet light and mitomycin-C. *Mutat Res* 1980;70:241–250.
295. Lynch HT, Lynch PM, Albano WA, Lynch JF. The cancer syndrome: a status report. *Dis Colon Rectum* 1981;24:311–322.
296. Mecklin JP, Jarvinen HJ. Clinical features of colorectal carcinoma in cancer family syndrome. *Dis Colon Rectum* 1986;29:160–164.
297. Vasen HFA, den Hartog Jager FCA, Menko FH, Nagengast FM. Screening for hereditary nonpolyposis colorectal cancer. A study of twenty-two kindreds in the Netherlands. *Am J Med* 1989;86:278–281.
298. Boland CR, Troncale FJ. Familial colonic cancer in the absence of antecedent polyposis. *Ann Intern Med* 1984;100:700–701.

299. Danes BS, Alm T, Bulow S, Svendsen LB. *In vitro* family studies of heritable colon cancer. In: Lynch PM, Lynch HT, eds. *Colon cancer genetics*. New York: Van Nostrand Reinhold; 1985: 157–175.
300. Lynch PM, Wargovich MJ, Lynch MT, et al. A follow-up study of colonic epithelial proliferation as a biomarker in a native-American family with hereditary nonpolyposis colon cancer. *J Natl Cancer Inst* 1991;83:951–954.
301. Lennard-Jones JE, Melville DM, Morson BC, Ritchie JK, Williams CB. Precancer and cancer in extensive ulcerative colitis: findings among 401 patients over 22 years. *Gut* 1990;31:800–806.
302. Ekbom A, Helmick C, Zack M, Adami HO. Ulcerative colitis and colorectal cancer: a population-based study. *N Engl J Med* 1990;323:1228–1233.
303. Bromstrom O. Ulcerative colitis and colon cancer: the role of surveillance. *Ann Med* 1989;21:309–311.
304. Sugita A, Sacher DB, Bodian C, Ribeiro MB, Aufses AH Jr, Greenstein AJ. Colorectal cancer in ulcerative colitis. Influence of anatomical extent and age at onset on colitis-cancer interval. *Gut* 1991;32:167–169.
305. Greenstein AJ, Sachar DB, Smith H, et al. Cancer in universal and left-sided ulcerative colitis: factors determining risk. *Gastroenterology* 1979;77:290–294.
306. Devroede G. Risk of cancer in inflammatory bowel disease. In: Winawer S, Schottenfeld D, Sherlock P, eds. *Colorectal cancer: prevention, epidemiology, and screening*. New York: Raven Press; 1989:325–334.
307. Prior P, Gyde SN, Macartney JC, Thompson H, Waterhouse JAH, Allan RN. Cancer morbidity in ulcerative colitis. *Gut* 1982;23:490–497.
308. Lashner BA, Silverstein MD, Hanauer SB. Hazard rates for dysplasia and cancer in ulcerative colitis. Results from a surveillance program. *Dig Dis Sci* 1989;34:1536–1541.
309. Dobbins WO. Current status of the precancer lesion in ulcerative colitis. *Gastroenterology* 1977;73:1431–1433.
310. Devroede GJ, Taylor WF, Sauer WG, Jackman RJ, Stickler GB. Cancer risk and life expectancy of children with ulcerative colitis. *N Engl J Med* 1971;285:17–21.
311. Morson BC, Pang LSC. Rectal biopsy as an aid to cancer control in ulcerative colitis. *Gut* 1967; 8:423–434.
312. Lennard-Jones JE, Morson BC, Ritchie JK, Williams CB. Cancer surveillance in ulcerative colitis. *Lancet* 1983;2:149–152.
313. Nugent FW, Haggitt RC. Results of a longterm prospective surveillance program for dysplasia in ulcerative colitis. *Gastroenterology* 1984;86:1197(abst).
314. Blackstone MO, Ridell RH, Rogers BHC, Levin B. Dysplasia-associated lesion or mass (DALM) detected by colonoscopy in long-standing ulcerative colitis: an indication for colectomy. *Gastroenterology* 1981;80:366–374.
315. Greenstein AJ, Sachar DB, Smith H, Janowitz HD, Aufses AH. A comparison of cancer risk in Crohn's disease and ulcerative colitis. *Cancer* 1981;48:2742–2745.
316. Gyde SN, Prior P, Macartney JC, Thompson H, Waterhouse JAH, Allan RN. Malignancy in Crohn's disease. *Gut* 1980;21:1024–1029.
317. Korelitz BI. Considerations of surveillance, dysplasia, and carcinoma of the colon in the management of ulcerative colitis and Crohn's disease. *Med Clin North Am* 1990;74:189–199.
318. Shamsuddin AKM, Phillips RM. Preneoplastic and neoplastic changes in colonic mucosa of Crohn's disease. *Arch Pathol Lab Med* 1981;105:283–286.
319. Delpre G, Kadish U, Wolloch Y. Colorectal cancer and colonic Crohn's disease. A matter for analysis and reflection. *Gastroenterol Clin Biol* 1989;13:45–50.
320. Ekbom A, Helmick C, Zack M, Adami H-O. Increased risk of large-bowel cancer in Crohn's disease with colonic involvement. *Lancet* 1990;336:357–359.
321. Slaughter DP, Southwick HW. Mucosal carcinoma as a result of irradiation. *Arch Surg* 1957;74: 420–429.
322. Day NE, Boice JD. Second cancer in relation to radiation treatment for cervical cancer. From the International Radiation Study Group on Cervical Cancer. *IARC Sci Publ* 1983;52:137–162.
323. Hanley JM, McGarity WC. Ureterosigmoidostomy and neoplasms of the colon. *Arch Surg* 1971; 103:69–72.
324. Lasser A, Acosta AE. Colonic neoplasms complicating ureterosigmoidostomy. *Cancer* 1975;35: 1218–1222.
325. Badalament RA, Cirulli C, Zerick W, Lucas JG, Drago JR. Colon carcinomas associated with ureterosigmoidostomy. *J Surg Oncol* 1990;45:207–211.

326. Kalble T, Tricker AR, Friedl P, et al. Ureterosigmoidostomy: long-term results, risk of carcinoma and etiological factors for carcinogenesis. *J Urol* 1990;144:1110–1114.
327. Sohn M, Fuzesi L, Deutz F, Lagrange W, Kirkpatrick JC, Braun JC. Signet ring cell carcinoma in adenomatous polyp at site of ureterosigmoidostomy 16 years after conversion to ileal conduit. *J Urol* 1990;143:805–807.
328. Crissey MM, Steale GD, Gilles RF. Rat model for carcinogenesis in ureterosigmoidostomy. *Science* 1980;207:1079–1080.
329. Tancer ML, Lasser D, Rosenblum N. Rectovaginal fistula or perineal and anal sphincter disruption, or birth, after vaginal delivery. *Surg Gynecol Obstet* 1990;171:43–46.
330. Morrison JG, Gathright JB Jr, Ray JE, Ferrari BT, Hicks TC, Timmcke AE. Results of operation for rectovaginal fistula in Crohn's disease. *Dis Colon Rectum* 1989;32:497–499.
331. Cohen JL, Stricker JW, Schoetz DJ Jr, Coller JA, Veidenheimer MC. Rectovaginal fistula in Crohn's disease. *Dis Colon Rectum* 1989;32:825–828.
332. En-Sheng Z. Cancer of the colon and schistosomiasis. *J R Soc Med* 1981;74:645.
333. Tanner M, Degrenant A, Monitoring and evaluation of schistosomiasis control with a primary health care program. *Trop Med Parasitol* 1986;37:220–223.
334. Cheevers AW. Schistosomiasis and neoplasia. *J Natl Cancer Inst* 1978;61:13–18.
335. Ming-Chai C, Chi-Yuan C, Pei-Yu C, Jen-Chun H. Evolution of colorectal cancer in schistosomiasis. *Cancer* 1980;46:1661–1675.
336. Ming-Chai C, Chi-Yuan C, Fu-Pan W, Yang-Chuan T, Shun-Chuan C. Colorectal cancer and schistosomiasis. *Lancet* 1981;1:971–973.
337. Ming-Chai C, Jen-Chun H, Pei-Yu C, Chi-Yuan C, et al. Pathogenesis of carcinoma of the colon and rectum in schistosomiasis japonica. *Chin Med J* 1965;84:513–525.
338. Sonntag SJ, Schnell T, Cheijfec G, Chintam R, Wanner J. Barrett's esophagus and colonic tumor. *Lancet* 1985;1:946–949.
339. Bremmer CG, Mamilton DG. Barrett's esophagus: controversial aspects. In: De Meester TR, Skinner DB, eds. *Esophageal disorders: pathophysiology and therapy.* New York: Raven Press; 1985: 233–239.
340. Robertson DA, Ayres RC, Smith CL. Screening for colonic cancer in patients with Barrett's oesophagus. *Br Med J* 1989;298(6674):6505.
341. Pero RW, Miller GD, Lipkin M, et al. Reduced capacity for DNA repair synthesis in patients with or genetically predisposed to colorectal cancer. *J Natl Cancer Inst* 1983;70:867–875.
342. Shamsuddin AKM. Morphogenesis of colonic carcinoma: ultrastructural features of azoxymethane-induced early lesions in colon epithelium of Fischer 344 rats. *Arch Pathol Lab Med* 1982; 106:140–144.
343. Shamsuddin AKM. Normal and pathological anatomy of the large intestine. In: Moyer MP, Poste GH, eds. *Colon cancer cells.* New York: Academic Press; 1990:15–40.
344. Neutra MR, O'Malley LF, Apecian RD. Regulation of intestinal goblet cell secretion. II. A survey of potential secretagogues. *Am J Physiol* 1982;242:G380–G387.
345. Specian RD, Neutra MR. Regulation of intestinal goblet cell secretion. I. Role of parasympathetic stimulation. *Am J Physiol* 1982;242:G370–G379.
346. Mantle M, Allen A. Gastrointestinal mucus. In: Davison JS, ed. *Gastrointestinal secretion.* London: Wright; 1989:202–229.
347. McKenzie KM, Purnell DM, Shamsuddin AKM. Expression of carcinoembryonic antigen, T-antigen, and oncogene products as markers of neoplastic and preneoplastic colonic mucosa. *Hum Pathol* 1987;18:1282–1286.
348. Bettetini D, Garrouste F, Remacle-Bonnet M, Culoascou J-M, Marvaldi J, Pommier G. Enhancement of production of superoxide anion by polymorphonuclear leukocytes exposed to products of the HT-29 human colonic adenocarcinoma cell line. *J Natl Cancer Inst* 1986;77:1225–1234.
349. Shamsuddin AKM, Sugano H, Trump BF. Morphogenesis of large intestinal carcinoma: its significance in early detection. *Gann Monogr Cancer Res* 1986;31:59–66.
350. Shamsuddin AKM. Perspectives on large intestinal cancer: animal models and human disease [Guest editorial]. *Hum Pathol* 1986;17:451–453.
351. Shamsuddin AKM, Trump BF. Colon epithelium. II. *In vivo* studies of colon carcinogenesis. Light microscopic, histochemical, and ultrastructural studies of histogenesis of azoxymethane-induced colon carcinoma in Fischer 344 rats. *J Natl Cancer Inst* 1981;66:389–401.
352. Shamsuddin AKM, Weiss L, Phelps PC, Trump BF. Colon epithelium. IV. Human colon carcinogenesis. Changes in human colon mucosa adjacent to and remote from carcinomas of the colon. *J Natl Cancer Inst* 1981;66:413–419.

353. Trump BF, Phelps PC, Shamsuddin AKM. Cellular pathobiology of human large intestine. *Prog Cancer Res Ther* 1984;29:23–49.
354. Ngoi SS, Staiano-Coico L, Godwin TA, Wong RJ, DeCosse JJ. Abnormal DNA ploidy and proliferative patterns in superficial epithelium adjacent to colorectal cancer. *Cancer* 1990;66:953–959.
355. Shamsuddin AM, Elsayed AM. A test for detection of colorectal cancer. *Hum Pathol* 1988;19:7–10.
356. Sakamoto K, Nakano G, Nagamachi Y. A pilot study on the usefulness of a new test for mass screening of colorectal cancer in Japan. *Gastroenterol Jpn* 1990;25:432–436.
357. Sakamoto K, Muratani M, Ogawa T, Nagamachi Y. Colon cancer screening by a new test. A prospective study of asymptomatic population. *Proc Am Assoc Cancer Res* 1991;32:168.
358. Lorenz E, Stewart HL. Intestinal carcinoma and other lesions in mice following oral administration of 1,2,4,6-dibenzanthracene and 20-methylcholanthrene. *J Natl Cancer Inst* 1941;1:17–40.
359. Evans JT, Shows TB, Sproul EE. Genetics of colon carcinogenesis in mice treated with 7,12-dimethylbenz[a]anthracene. *Cancer Res* 1977;37:134–136.
360. Walpole AL, Williams M, Roberts DC. The carcinogenic action of 4-aminodiphenyl and 3,2-dimethyl-4-aminodiphenyl. *Br J Ind Med* 1952;9:255–263.
361. Cleveland JC, Litvak SF, Cole JW. Identification of the route of action of the carcinogen 3,2'-dimethyl-4-aminobiphenyl in the induction of intestinal neoplasia. *Cancer Res* 1967;27:708–714.
362. Laqueur GL. Carcinogenic effect of cycad meal and cycasin, methylazoxymethanol glycoside, in rats and effects of cycasin in germ free rats. *Fed Proc* 1964;23:1386–1388.
363. Druckrey H, Preussmann R, Matzkies F. Selektive Erzeugung von Darmkrebs bei Ratten durch 1,2-Dimethylhydrazine. *Naturwissenschaften* 1967;54:285–286.
364. Druckrey H, Lange A. Carcinogenicity of azoxymethane dependent on age in SD rats. *Fed Am Soc Exp Biol* 1972;31:1482–1484.
365. Narisawa T, Sato M, Tani M, Kudo T, Takahashi T, Goto A. Inhibition of development of methylnitrosourea-induced rat colon tumors by indomethacin treatment. *Cancer Res* 1981;41:1954–1957.
366. Narisawa T, Magadia NE, Weisburger JH, Wynder EL. Promoting effect of bile acids on colon carcinogenesis after intrarectal instillation of N-methyl-N'-nitro-N-nitrosoguanidine in rats. *J Natl Cancer Inst* 1974;53:1093–1097.
367. Hinzman MJ, Novotny C, Ullah A, Shamsuddin AM. Fecal mutagen fecapentaene-12 damages mammalian colon epithelial DNA. *Carcinogenesis* 1987;8:1457–1479.
368. Drinkwater NR, Bennett LM. Genetic control of carcinogenesis in experimental animals. In: Ito N, Sugano H, eds. *Progress in experimental tumor research*. Vol 33. *Modification of tumor development in rodents*. Basel: S Karger; 1991:1–20.
369. Pozharisski K. The significance of nonspecific injury for colon carcinogenesis in rats. *Cancer Res* 1975;35:3824–3830.
370. Okayasu I, Hatakeyama S, Yamada M, Ohkusa T, Inagaki Y, Nakaya R. A novel method in the induction of reliable experimental acute and chronic ulcerative colitis in mice. *Gastroenterology* 1990;98:694–702.
371. Nigro ND, Bhadrachari N, Chomchai C. A rat model for studying colon cancer. Effect of cholestyramine on induced tumors. *Dis Colon Rectum* 1973;16:438–443.
372. Reddy B, Watanabe K, Weisburger J. Effect of high-fat diet on colon carcinogenesis in F344 rats treated with 7,12-dimethylbenz[a]anthracene, methylazoxymethanol acetate, or methylnitrosourea. *Cancer Res* 1977;37:4156–4159.
373. Reddy B, Weisburger J, Wynder E. Effect of dietary fat level and dimethylhydrazine on fecal acid and neutral sterol excretion and colon carcinogenesis in rats. *J Natl Cancer Inst* 1974;52:507–511.
374. Bull AW, Soullier BK, Wilson PS, Hayden MT, Nigro N. Promotion of azoxymethane-induced intestinal cancer by high-fat diet in rats. *Cancer Res* 1979;39:4956–4959.
375. Reddy B, Narisawa T, Weisburger J. Colon carcinogenesis in germ-free rats with intrarectal 1,2-dimethylhydrazine and subcutaneous azoxymethane. *Cancer Res* 1975;36:2874–2876.
376. Chomchai C, Bhadrachari N, Nigro N. The effect of bile on the induction of experimental intestinal tumors in rats. *Dis Colon Rectum* 1974;17:310–312.
377. Rogers AE, Newberne PM, Dietary effect on chemical carcinogenesis in animal models for colon and liver tumors. *Cancer Res* 1975;35:3427–3431.
378. Newberne PM, Schrager T. Promotion of gastrointestinal tract tumors in animals: dietary factors. *Environ Health Perspect* 1983;50:71–83.
379. Ward JM, Yamamoto RS, Weisburger JH. Cellulose dietary bulk and azoxymethane-induced intestinal cancer. *J Natl Cancer Inst* 1973;51:713–715.

380. Cameron IL, Ord VA, Hunter KE, Heitman DW. Colon carcinogenesis: modulation of progression. In: Moyer MP, Poste GH, eds. *Colon cancer cells*. New York: Academic Press; 1990:63–84.
381. Heitman DW, Ord VA, Hunter KE, Cameron IL. Effect of dietary cellulose on cell proliferation and progression of 1,2-dimethylhydrazine-induced colon carcinogenesis in rats. *Cancer Res* 1989; 49:5581–5585.
382. Iishi H, Baba M, Tatsuta M, Okuda S, Taniguchi H. Inhibition by the dopamine antagonist haloperidol of experimental carcinogenesis induced by azoxymethane in rat colon. *Cancer Res* 1991; 51:6150–6152.
383. Fiala ES, Joseph C, Sohn OS, el-Bayoumy K, Reddy BS. Mechanism of benzylselenocyanate inhibition of azoxymethane-induced colon carcinogenesis in F344 rats. *Cancer Res* 1991;51:2826–2830.
384. Rao CV, Nayini J, Reddy BS. Effect of oltipraz [5-(2-pyrazinyl)-4-methyl-1,2-dithiol-3-thione] on azoxymethane-induced biochemical changes related to early colon carcinogenesis in male F344 rats. *Proc Soc Exp Biol Med* 1991;197:77–84.
385. Tatsuta M, Iishi H, Baba M, Taniguchi H. Enhancement by neurotensin of experimental carcinogenesis induced in rat colon by azoxymethane. *Br J Cancer* 1990;62:368–371.
386. Kumar SP, Roy SJ, Tokumo K, Reddy BS. Effect of different levels of calorie restriction on azoxymethane-induced colon carcinogenesis in male F344 rats. *Cancer Res* 1990;50:5761–5766.
387. Tatsuta M, Iishi H, Baba M, Taniguchi H. Enhancement of azoxymethane-induced colon carcinogenesis in spontaneously hypertensive rats. *Int J Cancer* 1990;45:957–960.
388. Tatsuta M, Iishi H, Baba M, Taniguchi H. Tissue norepinephrine depletion as a mechanism for cysteamine inhibition of colon carcinogenesis induced by azoxymethane in Wistar rats. *Int J Cancer* 1989;44:1008–1011.
389. Dwivedi C, Oredipe OA, Barth RF, Downie AA, Webb TE. Effects of the experimental chemopreventative agent, glucarate, on intestinal carcinogenesis in rats. *Carcinogenesis* 1989;10:1539–1541.
390. Tanaka T, Shinoda T, Yoshimi N, Niwa K, Iwata H, Mori H. Inhibitory effect of magnesium hydroxide on methlazoxymethanol acetate-induced large bowel carcinogensis in male F344 rats. *Carcinogenesis* 1989;10:613–616.
391. Andrianopoulos GD, Nelson RL, Misumi A, Bombeck CT, Nyhus LM. Effect of activity-stress on experimental rat colon carcinogenesis: early histopathologic changes and colon tumor induction. *Cancer Detect Prev* 1988;13:31–39.
392. Reddy BS, Sugie S, Lowenfels A. Effect of voluntary-exercise on azoxymethane-induced colon carcinogenesis in male F344 rats. *Cancer Res* 1988;48(24 Pt 1):7079–7081.
393. Tutton PJM, Barkla DH. The influence of adrenoceptor activity on cell proliferation in colonic crypt epithelium and in colonic adenocarcinomata. *Virchows Arch B* 1977;24:139–146.
394. Deschner EE, Raicht RF. The influence of bile on kinetic behavior of colonic epithelial cells of the rat. *Digestion* 1979;19:322–327.
395. Deschner EE. Kinetics of normal, preneoplastic, and neoplastic colonic epithelium. In: Moyer MP, Poste GH, eds. *Colon cancer cells*. New York: Academic Press; 1990:41–61.
396. Deschner EE, Cohen BI, Raicht RF. Acute and chronic effect of dietary choleic acid on colonic epithelial cell proliferation. *Digestion* 1981;21:290–296.
397. Burkitt DP. Epidemiology of cancer of the colon and rectum. *Cancer* 1971;28:3–13.
398. Barnes DS, Clapp NK, Scott DA, et al. Effect of wheat, rice, corn and soybean bran on 1,2-dimethylhydrazine-induced large bowel tumorigenesis in F344 rats. *Nutr Cancer* 1983;5:1–9.
399. Sporn M. Retinoids and cancer prevention. In: Slaga TJ, ed. *Carcinogenesis: A Comprehensive Survey*. Vol 5. *Modifiers of Chemical Carcinogenesis*. New York, Raven Press; 1980:99–109.
400. Craven PA, Saito R, DeRubertis FR. Role of local prostaglandin synthesis in the modulation of proliferative activity of rat colonic epithelium. *J Clin Invest* 1983;72:1365–1375.
401. Yamaguchi A, Ishida T, Nishimura G, Katoh M, Miyazaki I. Investigation of colonic prostaglandins in carcinogenesis in the rat colon. *Dis Colon Rectum* 1991;34:572–576.
402. Drasar BS, Irving D. Environmental factors and cancer of the colon and breast. *Br J Cancer* 1973; 27:167–172.
403. Armstrong B, Doll R. Environmental factors and cancer incidence and mortality in different countries with special reference to dietary practices. *Int J Cancer* 1975;15:617–631.
404. Howeli MA. Diet as an etiological factor in the development of cancers of the colon and rectum. *J Chronic Dis* 1975;28:67–80.

405. Wynder FI, Ilirayama T. Comparative epidemiology of cancers of the United States and Japan. *Prev Med* 1977;6:567–594.
406. Liu K, Stamler J, Moss D, Garside D, Persky V, Soltero I. Dietary cholesterol fat and fibre and colon cancer mortality. *Lancet* 1979;2:782–785.
407. International Agency for Research on Cancer Intestinal Microecology Group. Dietary fibre, transit-time faecal bacteria, steroids and colon cancer in two Scandinavian populations. *Lancet* 1977; 2:207–211.
408. Jensen OM, MacLennan R, Wahrendore J (on behalf of the IARC large bowel cancer group). Diet, bowel function, fecal characteristics, and large bowel cancer in Denmark and Finland. *Nutr Cancer* 1982;4:5–19.

5
Renal Carcinogenesis

Noboru Konishi and Yoshio Hiasa

Second Department of Pathology, Nara Medical University, Kashihara, Nara, 634 Japan

Despite the relatively low incidence of renal cell tumors in humans, they are of great importance clinically and deserve considerable emphasis. For the clinician, there is much attention to renal cancer for determining their etiology, risk factors, and early diagnosis (1). A number of chemical and biological agents have induced renal tumors in rodents, including various chemical carcinogens, hormones, viruses, radiation, and dietary deficiencies (2).

However, few of these agents are potential carcinogens in humans. Epidemiologic studies show a significantly greater frequency of renal adenocarcinoma in cigar smokers and in cadmium workers who smoke (3,4). Recently, increased numbers of deaths from primary renal tumors have been noted among workers in the petroleum industry. Moreover, two cases of renal cancer in lead workers have been noted (5–7). These facts seem to link experimental renal carcinogenesis in rodents, although conclusive evidence has not been established. Lead salts have been found to produce renal tumors in experimental studies (8,9). Unleaded gasoline has also been shown to induce nephropathy, associated with an increased incidence of renal adenomas and adenocarcinomas in rats (10,11). Therefore, experimental carcinogenesis models provide a mechanism for elucidating their pathogenesis and etiology. Among environmental factors associated with cancer in humans, nephrotoxic agents are one of the most important factors for renal carcinogenesis. Several nephrotoxic chemicals, such as unleaded gasoline, have demonstrated carcinogenic potential in chronic assays (12,13). Some are metabolized to reactive intermediates that have been implicated in cytotoxicity and in tumor formation. In response to these toxic effects, increased cell proliferation occurs in such degenerative and regenerative tissues.

In this chapter, we describe rat renal tumorigenesis primarily, because of high susceptibility of the rat kidney to tumor induction by chemical carcinogens. Also described are renal tumor promoters and the relation between nephrotoxicity and nephrocarcinogenicity.

MORPHOLOGY OF RENAL TUMORS

Epithelial Tumors

Based on their cellular composition, epithelial tumors can be divided into two categories: cortical tubular cell tumors and pelvic epithelial tumors. It is generally accepted that cortical epithelial tumors originate in tubular epithelium. Rat tumors are designated as adenomas, adenocarcinomas, or carcinomas. Adenomas and adenocarcinomas are distinguished according to their size, invasive growth to the adjacent tissue, cellular pleomorphism, prominent mitotic figures, and other histologic characters, such as foci of necrosis or hemorrhage (Fig. 1).

However, the distinction is not easy (14) because renal adenocarcinomas often lack mitotic figures and atypism (Fig. 2). Tumor size is not a good indicator for malignancy, although necrosis and hemorrhage are seen even in small tumors below

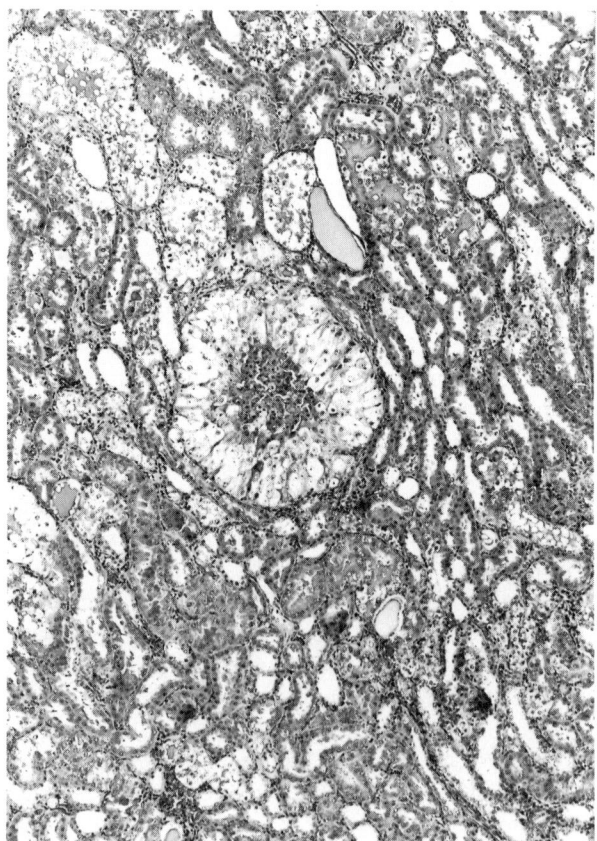

FIG. 1. Rat kidney. Renal cell tumor with necrosis in the central area. Some small adenomas are also seen. H&E, ×100.

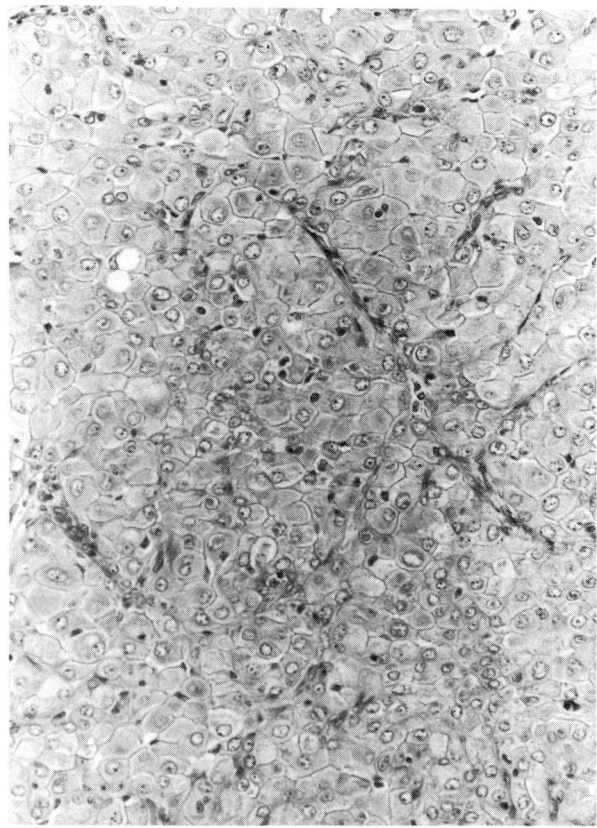

FIG. 2. Rat kidney. Renal cell carcinoma, showing a few mitotic figures and scant fibrous tissue stroma. H&E, ×200.

a diameter of 0.4 cm. Suggestive features of malignancy, occasionally seen in renal neoplasms, do not always reflect their biological behavior. Several factors must be taken into consideration. It is inappropriate to propose a rigid distinction between adenomas and adenocarcinomas or carcinomas. It is important to evaluate the numbers or sizes of these lesions to distinguish adenomas from carcinomas in certain experimental studies. This evaluation seems to correlate with the tumorigenic potential of the test chemicals. Distant metastases of renal cell carcinomas are rare in rats, usually observed in lungs or lymph nodes (15).

In macroscopic findings, cortical epithelial tumors usually appear as round, well-circumscribed masses grayish white or grayish yellow in color, projecting from the cortex. The red spots within tumors indicate hemorrhagic or necrotic change. Occasionally, cystic tumors are observed, and in some parts, the walls have numerous diverticulae. Tumors are identifiable at the kidney surface when they reach 2 to 5 mm in diameter. Small neoplasms are confined primarily to the cortical area, but larger tumors extend beyond the cortex.

Microscopically, renal tubular cell tumors are composed of irregularly arranged cells forming solid, tubular, lobular, cystic, papillary, or alveolar patterns (Figs. 3 and 4). From the morphological standpoint, the structures vary tumor including cells forming tubular arrangements, ill-defined tubules, and solid patterns without lumens. Cytologically, the tumor cells are divided into eosinophilic (acidophilic), basophilic, and clear cytoplasmic phenotype in their staining patterns (Fig. 5). Acidophilic cells, sometimes intermingled with clear cells, often contain abundant mitochondria. Although the basophilic cells have an abundance of free and membrane-bound ribosomes (16,17), the clear, vacuolated appearance of the tumor cells is due to their high glycogen content. Oncocytic phenotypes characterized by excess numbers of mitochondria are observed with swollen finely granular acidophilic cy-

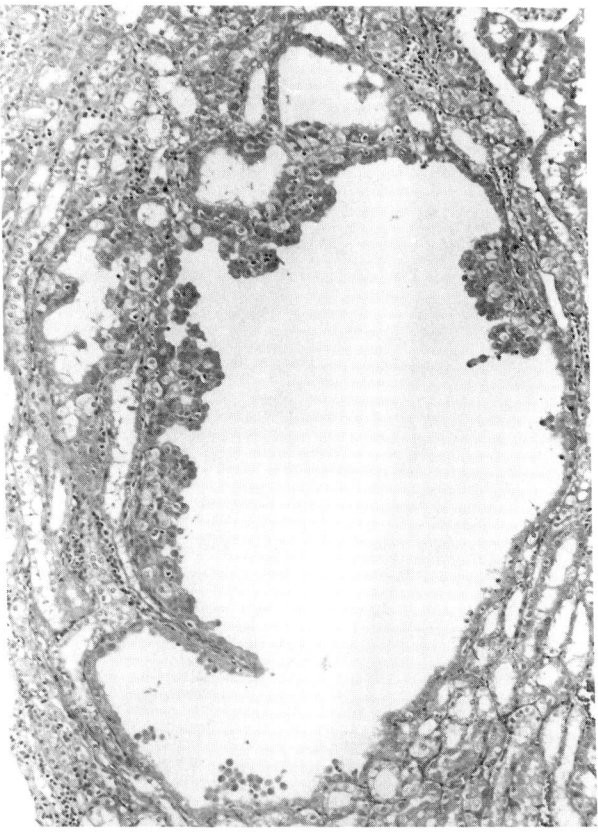

FIG. 3. Rat kidney. Cortical adenoma showing that cystic–papillary growth has compressed adjacent area. H&E, ×100.

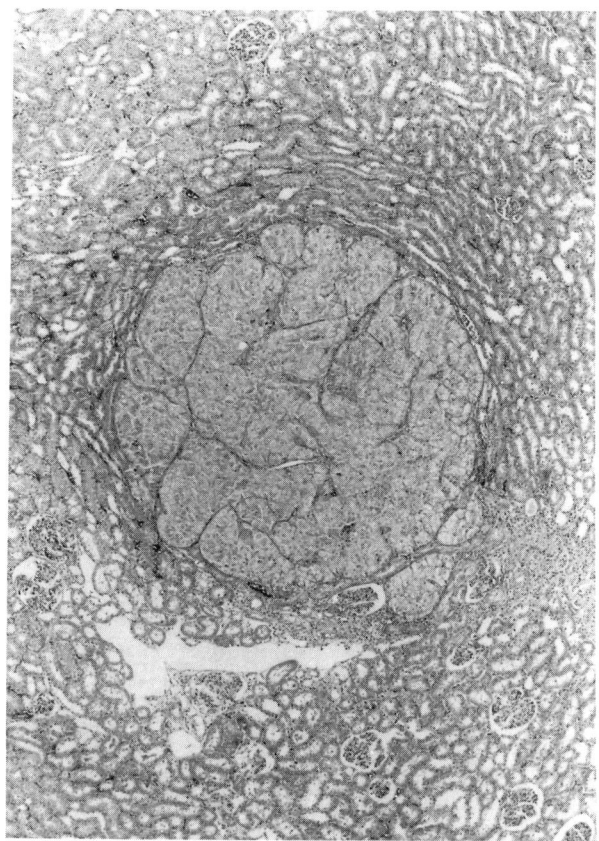

FIG. 4. Rat kidney. A solid renal adenoma composed with a tubular or alveolar pattern. H&E, ×40.

toplasm. In cortical epithelial tumors examined by electron microscopy, brush border and basement membrane formations were observed, suggesting proximal tubular cell origin (18,19).

Transitional and squamous cell carcinoma of renal pelvis are relatively rare. The former arises from pelvic transitional epithelium and resembles the transitional cell tumors of the bladder (Fig. 6). Most of these tumors demonstrate exophytic, papillary growth and are referred to as transitional cell papillomas when exhibiting a complex branching of papillary growth. Squamous cell carcinomas of renal pelvic origin are often associated with infections and mineralization, which cause chronic irritation of transitional epithelium. Foci of squamous metaplasia can be seen in transitional cell tumors. Spontaneous pelvic tumors in the rat are extremely rare (20). Early preneoplastic lesions of renal epithelial tumors are referred to later in the section on preneoplastic lesions.

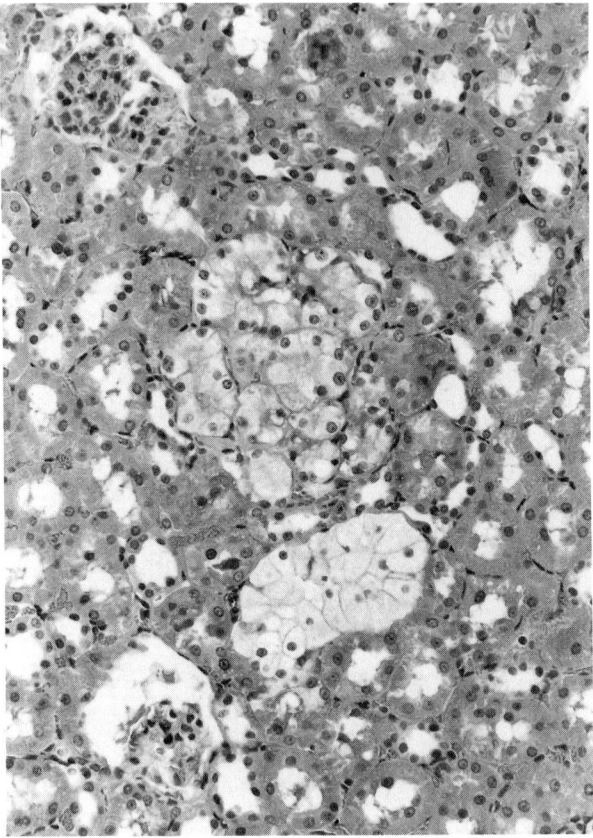

FIG. 5. Rat kidney. Simple hyperplasia, composed of cells with clear cytoplasm. H&E, ×200.

Nonepithelial Tumors

Renal mesenchymal tumors consist of spindle cells which may be of renal interstitial connective tissue cell origin. The spindle cells may differentiate and demonstrate mesenchymal elements such as fibrous tissue (Fig. 7), hemangiomatous tissue, smooth muscle, striated muscle, cartilage, and osteoid (Fig. 8). The predominant histologic type of the tumor may be fibrosarcomatous, hemangiosarcomatous, leiomyosarcomatous, rhabdomyosarcomatous, chondrosarcomatous, and osteosarcomatous. There has been confusion in the diagnosis of renal mesenchymal tumors, some of which are misdiagnosed as nephroblastomas (21–23). Nephroblastoma is an embryonal tumor originating in metanephrogenic blastema, representing bipotential neoplastic differentiation into both epithelium and secondary mesenchyme.

As is rare, collision tumors of renal adenocarcinoma with renal mesenchymal tumors are observed (23) and should be distinguished from the nephroblastoma. In

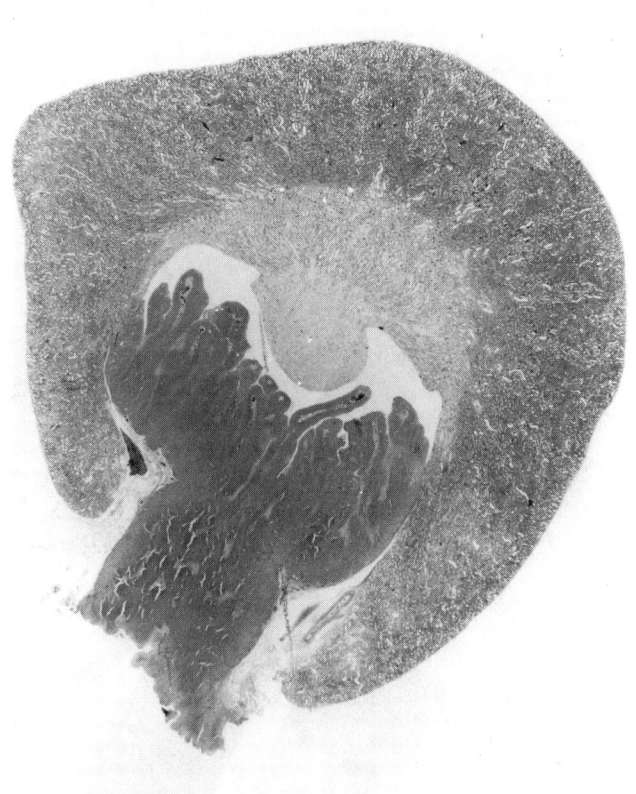

FIG. 6. Rat kidney. Transitional cell carcinoma; the papillary mass is composed of transitional cells arising from renal pelvic epithelium. H&E, ×20.

most mesenchymal tumors, spindle cells vary considerably in cellularity, including hypercellular and densely packed areas and less cellular, loosely textured myxoid areas. Small amounts of interstitial collagen or fibrillar material are found in less cellular areas.

Ultrastructurally, the basic spindle cell resembles an active fibroblast, characterized by abundant, anastomosing channels of rough endoplasmic reticulum and bundles of actin-like microfilaments (18). Fibrosarcomatous areas have in common a rather uniform and often fasciculated growth pattern, occasionally showing characteristic features of a herringbone pattern. Smooth muscle or striated muscle fibers and rich blood vessels are intermingled in such parenchymal areas.

By contrast, lipomatous tumors and hemangiomatous tumors are distinguished from renal mesenchymal tumors in rats because of the presence of neoplastic differentiation to the lipocytes, lipoblasts, and vascular spaces (hemangioma, heman-

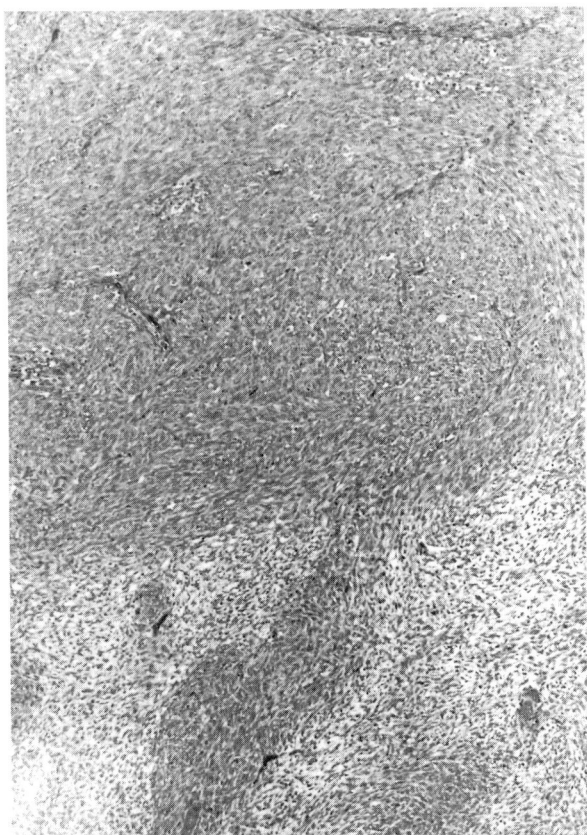

FIG. 7. Rat kidney. Renal mesenchymal tumor, exhibiting a fibrosarcomatous area showing a fascicular pattern of spindle cells. H&E, ×100.

giosarcoma, and hemangioendothelioma). Lipomatous tumors have been referred to as renal or lipomatous hamartoma (24,25) and mixed tumor of the kidney (26).

Another distinction between lipomatous tumors and mesenchymal tumors is a positive reaction for oil red O or sudan black stains, whereas mesenchymal tumors obviously do not differentiate into lipocytes and are negative for fat (27). However, it is doubtful whether lipomatous and hemangiomatous tumors constitute separate and distinct entities from renal mesenchymal tumors. Broadly, these tumors may be under the category of mesenchymal tumors if spindle cells are the stem cell of origin. They are often induced, however, by different chemical carcinogens.

Embryonal Tumors

Nephroblastoma, thought to be one of the embryonal tumors, is referred to as Wilms' tumor in humans and are found in rats. The tumors are invariably unilateral

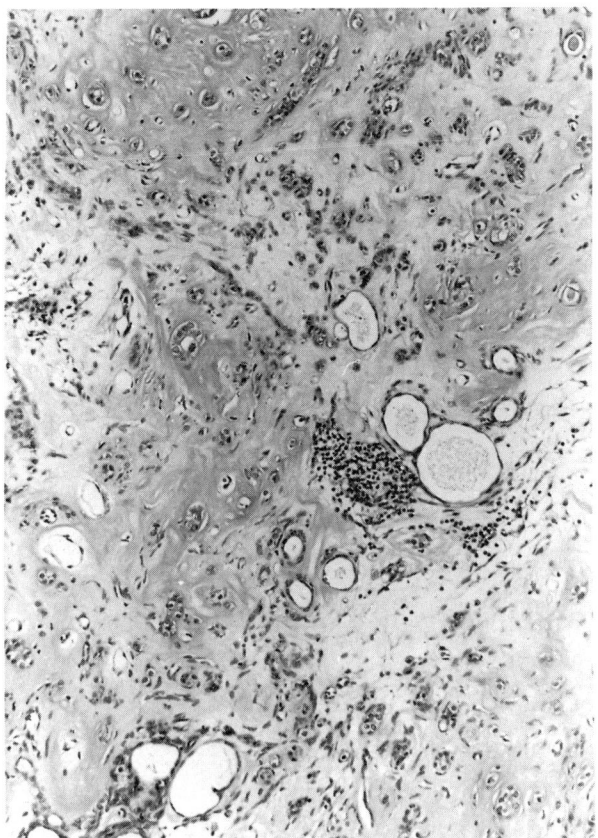

FIG. 8. Rat kidney. Renal mesenchymal tumor, exhibiting cartilagenous and myxoid lesions with progressive sequestration of tubules. H&E, ×100.

and may be found at one pole of the kidney. A variety of cell types corresponding to blastemal, epithelial, or stromal categories are usually present (Fig. 9).

Most of the differentiating elements in tumors appear to replicate various elements in renal embryogenesis. Unlike human nephroblastomas, differentiation into mesenchymal elements such as a fibrosarcomatous component, muscular tissue, and cartilagenous and osteoid tissue does not appear in the rat. The blastemal cells having oval-to-round nuclei with basophilic cytoplasm are densely packed into clusters. These cells exhibit epithelial differentiation such as tubular, papillary, and cystic structures, which correspond to the embryonic development of the kidney (Fig. 10). Cell nests are seen scattered throughout a relatively scanty connective tissue stroma. Organoid structures differentiating into primitive tubules or glomerular structures are often observed.

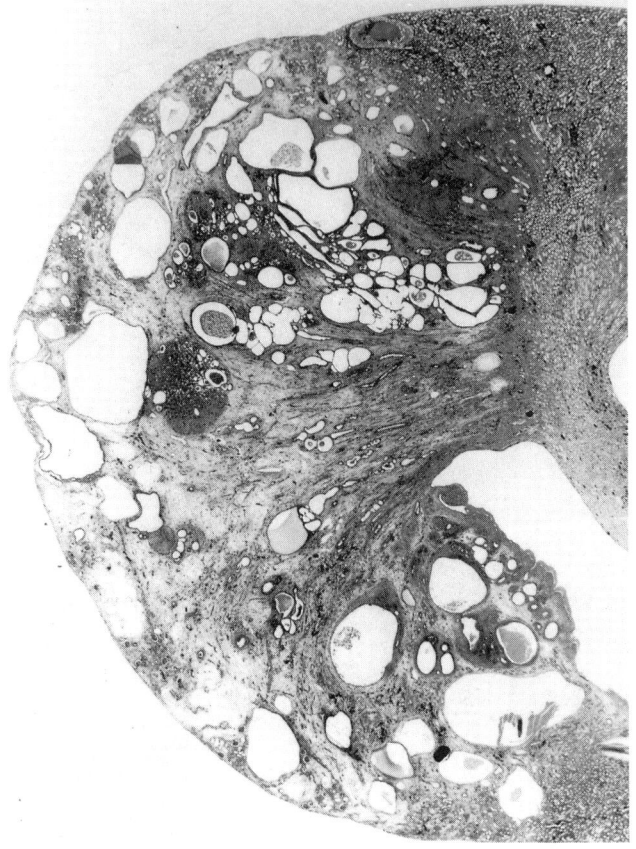

FIG. 9. Rat kidney. Large nephroblastoma, involving and destroying the kidney, with poorly defined tumor margins. H&E, ×40.

TUMOR INDUCTION

Chemical Carcinogens

Chemical induction of renal tumors in animals provides models for investigating the pathogenesis and mechanisms of renal tumorigenesis. Human renal cell tumors were also suggested to be associated with chemical exposures (28,29). There are many reports (Table 1) on experimentally induced renal tumors in animals, with probably more than 100 renal carcinogens (2,30–32). Carcinogenesis develops in renal and other epithelia through a multistage process (33–36). In animal models, tumor initiation and promotion are successive events in two-stage carcinogenesis in at least some epithelia (37,38). Some of renal carcinogens and tumor promoters are listed in Table 1 (39–90).

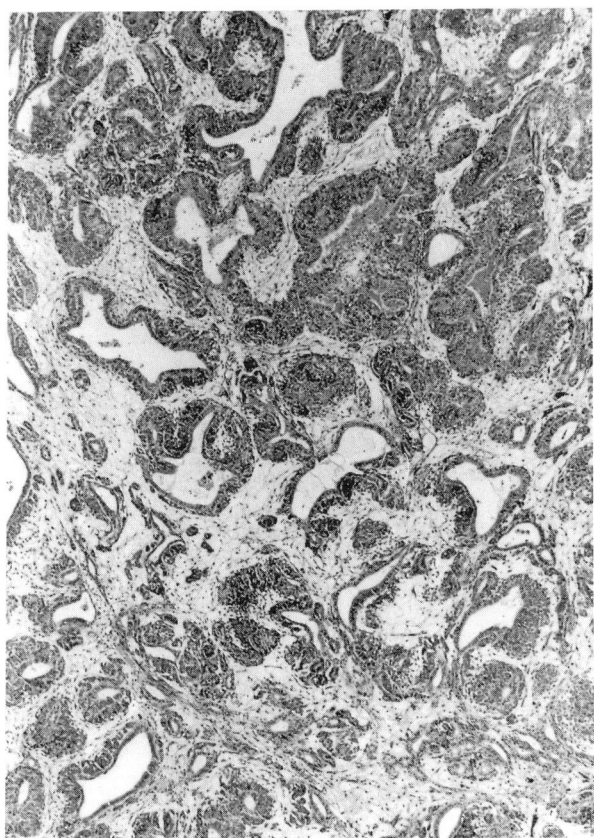

FIG. 10. Rat kidney. Nephroblastoma, exhibiting a blastomatous pattern and differentiation into tubule profiles of varying maturation. H&E, ×100.

Renal epithelial tumors are the most frequent kidney tumors induced by chemical carcinogens in rats. Representative agents following N-nitroso compounds have made possible the relatively specific induction of cortical epithelial tumors. These compounds include N-nitrosodimethylamine (DMN) (60,91–93), N-nitrosomorpholine (NNM) (61,94–96), and N-ethyl-N-hydroxyethylnitrosamine (EHEN) (55, 97). Based on electron microscopic studies, the majority of these renal epithelial tumors arise from the proximal convoluted tubular epithelium. Treatment with NNM induced oncocytic tubules in 66% and oncocytic microadenomas in 36% of Sprague–Dawley rats (98). The development of renal tumors could be followed from hyperplasia of individual tubules to areas of hyperplasia, nodules of hyperplasia, carcinoma in situ, small carcinoma, and later to large well-developed carcinomas.

N-(4'-Fluro-4-biphenylyl) acetamide (FBPA) provides a useful model for the sequential study of renal carcinogenesis (19). The carcinogenic effects of fungal me-

TABLE 1. Some renal carcinogens and tumor promoters in rats

	Ref.		Ref.
Renal epithelial tumors		Renal mesenchymal tumors	
Aflatoxin	39	Cycasin	70
1-Amino-2-methylanthraquinone	40	1,2-Dimethylhydrazine	71
Azoxymethane	41	N-Bis(2-hydroxypropyl)nitrosamine (DHPN)	72
Bromodichloromethane	42		
Chlorinated paraffins: C12, 60% chloride	43	N-Nitrosodimethylamine (DMN)	60
		N-Nitrosoethylurea (ENU)	73
Chloroform	44	N-Nitrosomethylurea (MNU)	74
Chlorothalonil	45		
Cinnamyl anthranilate	46		
Daunomycin	47	Renal pelvic tumors	
Dichloroacetylene (DCA)	48	o-Anisidine hydrochloride	75
1,4-Dichlorobenzene	49	Bis-(2-oxopropyl)nitrosamine (BOPN)	76
1,1-Dimethylhydrazine	50		
Hexachlorobutadiene	51	4,6-Dimethyl-2-(5-nitro-2-furyl)pyrimidine (nitrofuran)	77
4-Hydroxyaminoquinoline (4NQO)	52		
Isophorone	53	N-[4-(5-Nitro-2-furyl)-2-thiazolyl]formamide (FANFT)	78
Lead acetate	54		
N-Ethyl-N-hydroxyethylnitrosamine (EHEN)	55	Phenacetine	79
		Phenazone	79
N-(4'-Fluoro-4-biphenylyl)acetamide (FBPA)	56	o-Phenylphenate	80
		Sodium barbital	81
Nickel subsulfate	57		
1-Nitroso-1-hydroxyethyl-3-chloro-ethylurea	58		
		Tumor promoters	
N-Nitrosodiethylamine (DEN)	59	Acetaminophen	82
N-Nitrosodimethylamine (DMN)	60	p-Aminophenol	82
N-Nitrosomorpholine (NNM)	61	β-Cyclodextrin	83
N-(N-Methyl-N-nitrosocarbamoyl)-1-ornithine	62	DL-Serine	84
		D-Limonene	85
Ochratoxin A	63	Folic acid	86
Phenacetin	64	Lead acetate (LA)	9
Potassium bromate (KBrO$_3$)	65	Nicotinamide	87
Tetrachloroethylene	66	Potassium bromate (KBrO$_3$)	88
Tris(2,3-dibromopropyl)phosphate (TBP)	67	Sodium barbital	89
Trisodium nitrilotriacetate (NTA)	68	Trisodium nitrilotriacetate (NTA)	90
Streptozotocin	69	Unleaded gasoline	13

tabolites, aflatoxins B_1 and G_1, have been reported in rats (39). Some iatrogenic compounds including daunomycin (47), adriamycin (99), niridazole (100), and streptozotocin (69,89,101) also induce renal neoplasias. Steptozotocin [2-deoxy-2-(3-methyl-3-nitrosoureido)-D-glucopyranose] is an antibiotic isolated from *streptomyces achromogenes*, related to DMN and has been found to be diabetogenic in rats and dogs. Some hydrocarbons, including unleaded gasoline, have been shown to induce α_{2u}-globulin nephropathy and to be associated with renal carcinogenic effect in rats (13). These nongenotoxic agents have also provided good models to link nephrotoxicity and nephrocarcinogenecity. Hiasa and Ito reviewed the renal carcinogens mentioned above by animal strain, dosage used, experimental duration, and the incidences of renal tumors (2).

The chemical carcinogens that induce renal tumors are divided into two groups. One group consists of relatively strong carcinogens, such as EHEN, NNM, FBPA, DEN, and DMN. These carcinogens induce renal epithelial tumors when given at low dosages for a single injection, or for up to 10 weeks in the diet or water, and the tumors appear after relatively short latent periods.

The other group consists of "weak" carcinogens, which induce renal tumors only when given at high dosages and for longer times (usually, more than 1 year). These carcinogens, which include lead acetate (LA), trisodium nitrilotriacetate (NTA), and potassium bromate ($KBrO_3$) have renal tumor-promoting effects. There is some evidence that most target organ–specific tumor promoters are at least weak carcinogens in that a 2-year exposure to these agents alone often elicits a low incidence of tumors in the target organ (102). For renal promoters, this activity has usually been demonstrated by an increase in tumor incidence and not an increase in the numbers or sizes of putative preneoplastic lesions (13).

From the viewpoint of gap junctional intercellular communication, tumor promoters were found to inhibit cell–cell communication (103,104). At the same time it has been reported that transformed cells *in vitro* showed a selective lack of intercellular communication between transformed cells and surrounding normal cells, whereas transformed cells communicated among themselves (105). Therefore, it is hypothesized that tumor promoters help initiated cells to escape from the growth-regulatory influence of adjacent noninitiated cells by blocking communication between initiated cells and surrounding cells (102). Thus, initiated cells can be allowed to expand clonally to a critical mass necessary for phenotypic expansion of malignancy (106).

Chemically induced renal tumors in animals develop rarely within 40 weeks, usually by 50 weeks, or sometimes longer periods are required (107,108). Studies with DMN, renal cell tumors could first be observed at 26 experimental weeks (109). In two-stage carcinogenesis model of the kidney, however, 32 experimental weeks are usually sufficient time for the development of tumors and to identify tumor promoters.

For instance, the incidences of renal cell tumors at week 32 were 100% in rats treated with β-cyclodextrin (450 mg/kg s.c. for 1 week), 1,000 ppm LA, and 10,000 ppm NTA in the diet as a promoter when 1,000 ppm EHEN was used as an initiator for 2 weeks (21,83,90). Tumor incidences of 95% and 47% were observed in rats administered with DL-serine (1,000 mg/kg three times s.c.) and 1,000 ppm $KBrO_3$ in drinking water, respectively, in the same system (2,84).

Tumor promoters used in renal carcinogenesis studies consist of two operational types: (a) short-term treatment with β-cyclodextrin or DL-serine with a long latent period, and (b) those that are effective only when given for a long period at low dosage. LA induces degeneration of the proximal convoluted tubules at a high dose for short-term treatment, but promotes renal cell tumors at a low dose during long-term treatment.

It should be considered that tumor promoters given to animals at mild or moderately toxic doses only induce degenerative changes, hyperplastic lesions, and promote tumors among such initiated damaged tubules. Tumor promoters may target chemically or spontaneously initiated cells, which have different growth control mechanisms from noninitiated renal tubular cells. In other words, promoting effects may result from clonal expansion of initiated cells.

Distant metastases from primary renal tumors induced by chemicals involve lungs primarily, and sometimes liver. Metastases, however, are rare. For the chemical induction of renal mesenchymal tumors, DMN has been studied extensively. The dose response for tumor induction by a single dose of DMN in rats has been found associated with increases of DNA alkylation in the kidney. Low-protein diets altered the metabolic rate of DMN. Epithelial and mesenchymal tumors were produced in the approximate ratio 2:1 (110,111). N-Bis(2-hydroxypropyl)nitrosamine (DHPN) has tumorigenic effects on the lungs and thyroids, in addition to kidneys inducing various histologic types, such as renal epithelial cell tumors, transitional cell tumors, mesenchymal tumors, and nephroblastomas (72). Streptozotocin also induced renal mesenchymal tumors and epithelial tumors (89). Cycasin (β-D-glucosyloxyazoxymethane) (70). 1,2-dimethylhydrazines (71). N-nitrosomethylurea (MNU) (74), and transplacentally administered N-nitrosoethylurea (ENU) (22) induced mesenchymal tumors at relative high incidences.

True nephroblastoma, which is distinct from the renal mesenchymal tumor, has been found after 7,12-dimethylbenzanthracene (DMBA) administration under an immunodepressive state induced by antilymphocyte serum (112). Intragastric administration of DMBA to young rats also induced nephroblastomas in ovariectomized animals (113). Transplacental exposure to a single dose of ENU is a unique experimental model for the development of nephroblastoma in mice, rats, rabbits, and dogs (114–117).

Renal pelvic tumors, which usually consist of transitional cell carcinomas, have been induced by several urinary bladder carcinogens. Among the group of carcinogenic nitrofurans, N-[4-(5-nitro-2-furyl)-2-thiazolyl]formamide (FANFT) is a potent carcinogen that selectively induces transitional cell carcinomas of the urinary tract (78). Bis(2-oxopropyl)nitrosamine (BOPN) is carcinogenic for pelvic transitional epithelium (118). Long-term feeding of phenacetin or phenazone produces hyperplastic urothelium, leading to tumor development (79).

Viruses

Oncogenic effects of polyoma virus have been described in rodents (119). Eddy et al. induced renal angiosarcomas with tissue-cultured polyoma virus injected subcutaneously into neonatal rats of the Sprague–Dawley strain (120). Multiple mesenchymal tumors of the kidneys, bones, blood vessels, and adipose tissue were observed in Wistar rats given injections of leukemic AKR mouse cells containing the polyoma virus (119). The oncogenic activity of the virus was investigated for strain differences in susceptibility, tumor frequency, survival times, and histologic types of polyoma tumors. Increased tumor frequency and decreased survival times with increasing virus dose were observed. However, injection of low doses of virus was the most effective method for inducing a high incidence of renal sarcoma. There were no strain differences. Susceptibility of rats to oncogenesis by polyoma virus ceased after the seventh day postpartum (121).

For *in vitro* models, viral transformation of the proximal tubular epithelia was generated by transfection with SV40 viral genome or by direct infection with adenovirus. The transformants expressed low levels of proximal tubule markers, suggesting that dedifferentiation is associated with transformation (122). However, oncogenic effects of these viruses are not reported *in vivo*.

Hormones

Renal tumors are generated by the injection or subcutaneous implantation of natural estrogens, synthetic estrogenic products, and estrogenic substances in the male or the castrated female Syrian golden hamster (123–125). No renal tumors can be induced by estrogens in rats or mice. Although the detailed mechanisms underlying the induction of renal tumors by estrogens are still unknown, recent studies have demonstrated potential hormonal cell-proliferative chemical and molecular events.

Li et al. reported the presence of steroid receptors for estrogen, progesterone, androgen, and glucocorticoids in the hamster renal cortex (124–126). The findings suggest, at the least, that hamster kidney is a hormone-sensitive tissue. However, there is evidence that the hormonal activity of estrogens solely is not sufficient for nephrocarcinogenesis (127,128). Estrogens require enzymatic activation to exert their carcinogenic activities, particularly in quinone chemistry. Quinone formation was postulated to play a role in the carcinogenic process initiated by synthetic or natural estrogens (129) because it generates superoxide anion radicals, contributing to hydrogen peroxide generation. Reactive oxygen may damage enzymes and act as a mutagen (130,131). Recent studies using the highly sensitive postlabeling technique demonstrated the formation of covalent DNA addition products (adducts) in premalignant kidneys exposed to a synthetic estrogen (diethylstilbestrol), a natural hormone (17β-estradiol), and several synthetic steroids (132,133).

The histogenesis of estrogen-induced renal tumors is still controversial. A heterogeneous histologic pattern inducing epithelial and dysembryomatous (blastemic) components has been identified in various ratios, depending on the type of estrogen used (134). It has been suggested that the tumors are of carcinomatous appearance and arise in the proximal convoluted tubules (126,135–137) even if stromal components or embryonal rest are still possible precursors (135,138,139). Although estrogen-mediated nephrocarcinogenesis remains to be clarified, estrogen metabolism is postulated to play a key role in hormonal carcinogenesis.

Other Factors

X-irradiation and neutrons induce renal tumors in rats (140–142). A single injection with a radioisotope of polonium also produced renal tumors (143). The morphology of these tumors is the same as adenomas and adenocarcinomas induced after chemical carcinogen exposures. Unilateral nephrectomy also influenced renal tumorigenesis in rodents (108,144–146). Unilateral hydronephrosis induced by ligation of the ureter had enhancing effects on DMN-induced tumors in the remaining kidney (147). There have been reports of increased risk of various cancer development in patients with chronic renal failure or long-term hemodialysis (148,149). These data suggest that chronic repair or unknown factors may increase the susceptibility to the tumor induction not only in the compensatory kidney but in the extrarenal organs.

Sufrin et al. showed that unilateral nephrectomy enhances the growth of transplantable Wistar/Furth Wilms' tumors in the subcutaneous tissue of the same rats (150). This operation increased the tumor weight and DNA synthesis. The rate of cell proliferation was significantly higher in animals with unilateral nephrectomy than in sham-operated rats. One explanation is a release of growth factors in response to the loss of renal parenchyma (150). Under the same conditions using parabiotic rats, it was hypothesized that a humoral growth factor is released by a parabiont in response to nephrectomy (151). This may be the same factor responsible for compensatory renal hypertrophy.

PRENEOPLASTIC LESIONS

Morphology

The histogenesis of early renal neoplastic lesions is still not understood, although many studies dealing with chemically induced renal cell tumors have been reported. Morphological studies using electron microscopy, histochemistry, immunohistochemistry, and biochemical methods have indicated that the proximal convoluted tubular epithelium is most commonly involved in the histogenesis of renal cell tumors (Fig. 11). The steps in tumor development might proceed via hyperplastic tubules and dysplastic lesions (Fig. 12). These terms probably correspond to dysplastic tubular epithelium (152), proliferating tubules (153), focal areas of dysplastic tubular epithelium (93), cellular proliferation with dysplasia (107), adenomatous hyperplasia (154,155), dysplastic lesions (55), and atypical cell foci (13). Renal adenomas and adenocarcinomas can obviously be categorized as neoplastic lesions; however, the dysplastic lesions listed above might include reversible hyperplastic epithelium. Some of these lesions must develop to gross tumors with histological features of adenomas and then adenocarcinomas.

In studies with NTA by Alden et al., hyperplasia of proximal tubules was classified into simple tubular hyperplasia, tubular hyperplastic nodules, and adenomatous hyperplasia (154), and two pathways leading to tumor formation were postulated. One pathway is specific for the NTA-induced lesion, which represents vacuolation of the proximal tubules. Another pathway to tumor formation is associated with a proliferative response in kidneys associated with severe age-related nephrosis. Both

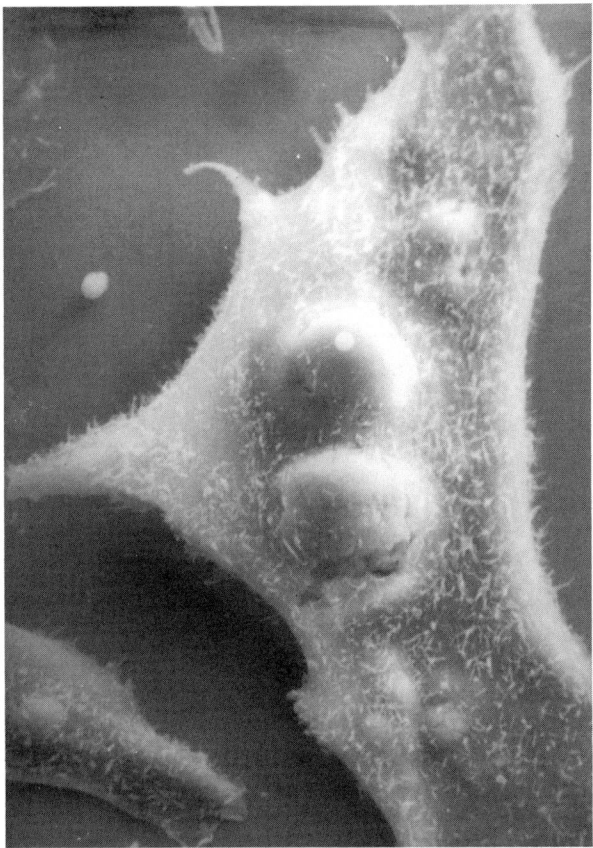

FIG. 11. Scanning electron micrograph showing numerous microvilli on the surface of a renal cell carcinoma cell *in vitro*; tumor originated in a rat treated with EHEN. ×3,000.

pathways are fundamentally concomitant. Tubular cell neoplasia might arise after such proliferative lesions attain an adenomatous character if cell injuries or toxic effects continue (156). These hyperplasias can be reversible lesions unless toxic injury persists (155). The diagnosis of hyperplasia versus neoplasia is probably the most critical issue in the classification of early preneoplastic lesions. Theoretically, the tubular hyperplastic response should increase the chance for expression of spontaneously growing cells, reflected in an increased incidence of neoplasia.

No definite morphological criteria have been shown to differentiate hyperplastic lesions (reversible) from early (small) adenomas (irreversible). With little or no cellular atypism, preneoplastic or neoplastic lesions are considered to be irreversible and progressive. The differentiation between hyperplasia and preneoplasia is based on morphology, cytology, cellular atypia, and growth pattern.

Early histological preneoplastic lesions in the kidney are classified as simple and

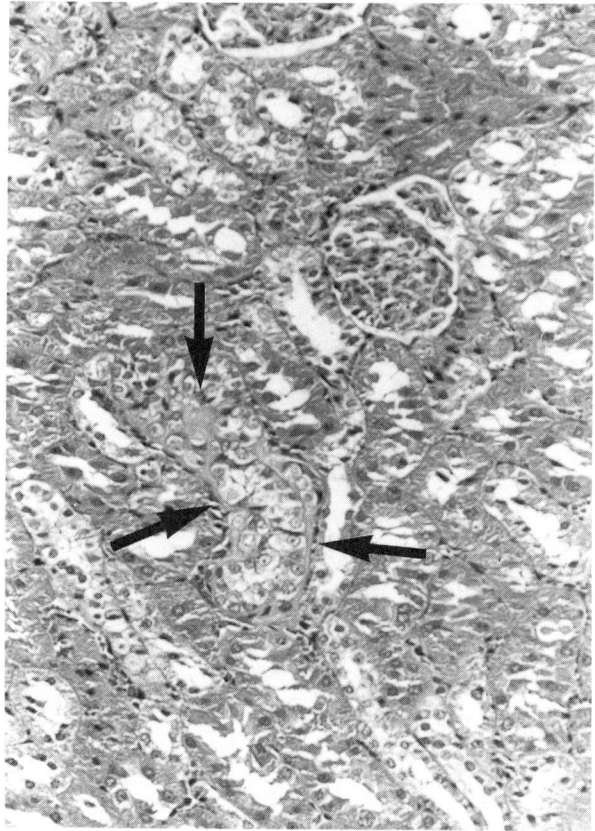

FIG. 12. Rat kidney. Simple hyperplasia (*arrow*), still within the confines of a tubule, with more abundant cytoplasm characterized by basophilia than in normal tubular epithelium. H&E, ×200.

adenomatous hyperplasias. Simple hyperplasias are composed of proliferative epithelium with clear cells or basophilic cells (Fig. 5). Proliferation of the epithelial cells is not marked, and therefore the tubular structure is retained. The lesions probably contain regenerative, and therefore, reversible tubular epithelium. By contrast, adenomatous hyperplasias are often delineated from the surrounding parenchyma and extend in a nodular fashion beyond the limits of a single tubule. Cells in these foci are hyperchromatic, with slight or no cellular atypia. They are differentiated from adenomas by lack of compression of adjacent parenchyma and lack of production of abnormal tubular structures.

Histochemistry and Enzyme Alterations

Histochemical studies have been made on the activities of a broad spectrum of enzymes in preoplastic and neoplastic renal lesions induced by chemical carcinogens (35,97,157,158). There are some renal tubular enzymatic functions that represent not only detoxification reaction but also metabolic activation of xenobiotics (159). Enzyme alterations are therefore interpreted as indicating the histogenesis of lesions from the proximal tubular epithelium. The increasing activity of glucose-6-phosphate dehydrogenase (G6PDH) seen in chemically induced renal cell tumors indicates a marked shift of energy metabolism from oxidative pathways toward the glycolytic production of ATP with a corresponding reduction in mitochondrial respiration. Enzyme activities of alkaline phosphatase (ALP), 5' nucleotidase, and γ-glutamyltranspeptidase (γ-GT) are related to brush border of the proximal convoluted tubules, and reduction of these enzyme activities represents a simplification of overall plasma membrane specialization.

Enzyme alterations of glutathione S-transferase placental form (GST-P) are observed in preneoplastic rat liver (160–162). The various forms (A, B, C, D, and P) of GST have also been compared with the activities of G6PDH and γ-GT during the early stages of renal tumorigenesis (97). In preneoplastic lesions designated as altered tubules and microadenomas induced by EHEN (55), the absence of γ-GT, ALP, and GST-B was considered as reflecting a loss of the normal activity in the proximal tubules. On the other hand, GST-A, which is a positive marker for distal straight segments, appears to be a comparative positive marker for altered tubules and microadenoma (Fig. 13). A single altered tubule, which is clearly distinguishable from adjacent tubules, also reacted strongly with the GST-A antibody. The presence of a PAS-positive brush border was seen at the apical surface of cells within these lesions (Fig. 14). The reduction in histochemically detectable enzyme of the proximal tubular brush border, such as γ-GT and ALP, may indicate dedifferentiated cells (35). There have been many reports that ultrastructural studies demonstrated well-developed brush borders on renal tumor surfaces (17,19,93, 153). The same structure is often observed on the surface of culture cells derived from rat renal carcinoma (Fig. 11). These histochemical and immunohistochemical investigations demonstrated that the alterations in enzyme phenotype occur during the early stages of neoplastic development in renal tumorigenesis.

For oncocytomas, the histochemical pattern differs fundamentally from that of other renal tubular epithelial tumors, suggesting that this tumor type develops from distal segments of the nephron (35). Cytochrome c oxidase can act as a specific marker for renal oncocytes (163). Some enzymatic metabolism may be associated with certain renal carcinogens. Cytochrome P450 monooxygenase is related to the activation of DMN in rat kidney (60). Although little is known about the metabolic pathway of renal carcinogens, these enzyme alterations may be actual preneoplastic markers in renal tumorigenesis.

Tumor-Associated Antigen

Study of the origin of early lesions during renal tumorigenesis has been seriously hampered by the lack of specific tumor markers. There have been few reports on tumor-specific antigens in chemically induced renal tumors. Transplantable renal

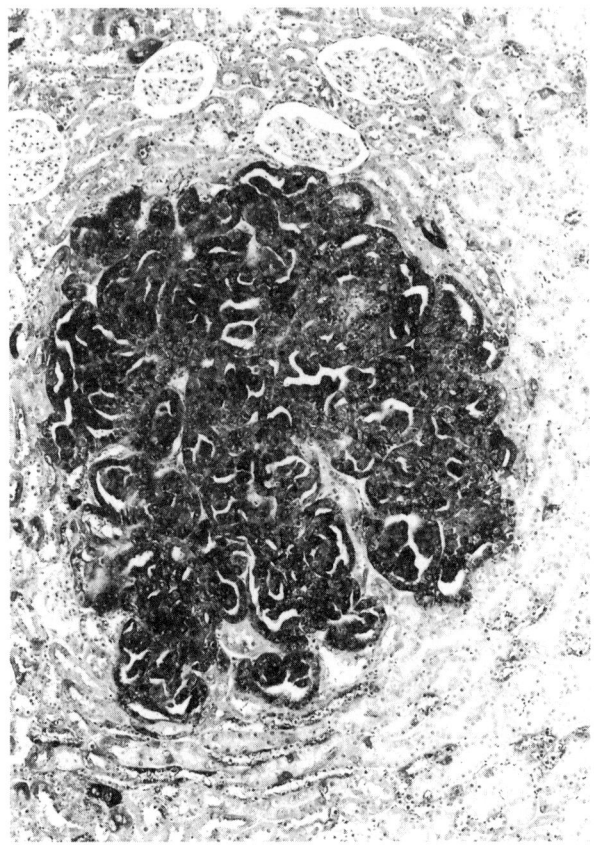

FIG. 13. Rat kidney. Renal adenoma exhibiting immunoreactivity for GST-A, using the avidin–biotin–peroxidase complex (ABC) method, counterstained with hematoxylin. ×100.

adenocarcinomas initiated by EHEN followed by promotion with β-cyclodextrin demonstrated high metastatic potential to other organs (164). Electrophoretic analysis of cellular proteins in polyacrylamide gels revealed that tumor tissues exhibited five polypeptides that were either lacking or undetectable in the nontumorous areas and control kidneys. Since the tumor-associated antigens might include these polypeptides, a monoclonal antibody against these polypeptides has been developed (165). We have purified one of the antigenic components through sequential chromatography and produced monoclonal antibodies to each polypeptide. Immunohistochemical analysis indicated that this tumor-associated antigen (polypeptide of 81,000 Da) was expressed in simple hyperplasia, adenomatous hyperplasia (Fig. 15), and in renal cell tumors induced by EHEN and NTA. It was strongly suggested that these hyperplastic lesions eventually achieve autonomous growth and lead to renal tubular cell tumors. The antibody demonstrated positive binding not only in

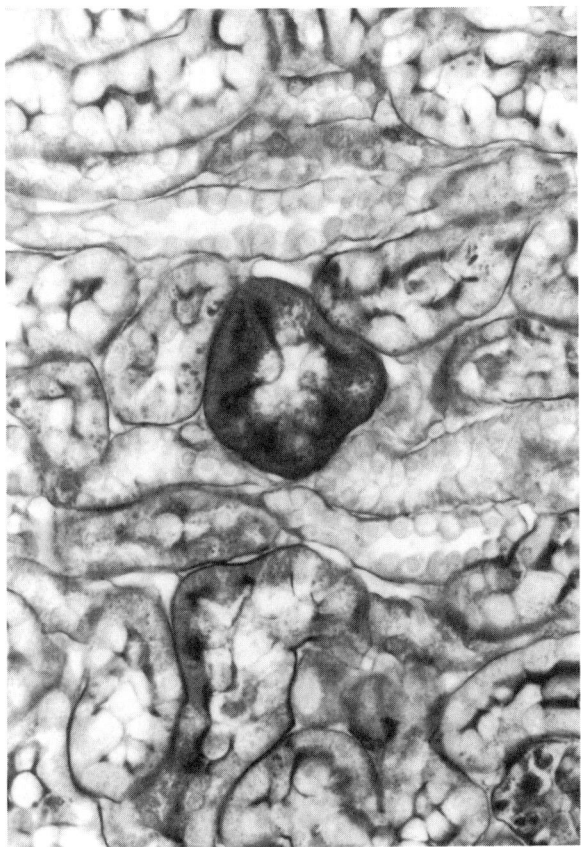

FIG. 14. Rat kidney. Enzyme-altered tubule, showing positive staining for GST-A. Note the presence of PAS-positive brush border at the apical surface of cells. PAS-GST-A double staining, ×200.

clear and basophilic cell types of simple hyperplasia but also in proximal tubules of nontumorous areas (Fig. 16). It was also suggested that different histological types of hyperplastic tubules may arise from the proximal tubules. Thus the enzyme phenotype in rat altered tubules reported by Tsuda et al. (35) and the expression of tumor-associated antigens in the initiated cells of early preneoplastic lesions may be detectable in similar human cases.

CELL INJURY, PROLIFERATION, AND CARCINOGENICITY

Toxic Responses Followed by Cell Injury

The kidney plays an important role in the regulation of total body homeostasis. It excretes the waste products of metabolism, regulates the concentration of electro-

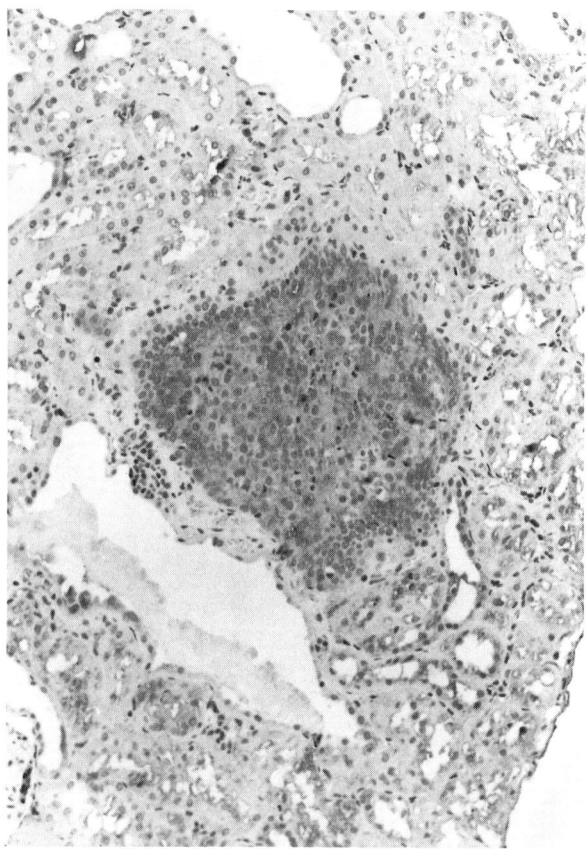

FIG. 15. Rat kidney. Immunoreactivity of adenomatous hyperplasia with an antibody to a rat renal tumor antigen. ABC method, ×100.

lytes precisely, controls acid–base balance, and serves as an endocrine organ, secreting such hormones as erythropoietin, renin, vasoactive prostaglandins, and kinins. These functions are carried out by a high degree of structural complexity. Therefore, it is important to understand the functional anatomy. The structural unit of the kidney, the *nephron*, consists primarily of the glomerulus and the tubular elements. The tubular part of the nephron consists of the proximal convoluted tubule, the loop of Henle, and the distal convoluted tubules. Among each segment of the nephron, the tubular elements are influenced by nephrotoxins. Histologically, the proximal convoluted tubule fills a major part of the renal cortex and is subdivided into three segments (P_1, P_2, and P_3), based on ultrastructural, anatomical, and functional differences (166).

Although a number of chemicals produce nephrotoxicity in humans and animals, there are several reasons for the unique susceptibility of the kidney. The blood is

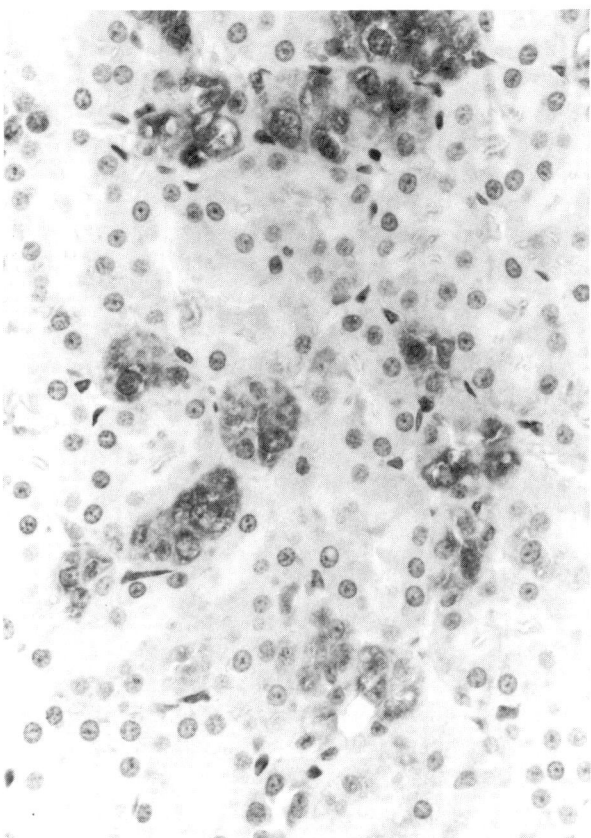

FIG. 16. Rat kidney. Immunoreactivity of renal proximal tubular epithelium with an antibody to a rat renal tumor cell antigen. ABC method, ×200.

delivered in relatively high volumes to the kidney. Approximately one-fourth of the whole blood reaching this organ is filtered through the glomeruli and reabsorbed in the proximal tubules. Thus drugs or chemicals in the blood are concentrated and become toxic in the kidney even if they are nontoxic in any other organs. The proximal tubular epithelium is supposed to be the first affected renal site in this process. The chemical agents accumulate within the tubular epithelium in concentrations higher than in plasma. In addition, active secretion of compounds occurs in the proximal tubule, with a high concentration of some agents in the tubular lumen. In contrast to the cortex, the medulla of the kidney is less susceptible to toxic agents because of the low blood flow and lower concentration of toxicants. Except for specific nephrotoxic agents, the proximal convoluted tubule is the primary site of action for many nephrotoxins (167).

Histologically, the affected tubules are variable in appearance, some having dilated lumens and others without lumens. Tubular epithelium often shows vacuolation (168,169), hyaline droplets (170), and cytoplasmic degeneration. Nephrotoxic tubular necrosis occurs principally in the proximal convoluted segments of the nephron. Morphological evidence of tubular necrosis tends to be extensive along proximal tubule segments (171). The toxic agents also induce nuclear changes such as karyomegary (172). Protein casts, crystals, and stones can provide information concerning nephrotoxicity of a chemical. Electron microscopic examination of cell damage could demonstrate subcellular localization of alterations of the nuclei, mitochondria, endoplasmic reticulum, and other organelles. Histochemistry, including staining by PAS (periodic acid–Schiff), is useful to identify brush borders in the proximal tubular cells. Other histochemical techniques are also available to evaluate renal responses to toxicants.

Nephrotoxic damage of renal tubular cells by chemical agents may be interpreted according to three possible mechanisms (173). Most heavy metals, including mercuric chloride, interfere directly with an essential functional or metabolic process (174). Mercury will combine with sulfhydryl groups and inhibit several enzyme systems. A second mechanism of toxicity is the covalent binding to protein or initiation of lipid peroxidation (e.g., acetaminophen) (175). A third mechanism may be due to induction of renal enzymes such as β-lyase (e.g., hexachloro-1,3-butadiene) (176).

As mentioned above, sites of action of many nephrotoxins are limited to the proximal tubule whether or not the compounds are specific. However, there are some site-specific nephrotoxins in the kidney. For example, the distal convoluted tubule is affected by amphotericin, which has been shown to influence the ability of the kidney to acidify the urine. Some analgesic mixtures (aspirin and phenacetin) influence the loop of Henle. The glomerulus may be injured by a variety of factors, including immunologic diseases, vascular disorders, metabolic diseases, and some hereditary conditions. However, few nephrotoxins induce renal cell tumors, which are believed to originate from tubular epithelium, which are targets of nephrotoxins.

Cell Injury and Cell Proliferation

As a result of nephrotoxic responses in the kidney leading to cell injury, cell proliferation may occur to repair tissue damage. Such tubular regeneration is often accompanied by proliferation of mesenchymal tissues as fibroblasts and capillaries. Tubular hyperplasia could be seen in these degenerative areas. The pathologic term *hyperplasia* constitutes an increase in the number of cells in an organ or tissue. Therefore, it will take place if the cellular population is capable of synthesizing DNA, thus permitting mitotic activity. Chronic tissue damage is usually associated with hyperplasia and increased levels of cell proliferation (177,178). This hyperplasia responds to regular growth control of cells since it stops or regresses when the stimulus has ceased. However, it should be stressed that hyperplasia constitutes an important soil in which tumorous proliferation may eventually arise. Many naturally occurring human and animal tumors are associated with chronic tissue damage (179–181), possibly due to the increased cell proliferation.

Cell Proliferation in Nephropathy

Based on levels of DNA synthesis using [^{3}H]thymidine autoradiography or Brdu immunohistochemistry, renal tubular cell kinetics in chemically induced nephrotoxicity and nephropathy has been reported (11,182–184). Toxic nephropathy may also occur from the secondary effect of several pharmacologic agents (185). Nephropathy defines degenerative and hyperplastic changes of the proximal tubules with proteinaceous casts in tubules, sometimes associated with lymphocyte infiltration and thickening of glomerular, Bowman's capsular, and tubular basement membranes (186). Aging nephropathy in rats, probably affected by dietary, hormonal, and genetic factors, is associated with increased DNA synthesis, especially in hyperplastic renal tubules (187). These hyperplastic tubules may provide a promoting or copromoting stimulus for nongenotoxic carcinogens. In a study of increased susceptibility of the kidney to a renal carcinogen, N-4(4'-fluorobiphenyl)acetamide, older rats developed more renal tumors than did young rats (188). The hyperplasia of aging nephropathy may serve as a promoter of chemically induced renal carcinogenesis, possibly due to the increased levels of DNA synthesis in target cells.

Cell Proliferation in Renal Carcinogenesis

The major site of increased cell proliferation after chemically induced toxic renal lesions was shown to be the outer stripe of the outer medulla, or the P_2 segment of the proximal tubules in rats (11). A similar pathogenesis may be hypothesized for tumor promotion by these nongenotoxic chemicals (13). Transformation leading to carcinogenesis occurs in a proliferative environment in which initiated cells are selected. The hypothesis that epigenetic or nongenotoxic events play a role in transformation arose in part as an attempt to explain the role of wounding in cancer (122).

Chronic exposure to S-(1,2-dichlorovinyl)-L-cysteine (DCVC) induces regenerative cells of the P_2 segment in the proximal tubule, in which there is increased rate of cell proliferation, a decrease in differentiation, and an increase in markers more characteristic of embryonic kidney (122,189). Thus the nephrogenic repair response induces not only cell proliferation but also a dedifferentiated state of renal tubules.

On the other hand, intracellular calcium homeostasis is closely related to cell injury. The increased accumulation of calcium in chemically induced toxicity is important in causing coagulative necrosis (190). Cells treated with tumor promoters may alter their response to change calcium concentration (191). Calcium may also regulate indirectly by alkalinization of the cytoplasm via protein kinase C and phosphatidyl inositol pathway. The calcium-mediated events may be induced by several tumor promoters (192).

It is well known that these tumor promoters decrease gap junctional intercellular communication during the cause of neoplastic transformation. This is probably due to the increased calcium in the cytoplasm. Gap junctions play an important role in maintaining tissue homeostasis and in regulating cell proliferation and differentiation (193).

Culture cell lines derived from rat kidneys have been examined for cell proliferation and gap junction dysfunction under influences of renal carcinogens and tumor promoters (e.g., streptozotocin, sodium barbital, and NTA). The effects of these chemicals on intercellular communication were generally correlated with their reported tumorigenic capability in the kidney (194).

Nephrotoxicity and Nephrocarcinogenicity

Although the renal carcinogenic process has not been clearly defined, a simplified classification of carcinogens may induce these carcinogens with genotoxic activity and those with evidence of genotoxicity. It is commonly observed that exposure to genotoxic carcinogens may cause DNA damage and that the DNA interaction in the kidney may initiate tumor formation (195). Tumor-initiating agents in renal two-stage carcinogenesis, especially with N-nitroso compounds, may act via a direct genotoxic mechanism (e.g., interaction with DNA in target cells). As mentioned previously, tumor promoters are commonly weak carcinogens, usually with nongenotoxic chemicals, producing tumors primarily via a potential extranuclear, epigenetic pathway. A recent well-documented example of this phenomenon concerns NTA and unleaded gasoline (11,13,154,155).

However, the role of genotoxicity versus epigenetic effects on the nephrocarcinogenicity of compounds that are intermediates between the two categories (i.e., compounds that are weak genotoxins and potent nephrotoxins) is still unclear. A number of factors can be identified that contribute to the mechanism of carcinogenesis. These include the toxicodynamics, metabolism, DNA alteration, and cell proliferation associated with chemical exposure (196). The toxicity changes with the magnitude of an individual dose, the rate and duration of dosing, and the route of exposure. The toxic effects induced by nongenotoxic compounds play an important role in their renal carcinogenicity. Metabolism often contributes to the enzyme-mediated biotransformation of a compound to a derivative that is chemically reactive. DNA alterations occur by a number of different mechanisms.

Cell proliferation may occur to repair tissue damage or as a direct mitogenic effect of the chemical. The early part of the S phase is extremely sensitive to carcinogen damage and ultimate carcinogenesis (197). Control of this proliferation, in part, appears to be mediated by gap junctional intercellular communication between cells and can be interrupted by tumor promoters (194).

A considerable amount of data has accumulated on the nephrotoxicity of carcinogens. It has become increasingly evident that most renal carcinogens induce toxicity in proximal tubular epithelium and that the toxic lesions precede and occur along with tumor development (198). For instance, halogenated alkenes such as hexachloro-1,3-butadiene (HCBD) and tetrafluoroethylene (TFE) are catalyzed by hepatic glutathione-S-transferase, then metabolized by renal γ-glutamyltransferase and dipeptidases to their cysteine S-conjugate. Cysteine conjugates may be direct-acting nephrotoxins or may undergo bioactivation mediated by the cysteine conjugate β-lyase (178). HCBD demonstrated some mutagenic potential due to its primary metabolism via glutathione conjugation, and this may be responsible for the development of renal tumors (199). Perchloroethylene induces a slightly increased incidence of renal tumors in male F344 rat (200), suggesting that the cysteine conjugate of this compound could account for the tumor formation (201). Moreover, perchloroethylene causes hyaline droplets consisting of α_{2u}-globulin in the P_2 segment of the proximal tubules, similar to the case of petroleum hydrocarbons (202). Acute and chronic cytotoxic injury induced by unleaded gasoline is associated with increased cell proliferation in the P_2 segment of the tubules (11,13,203). These changes have been linked to the binding of the hydrocarbon or its metabolites to α_{2u}-globulin. A similar pathogenesis may be hypothesized for tumor promotion by some other nongenotoxic nephrotoxins.

Whether renal neoplasms develop from nongenetic events, toxic effects, or interactions of reactive intermediates with DNA, morphological evidence has been made for the sequence of tumorigenic events of the kidney. Figure 17 shows that the steps in tumor development may proceed via hyperplastic and dysplastic renal tubules to gross tumors designated as adenomas, carcinomas, or adenocarcinomas (184). Degenerative and regenerative changes of the tubules indicative of acute or chronic toxicity may also precede this proliferative sequence. Cell proliferation at a specific site of origin may depend on the individual chemical. For example, the specific site for cell proliferation induced by DMN is probably the P_1 or P_2 segment (109), while FBPA-induced tumors may arise from the P_3 segment (107), and LA or DEN appears to induce tumors in both the P_2 and P_3 segments of the proximal tubules (204). This target affinity for genotoxic chemicals might be due to a hot spot in DNA, where the reactivity is greater than expected by chance alone, and another where mutation occurs more frequently. However, the reason for susceptibility of the proximal tubules for most nongenotoxic carcinogens may be exposure of the tubular cells to high concentrations of chemicals.

There are very few reports on the molecular events in renal carcinogenesis that may initiate the conversion of normal to neoplastic cells. Recently, activation of the K-*ras* (40%) and N-*ras* (4%) oncogenes were detected in *N*-methyl-*N*-methoxymethylnitrosamine-induced renal mesenchymal tumors in rats but not in renal tubular cell tumors (205). In their activated forms oncogenes have been present in many other tumors induced by chemical carcinogens (196). Therefore, long-term chronic exposure to a carcinogen is capable of reproducibly activating oncogenes similar to those observed in both single-dose and two-step carcinogenesis. In human renal carcinomas, chromosomal abnormalities have been reported (206). Moreover, normal human kidney proximal tubular cells *in vitro* with an inserted mutated *ras* oncogene undergo transformation characteristic of renal carcinomas (207). Thus renal carcinogenesis in experimental animals is affected by a variety of factors, including natural products, chemical carcinogens, nephrotoxins, hormones, virus, radiation, and molecular events. They may provide a linkage between nephrocarcinogenicity in rodents and humans.

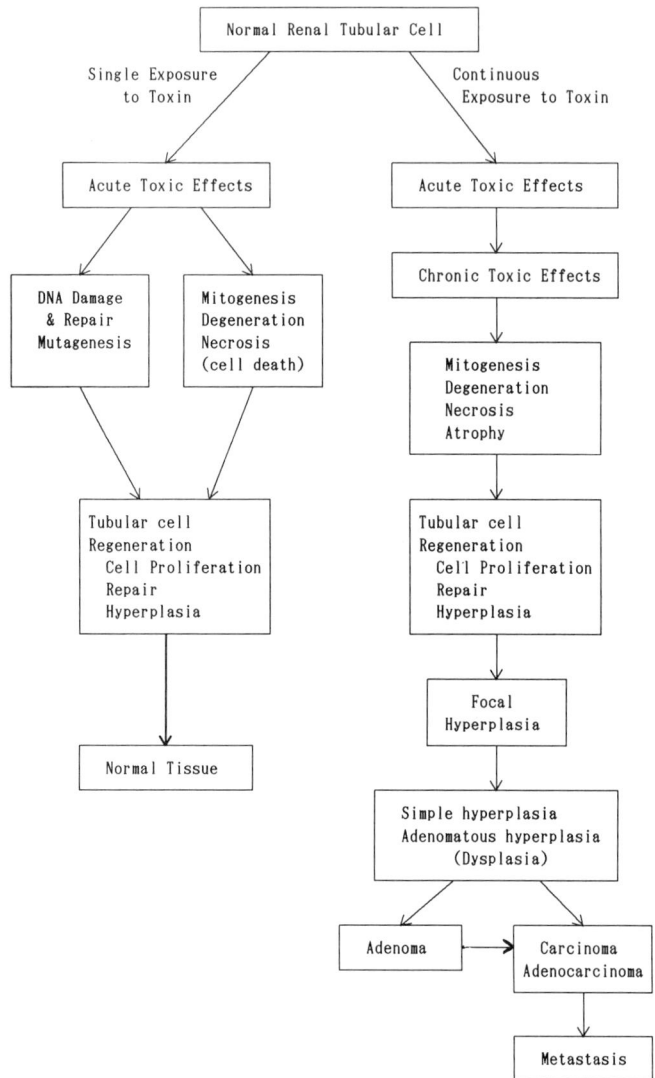

FIG. 17. Pathological sequence of events in tubular damage caused by nephrotoxins, including renal carcinogens or tumor promoters. [Modified from Ward et al. (184).]

ACKNOWLEDGMENTS

The authors wish to thank Dr. Hiroyuki Tsuda, Department of Pathology, Fujita Health University School of Medicine, for contributing immunohistochemical photographs, and Mr. Yoshiteru Kitahori for photomicrography. We also thank Dr. Jerrold M. Ward, Laboratory of Comparative Carcinogenesis, National Cancer Institute, Frederick, Maryland, for his advice and generous support, and for Fig. 17.

REFERENCES

1. Brodsky GL, Garnick MB. Renal tumors in the adult patient. In: Tisher CG, Brenner BM, eds. *Renal pathology with clinical and functional correlations*. Vol II. Philadelphia: JB Lippincott; 1989:1467–1504.
2. Hiasa Y, Ito N. Experimental induction of renal tumors. *CRC Crit Rev Toxicol* 1987;17:279–343.
3. Bennington JL. Cancer of the kidney—etiology, epidemiology and pathology. *Cancer* 1973;32:1017–1029.
4. Kolonel LN. Association of cadmium with renal cancer. *Cancer* 1976;37:1782–1787.
5. Baker EL, Boyer RA, Fowler BA, et al. Occupational lead exposure, nephropathy and renal cancer. *Am J Ind Med* 1980;1:139–148.
6. Lilis R. Long-term occupational lead exposure: chronic nephropathy and renal cancer: a case report. *Am J Ind Med* 1981;2:293–297.
7. Hanis NM, Holmes TM, Shallenberger LG, Jones KE. Epidemiologic study of refinery and chemical workers. *J Occup Med* 1982;24:203–212.
8. Roe FJC, Boyland E, Dukes CE, Mitchley BCV. Failure of testosterone or xanthopterin to influence the induction of renal neoplasms by lead in rats. *Br J Cancer* 1965;19:860–866.
9. Hiasa Y, Ohshima M, Kitahori Y, Fujita T, Yuasa T, Miyashiro A. Basic lead acetate: promoting effect on the development of renal tubular cell tumors in rats treated with N-ethyl-N-hydroxyethylnitrosamine. *J Natl Cancer Inst* 1983;70:761–765.
10. Kitchen DN. Neoplastic renal effects of unleaded gasoline in Fischer F344 rats. In: Mehlman, MA, ed. *Renal effects of petroleum hydrocarbons*. Vol 7. Princeton, NJ: Princeton Scientific Publishing; 1984:65–71.
11. Short BG, Burnett VL, Cox MG, Bus JS, Swenberg JA. Site-specific renal cytotoxicity and cell proliferation in male rats exposed to petroleum hydrocarbons. *Lab Invest* 1987;57:564–577.
12. Kluwe WM, Abdo KM, Huff J. Chronic kidney disease and organic chemical exposures: evaluations of causal relationships in humans and experimental animals. *Fundam Appl Toxicol* 1984;4:889–901.
13. Short BG, Steinhagen WH, Swenberg JA. Promoting effects of unleaded gasoline and 2,2,4-trimethylpentane on the development of atypical cell foci and renal tubular cell tumors in rats exposed to N-ethyl-N-hydroxyethylnitrosamine. *Cancer Res* 1989;49:6369–6378.
14. Ito N. Experimental studies on tumors of the urinary system of rats induced by chemical carcinogens. *Acta Pathol Jpn* 1973;23:87–109.
15. Hard GC. Tumors of the kidney, renal pelvis and ureter. In: Turusov VS, Mohr U, eds. *Pathology of tumours in laboratory animals. vol 1. Tumours of the rats*. Lyon, France: International Agency for Research on Cancer; 1990:301–324.
16. Bannasch P, Krech R, Zerban H. Morphogenese und Mikromorphologie epithlialer Nierentumoren bei Nitrosomorphalin-vergifteten Ratten. II. Tubuläre Glykogenose und die Genese von Klar oder acidophilzelligen Tumoren. *Z Krebsforsch* 1978;92:63–86.
17. Bannasch P, Krech R, Zerban H. Morphogenese und Mikromorphologie epithelialer Nierentumoren bei Nitrosomorpholin-vergifteten Ratten. IV. Tubuläre Läsionen und basophile Tumoren. *J Cancer Res Clin Oncol* 1980;98:243–265.
18. Hard GC, Butler WH. Ultrastructural aspects of renal adenocarcinoma induced in the rat by dimethylnitrosamine. *Cancer Res* 1971;31:366–372.
19. Dees JH, Reuber MD, Trump BF. Adenocarcinoma of the kidney. I. Ultrastructure of renal adenocarcinomas induced in rats by N-(4'fluoro-4-biphenylyl)acetamide. *J Natl Cancer Inst* 1976;57:779–794.
20. Deerberg F, Rehm S. Spontaneous renal pelvic carcinoma in DA/Han rats. *Z Versuchstierk* 1985;27:33–38.
21. Hard GC, Butler WH. Cellular analysis of renal neoplasia. Induction of renal tumors in dietary-conditioned rats by dimethylnitrosamine with a reappraisal of morphological characteristics. *Cancer Res* 1979;30:2796–2805.
22. Turusov VS, Alexandrov VA, Timoshenko IV. Nephroblastoma and renal mesenchymal tumor induced in rats by N-nitrosoethyl- and N-nitrosomethylurea. *Neoplasia* 1980;27:229–235.
23. Hard GC. Mesenchymal tumor, kidney rat. In: Jones TC, Mohr U, Hunt RP, eds. *Urinary system*. Berlin: Springer-Verlag; 1986:61–71.
24. Crain RC. Spontaneous tumors in the Rochester strain of the Wistar rat. *Am J Pathol* 1958;34:311–335.

25. Snell KC. Renal disease of the rat. In: Cotchin E, Roe FJC, eds. *Pathology of laboratory rats and mice.* Oxford: Blackwell; 1967:105–147.
26. Goodman DG, Ward JM, Squire RA, Chu KC, Linhart MS. Neoplastic and nonneoplastic lesions in aging F344 rats. *Toxicol Appl Pharmacol* 1979;48:237–248.
27. Hard GC. Lipomatous tumors, kidney, rat. In: Jones TC, Mohr U, Hunt RP, eds. *Urinary system* Berlin: Springer-Verlag; 1986:80–87.
28. McLaughlin JK, Blot WJ, Mandel JS, Schuman LM, Mehl ES, Fraumeni JF. Etiology of cancer of the renal pelvis. *J Natl Cancer Inst* 1983;71:287–291.
29. McLaughlin JK, Mandel JS, Bolt WS, Schuman LM, Mehl ES, Fraumeni JF. A population-based case-control study of renal cell carcinoma. *J Natl Cancer Inst* 1984;72:275–284.
30. Hard GL. Renal carcinogenesis, Rat. In: Jones TC, Mohr U, Hunt RP, eds. *Urinary system.* Berlin: Springer-Verlag; 1986:45–49.
31. Gold LS, Slone TH, Manley NB, Bernstein L. Target organs in chronic bioassays of 533 chemical carcinogens. *Environ Health Perspect* 1991;93:233–246.
32. Huff J, Cirvello J, Haseman J, Bucher J. Chemicals associated with site-specific neoplasia in 1394 long-term carcinogenesis experiments in laboratory rodents. *Environ Health Perspect* 1991;93: 247–270.
33. Ward JM, Reznik G. Refinements of rodent pathology and the pathologist's contribution to evaluation of carcinogenesis bioassays. *Prog Exp Tumor Res* 1983;26:266–291.
34. Ward JM. Pathology of toxic, preneoplastic, and neoplastic lesions. In: Douglas JF, ed. *Carcinogenesis and mutagenesis testing.* Clifton, NJ: Humana Press; 1984:97–130.
35. Tsuda H, Hacker HJ, Katayama H, Masui T, Ito N, Bannasch P. Correlative histochemical studies on preneoplastic and neoplastic lesions in the kidney of rats treated with nitrosamines. *Virchows Arch B Cell Pathol* 1986;51:385–404.
36. Pitot HC. Progression: the terminal stage in carcinogenesis. *Jpn J Cancer Res* 1989;80:599–607.
37. Berenblum I. The carcinogenic action of croton resin. *Cancer Res* 1941;1:44–48.
38. Boutwell RK. Some biological aspects of skin carcinogenesis. *Prog Exp Tumor Res* 1964;4: 207–250.
39. Butler WH, Greenblatt M, Lijinsky W. Carcinogenesis in rats by aflatoxins B_1, G_1 and B_2. *Cancer Res* 1969;29:2206–2211.
40. Murthy AS, Russfield AB, Hagopian M, Monson R, Snell J, Weisburger EK. Carcinogenicity and nephrotoxicity of 2-amino-, 1-amino-2-methyl-, and 2-methyl-1-nitro-anthraquinone. *Toxicol Lett* 1979;4:71–78.
41. Lijinsky W, Reuber MD, Saavedra JE. The effect of deuterium substitution on carcinogenesis by azoxymethane. *Cancer Lett* 1984;24:273–80.
42. Dunnick JK, Eustin SL, Lilja HS. Bromodichloromethane, a trihalomethane that produces neoplasms in rodents. *Cancer Res* 1987;47:5189–5193.
43. Bucher JR, Alison RH, Montgomery CA, et al. Comparative toxicity and carcinogenicity of two chlorinated paraffins in F344/N rats and B6C3F1 mice. *Fundam Appl Toxicol* 1987;9:454–468.
44. Jorgenson TA, Meierhenry EF, Rushbrook CJ, Bull RJ, Robinson M. Carcinogenicity of chloroform in drinking water to male Osborne–Mendel rats and female B6C3F1 mice. *Fundam Appl Toxicol* 1985;5:760–769.
45. Carcinogenesis Testing Program. Bioassay of chlorothalonil for possible carcinogenicity. *Natl Cancer Inst Carcinog Tech Rep Ser* 1978;41:94.
46. Carcinogenesis Testing Program. Bioassay of cinnamyl anthranilate for possible carcinogenicity. *Natl Cancer Inst Carcinog Tech Rep Ser* 1980;196:92.
47. Sternberg SS, Philips FS, Cronin AP. Renal tumors and other lesions in rats following a single intravenous injection of daunomycin. *Cancer Res* 1972;32:1029–1036.
48. Reichert D, Spengler U, Romen W, Henschler D. Carcinogenicity of dichloroacetylene an inhalation study. *Carcinogenesis* 1984;5:1411–1420.
49. Bomhard E, Luckhaus G, Voigt WH, Loeser E. Induction of light hydrocarbon nephropathy by p-dichlorobenzene. *Arch Toxicol* 1988;61:433–439.
50. Toth B. 1,1-Dimethylhydrazine (unsymmetrical) carcinogenesis in mice. Light microscopic and ultrastructural studies on neoplastic blood vessels. *J Natl Cancer Inst* 1973;50:181–194.
51. Kociba RJ, Schwetz BA, Keyes DG, et al. Chronic toxicity and reproduction studies of hexachlorobutadiene in rats. *Environ Health Perspect* 1977;21:49–53.
52. Tucker MJ. Carcinogenic action of quinoxaline 1,4-dioxide in rats. *J Natl Cancer Inst* 1975;55: 137–146.

53. Bucher JR, Huff J, Kluwe WM. Toxicology and carcinogenesis studies of isophorone in F344 rats and B6C3F1 mice. *Toxicology* 1986;39:207–219.
54. Boyland E, Dukes CE, Grover PL, Mitchley BCV. The induction of renal tumors by feeding lead acetate to rats. *Br J Cancer* 1962;16:283–288.
55. Hiasa Y, Ohshima M, Iwata C, Tanikake T. Histopathological studies on renal tubular cell tumors in rat treated with N-ethyl-N-hydroxyethylnitrosamine. *Gann* 1979;70:817–820.
56. Hinton DE, Heatfield BM, Lipsky MM, Trump BF. Animal model of human disease: renal tubular carcinomas. *Am J Pathol* 1980;100:317–320.
57. Jasmin G, Riopelle JL. Renal carcinomas and erythrocytosis in rats following intrarenal injection of nickel subsulfate. *Lab Invest* 1976;35:71–78.
58. Lijinsky W, Kovatch RM, Singer SS. Carcinogenesis in F344 rats induced by nitrosohydroxyalkylchloroethylureas. *J Cancer Res Clin Oncol* 1986;112:211–228.
59. Mohr U, Hilfrich J. Brief communication: effect of a single dose of N-diethylnitrosamine on the rat kidney. *J Natl Cancer Inst* 1972;49:1729–1731.
60. Hard GC. High frequency, single-dose model of renal adenoma/carcinoma induction using dimethylnitrosamine in Crl:(W) BR rats. *Carcinogenesis* 1984;5:1047–1050.
61. Bannasch P. Sequential cellular changes during chemical carcinogenesis. *J Cancer Res Clin Oncol* 1984;108:11–22.
62. Longnecker DS, Curphey TJ, Lilja HS, French JI, Daniel DS. Carcinogenicity in rats of the nitrosourea amino acid N-delta-(N-methyl-N-nitroscocarbamoyl)-1-ornithine. *J Environ Pathol Toxicol* 1980;4:117–129.
63. Dietrich DR, Swenberg JA. Preneoplastic lesions in rodent kidney induced spontaneously or by non-genotoxic agents: predictive nature and comparison to lesions induced by genotoxic carcinogens. *Mutat Res* 1991;248:239–260.
64. Nakanishi K, Kurata Y, Oshima M, Fukushima S, Ito N. Carcinogenicity of phenacetin: long term feeding study in B6C3F1 mice. *Int J Cancer* 1982;29:439–444.
65. Kurokawa Y, Hayashi Y, Maekawa A, Takahashi M, Kokubo T, Odashima S. Carcinogenicity of potassium bromate administered orally to F344 rats. *J Natl Cancer Inst* 1983;71:965–972.
66. Goldsworthy TL, Lyght O, Burnett VL, Popp JA. Potential role of α_{2u}-globulin, protein droplet accumulation, and cell proliferation in the renal carcinogenicity of rats exposed to trichloroethylene, perchloroethylene, and pentachloroethane. *Toxicol Appl Pharmacol* 1988;92:367–379.
67. Reznik G, Ward JM, Hardisty JF, Russfield A. Renal carcinogenic and nephrotoxic effects of the flame retardant tris(2,3-dibromopropyl)phosphate on F344 rats and (C57BL/6N X C3H/HEN)F1 mice. *J Natl Cancer Inst* 1979;63:205–212.
68. Goyer FA, Falk HL, Hogan M, Feldmen DD, Richter W. Renal tumors in rats given trisodium nitrilotriacetic acid in drinking water for 2 years. *J Natl Cancer Inst* 1981;66:869–880.
69. Horton L, Fox CC, Corrin B, Sonksen H. Streptozotocin-induced renal tumors in rats. *Br J Cancer* 1977;36:692–699.
70. Fukunishi R, Kadota A, Yoshida A, Hirota N. Induction of tumors with cycasin in newborn and preweaning rats. *J Natl Cancer Inst* 1985;74:1275–1281.
71. Turusov VS. Role of host factors in carcinogenesis induced in mice by 1,2-dimethylhydrazine. *IARC Sci Publ* 1983;51:39–48.
72. Shirai T, Kurata Y, Fukushima S, Ito N. Dose-related induction of lung, thyroid and kidney tumors by N-bis(2-hydroxypropyl)nitrosamine given orally to F344 rats. *Gann* 1984;75:502–507.
73. Vesselinovitch SD, Itze L, Mihailovich N, Rao KV, Manojlovski B, Role of hormonal environment, partial hepatectomy, and dose of ethylnitrosourea in renal carcinogenesis. *Cancer Res.* 1973; 33:339–341.
74. Leaver DD, Swann PF, Magee PN. The induction of tumours in the rat by a single oral dose of N-nitrosomethylurea. *Br J Cancer* 1969;23:177–187.
75. Carcinogenesis Testing Program. Bioassay of o-anisidine hydrochloride for possible carcinogenicity. *Natl Cancer Inst Car Tech Rep Ser* 1978;89:1–130.
76. Adolphs HD, Thiele J, Kiel H, Steffens E. Induction of transitional carcinoma of urinary bladder in rats by feeding N-[4-5(nitro-2-furyl)-2-thiazolyl]formamide. *Urol Res* 1978;6:19–27.
77. Cohen SM, Erturk E, Bryan GT. Comparative carcinogenicity of 5-nitrothiophenes and 5-nitrofurans in rats. *J Natl Cancer Inst* 1976;57:277–282.
78. Erturk E, Price JM, Morris JE, et al. The production of carcinoma of the urinary bladder in rats by feeding N-[4-(5-nitro-2-furyl)-2-thiazolyl]-formamide. *Cancer Res* 1967;27:1998–2002.

79. Johansson SL. Carcinogenicity of analgesics: long-term treatment of Sprague–Dawley rats with phenacetin, phenazone, caffeine and paracetamol (acetamidophen). *Int J Cancer* 1981;27:521–529.
80. Hiraga K, Fujii T. Induction of tumors of the urinary system in F344 rats by dietary administration of sodium *o*-phenylphenate. *Food Cosmet Toxicol* 1981;19:303–310.
81. Diwan BA, Ohshima M, Rice JM. Promotion by sodium barbital of renal cortical and transitional cell tumors, but not intestinal tumors, in F344 rats given methyl(acetoxymethyl)nitrosamine, and lack of effect of phenobarbital, amobarbital, or barbituric acid on development of either renal or intestinal tumors. *Carcinogenesis* 1989;10:183–188.
82. Kurata Y, Tsuda H, Sakata T, Yamashita T, Ito N. Reciprocal modifying effects of isometic forms of aminophenol on induction of neoplastic lesions in rat liver and kidney initiated by *N*-ethyl-*N*-hydroxyethylnitrosamine. *Carcinogenesis* 1987;8:1281–1285.
83. Hiasa Y, Ohshima M, Kitahori Y, Konishi N, Fujita T, Yuasa T. β-Cyclodextrin: promoting effect on the development of renal tubular cell tumors in rat treated with *N*-ethyl-*N*-hydroxyethylnitrosamine. *J Natl Cancer Inst* 1982;69:963–967.
84. Hiasa Y, Enoki N, Kitahori Y, Konishi N, Shimoyama T. DL-Serine: promoting activity on renal tumorigenesis by *N*-ethyl-*N*-hydroxyethylnitrosamine in rats. *J Natl Cancer Inst* 1984;73:297–299.
85. Dietrick DR, Swenberg JA. The presence of α_{2u}-globulin is necessary for D-limonene promotion of male rat kidney tumors. *Cancer Res* 1991;51:3512–3521.
86. Shirai T, Ohshima M, Masuda A, Tamano S, Ito N. Promotion of 2-(ethylnitrosamino)ethanol-induced renal carcinogenesis in rats by nephrotoxic compounds: positive responses with folic acid, basic lead acetate, and *N*-(3,5-dichlorophenyl)succinimide but not with 2,3-dibromo-l-propanol phosphate. *J Natl Cancer Inst* 1984;72:477–482.
87. Rosenberg MR, Novicki DL, Jirtle RL, Novotny A, Michalopoulos G. Promoting effect of nicotinamide on the development of renal tubular cell tumors in rats initiated with diethylnitrosamine. *Cancer Res* 1985;45:809–814.
88. Kurokawa Y, Aoki S, Imazawa T, Hayashi T, Matsushima Y, Takamura N. Dose-related enhancing effect of potassium bromate on renal tumorigenesis in rats initiated with *N*-ethyl-*N*-hydroxyethylnitrosamine. *Jpn J Cancer Res* 1985;76:583–589.
89. Konishi N, Diwan BA, Ward JM. Amelioration of sodium barbital–induced nephropathy and regenerative tubular hyperplasia after a single injection of streptozotocin does not abolish the renal tumor promoting effect of barbital sodium in male F344/NCr rats. *Carcinogenesis* 1990;11:2149–2156.
90. Hiasa Y, Kitahori Y, Konishi N, Enoki N, Shimoyama T, Miyashiro A. Trisodium nitrilotracetate monohydrate: promoting effects on the development of renal tubular cell tumors in rats treated with *N*-ethyl-*N*-hydroxyethylnitrosamine. *J Natl Cancer Inst* 1984;72:483–489.
91. Magee PN, Barnes JM. Induction of kidney tumors in the rat with dimethylnitrosamine (*N*-nitrosodimethylamine). *J Pathol Bacteriol* 1962;84:18–31.
92. Murphy GP, Mirand EA, Johnston GS, Schmidt JD, Scott WW. Renal tumors induced by a single dose of dimethylnitrosamine: morphologic, functional, enzymatic and hormonal characterization. *Invest Urol* 1966;4:39–50.
93. McGiven AR, Ireton HJC. Renal epithelial dysplasia and neoplasia in rats given dimethylnitrosamine. *J Pathol* 1972;108:187–190.
94. Druckrey H, Preussmann R, Ivankovic S, Schmahl D. Organotrope carcinogene Wirkungen bei 65 verschiedenen *N*-Nitroso-Verbindungen an BD-Ratten. *Z Krebsforsch* 1967;69:103–201.
95. Bannasch P, Schacht U, Storch E. Morphogenese und Mikromorphologie epithelialer Nierentumoren bei Nitrosomorpholin-vergifteten Ratten. I. Induktion und Histologie der Tumoren. *Z Krebsforsch* 1974;81:311–331.
96. Bannasch P, Mayer D, Krech R. Neoplastische und praeoplastische Veränderungen bei Ratten nach einmaliger oraler Applikation von *N*-Nitrosomorpholin. *J Cancer Res Clin Oncol* 1979;94:233–248.
97. Tsuda H, Moore MA, Asamoto M, et al. Comparison of the various forms of glutathione *S*-transferase with glucose-6-phosphate dehydrogenase and γ-glutamyltranspeptidase as markers of preneoplastic and neoplastic lesions in rat kidney induced by *N*-ethyl-*N*-hydroxyethylnitrosamine. *Gann* 1985;76:919–929.
98. Bannasch P, Krech R, Zerban H. Morphogenese und Mikromorphologie epithelialer Nierentumoren bei Nitrosomorpholin-vergifteten Ratten. III. Onkocytentubuli und Onkocytome. *Z Krebsforsch* 1978;92:87–104.
99. Jang JJ, Takahashi M, Hasegawa R, et al. Mammary and renal tumor induction by low doses of adriamycin in Sprague–Dawley rats. *Carcinogenesis* 1987;8:1149–1153.

100. Bulay O, Clayson DB, Shubik P. Carcinogenic effects of niridazole in rats. *Cancer Lett* 1978;4: 305–310.
101. Mauer SM, Lee CS, Najarian JS, Brown DM. Induction of malignant kidney tumors in rats with streptozotocin. *Cancer Res* 1974;34:158–160.
102. Yamasaki H. Tumor promotion: from the view point of cell society. In: Inversen OH, ed. *Theories of carcinogenesis*. Washington, DC: Hemisphere; 1988:143–157.
103. Murray AW, Fitzgerald DJ. Tumor promoters inhibit metabolic cooperation in cocultures of epidermal and 3T3 cells. *Biochem Biophys Res Commun* 1979;91:395–401.
104. Yotti LP, Chang C, Trosko JE. Elimination of metabolic cooperation in Chinese hamster cells by a tumor promoter. *Science* 1979;206:1089–1091.
105. Enomoto T, Yamasaki H. Lack of intercellular communication between chemically transformed and surrounding nontransformed BALB/c 3T3 cells. *Cancer Res* 1984;44:5200–5203.
106. Trosko JE, Chang C, Netzloff M. The role of inhibited cell–cell communication in teratogenesis. *Teratogenesis Carcinog Mutagen* 1982;2:31–45.
107. Dees JH, Heatfield BM, Reuber MD, Trump BF. Adenocarcinoma of the kidney III. Histogenesis of renal adenocarcinomas induced in rats by *N*-(4'-fluoro-4-biphenylyl)acetamide. *J Natl Cancer Inst* 1980;64:1537–1545.
108. Tsuda H, Sakata T, Tamano S, Okumura M, Ito N. Sequential observations on the appearance of neoplastic lesions in the liver and kidney after treatment with *N*-ethyl-*N*-hydroxyethylnitrosamine followed by partial hepatectomy and unilateral nephrectomy. *Carcinogenesis* 1983;4:523–528.
109. Hard GC, Butler WH. Morphogenesis of epithelial neoplasms induced in the rat kidney by dimethylnitrosamine. *Cancer Res* 1971;31:1496–1505.
110. Swann PF, Kaufman DG, Magee PN, Mace R. Induction of kidney tumours by a single dose of dimethylnitrosamine: dose response and influence of diet and benzo(*a*)pyrene pretreatment. *Br J Cancer* 1980;41:285–294.
111. Driver HE, White INH, Butler WH. Dose-response relationships in chemical carcinogenesis: renal mesenchymal tumours induced in the rat by single dose dimethylnitrosamine. *Br J Exp Pathol* 1987;68:133–143.
112. Bourgoin JJ, Cueff J, Bailly C, Dargent M. Incidence de néphroblastomes chez le rat Sprague–Dawley immundeprime soumis au DMBA. *Bull Cancer (Paris)* 1972;59:429–434.
113. Jasmin G, Riopelle JL. Nephroblastomas induced in ovariectomized rats by dimethylbenzanthracene. *Cancer Res* 1970;30:321–326.
114. Vesselinovitch SD, Koka M, Rao KV, Mihailoivh N, Rice JM. Prenatal multicarcinogenesis by ethylnitrosourea in mice. *Cancer Res* 1977;37:1822–1828.
115. Napalkov NP, Alexandrov VA, Anisimov VN. Transplacental carcinogenic effect of *N*-nitrosoethylurea in dogs. *Cancer Lett* 1981;12:161–167.
116. Fox RR, Meier H, Bedigian HG, Crary DD. Genetics of transplacentally induced teratogenic and carcinogenic effects in rabbits treated with *N*-nitroso-*N*-ethylurea. *J Natl Cancer Inst* 1982;69: 1411–1417.
117. Hard GC. Differential renal tumor response to *N*-ethylnitrosourea and dimethylnitrosamine in the Nb rat: basis for a new rodent model of nephroblastoma. *Carcinogenesis* 1985;6:1551–1558.
118. Reznik G, Mohr U. Induction of renal pelvic tumours in Sprague–Dawley rats by di-isopropanolnitrosamine. *Cancer Lett* 1976;2:87–92.
119. Kirsten WH, Anderson DG, Platz CE, Crowell EB. Observations on the morphology and frequency of polyoma tumors in rats. *Cancer Res* 1962;22:484–491.
120. Eddy BE, Stewart SE, Stanton MF, Marcotte JM. Induction of tumors in rats by tissue culture preparation of SE polyoma virus. *J Natl Cancer Inst* 1959;22:161–171.
121. Flocks JS, Weis TP, Kleiman DC, Kirsten WH. Dose-response studies to polyoma virus in rats. *J Natl Cancer Inst* 1965;35:259–284.
122. Stevens JL, Jones TW. The role of damage and proliferation in renal carcinogenesis. *Toxicol Lett* 1990;53:121–126.
123. Kirkman H, Bacon RL. Malignant renal tumors in male hamsters (*Cricetus auratus*) treated with estrogens. *Cancer Res* 1950;10:122–124.
124. Li JJ, Li SA, Klicka JK, Parsons JA, Lam LKT. Relative carcinogenic activity of various synthetic and natural estrogens in the Syrian hamster kidney. *Cancer Res* 1983;43:5200–5204.
125. Li JJ, Li SA. Estrogen-induced tumorigenesis in hamsters: roles for hormonal and carcinogenic activities. *Arch Toxicol* 1984;55:110–118.
126. Li JJ, Cuthbertson TL, Li SA. Inhibition of estrogen tumorigenesis in the Syrian golden hamster kidney by antiestrogens. *J Natl Cancer Inst* 1980;64:795–800.

127. Liehr JG, Stancel GM, Chorich LP, Bousfield GR, Ulubelen AA. Hormonal carcinogenesis: separation of etrogenicity from carcinogenicity. *Chem Biol Interact* 1986;59:173–184.
128. Metzler M. Nephrocarcinogenicity of estrogens. *Toxicol Letter* 1990;53:111–114.
129. Metzler M, McLachlan JA. Oxidative metabolism of diethylstilbestrol and steroidal estrogens as a potential factor in their fetotoxicity. In: Neuberr D, Merker HJ, Nau H, Langman J, eds. *Role of pharmacokinetics in prenatal and perinatal toxicology*. Stuttgart; Germany: Georg Thieme; 1978; 157–164.
130. Ames BN. Dietary carcinogens and anticarcinogens. *Science* 1983;221:1256–1264.
131. Cerutti P. Prooxidant states and tumor promotion. *Science* 1985;227:377–381.
132. Liehr JG, Randerath K, Randerath E. Target organ-specific covalent DNA damage preceding diethylstilbestrol-induced carcinogenesis. *Carcinogenesis* 1985;6:1067–1069.
133. Liehr JG, Avitts TA, Randerath E, Randerath K. Estrogen-induced endogenous DNA adduction: possible mechanism of hormonal cancer. *Proc Natl Acad Sci USA* 1986;83:5301–5305.
134. Llombart-Bosch A, Peydro A. Morphological histochemical and ultrastructural observations of diethylstilbestrol-induced kidney tumors in the Syrian golden hamster. *Eur J Cancer* 1975;11:403–412.
135. Kirkman H, Robbins M. Estrogen-induced tumors of the kidney. V. Histology and histogenesis in the Syrian hamster. *Natl Cancer Inst Monogr* 1959;1:93–139.
136. Hamilton JM, Flaks A, Saluja PG, Maguire S. Hormonally induced renal neoplasia in the male Syrian hamster and the inhibitory effect of 2-bromo-α-ergocryptine methanesulfonate. *J Natl Cancer Inst* 1975;54:1385–1400.
137. Goldfarb S, Pugh TH. Morphology and anatomic localization of renal microneoplasms and proximal tubule dysplasias induced by four different estrogens in the hamster. *Cancer Res* 1990;50:113–119.
138. Hacker HJ, Bannasch P, Liehr J. Histochemical analysis of the development of estradiol-induced kidney tumors in male Syrian hamsters. *Cancer Res* 1988;48:971–976.
139. Gonzales A, Oberley TD, Li JJ. Morphological and immunohistochemical studies of the estrogen-induced Syrian hamster renal tumor: probable cell of origin. *Cancer Res* 1989;49:1020–1028.
140. Rosen VJ, Castanera TJ, Kimeldorf DJ, Jones DC. Renal neoplasms in the irradiated and nonirradiated Sprague–Dawley rat. *Am J Pathol* 1961;38:359–369.
141. Rosen VJ, Castanera TJ, Kimeldorf DJ, Jones DC. Pancreatic islet-cell tumors and renal tumors in the male rat following neutron exposure. *Lab Invest* 1962;11:204–210.
142. Berdjis CC. Kidney tumours and irradiation pathogenesis of kidney tumours in irradiated rats. *Oncologia (Basel)* 1963;16:312–324.
143. Sanotskii VA, Erleksova EV. Morphological changes in rats at long intervals after administration of Po^{210}. *Fed Proc* 1964 [23 Trans Suppl];785–788.
144. Ito N, Hiasa Y, Tamai A, Yoshida K. Effect of unilateral nephrectomy on the development of kidney tumor in rats treated with *N*-nitrosodimethylamine. *Gann* 1969;60:319–327.
145. Williams PD, Bhanalaph T, Murphy GP. Unilateral nephrectomy. Its effects on primary murine renal adenocarcinoma. *Urology* 1973;2:619–622.
146. Murphy GP, Sufrin G, Williams PD. Effect of unilateral nephrectomy on tumor growth of the murine renal cell adenocarcinoma and neuroblastoma. *Oncology* 1984;41:417–419.
147. Ohmori T. Enhancing effect on *N*-nitrosodimethylamine-induced tumorigenesis by unilateral hydronephrosis. *J Natl Cancer Inst* 1984;73:951–957.
148. Matas B, Simmon RL, Lkjellstrand LM, Buselmeter TJ, Majarian JS. Increased incidence of malignancy during chronic renal failure. *Lancet* 1975;1:883–886.
149. Ohmori T, Sekigawa S, Sunagawa M, et al. Confirmation of the development of multiple renal cell tumors in end-stage long-term hemodialysis kidney revealing typical acquired cystic transformation. *Acta Pathol Jpn* 1981;31:1097–1104.
150. Sufrin G, Green D, Pontes JE, Williams PD, Murphy GP. Effect of unilateral nephrectomy on growth of the Wistar/Furth Wilms' tumor. *J Urol* 1984;131:378–382.
151. Trindade JCS, Rangel MC, Ross JH, et al. Influence of nephrectomy on the growth of a murine Wilms tumor: a study using parabiotic rat. *J Urol* 1990;144:418–421.
152. Riopelle JL, Jasmin G. Nature, classification and nomenclature of kidney tumors induced in the rat by dimethylnitrosamine. *J Nalt Cancer Inst* 1969;42:643–662.
153. Hard GC, Butler WH. Ultrastructural analysis of renal mesenchymal tumor induced in the rat by dimethylnitrosamine. *Cancer Res* 1971;31:348–365.
154. Alden CL, Kanerva RL. The pathogenesis of renal cortical tumor in rats fed 2% trisodium nitrilotriacetate monohydrate. *Food Chem Toxicol* 1980;20:441–450.

155. Alden CL, Kanerva RL, Anderson RL, Adkins AG. Short-term effects of dietary nitrilotriacetic acid in the male Charles River rat kidney. *Vet Pathol* 1981;18:549–559.
156. Myers MC, Kanerva RL, Alden CL, Anderson RL. Reversibility of nephrotoxicity induced in rats by nitrilotriacetate in subchronic feeding studies. *Food Chem Toxicol* 1982;20:925–934.
157. Jasmin G, Riopelle JL. Renal adenomas induced by dimethylnitrosamine. Enzyme histochemistry in the rat. *Arch Pathol* 1968;85:298–305.
158. Heatfield BM, Hinton DE, Trump BF. Adenocarcinoma of the kidney. II. Enzyme histochemistry of renal adenocarcinoma induced in rat by N-(4-fluoro-4-biphenylyl)acetamide. *J Natl Cancer Inst* 1976;57:795–808.
159. Ford SM, Hook JB. Biochemical mechanisms of toxic nephropathies. *Semin Nephrol* 1984;4:88–106.
160. Kitahara A, Satoh K, Sato K. Properties of the increased glutathione S-transferase A form in rat preneoplastic hepatic lesions induced by chemical carcinogens. *Biochem Biophys Res Commun* 1983;112:20–28.
161. Kitahara A, Satoh K, Nishimura K, et al. Changes in molecular forms of rat hepatic glutathione S-transferase during chemical hepatocarcinogenesis. *Cancer Res* 1984;44:2698–2703.
162. Sato K, Kitahara A, Satoh K, Ishikawa T, Tatematsu M, Ito N. The placental form of glutathione S-transferase as a new marker protein for preneoplasia in rat chemical hepatocarcinogenesis. *Gann* 1984;75:199–202.
163. Mayer D, Weber E, Kadenbach B, Bannasch P. Immunocytochemical demonstration of cytochrome c oxidase as a marker for renal oncocytes and oncocytomas. *Toxicol Pathol* 1989;17:46–49.
164. Hiasa Y, Lin JC, Konishi N, Kitahori Y, Enoki N, Shimoyama T. Histopathological and biochemical analyses of transplantable renal adenocarcinoma in rats induced by N-ethyl-N-hydroxyethylnitrosamine. *Cancer Res* 1984;44:1664–1670.
165. Konishi N, Kitahori Y, Shimoyama T, Lin JC, Hiasa Y. Monoclonal antibody against rat renal cell tumor-associated antigen as a new tool for the analysis of renal tumorigenesis. *Jpn J Cancer Res* 1989;80:771–777.
166. Maunsbach AB. Observations on the segmentation of the proximal tubules in the rat kidney. Comparison of results from phase contrast, fluorescence and electron microscopy. *J Ultrastruct Res* 1966;16:239–258.
167. Doull J, Klaassen CD, Amdur MO, eds. *Casarett and Doull's toxicology: the basic science of poisons*. 2nd ed. New York: Macmillan; 1980.
168. Merski JA. Acute structural changes in renal tubular epithelium following administration of nitrilotriacetate. *Food Chem Toxicol* 191;19:463–470.
169. Merski JA, Meyers MC. Light- and electron-microscopic evaluation of renal tubular cell vacuolation induced by administration of nitrilotriacetate or sucrose. *Food Chem Toxicol* 1985;23:923–930.
170. Halder CA, Holdsworth CE, Cockrell BY, Piccirillo VJ. Hydrocarbon nephropathy in male rats: identification of the nephrotoxic components of unleaded gasoline. *Toxicol Ind Health* 1985;1:67–87.
171. Oliver J, MacDowell M, Tracy A, et al. The pathogenesis of acute renal failure associated with traumatic and toxic injury, renal ischemia, nephrotoxic damage and the ischemic episode. *J Clin Invest* 1951;30:1307–1439.
172. Woodard JC, Alvarez MR. Renal lesions in rats fed diets containing alpha protein. *Arch Pathol* 1967;84:153–162.
173. Rush GF, Smith JH, Newton JF, Hook JB. Chemically induced nephrotoxicity: role of metabolic activation. *CRC Crit Rev Toxicol* 1984;13:99–160.
174. McDowell EM, Nagle RB, Zalure RC, McNeil JS, Flanenbaum W, Trump BF. Studies on the pathophysiology of acute renal failure. I. Correlation of ultrastructure and function in the proximal tubule of the rat following administration of mercuric chloride. *Virchows Arch B Cell Pathol* 1976;22:173–196.
175. McMurtry RJ, Snodgrass WR, Mitchell JR. Renal necrosis, glutathione depletion, and covalent binding after acetaminophen. *Toxicol Appl Pharmacol* 1978;46:87–100.
176. Nash JA, King LJ, Lock EA, Green T. The metabolism and disposition of hexachloro-1,3-butadiene in the rat and its relevance to nephrotoxicity. *Toxicol Appl Pharmacol* 1984;73:124–137.
177. Laurent G, Toubeau G, Heuson-Stiennon JA, Tulkens P, Maldague P. Kidney tissue repair after nephrotoxic injury. Biochemical and morphological characterization. *Crit Rev Toxicol* 1988;19:147–183.

178. Lock EA. Studies on the mechanism of nephrotoxicity and nephrocarcinogenicity of halogenated alkenes. *Crit Rev Toxicol* 1988;19:23–42.
179. Grasso P. Persistent organ damage and cancer production in rats and mice. *Arch Toxicol Suppl* 1987;11:75–83.
180. Clayson DB. Can a mechanistic rationale be provided for non-genotoxic carcinogens identified in rodent bioassays? *Mutat Res* 1989;221:53–67.
181. Clayson DB, Nera EA, Lok E. The potential for the use of cell proliferation studies in carcinogen risk assessment. *Regul Toxicol Pharmacol* 1989;9:284–295.
182. Wachsmuth ED. Chemcially induced cell turnover in the kidney and its possible role in carcinogenesis. In: Butterworth BE, Slaga TJ, eds. *Banbury report 25: nongenotoxic mechanims in carcinogenesis*. Cold Spring Harbor, NY: Cold Spring Harbor Laboratory; 1987:137–150.
183. Seifert J, Mostecka H. Effect of nafenopin and clofibrate on uptake and utilization of labeled thymidine for DNA synthesis in rat liver and kidney. *Carcinogenesis* 1988;9:3–8.
184. Ward JM, Weghorst BA, Diwan BA, Konishi N, Lubet RA, Henneman JR, Devor DE. Evaluation of cell proliferation in the kidney of rodents with bromodeoxyuridine immunohistochemistry or tritiated thymidine autoradiography after exposure to renal toxins, tumor promoters and carcinogens. *Prog Clin Biol Res* 1991;369:369–388.
185. Maher JF. Toxic neophropathy. In: Brenner BM, Rector FC Jr, eds. *The kidney*. Philadelphia: WB Saunders; 1976.
186. Coleman GL, Barthold SW, Osbaldiston GW, Foster ST, Jonas AM. Pathological changes during aging in barrier-reared Fischer 344 male rats. *J Gerontol* 1977;32:258–278.
187. Konishi N, Ward JM. Increased levels of DNA synthesis in hyperplastic renal tubules of aging nephropathy in female F344/NCr rats. *Vet Pathol* 1989;26:6–10.
188. Reuber MD. Hyperplastic and neoplastic lesions of the kidney in Buffalo rats of varying ages ingesting N-4-(4'-fluorobiphenyl)acetamide. *J Natl Cancer Inst* 1975;54:427–429.
189. Jaffe DR, Gandolfi AJ, Brendel K. Chronic toxicity of *S-trans*-(1,2-dichlorovinyl)-L-cysteine in mice. *J Appl Toxicol* 1985;4:315–319.
190. Farber JL. Biology of disease: membrane injury and calcium homeostasis in the pathogenesis of coagulative necrosis. *Lab Invest* 1982;47:114–123.
191. Vamvakas S, Anders MW. Perturbation of calcium homeostasis as a link between acute cell injury and carcinogenesis in the kidney. *Toxicol Lett* 1990;53:115–120.
192. Trump BG, Berezesky J. Ion regulation, cell injury and carcinogenesis. *Carcinogenesis* 1987;8:1027–1031.
193. Loewenstein WR. Junctional intercellular communication and the control of growth. *Biochim Biophys Acta* 1979;560:1–65.
194. Konishi N, Donovan PJ, Ward JM. Differential effects of renal carcinogens and tumor promoters on growth promotion and inhibition of gap junctional communication in two rat renal epithelial cell lines. *Carcinogenesis* 1990;11:903–908.
195. Henschler D, Dekant W. Nephrocarcinogenic xenobiotics. *Toxicol Lett* 1990;53:105–110.
196. Diwan BA, Rice JM. Organ and species specificity in chemical carcinogenesis and tumor promotion. In: Sirica AE, ed. *The pathobiology of neoplasia*. New York: Plenum; 1989:149–171.
197. Kaufmann WK, Rice JM, Wenk ML, Devor D, Kaufman DG. Cell cycle-dependent initiation of hepatocarcinogenesis in rats by methyl(acetoxymethyl)nitrosamine. *Cancer Res* 1987;47:1263–1266.
198. Lipsky MM, Trump BF. Chemically induced renal epithelial neoplasia in experimental animals. In: Richter GW, ed. *International review of experimental pathology, kidney diseases*. Vol 30. San Diego, CA: Academic Press; 1987:357–383.
199. Reichert D, Neudlecker T, Schutz S. Mutagenicity of hexachlorobutadiene, perchlorobutenoic acid and perchlorobutenoic acid chloride. *Mutat Res* 1984;137:89–93.
200. *Toxicology and carcinogenesis studies of tetrachloroethylene (perchloroethylene) in F344/N rats and B6C3F1 mice (inhalation studies)*. NTP Technical Report 311. Research Triangle Park, NC: National Toxicology Program, 1986.
201. Dekant W, Metzler M, Henschler D. Identification of S-1, 2, 2-trichlorovinyl-N-acetylcysteine as a urinary metabolite of tetrachloroethylene: bioactivation through glutathione conjugation as a possible explanation of its nephrocarcinogenicity. *J Biochem Toxicol* 1986;1:57–72.
202. Green T, Odum J, Foster JR, Hext PM. Perchloroethylene induced hepatic peroxisome proliferation in mice and renal hyaline droplet formation in rats. *Toxicologist* 1986;6:314.
203. Goldsworthy TL, Lyght O, Popp JA. Relationship between alpha-2u-globulin, protein droplet accumulation and cell replication in male and female rats exposed to chlorinated hydrocarbons. *Proc Am Assoc Cancer Res* 1987;28:87(343).

204. Nogueira E. Rat renal carcinogenesis after chronic simultaneous exposure to lead acetate and N-nitrosodiethylamine. *Virchows Arch B Cell Pathol* 1987;53:365–374.
205. Sukumar S, Perantoni A, Reed C, Rice JM, Wenk M. Activated K-*ras* and N-*ras* oncogenes in primary renal mesenchymal tumors induced in F344 rats by methyl(methoxymethyl)nitrosamine. *Mol Cell Biol* 1986;6:2716–2720.
206. Zbar BH, Brauch C, Talmadge M, Linehan WM. Loss of alleles of loci on the short arm of chromosome 3 in renal cell carcinoma. *Nature (London)* 1987;327:721–724.
207. Nanus DM, Ebrahim SAD, Bander NH. Transformation of human kidney proximal tubule cells by *ras*-containing retroviruses. *J Exp Med* 1989;169:953–972.

Carcinogenesis, edited by
M.P. Waalkes and J.M. Ward.
Published by Raven Press, Ltd.,
New York, 1994.

6
Urinary Bladder Carcinogenesis in the Rodent

Charles H. Frith, *David L. Greenman, and †Samuel M. Cohen

*Toxicology Pathology Associates, Little Rock, Arkansas 72211;
Office of Director and Scientific Coordination, National Center for Toxicology Research, Jefferson, Arkansas 72079; †Departments of Pathology and Microbiology, University of Nebraska Medical Center, Omaha, Nebraska 68198

One of the major problems in the study of experimental carcinogenesis is that of organ specificity. Review of data reveals that not all tissues of the mouse and rat are equally at risk for neoplasia. Spontaneous neoplasms of the rodent urinary bladder are rare (1,2); however, the urinary bladder of the rodent serves as an excellent target for urinary bladder carcinogenesis, as evidenced by the induction of urinary bladder tumors in both rats and mice with a variety of carcinogens (3–7). The primary metabolically active cells of the urinary bladder are the transitional epithelial cells that line the entire lower urinary tract. These cells have a very low normal mitotic index in the postweaning animal. However, they readily respond to stimuli such as crystals, calculi, and chemicals (8–10) within the urine and are susceptible to injury because of their location. The urinary bladder is the most susceptible area of the lower urinary tract, apparently because of its storage function and extended exposure time to urinary toxicants.

Hyperplasia and neoplasia of the urinary bladder have been studied extensively in these species with model compounds such as 2-acetylaminofluorene (2-AAF) (11, 12) and *N*-[4-(5-nitro-2-furyl)-2-thiazolyl]formamide (FANFT) (13,14). Although the diagnosis of urinary bladder neoplasms is fairly straightforward, a consensus cannot always be reached on equivocal lesions (15). The purpose of this chapter is to present an overview of urinary bladder carcinogenesis in rats and mice, including anatomy, preparation for microscopic evaluation, a classification of proliferative lesions, comparison with other species, and factors modulating tumor development in the urinary bladder.

ANATOMY OF THE URINARY BLADDER

Gross Appearance

The urinary bladder of both the mouse and rat is a muscular pear-shaped structure located in the posterior abdominal cavity in the midline of the body ventral to the colon. The size of the urinary bladder and the thickness of the smooth muscle wall vary with the amount of urine in the bladder (16). The ureters, which originate from the renal pelvis of the kidneys, extend from the hilus of the kidneys to the dorsal neck of the urinary bladder. An intramural part of the ureter courses through the bladder musculature. The area of the urinary bladder where the ureters enter is called the *trigone*. Posteriorly, the bladder neck is continuous with the urethra. The urinary bladder can be divided into dorsal and ventral areas as well as the blind dome, which is referred to as the *fundus* or *vertex*. The urinary bladder is attached to the ventral body wall by the ventral ligament.

Microscopic Features

Light Microscopy

The urinary bladder is a muscular hollow organ, lined by a mucosa resting on a basement membrane which is separated from the smooth muscle by a layer of connective tissue. The mucosa of the renal pelvis, ureters, urethra, and urinary bladder is composed of a multilayered transitional epithelium, which is also referred to as *urothelium*. The transitional epithelium of the urinary bladder of both the mouse and the rat consists of three distinct layers (Fig. 1). Using light microscopy and depending on the distension of the urinary bladder, the epithelium may appear to be only one or two cells thick; however, with transmission electron microscopy, the epithelium is definitely three cell layers thick (9,17,18). The surface cells, which contact the urine, are extremely large, with prominent eosinophilic cytoplasm and may be multinucleated or polyploid. These cells have been referred to as *umbrella cells* since they cover the underlying intermediate cells, which are somewhat smaller and are generally round to oval with a centrally placed nucleus and a moderate amount of cytoplasm. The basal cells are similar in appearance but somewhat smaller than the intermediate cells and rest against a thin basement membrane interposed between the epithelium and lamina propria. The lamina propria is vascular and sometimes contains foci of lymphocytes, especially in the mouse. The lamina propria has

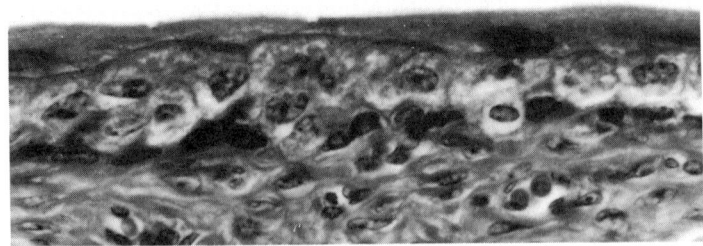

FIG. 1. Light photomicrograph of normal urinary bladder epithelium of a mouse. H&E, ×555.

been designated by some as submucosa and by others as subepithelial connective tissue. The musculature is composed of smooth muscle bundles of irregular size separated by collagen. Around the neck of the bladder, the muscle bundles are arranged circularly to form the bladder sphincter.

Electron Microscopy

The transitional epithelium of the rodent assumes the normal adult ultrastructural pattern by 3 to 4 weeks of age, when three distinct cell layers become readily visible (18). One group of investigators (18) studied bladders from fetal and neonatal BALB/c mice and Sprague–Dawley rats with scanning and transmission electron microscopy to establish the sequence of events in their morphological development. On fetal day 18 or 19, the epithelium from the mouse and the rat displayed two or three distinct layers. With transmission electron microscopy, a starlike contraction of the cell surface was seen in the mouse urinary bladder but was not seen in the developing rat urinary bladder. The significance of this starlike contraction of the cell surface is not known. In both the rat and the mouse, some of the superficial cells sloughed between fetal day 18 or 19 and the day of birth. On the day of birth, the epithelium was composed of only two layers. Three weeks after birth, the epithelium was three cell layers thick and appeared as the adult pattern with both scanning (Fig. 2) and transmission electron microscopy (Fig. 3).

Cohen et al. (19) found similar appearances in the developing rat bladder, and also examined earlier periods of development. At days 11 and 12 of gestation, the bladder epithelium consists of a single layer of cuboidal cells which are frequently dividing. By day 13, their surface is covered by numerous uniform microvilli and single, central cilia appear which are present until approximately gestation day 17. The large, polygonal superficial cells of the adult urothelium appear at approximately 17 days of gestation.

The luminal surface epithelial cells contain a unique membrane system referred to as the asymmetric membrane. This membrane system is believed to allow for the expansion of the urinary bladder as it fills with urine, and the quantity of the membrane system decreases as the bladder fills with urine. With scanning electron microscopy, the luminal surface contains fine microridges formed by regularly arranged polygonal cells (18).

PREPARATION OF THE URINARY BLADDER FOR MICROSCOPIC EVALUATION

Technical preparation of the urinary bladder for proper microscopic evaluation is of extreme importance for facilitating proper histopathological diagnosis (5,20). Inflation of the urinary bladder with fixative and trimming and sectioning are all important.

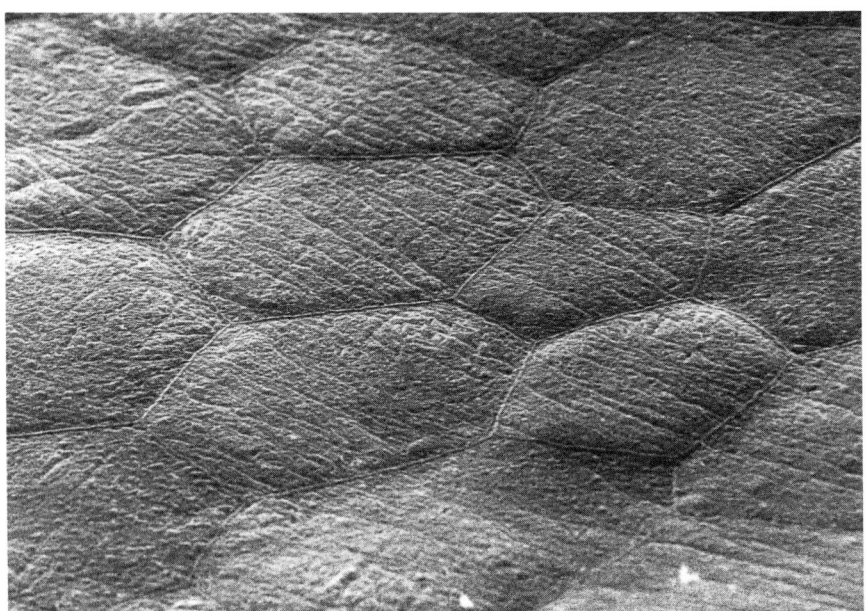

FIG. 2. Scanning electron micrograph of normal urothelium of an adult mouse. Note the hexagonal shape. Uranyl acetate–lead citrate, ×1,050. [Reprinted from Frith et al. (9), with permission.]

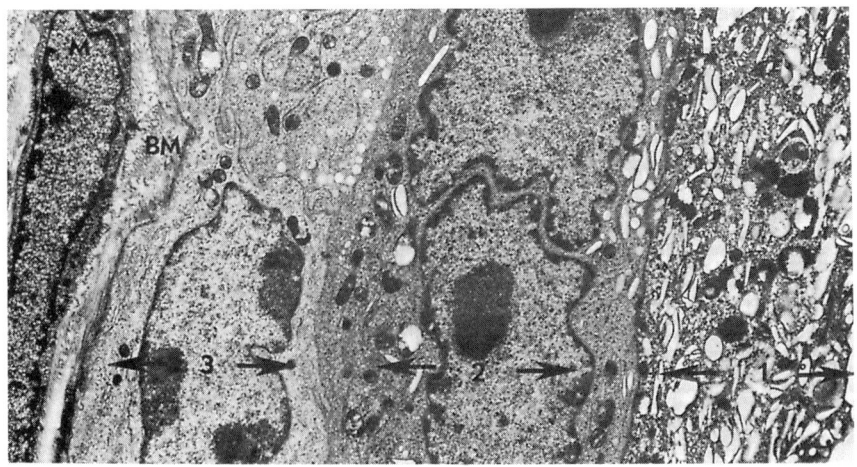

FIG. 3. Transmission electron micrograph of normal urothelium of an adult mouse. Note three cell layers: (1) superficial layer, (2) intermediate layer, (3) basal layer. BM, basement membrane. Uranyl acetate–lead citrate, ×7,800. [Reprinted from Frith et al. (16), with permission.]

Inflation of the Urinary Bladder

Pathologists with experience in the microscopic evaluation of rodent urinary bladders can readily assess the inflated or uninflated urinary bladder mucosa for hyperplasia. However, the inexperienced pathologist may interpret the normal thickness and artifactual folds of the uninflated urinary bladder mucosa to be hyperplasia. The urinary bladder of rodents can be inflated via two methods. The first and less effective of the two is to inject the fixative into the lumen through the muscular wall with a small-gauge (24 to 26 gauge) needle. This sometimes results in deposition of the fixative into the bladder wall rather than the lumen, resulting in microscopic distortion of the bladder epithelium and making interpretation of the urothelium difficult. The second and preferred method is inflation through the urethra with a blunt needle. In either case, the bladder should be filled to normal size but should not be overinflated. If the urinary bladder is already full of urine, the urine can be withdrawn by either method and the bladder refilled with fixative. The urinary bladder will stay inflated in males if the coagulating glands and seminal vesicles are removed *in toto* with the urinary bladder. It may be necessary to place a ligature around the neck of the bladder to prevent the fixative from leaking. The distended bladder should be immersed in fixative after proper inflation. For electron microscopy, fixation may be better if the urinary bladder is divided longitudinally into halves after 1 h of fixation. For light microscopy, the urinary bladder may be inflated with a fixative such as 10% neutral buffered formalin; for electron microscopy, it is better to inflate with a fixative such as glutaraldehyde. If orientation of the urinary bladder is important, the ventral or other surface of the urinary bladder can be identified with a dot of India ink at the time of necropsy. The ink will remain on the bladder wall during processing and can be visualized with the microscope.

Trimming and Sectioning of the Urinary Bladder

For most routine studies where no histopathology of the urinary bladder is anticipated, the inflated urinary bladder can be removed from the fixative and divided sagittally into two halves. These halves may be embedded into a single paraffin block with the luminal side down, and a single section may be taken for two complete sagittal sections of the urinary bladder. If the urinary bladder is a target organ or bladder lesions are expected, the urinary bladder should be divided and the mucosa should be examined carefully with a dissecting microscope. Suspect lesions can be identified and the urinary bladder can be trimmed to include the suspect lesions for sectioning. A second method of trimming the urinary bladder, which provides more mucosal surface for microscopic examination, includes dividing each bladder half into three to five strips and embedding the strips on end in a single paraffin block for sectioning (2). Since the lesions in the urinary bladder mucosa may be extremely small and multifocal, serial sectioning (sectioning completely through the bladder) may be necessary and has been shown to increase significantly the identification of microscopic lesions (20). Of a total of 517 BALB/c mice with transitional cell carcinomas, serial sectioning was found to increase significantly the diagnosis of bladder tumors. Sixty-two (12%) of the 517 bladder carcinomas would not have been diagnosed if only one section per bladder half had been examined rather than serial sections.

PROLIFERATIVE LESIONS OF THE URINARY BLADDER

Spontaneous Lesions

Hyperplasia

Hyperplasia usually precedes the development of neoplasia (21) and may occur as a spontaneous lesion in both rats and mice. Hyperplasia may be classified as simple, nodular, or papillary, and may be either a focal, multifocal, or diffuse lesion (1). These lesions are described fully in the section on induced lesions. Spontaneous hyperplasia usually occurs as simple hyperplasia, but nodular and papillary hyperplasia are sometimes seen. The spontaneous lesions may occur without evidence of an etiology, but most often is associated secondarily with either urinary bladder calculi or inflammation of the urinary bladder (cystitis) (Fig. 4). Focal hyperplasia may occur as a response to submucosal infiltrates of neoplastic cells such as those observed with disseminated hematopoietic neoplasms. An association with calculi or crystalluria can occasionally be suggested by observing increased calcification in tissues (possibly using a special stain for calcium, such as the von Kossa stain) or by screening urine by light or scanning electron microscopic observations (22).

Neoplasia

Spontaneous bladder neoplasms are extremely rare in the mouse (23) but are noted occasionally in rats (24). In one study involving 3,000 virgin and 800 retired breeder BALB/c and C57BL/6 mice, untreated and of both sexes, no urinary bladder tumors were seen (25). In the large ED_{01} study conducted at the National Center for Toxicological Research in Jefferson, Arkansas, where over 20,000 BALB/c female mice were administered either a control diet or a diet containing one of seven dose levels of 2-acetylaminofluorene, no spontaneous bladder carcinomas were seen (6). Initially, a small number of bladder tumors were diagnosed in the control group, but reevaluation of these lesions by one of the authors (CHF) resulted in a diagnosis of chronic cystitis and nodular hyperplasia (26).

In a large study performed at International Research and Development Corporation (IRDC) in Mattawan, Michigan, involving the evaluation of the dose response and *in utero* exposure to saccharin in the Sprague–Dawley rat, 2,500 second-generation male rats were administered a control diet or a diet with one of six dose levels of saccharin (2). No bladder tumors were seen in the control group, but five bladder

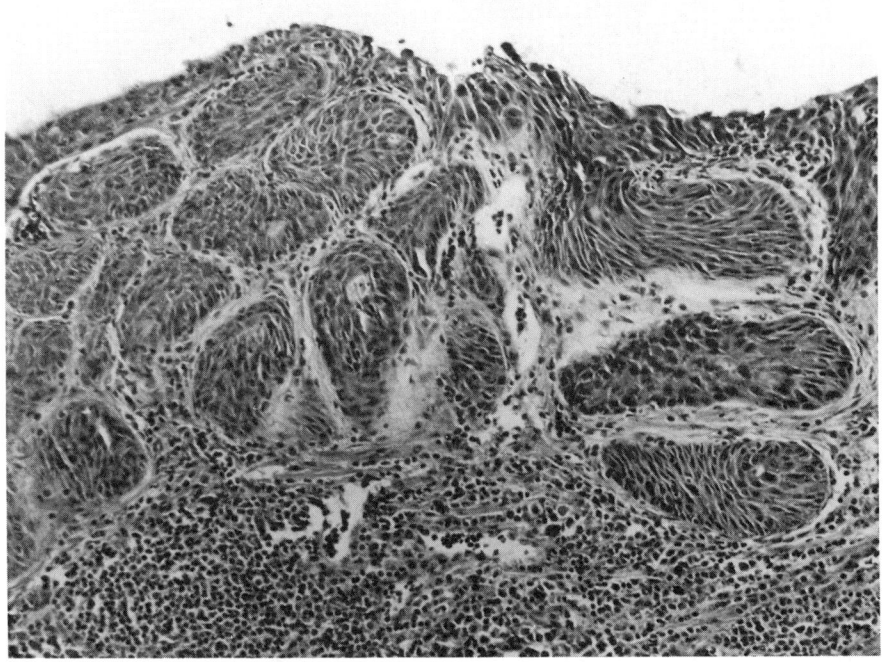

FIG. 4. Chronic inflammation and nodular hyperplasia in a control mouse. H&E, ×140.

neoplasms (four papillomas and one carcinoma) were seen in the 1% sodium saccharin group. Some of these were believed to have been spontaneous tumors since the background historical incidence of spontaneous bladder tumors at IRDC in male Sprague–Dawley rats was 0.8%. Lymphomatous and/or leukemic infiltrates occur in the urinary bladder, especially in the submucosa, and most commonly in strains of mice with high spontaneous incidences of lymphoma or leukemia (22).

Induced Lesions

Hyperplasia

Hyperplasia of the transitional epithelium is an uncommon spontaneous lesion, but it is a common finding in animals treated with bladder carcinogens and certain other compounds and may be either focal, multifocal, or diffuse (Figs. 5 and 6) and simple, papillary, or nodular (Table 1) (1,27,28,77). Urothelial hyperplasia is a primary response to many urothelial carcinogens but may also be associated secondarily with chronic cystitis or calculus formation induced by such compounds as cyclophosphamide or 4-ethylsulfonylnaphthalene-1-sulfonamide (ENS) (8,9,29,30). Simple hyperplasia may be quantitated as mild, moderate, or marked. Lesions have

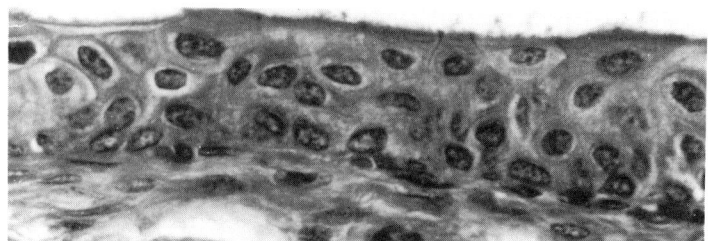

FIG. 5. Diffuse simple hyperplasia. H&E, ×555.

been classified as mild hyperplasia when the urothelium averages four transitional cell layers thick, as moderate when it averages five to six cell layers, and as marked when it averages seven or more cell layers. Mild hyperplasia, particularly if focal, may require extensive serial sectioning of the bladder to detect it or even scanning electron microscopy or labeling index analyses with tritiated thymidine or bromodeoxyuridine (22). Table 2 lists a variety of chemically induced toxic and neoplastic changes induced in the rodent urinary bladder.

Papillary hyperplasia (Fig. 7) differs from simple hyperplasia in that the urothelial surface is irregular due to papillary projections, rather than flattened or squa-

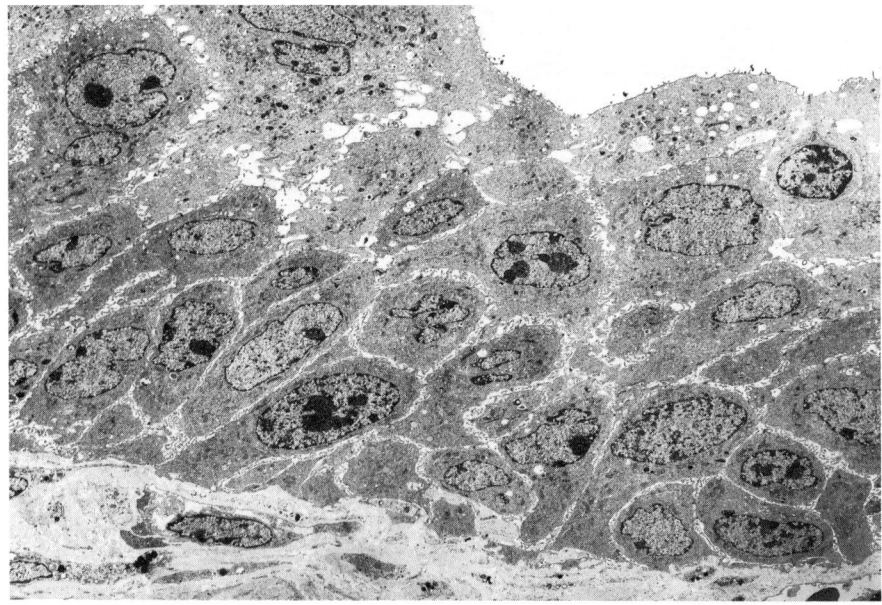

FIG. 6. Transmission electron micrograph of simple hyperplasia of a mouse urinary bladder. Uranyl acetate–lead citrate, ×1,400. [Reprinted from Frith et al. (9), with permission.]

TABLE 1. *Morphological classification of proliferative lesions of the urinary bladder of rodents*

Hyperplasia
  Simple
  Papillary
  Nodular
Diverticula
Neoplasia
  Primary epithelial neoplasms
    Benign: papilloma
    Malignant: carcinoma
      By histological pattern
        Papillary
        Nonpapillary
      By histologic cell type
        Transitional
        Transitional with squamous differentiation
        Squamous cell
        Undifferentiated
        Adenocarcinoma
      By depth of invasion
        Stage 0: noninfiltrative (carcinoma in situ)
        Stage A: invasion into submucosa
        Stage B: early invasion into muscle wall
        Stage C: deep invasion into muscle wall
        Stage D: invasion by local extension or distant metastasis
  Primary mesenchymal neoplasms
    Vascular tumors
      Hemangioma
      Hemangiosarcoma
    Muscular tumors
      Leiomyoma
      Leiomyosarcoma
      Rhabdomyosarcoma
    Fibrous connective tissue tumors
      Fibroma
      Fibrosarcoma
    Others
      Undifferentiated sarcoma
      Hematopoietic neoplasms
      Lymphoma
      Mixed sarcoma–carcinoma
  Metastatic tumors

Modifed from Frith (1).

mous. Papillary hyperplasia occurs much more frequently in rats than in mice both as a spontaneous and as an induced lesion. Nodular hyperplasia (Fig. 8) (epithelial downgrowths) may occur in conjunction with either simple or papillary hyperplasia. These nodular downgrowths exist as solid islands or cords of transitional epithelial cells that extend into the lamina propria. Acute and/or chronic inflammation often accompanies the hyperplasia, which may be focal, multifocal, or diffuse. Nodular hyperplasia is comparable morphologically to von Brunn's nests or to cystitis cys-

TABLE 2. *Examples of chemically induced toxic and neoplastic changes of the urinary bladder*

Compound	Histopathology[a]	Refs.
ENS	Crystalluria/nodular hyperplasia	8,29
FANFT	Transitional cell carcinomas	14
ENS	Calculi	8,29
Melamine	Calculi and transitional carcinomas	10
Benzidine dihydrochloride	Vacuolization	95,96
ENS	Hyperplasia/pleomorphic microvilli (EM)	9
FANFT	Pleomorphic microvilli (EM)	13
2-AAF[b]	Hyperplasia	11
OTOS[c]	Neoplasia	97
2-AAF	Hyperplasia/neoplasia	37
BBN[d]	Papillomas/carcinomas	7
Sodium saccharin	Hyperplasia/neoplasia	2

From Alden and Frith (94).
[a]EM, ultrastructural change.
[b]2-AAF, 2-acetylaminofluorene.
[c]OTOS, *N*-oxydiethylene thiocarbamyl-*N*-oxydiethylene sulfenamide.
[d]BBN, *N*-butyl-*N*-(4-hydroxybutyl)nitrosamine.

tica in humans. The inexperienced pathologist may diagnose nodular hyperplasia as carcinoma. Depending on sectioning, focal areas of nodular hyperplasia may appear to be invading the lamina propria and have no connection to the mucosa. If serial sections are examined, however, areas of nodular hyperplasia are continuous with the mucosa. Also, in contrast to carcinomas, nodular hyperplasia does not have cellular atypia or dysplasia.

One study compared experimental and spontaneously occurring hyperplasia in BALB/c mice administered 2-acetylaminofluorene (2-AAF) or 4-ethylfulfonylnaphthalene-1-sulfonamide (ENS) (21). Nodular hyperplasia was located more commonly in the vertex of the bladder of the 2-AAF-treated mice but was more commonly located in the neck region of the urinary bladder in ENS and control mice. The 2-AAF-induced hyperplasia appeared to be capable of regression or progression to neoplasia. The ENS-induced and spontaneously occurring nodular hyperplasia appeared to be secondary to chronic cystitis and did not appear to progress to neoplasia.

Pleomorphic Microvilli

Changes induced by urinary toxicants as shown by scanning electron microscopy (SEM) include a number of nonspecific changes, including irregularity in the shape and size of the transitional epithelial cells, sloughing of epithelial cells, and the presence of pleomorphic microvilli. Pleomorphic microvilli have been identified in rats given various urinary bladder carcinogens as early as 8 weeks after beginning of exposure. They also have been observed in other experimental cancer models as

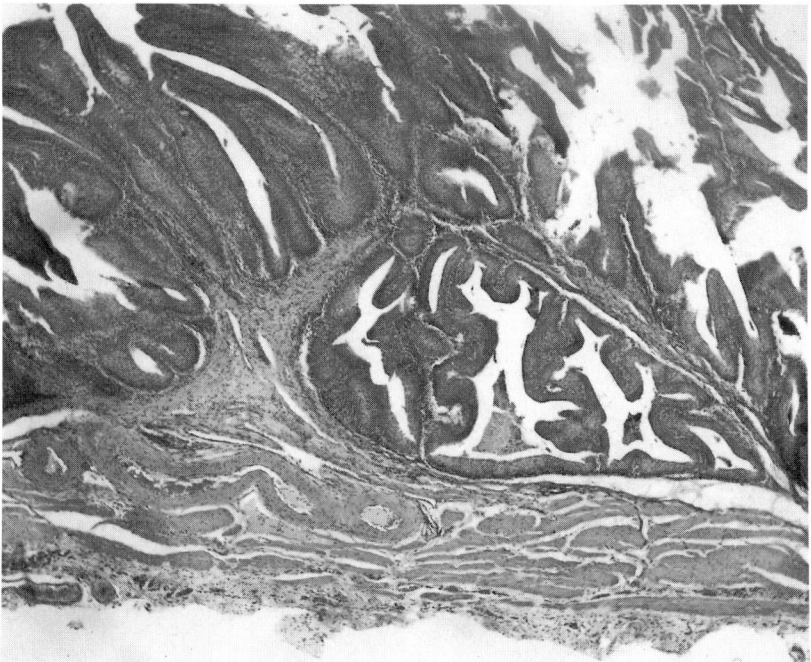

FIG. 7. Papillary hyperplasia in a rat. H&E, ×40.

well as in humans. Thus a strong correlation had been suggested between the presence of pleomorphic microvilli and bladder cancer. However, in more recent studies in rats and mice (9), pleomorphic villi were induced within 4 days but disappeared 3 days later. This suggests that they are indicative of increased proliferation which occurs as part of an acute or chronic toxic response and may not necessarily indicate a preneoplastic change (34,35).

Diverticulum

Diverticuli consist of downgrowths of the transitional epithelium into the muscular tissue. They have been described in both the ureter and the urinary bladder and have been mistaken as transitional cell carcinomas because of their location within the muscularis. The lesion exists as a downgrowth into either the urinary bladder or the ureteral wall (Fig. 9), and the surface epithelium may extend through the muscularis into the adventitia. Distinguishing diverticuli from carcinoma may be difficult, but the epithelium in diverticuli is normal or hyperplastic but without dysplasia. The lesion appears to be associated with chronic irritation as a result of crystalluria or calculi (36). It is also related to the genotype.

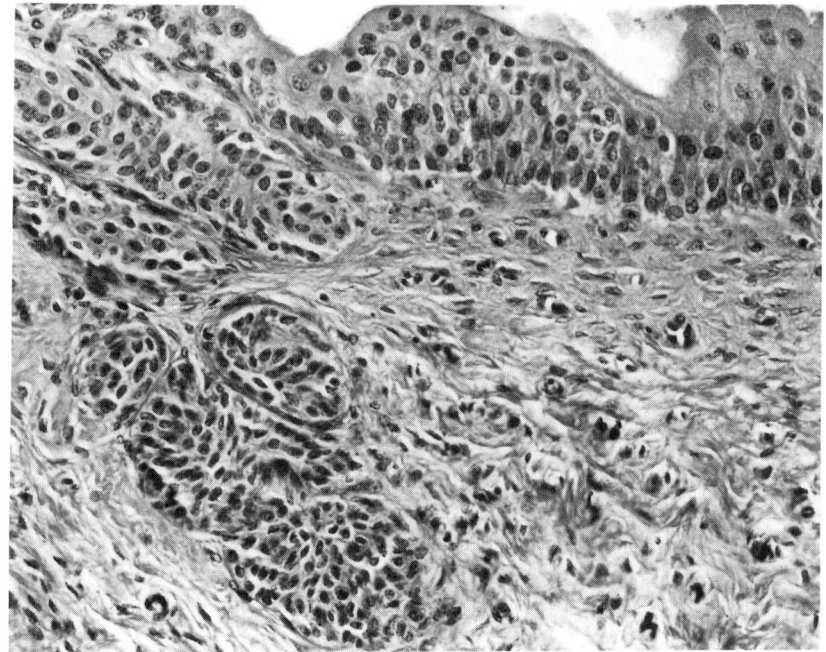

FIG. 8. Nodular hyperplasia in a mouse. H&E, ×350.

Neoplasia

Urinary bladder tumors induced in both rats and mice develop most commonly in the vertex or fundus of the urinary bladder. Such is the case with tumors induced in mice with 2-AAF (37) and in rats with sodium saccharin (2). This area would probably be in longer contact with urine containing urinary toxicants or their metabolites, due to the anatomical position of the urinary bladder.

Papillomas occur as papillary formations projecting into the lumen (Figs. 10 and 11). The epithelium shows no pleomorphism, atypia, or anaplasia and is well differentiated. Papillomas may have a slender narrow stalk (pedunculated) or a broad base (sessile). Ito and Shirai (38) stated that a characteristic that distinguishes a papilloma from papillary hyperplasia is the presence of a fibrovascular core that has a complex branching of secondary or tertiary stalks. Diffuse papillomatosis is frequently observed in association with urinary calculi, which are reversible if the calculi can be removed (36,39).

Experimentally induced malignant neoplasms of the urothelium are classified according to histologic pattern, cell type, and depth of invasion (Table 1) (1,27,40). Malignant epithelial lesions classified by histologic pattern may be divided into papillary and nonpapillary carcinomas. Transitional cell carcinomas may project

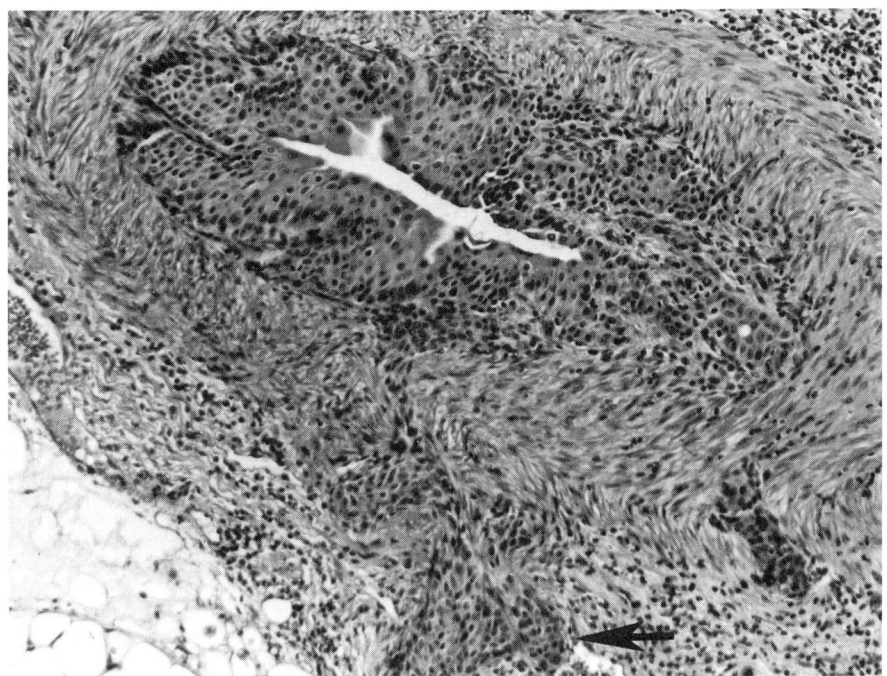

FIG. 9. Diverticulum (*arrow*) in the ureter of a mouse administered 4-ethylsulfonyl-naphthalene-1-sulfonamide (ENS). H&E, ×140. [Reprinted from Frith (40), with permission.]

into the lumen as exophytic growths (Figs. 12 and 13) or they may grow into the subepithelial tissue as endophytic growths (Fig. 13). The diagnosis of carcinoma can be made on morphology alone and invasion need not be present. One group of investigators (41) described the sequential morphogenesis of urinary bladder tumors in BALB/c female mice administered 2-acetylaminofluorene. The study indicated two distinct patterns. The first was a focal neovascularization of the transitional epithelium, resulting initially in exophytic nodules which appeared more likely to develop into papilloma. The second was a nodular downgrowth of the transitional epithelium, resulting initially in endophytic tumors which progressed to endophytic and exophytic carcinomas.

Bladder carcinomas classified according to histologic cell type are divided into transitional cell (Fig. 14), transitional cell with squamous differentiation (Fig. 15), squamous cell (Fig. 16), undifferentiated (Fig. 17), and adenocarcinoma types (1). Occasionally, tumors of mixed type occur. The most common induced type is the transitional cell carcinoma, but this may depend on the type and dose level of the carcinogen. Transitional cell carcinoma with squamous differentiation and squamous cell carcinomas tend to be more aggressive and infiltrative than transitional cell carcinomas, especially in the mouse (1,42). Urinary bladder carcinomas com-

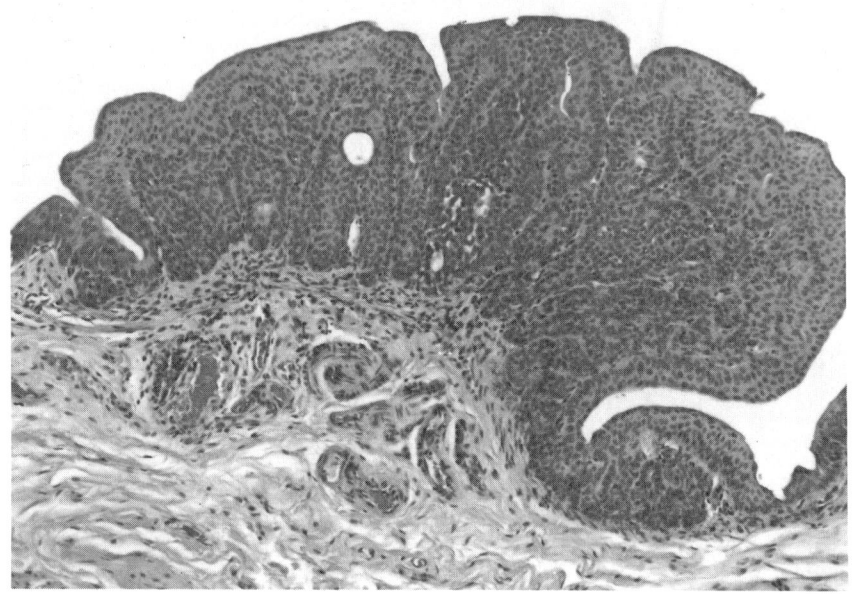

FIG. 10. Small exophytic papilloma in the urinary bladder of a rat. H&E, ×115.

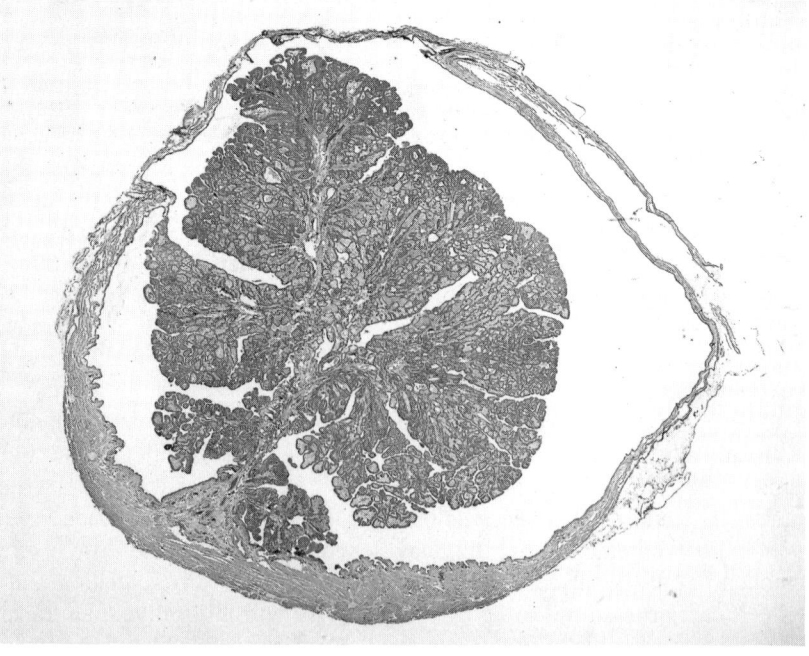

FIG. 11. Large pedunculated papilloma in the urinary bladder of a rat. H&E, ×7.

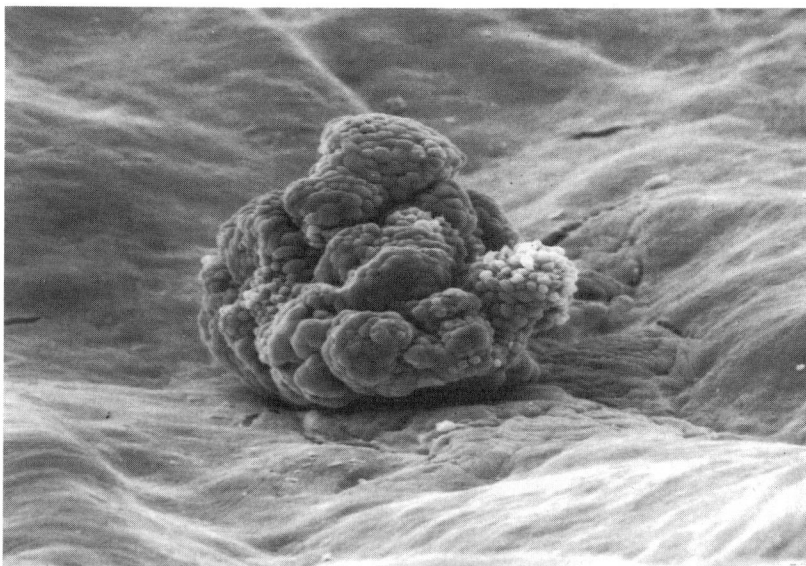

FIG. 12. Scanning electron micrograph of a transitional cell carcinoma in the urinary bladder of a rat. Uranyl acetate–lead citrate, ×150. Reprinted from Frith (40), with permission.]

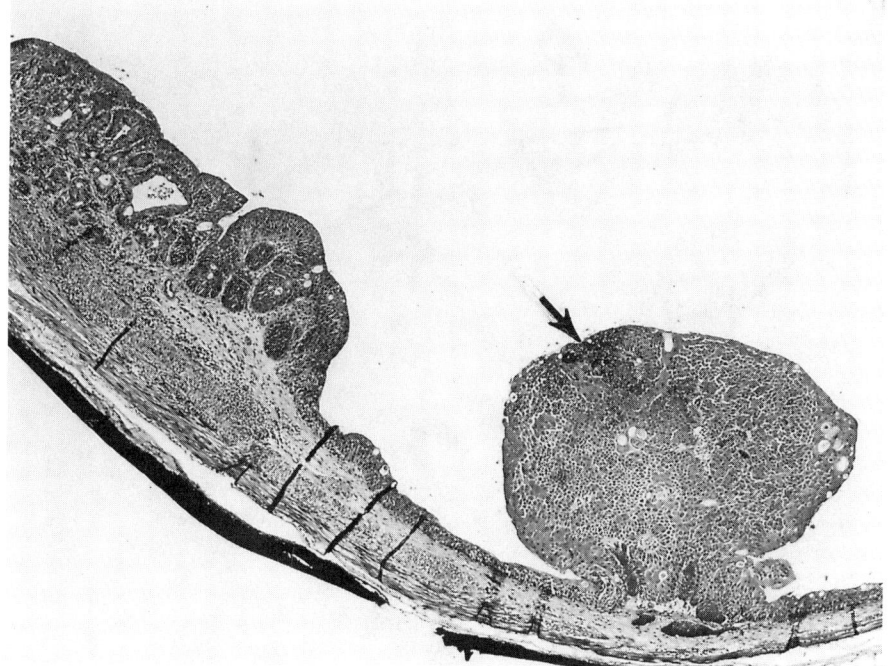

FIG. 13. Exophytic tumor (*arrow*) and endophytic tumor in the urinary bladder of a mouse administered 2-acetylaminofluorene. Note India ink which has been used to mark the ventral surface of the urinary bladder. H&E, ×56. [Reprinted from Frith (40), with permission.]

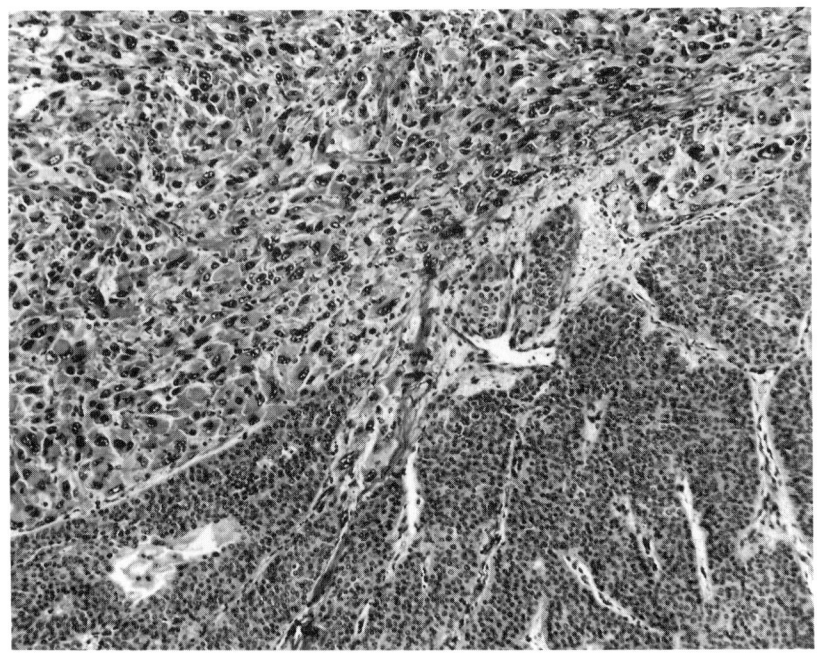

FIG. 14. Transitional cell carcinoma (**bottom**) adjacent to an undifferentiated carcinoma (**top**) in a mouse administered 2-acetylaminofluorene (2-AAF). H&E, ×140.

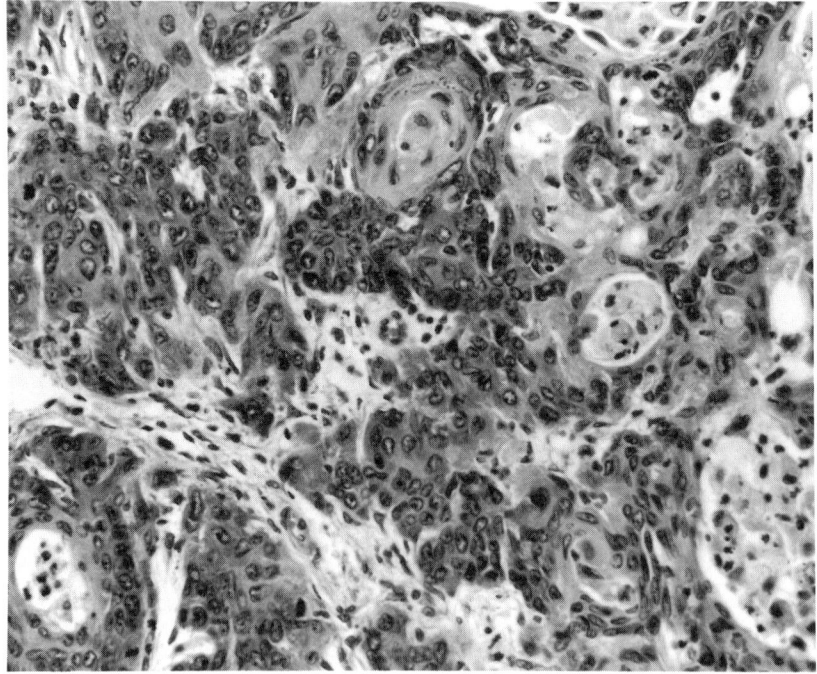

FIG. 15. Transitional cell carcinoma with squamous differentiation in a mouse administered 2-acetylaminofluorene (2-AAF). H&E, ×350. [Reprinted from Frith (40), with permission.]

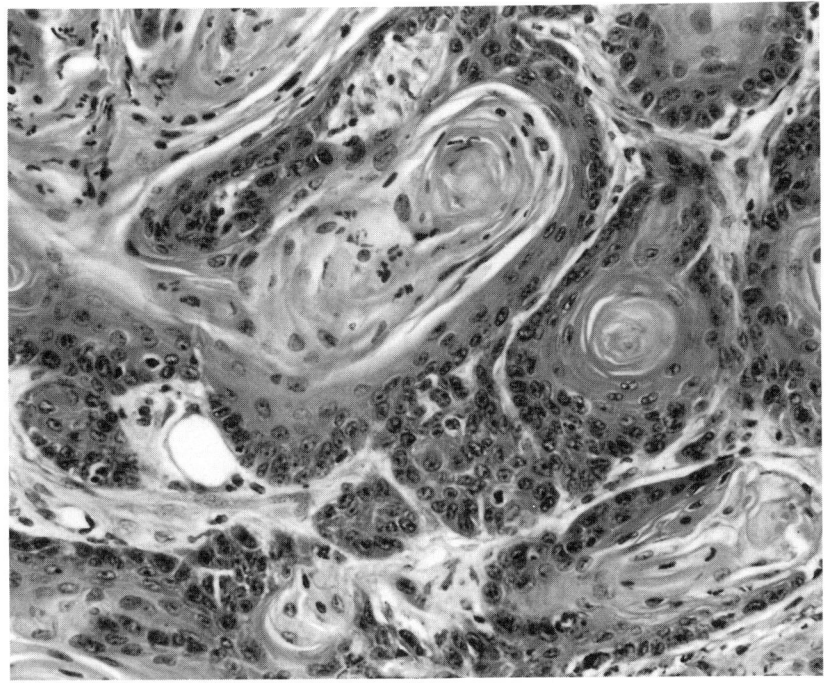

FIG. 16. Squamous cell carcinoma in the urinary bladder of a mouse. H&E, ×350. [Reprinted from Frith (40), with permission.]

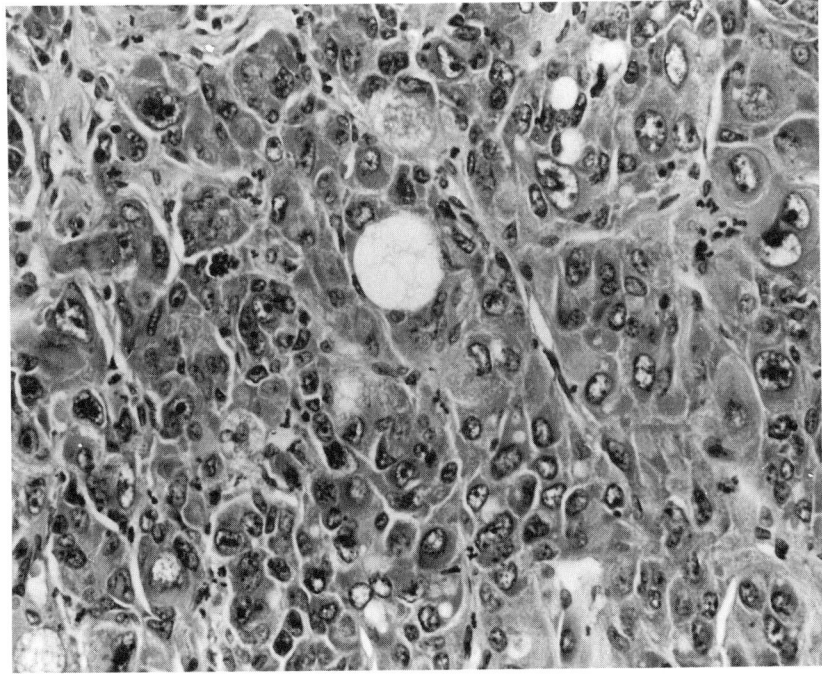

FIG. 17. Undifferentiated carcinoma in a mouse administered 2-acetylaminofluorene (2-AAF). H&E, ×350.

monly invade through the muscle wall (Fig. 18) and locally but only occasionally metastasize to the regional lymph nodes and the lungs (Fig. 19). Undifferentiated carcinomas are also rare. These may be difficult to distinguish from mesenchymal tumors; tumor giant cells and large eosinophilic neoplastic cells with large nuclei and prominent nucleoli may be seen.

Experimentally induced primary mesenchymal tumors of the rat and mouse urinary bladder occur much less freqently than do epithelial tumors. The most common are vascular tumors such as hemangioma (Fig. 20) and hemangiosarcoma (Fig. 21). Hemangiosarcomas may occasionally occur in conjunction with transitional cell carcinomas. Mesenchymal tumors of muscle origin are extrememly rare. Mesenchymal tumors with smooth muscle and/or pericyte differentiation (Figs. 22 and 23), confirmed by electron microscopic examination, have been reported as both an induced and a spontaneous lesion (43,44). In the mouse, the tumors occur in the subepithelial tissue of the urinary bladder and occur most commonly in the trigone area. The neoplastic cells are often large with prominent cytoplasm and bizarre nuclei. No tumor with similar appearance has been observed in rats or other experimental species nor in humans. Occasionally, tumors resembling sarcomas are seen, but if poorly differentiated they may be difficult to distinguish from undifferentiated carcinomas.

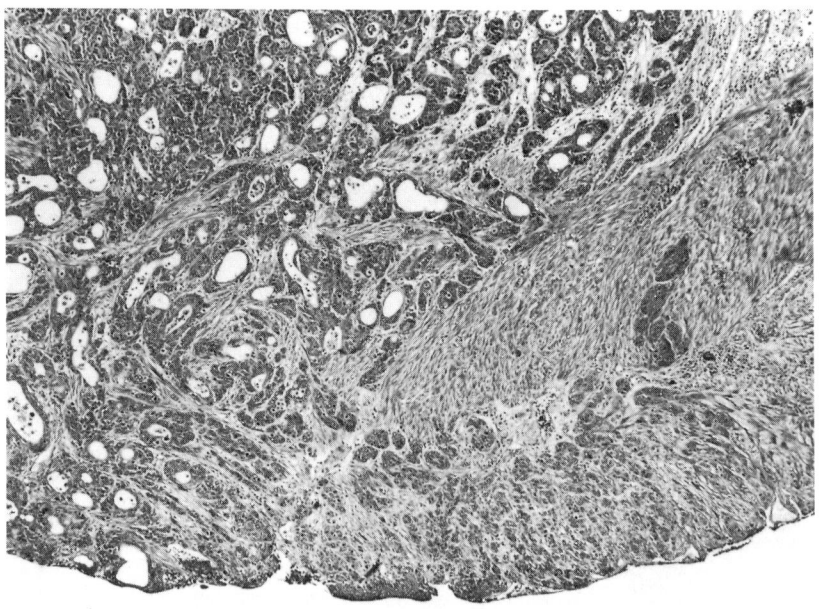

FIG. 18. Transitional cell carcinoma in a mouse which has invaded to the serosal surface. H&E, ×48. [Reprinted from Frith (40), with permission.]

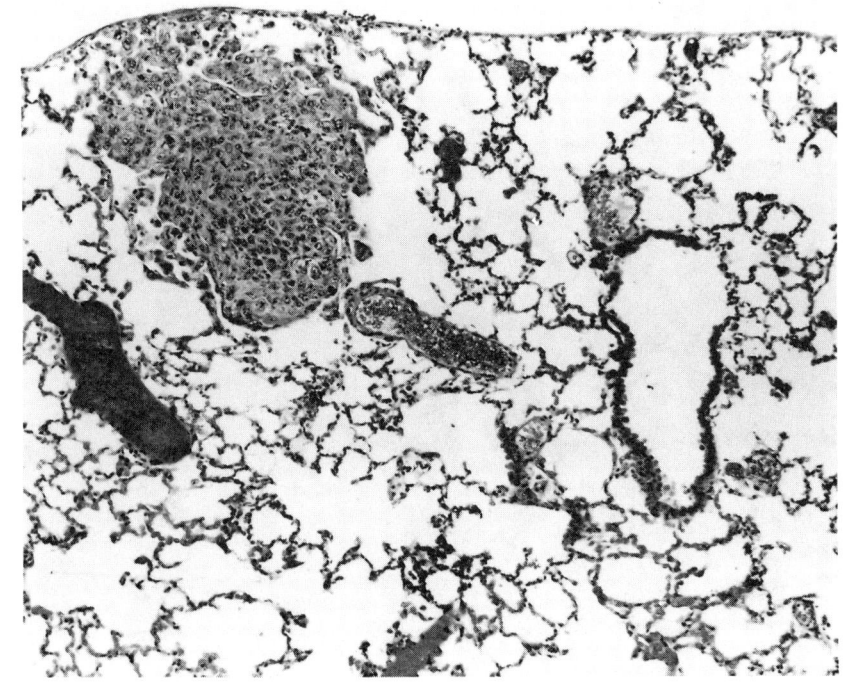

FIG. 19. Pulmonary metastasis of a transitional cell carcinoma in a mouse. H&E, ×140. [Reprinted from Frith (40), with permission.]

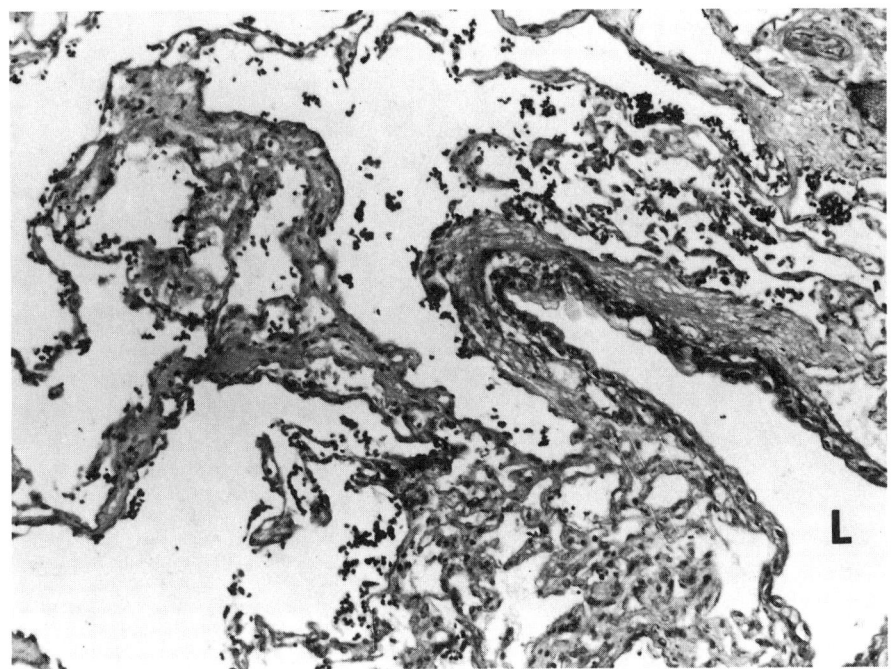

FIG. 20. Hemangioma in the submucosa of urinary bladder of a mouse. L, lumen. H&E, ×140.

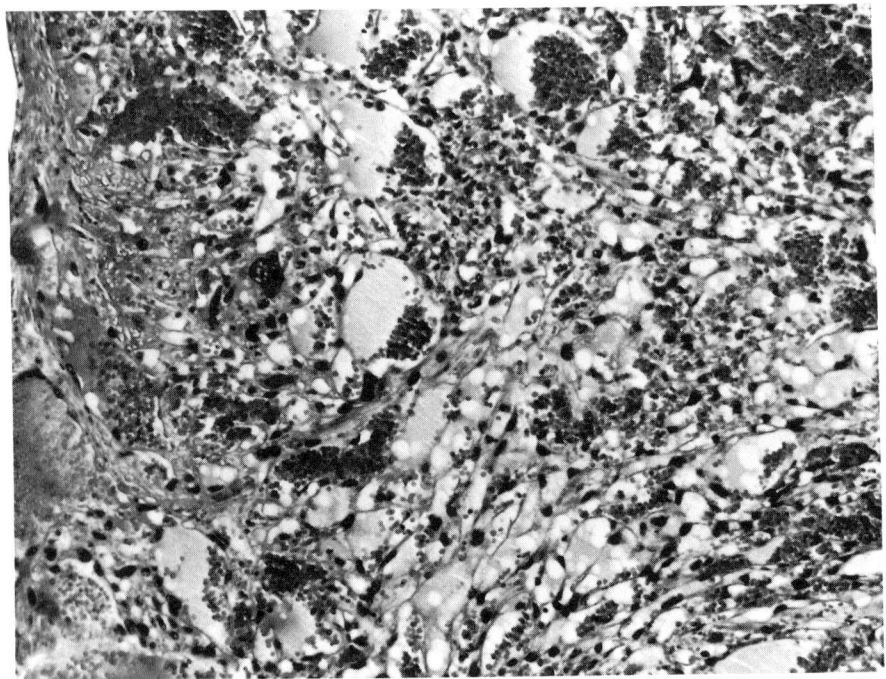

FIG. 21. Hemangiosarcoma in the submucosa of urinary bladder of a mouse. H&E, ×140.

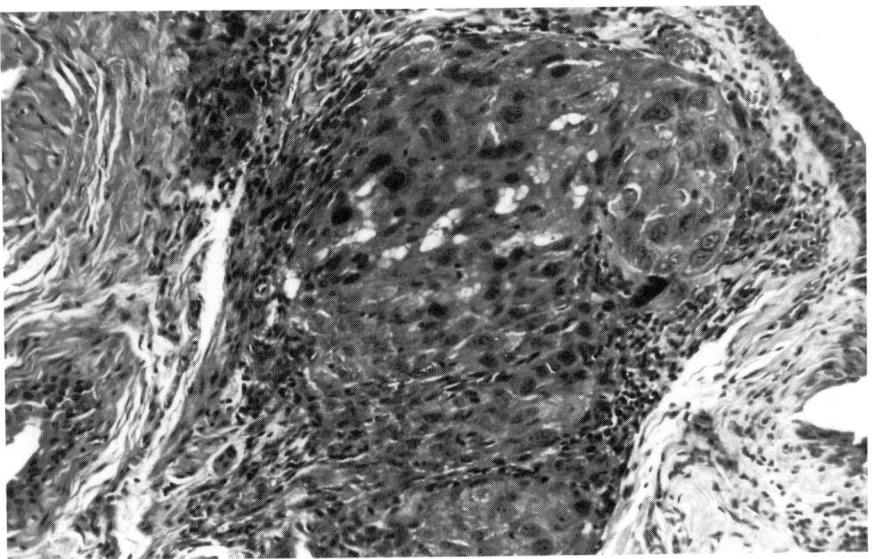

FIG. 22. Smooth muscle tumor occurring in the submucosa near the trigone of the urinary bladder of a mouse. H&E, ×400. [Reprinted from Chandra and Frith (44), with permission.]

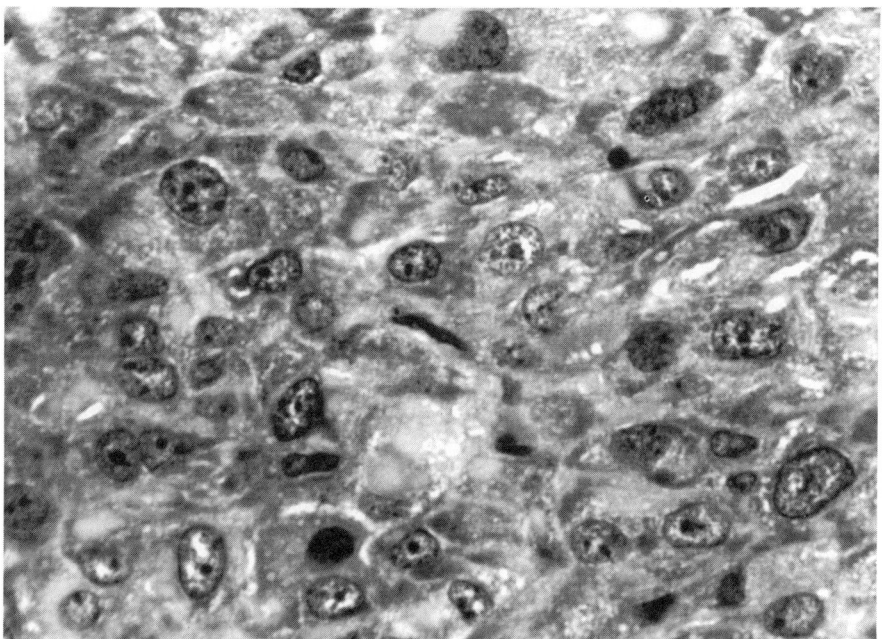

FIG. 23. Higher magnification of smooth muscle tumor showing large bizarre cells. H&E, ×620. [Reprinted from Chandra and Frith (44), with permission.]

COMPARISON WITH OTHER SPECIES

Since the light and ultrastructural characteristics of urothelium have been studied best in the mouse and rat, these two species have been used extensively as models for the study of urothelial toxicity and carcinogenesis. Many urinary bladder lesions in humans are similar in both morphology and behavior to those induced in the mouse and rat. While spontaneous urinary bladder tumors are not uncommon in humans, spontaneous urinary bladder neoplasms are rare in the rat and extremely rare in the mouse. Classification systems have been developed for both humans and experimental models and are similar in their approach and descriptions (1,27, 45,46). Urinary bladder tumors in humans are commonly graded or staged based on their degree of cellular atypia and their spread or depth of invasion. Similar schemes have been used for the mouse (1). Urinary bladder tumors in the mouse may undergo squamous differentiation, resulting in the development of squamous cell carcinomas. In the mouse, squamous cell carcinomas appear to be more malignant and invasive than does the typical transitional cell carcinoma. In both humans and experimental animals, urinary bladder carcinomas tend to invade adjacent organs, but distant metastases are uncommon.

URINARY BLADDER CARCINOGENESIS

Urinary bladder carcinogens are considered to induce bladder carcinomas most commonly by chemical formation of DNA adducts and an increased rate of mutations and genetic errors. Aromatic amines and amide compounds have been studied in detail in rodents in the experimental study of bladder carcinogenesis (3,4). Although a number of these have been identified to be specific urinary bladder carcinogens in humans, many of them will induce tumors of other organs in the mouse and the rat. For example, benzidine dihydrochloride is used in the commercial production of many dyes and is a known human urinary bladder carcinogen. In mice, benzidine causes an increased incidence of hepatocellular carcinomas, which is indicative of its carcinogenicity, but in the mouse it does not appear to be a urinary bladder carcinogen (47). One of the best studied urinary bladder carcinogens in the mouse is 2-acetylaminofluorene (2-AAF). In a large study in the BALB/c female mouse referred to as the ED_{01} (6), 2-AAF was administered at seven dietary concentrations, ranging from 30 to 150 ppm.

Hyperplasia During 2-AAF Carcinogenesis

The prevalence and severity of hyperplastic lesions may be highly dependent on dose and length of exposure to a given carcinogen. This is demonstrated in Table 3. In the ED_{01} study at NCTR (31) after 24 months of exposure to dietary 2-AAF, the prevalence of hyperplasia in BALB/c female control mice was 1.0%, at levels of 30 to 60 ppm it was less than 10%, and a dramatic increase in prevalence was noted between 75 and 150 ppm. Furthermore, 150 ppm 2-AAF induced hyperplasia in over 90% of the animals after only 12 months of exposure, while hyperplasia in lower-dose groups was significantly above controls at this time only in the 100-ppm group. In a separate study (32), only a 6-month exposure period was required for

TABLE 3. Influence of dietary 2-AAF on urinary bladder hyperplasia[a]

Dietary concentration (ppm)	Prevalence of bladder hyperplasia (%) at:				
	9 months	12 months	15 months	18 months	24 months
0	1	0	1	2	1
30	—	—	—	1	2
35	—	—	—	1	3
45	—	—	—	2	3
60	1	0	1	2	7
75	6	2	6	10	22
100	42	51	48	56	71
150	79	96	96	97	91

[a]BALB/c female mice were fed dietary 2-AAF for periods ranging from 9 to 24 months and killed immediately at the end of the exposure period. Prevalence is the percentage of the exposed population exhibiting either mild or moderate urothelial hyperplasia when sacrificed.

500 ppm dietary 2-AAF to induce hyperplasia in 100% of a population of female BALB/c mice. In the studies cited above, severity of hyperplasia was similarly dose and time dependent (Figs. 24 and 25). In the ED_{01} study (31), moderate hyperplasia was seldom observed at dietary concentrations below 75 ppm. At 75 ppm virtually all hyperplasia was mild until after 24 months of exposure to 2-AAF (Fig. 24). After 33 months of exposure the prevalence of moderate hyperplasia had risen to somewhat over 20% (Fig. 25). The prevalence of moderate hyperplasia began to rise somewhat earlier in mice exposed to 100 ppm 2-AAF but did not exceed 25% at 33 months. In mice exposed to 150 ppm 2-AAF the prevalence of moderate hyperplasia rose to a maximum of about 45% at 17 to 18 months but did not continue to rise after that (Fig. 25). When fed 500 ppm 2-AAF for only 6 months, 35% to 94% of BALB/c females developed moderate hyperplasia, depending on their age or other factors during exposure (32). In the dose range 75 to 150 ppm, mild hyperplasia always preceded and was much more prevalent than neoplasia, while moderate hyperplasia generally was a late occurring event, appearing at about the same time but generally more slowly than bladder neoplasia. Thus mild hyperplasia exhibited the character of a precursor to both moderate hyperplasia and neoplasia, but moderate hyperplasia did not appear to be an essential precursor to neoplasia (31)

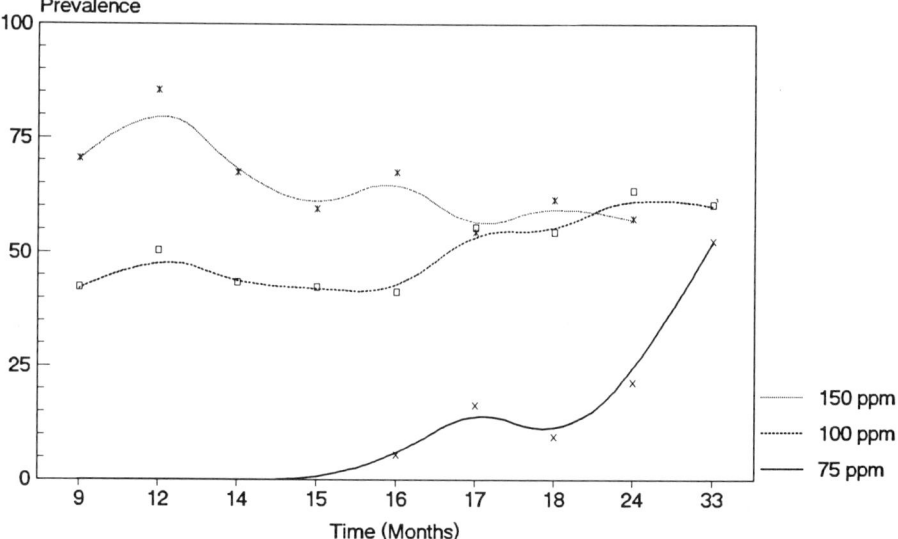

FIG. 24. Graph showing mild urothelial hyperplasia in the ED_{01} study induced by continuous exposure to dietary 2-AAF. BALB/c female mice were fed dietary 2-AAF continuously for periods of 9 to 33 months and killed immediately after terminating exposure. The prevalence is the percentage of the exposed population exhibiting mild urothelial hyperplasia when sacrificed. Dietary concentrations of 2-AAF were 75, 100, or 150 ppm.

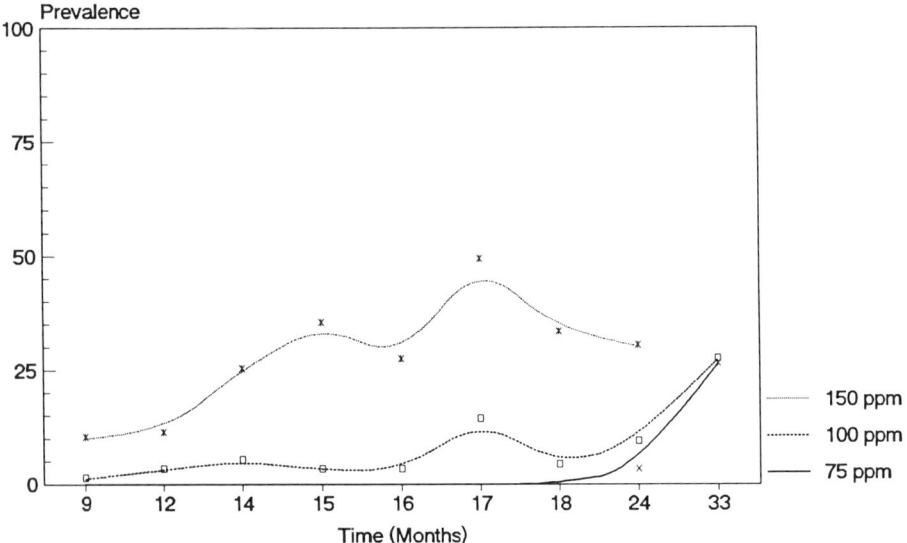

FIG. 25. Graph showing moderate urothelial hyperplasia in the ED_{01} study induced by continuous exposure to dietary 2-AAF. BALB/c female mice were fed dietary 2-AAF continuously for periods of 9 to 33 months and killed immediately after terminating exposure. The prevalence is the percentage of the exposed population exhibiting moderate urothelial hyperplasia when sacrificed. Dietary concentrations of 2-AAF were 75, 100, or 150 ppm.

Hyperplastic lesions induced by 2-AAF have been shown to regress to varying degrees when the carcinogenic stimulus was removed. The extent of regression was dependent on the dose level as well as the period of exposure. In the ED_{01} study (31), exposure of BALB/c females to dietary levels of 100 or 150 ppm 2-AAF for 9, 12, or 15 months followed by discontinuation of dosing resulted in only partial reversal of hyperplasia. The hyperplasia that persisted for longer than 3 months after discontinuing 2-AAF exposure was classified as persistent hyperplasia. Reversal after a given period of exposure was much more nearly complete for animals fed 100 ppm 2-AAF than for those fed 150 ppm (Fig. 26). Thus about 20% of mice fed 100 ppm for 15 months had persistent hyperplasia when examined 9 months later, while about 70% of those fed 150 ppm for that period had hyperplasia that did not disappear after a 9-month period of discontinuation. At a given dose level the reversal tended to be less complete the longer the period of exposure. For example, about 50% of the mice fed 150 ppm for 9 months developed persistent hyperplasia, while about 70% of those fed the same dose for 15 months developed persistent hyperplasia (Fig. 26). Hyperplasia persisting in nontumor animals was almost always mild, while in tumor-bearing animals tended to be evenly distributed between mild and moderate.

In this study the prevalence of persistent hyperplasia found after a given period of exposure was very closely predictive of the prevalence of bladder tumors that were

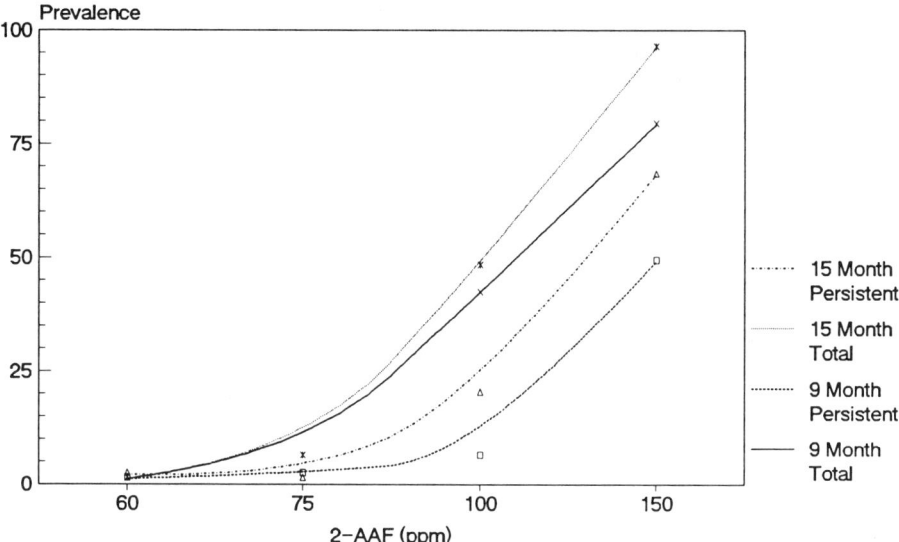

FIG. 26. Graph showing total and persistent urothelial hyperplasia in the ED_{01} study induced by continuous exposure to dietary 2-AAF. BALB/c female mice were fed dietary 2-AAF for periods of 9 or 15 months. They were killed immediately after terminating exposure or at least 3 months after discontinuing exposure. The prevalence is the percentage of the exposed population exhibiting urothelial hyperplasia (mild or moderate) when sacrificed immediately after discontinuing exposure at 9 or 15 months, or it is the hyperplasia persisting at least 3 months after discontinuing exposure at 9 or 15 months.

found if 2-AAF exposure were continued for an additional 9 months. In other words, the prevalence of bladder neoplasia after an 18-month exposure to 2-AAF was virtually identical to the prevalence of persistent hyperplasia induced by a 9-month exposure, and the persistent hyperplasia induced by 15 months of exposure closely predicted neoplasia found after a 24-month exposure. Based on this study it seems that persistent hyperplastic cells may be the target cells from which neoplasia arises when 2-AAF exposure is continued.

At least two additional studies have examined the persistence of hyperplasia after feeding 500 ppm 2-AAF for varying periods of time. Feeding BALB/c male mice 500 ppm of 2-AAF for 6 or 13 weeks induced urothelial hyperplasia in 99% to 100% of the animals in both groups, but when mice were sacrificed at periodic intervals after discontinuing the exposure, hyperplasia regressed faster and to a greater degree in animals treated for 6 weeks than those treated for 13 weeks (33). Only 4% of mice exposed for 6 weeks still had evidence of hyperplasia 7 or 20 weeks after 2-AAF feeding had been discontinued. However, 17% of the mice exposed for 13 weeks still had hyperplasia 26 weeks after 2-AAF discontinuation. A small number of bladder carcinomas were seen in the animals treated for 13 weeks and sacrificed at 26 and 39 weeks, suggesting that exposure to a high level of a carcinogen even for a relatively brief period may result in the development of carcinoma after cessation of exposure.

In a separate study (32), when BALB/c females were fed 500 ppm 2-AAF for 26 weeks, virtually 100% developed urothelial hyperplasia, which disappeared in only about half of the animals 3 to 6 months after discontinuing the exposure. While a 6-month exposure to 500 ppm 2-AAF generally induced a higher incidence of moderate than mild hyperplasia, discontinuation of exposure resulted in reversion to a constant level of primarily mild hyperplasia. Nevertheless, in contrast to the ED_{01} study (at much lower doses), hyperplasia persisting 6 months after discontinuing 2-AAF exposure had not all reverted to mild hyperplasia. Up to 30% of the persistent hyperplasia was moderate hyperplasia. Whether this moderate hyperplasia was associated only with neoplasia is unknown but possible, since in this study the prevalence of bladder neoplasia continued to increase markedly up to 6 months after discontinuation of 2-AAF exposure. This is in contrast to the ED_{01} study, where discontinuation of the lower doses resulted in little further development of neoplasia (31).

Neoplastic Dose Response to 2-AAF

In the ED_{01} study, the number of urinary bladder tumors increased with time at doses of 60 to 150 ppm, increasing sharply after 24 months. For animals killed at the end of an 18-, 24-, or 33-month exposure to 2-AAF, the prevalence of urinary bladder tumors was very clearly nonlinearly related to the dietary concentration of the compound across a dietary concentration range of 30 to 150 ppm (Fig. 27). At concentrations of 60, 75, and 100 ppm fed for 33 months, there was a very steep dose-response relationship, while those exposed to 30, 35, or 45 ppm had a very shallow to nonexistent dose-response relationship. On the other hand, the steep portion of the dose-response curve was highly time dependent. Thus in animals sacrificed at 18 or 24 months, the steep part of the curve involved only animals fed the 100- or 150-ppm concentrations. When 2-AAF administration was discontinued after 9, 12, or 15 months and the animals were fed the control diet until 24 months, the incidence of bladder tumors at the end of 24 months was only slightly greater than the incidence at the time the diet was discontinued. These results suggest the need for continued exposure to increase the incidence of bladder tumors and are consistent with a two-stage model for carcinogenesis (48).

Carcinogenesis studies done in BALB/c female mice at 2-AAF concentrations of 100, 250, or 500 ppm (49) are generally consistent with the ED_{01} study results. The higher doses (250 and 500 ppm) both resulted in a 100% prevalence of bladder neoplasia in animals sacrificed at 18 months, while only 28% of those fed 100 ppm 2-AAF had bladder tumors at that time. In addition, the time to death with bladder tumors was dose dependent. Those fed 500 ppm clearly died with bladder neoplasia sooner than did those fed 250 ppm and those fed 100 ppm. C57BL/6 females were somewhat less sensitive to 2-AAF but gave similar results. In this study male BALB/c mice were quite different from females. All three dose groups sacrificed at 18 months had a 94% to 100% prevalence of bladder tumors, but the time to death

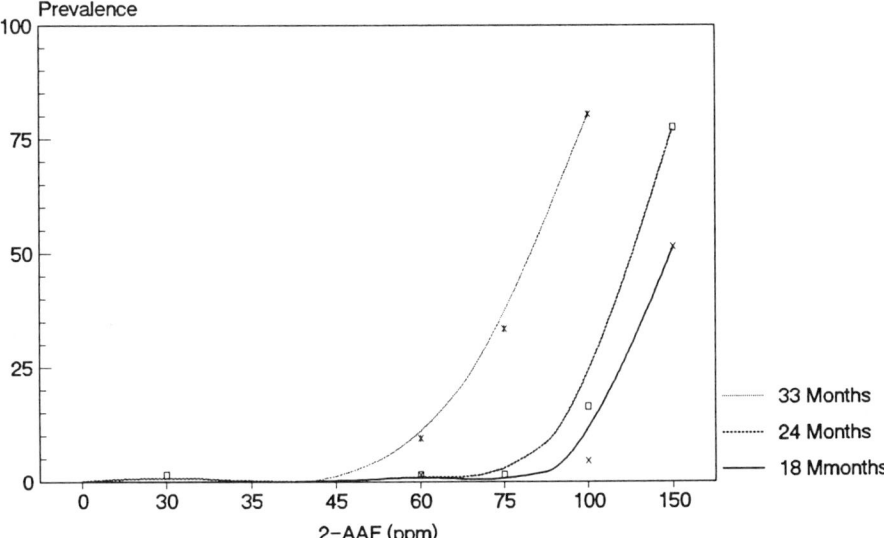

FIG. 27. Graph showing urinary bladder neoplasia in the ED_{01} study induced by continuous dietary exposure to 2-AAF. BALB/c female mice were fed dietary 2-AAF continuously at concentrations ranging from 30 to 150 ppm for periods of 18, 24, or 33 months and killed immediately after terminating exposure. The prevalence is the percentage of the exposed population with urinary bladder neoplasia when sacrificed.

with bladder tumors showed a biphasic relationship to dose, with those fed 250 ppm dying with tumors sooner than those fed either 100 or 500 ppm. Indeed, time to death with tumors was almost identical for the latter two groups. Similar observations were made in male C57BL/6 mice. These results seem to indicate that very high levels of 2-AAF may alter the pharmacokinetics of 2-AAF action and may have an antineoplastic effect, especially in males.

It has long been considered that the carcinogenicity of 2-AAF was related to its initial conversion to N-OH-2-AAF, which is equally carcinogenic toward the urinary bladder as 2-AAF, followed by the formation of reactive electrophiles that subsequently bind covalently to DNA (50). Studies in rat and mouse strains that are sensitive to the induction of liver neoplasia by 2-AAF have shown that N-OH-2-AAF gives rise to three major hepatic DNA adducts, two acetylated aminofluorene–deoxyguanosine adducts, and one aminofluorene–deoxyguanosine adduct. Several enzymes have been implicated in adduct formation. These include deacetylase activity for N-OH-2-AAF and sulfotransferase activity for N-OH-2-AAF, which is present in the liver of both species (50). Lai et al. (51) have suggested that N-sulfoxy-AF is the major ultimate electrophilic metabolite of N-OH-AAF that gives rise to the primary DNA adduct, N-(dG-8-yl)-AF in the liver of $B6C3F_1$ infant male mice, and Poirier et al. (52) have identified dG-C8-AF as the major DNA adduct found in bladder DNA of female BALB/c mice after feeding 2-AAF for 28 days.

This DNA adduct quantitatively was found to be linearly related to the dietary concentration of 2-AAF over the range 5 to 150 ppm in urinary bladder DNA. This linearity clearly deviated from the shape of the bladder tumor dose-response curve. Thus even when the DNA adduct level was substituted for the dietary 2-AAF concentration as the measure of exposure, the dose-response curve for bladder tumors was distinctly nonlinear, and this was interpreted as an indication of a multistage process involving more than one adduct-related event. Furthermore, using a biologically based model of two-event carcinogenesis that accounts for both genotoxic and nongenotoxic proliferative effects, Cohen and Ellwein (48) made use of the dose-related DNA adduct levels together with neoplastic and hyperplastic data discussed above to estimate model parameters. They demonstrated that tumor prevalence in the bladder could be explained by synergy between AAF toxicity affecting both genetic events and cellular proliferation at higher doses.

N-[4-(5-Nitro-2-furyl)-2-thiazolyl]formamide (FANFT) is one of several nitrofuran carcinogens (13,14). It is another well-studied urinary bladder carcinogen in the rodent but is the only one in this class that is highly specific for the urinary bladder in mice. N-Butyl-N-(4-hydroxybutyl)nitrosamine (BBN) is a metabolite of the symmetric dibutyl nitrosamine (DBN) (7). In rats and mice, both are urinary bladder carcinogens, with BBN being more specific than DBN toward the urothelium.

Numerous chemicals have been studied by direct implantation of pellets containing the suspected carcinogens (3). As mentioned earlier, the interpretation of the carcinogenicity of these compounds is suspect because of the occurrence of bladder carcinomas in mice in which a pellet of the carrier material alone, without added chemical, was implanted in the urinary bladder (53,54).

Gold et al. (55) studied interspecies extrapolation in carcinogenesis from rats to mice and from mice to rats. The Carcinogenic Potency Data Base, which includes 3,500 cancer tests conducted in rats or mice on 955 compounds, was used for analysis. For 392 chemicals tested in both species, 76% of the rat carcinogens were also positive in the mouse, and 70% of mouse carcinogens were also positive in the rat. Of a total of 341 chemicals evaluated as carcinogenic in the rat, 34 (10%) were urinary bladder carcinogens. Of a total of 278 chemicals evaluated as carcinogenic in the mouse, 11 (4%) were urinary bladder carcinogens.

Gold et al. (56) also studied target organs in chronic bioassays of 533 chemical carcinogens. The Carcinogenic Potency Data Base (CPDB) included a total of 3969 experiments, and chemical carcinogens were reported for 35 different target organs in rats or mice. More than 80% of the carcinogens in each of these species were positive in at least one of the eight most frequent sites: liver, lung, mammary gland, stomach, vascular system, kidney, hematopoietic system, and urinary bladder. Urinary bladder carcinogens for rats and mice from this study are listed in Table 4. These include NCI/NTP chemicals (57) as well as a number of other chemicals.

Huff et al. (57) evaluated chemicals associated with site-specific neoplasia in 1,394 long-term carcinogenesis experiments (300 chemicals) in laboratory rodents from NCI/NTP studies over the past 20 years. Out of the total 1,394 experiments,

TABLE 4. Urinary bladder carcinogens in rats and mice: NCI/NTP and other chemicals

Chemical	Species[a]	Refs.
Acetaminophen	R	56
2-Acetylaminofluorene (2-AAF)	M	6,26,31,32,56
Allyl isothiocyanate	R	56,57,92
4-Aminodiphenyl	M	56
4-Aminodiphenyl·HCl	M	56
2-Aminodiphenylene oxide	M	56
2-Amino-3-methylimidazo[4,5-b]quinoline·HCl	R	56
2-Amino-4-(5-nitro-2-furyl)thiazole	R	56
4-Amino-2-nitrophenol	R	56,57,90
11-Aminoundecanoic acid	R	56,57
o-Anisidine·Hcl	R, M	56,57,87
Aspirin, phenacetin, and caffeine	R	57
p-Benzoquinone dioxime	R	57
Bracken fern	R	81,82,83
CI Disperse Blue 1	R	56,57
N-Butyl-N-(4-hydroxybutyl) nitrosamine (BBN)	R	7,28,56,71,78,79
4-Chloro-4'-aminodiphenyl ether	M	56
4-Chloro-o-phenylenediamine	R	56,57
m-Cresidine	R	56,57
p-Cresidine	R, M	56,57
Cyclophosphamide	R	56
1,3-Dichloropropene	R	56
Diethylene glycol	R	56
4-Ethylsulfonylnaphthalene-1-sulfonamide (ENS)	M	56
Glycidol	R	57
N-Hydroxy-2-acetylaminofluorene	M	51,56
Melamine	R	10,56,57,93
2-Methoxy-3-aminodibenzofuran	R	56
Methylalkylnitrosamines	R	80
2-Naphthylamine	R	56,85
Nitrilotriacetic acid (NTA)	R	56,57,88
Nitrilotracetic acid, trisodium salt, monohydrate	R	56,57
N-[4-(5-Nitro-2-furyl)-2-thiazolyl]formamide (FANFT)	R, M	14,56,84
Nitrosodi-n-butylamine	R	58
Nitrosodihydroxypropylethanolamine	R	58
N-Nitroso-n-methyl-n-dodecylamine	R	55,58
Nitrosomethyl-n-hexylamine	R	58
N-Nitrosodiphenylamine	R	56,57,91
o-Nitrosotoluene	R	56
n-Oxydiethylene thiocarbamyl-n-oxydiethylene sulfenamide (OTOS)	R	56,97
Phenacetin	R, M	56
Phenazone	R	56
o-Phenylphenate, sodium	R	56
o-Phenylphenol	R	56
Quercetin	R	56,82
p-Quinone dioxime	R	56,86
Saccharin, sodium	R	2,56
o-Toluenesulfonamide	R	56
o-Toluidine·HCl	R	56,57,89
Telone II	M	56

[a]R, rat; M, mouse.

10 were urinary bladder carcinogens in male rats and 10 were positive in female rats. In mice, 3 were urinary bladder carcinogens in males and 3 were positive in females. The most common tumor site was the liver, followed in rank order by lung, hematopoietic system and kidneys, mammary glands, forestomach, thyroid glands, Zymbal's glands, urinary bladder, skin and uterus/cervix, and circulatory system and adrenal glands. Of a total of 379 positive studies, 104 (27%) were hepatic carcinogens in rats or mice compared to 16 chemicals (4%) that were urinary bladder carcinogens in rats or mice. Chemicals identified as urinary bladder carcinogens in rats or mice from this study are listed in Table 4.

Stula (24) tabulated a list of urinary bladder lesions in rats from feeding various chemicals. The lesions included hyperplasia, adenocarcinoma, squamous cell carcinoma, transitional cell carcinoma, transitional cell papilloma, and undifferentiated carcinoma. The chemicals are shown in Table 4. Lijinski (58) compared the carcinogenic action of approximately 50 N-nitroso compounds in rats and hamsters. The nitroso compounds resulting in bladder neoplasms in rats are included in Table 4.

MODULATING FACTORS IN URINARY BLADDER CARCINOGENESIS

Sex and strain differences in response to urinary bladder carcinogens are well known. Studies carried out with 2-AAF are especially informative in this regard. In a study of chronic dietary exposure to 2-AAF at concentrations of 100, 250, or 500 ppm it was clearly shown that BALB/c mice were more sensitive to 2-AAF than were C57BL/6 mice, and that males were more sensitive than females (59). In another genotype comparison it was noted that BALB/c mice were more sensitive to 2-AAF-induced bladder neoplasia than were $B6C3F_1$ mice; males were once again more sensitive than females (60,61).

In a large study done primarily to evaluate the effect of age on bladder tumor response to 2-AAF, female BALB/c mice were fed a dietary concentration of 500 ppm 2-AAF for a 6-month period beginning at 1, 7, or 13 months of age (32). These age groups were exposed to the carcinogen in tandem and in parallel (i.e., different age groups were exposed either sequentially or at the same time) to control for potential environmental variables. Although the neoplastic response to 2-AAF in one replicate of the youngest exposure group was very low (4.2%) compared to replicates of the two older exposure groups (12.3% to 19.0%), it was concluded that age had no detectable effect on the prevalence of neoplasia when subsequent replicates of the youngest exposure groups were examined and 13.5% and 19.5% prevalences were found. In contrast, it was clearly shown that age had an effect on the severity of hyperplasia, the youngest animals at the start of treatment were much less likely than older animals to have moderate as opposed to mild hyperplasia (<50% versus >90%). This lack of correlation of severity of hyperplasia and prevalence of neoplasia was consistent with conclusions drawn earlier by Littlefield et al. (31) that persistent mild hyperplasia was a more likely precursor to neoplasia than were either the combination of mild and moderate hyperplasia or moderate hyperplasia alone. Since replicates of the youngest age group that were exposed at different times (in tandem) showed a large variation (4.2% to 19.5%) in the neoplastic response to 2-AAF, several potential variables in the study were evaluated for their contribution to variation. The three replicates showing this variation had somewhat different populations with respect to litter size (1 to 16 pups), parity of the dam (first through eighth litters), and exact age (21 to 31 days) at the start of exposure. None of these variables had a significant impact on the response. Although one study in Sprague–Dawley rats has reported greater sensitivity in young than in older rats in bladder tumor response to 2-AAF, this study was done only in tandem, so that a firm conclusion could not be drawn (62) since the converse conclusion would have been made in the BALB/c study if age groups had been done only in tandem.

The concept of two-stage carcinogenesis is now well established for many organs, including the urinary bladder (63,64). Fukushima (65) examined the promoting activity of various chemicals on the development of bladder tumors in rats, and these are listed in Table 5.

TABLE 5. Classification of urinary bladder cancer promoters

Sodium or potassium salts
  Sodium saccharin
  Sodium L-ascorbate
  Sodium o-phenylphenate
  Sodium bicarbonate
  Sodium citrate
  Sodium erythorbate
  Sodium phenobarbital
  Sodium barbital
Urolithiasis-inducing chemicals
  Uracil
  Diphenyl
Antioxidants
  Butylated hydroxyanisole
  Butylated hydroxytoluene
  Ethoxyquin
  t-Butylhydroxyquinone
  2-t-Butyl-4-methylphenol
Anticancer agents
  Adriamycin
  Mitomycin
Amino acids
  DL-Tryptophan
  L-Leucine
  L-Isoleucine
Others
  Components of urine (fractions I and II)
  Allopurinol (?)
  Physical injury
  Partial cystotomy

From Fukushima (65).

Originally, sodium saccharin was found to increase the incidence of bladder tumors in rats by chronic feeding in a two-generation bioassay (66). Hicks et al. (67) demonstrated that prior instillation into the rat urinary bladder of a low dose of the bladder carcinogen MNU, followed by oral administration of sodium saccharin, resulted in a very high incidence of bladder tumors. Cohen et al. (68) confirmed that sodium saccharin has a strong promoting activity for bladder cancer by feeding 5% sodium saccharin to rats pretreated with FANFT.

The coexistence of carcinoma and calculi in the urinary bladder of rats and mice has been observed in many studies. The Brown Norway rat strain has a high incidence of spontaneous bladder tumors that are often associated with the presence of calculi (69). These findings indicate that tumor formation may be caused by the stimulation of proliferation by calculi or foreign body–associated trauma. It is likely that any foreign body in the bladder lumen, whether implanted as a pellet or generated as a calculus by administration of some agent, produces increased urothelial proliferation and ultimately carcinoma (53,54,63).

To examine the effects of urolithiasis on urinary bladder carcinogenesis, male rats were given 0.05% BBN in their drinking water for 4 weeks and then treated with uracil for a further 8 or 16 weeks (70). After cessation of the uracil treatment, rats were given a basal diet without uracil until week 28 of the experiment. The incidences of bladder cancer were 91% or 100% in the groups receiving 8 or 16 weeks of uracil exposure after initiation of BBN, whereas the respective value was only 6% for the BBN-alone animals. More recently, the carcinogenicity of uracil has been demonstrated like that of other calculus-forming chemicals (71).

Bladder cancers in rats can also be promoted with adriamycin (ADR) and mitomycin C (MMC), two anticancer agents (72). Female rats were given BBN and then after 1 week without treatment received weekly intravesical instillation of ADR or MMC for 12 weeks. The carcinoma incidences were significantly higher (61% in the group receiving 1 mg/mL of ADR, 42% after 0.5 mg/mL of ADR, and 50% with MMC) than the control value (4%).

Diet composition may be an important modulator of bladder carcinogenesis. In studies involving two mouse stocks (BALB/c and $B6C3F_1$) this has been clearly demonstrated for 2-AAF (60,61). The bladder tumor response to 2-AAF was evaluated in both sexes of these two mouse stocks when this carcinogen was administered as an admixture with a purified diet (AIN-76A) or a cereal-based diet (NIH-07). Although no difference was noted in the bladder response of female BALB/c mice receiving the same three dietary concentrations of 2-AAF in the two diets, male BALB/c and male and female $B6C3F_1$ mice were clearly more sensitive to the bladder tumorigenic effect of 2-AAF administered with AIN-76 than with NIH-07 diet. Thus in three out of four instances the purified diet tended to enhance bladder carcinogenesis compared to the cereal-based diet.

Dietary protein and fat levels have been shown to affect the incidence of urinary bladder neoplasms induced with 2-acetylaminofluorene in mice (73). Mice were continuously fed diets containing combinations of 12% or 24% protein, 4% or 24% fat, and 500 ppm 2-acetylaminofluorene for 78 weeks. Mice on the high-fat diets demonstrated a significant increase in the incidence of urinary bladder carcinomas. The incidence of bladder tumors was less in the mice fed low-fat and low-protein diets compared to the other three diets. The protein levels alone appeared to have no effect on the incidence of bladder tumors. Mice fed the diet with lower levels of fat and protein showed a significantly lower incidence of bladder carcinomas compared to the mice fed the higher levels of fat and protein.

There have been a number of reports concerning the relationship between vitamins and cancer development. Vitamin C has been suggested as a possible preventive agent for urinary bladder cancer (74), yet sodium ascorbate at high doses promotes bladder cancer in rats (65). Anticarcinogenic effects of various retinoids have also been observed (64).

Antioxidants have been widely used as additives in various processed foods. The use of these compounds has generally been thought to be without hazard. Antioxidants have even been demonstrated to have anticarcinogenic activities when given before and/or together with carcinogens (75). Recent reports, however, have demonstrated their enhancement of tumor formation in animals (65,76).

SUMMARY

Since the light microscopic and ultrastructural characteristics of the urothelium of the urinary bladder of the mouse and the rat have been studied and characterized extensively and since many urinary bladder lesions in humans are similar in both morphology and behavior to those induced in the mouse and the rat, these two species make excellent models for studying urinary bladder carcinogenesis. Furthermore, urinary bladder toxicity and neoplasia can be induced with a variety of chemicals in both the mouse and the rat. Because of extensive studies of the morphology and character of preneoplastic and neoplastic progression and the wealth of dose-response information already available, this target organ provides one of the best models for study of the mechanism of carcinogenesis.

REFERENCES

1. Frith CH. Morphological classification of inflammatory, nonspecific, and proliferative lesions of the urinary bladder of mice. *Invest Urol* 1979;16:435–444.
2. Schoenig GP, Goldenthal EI, Geil RG, Frith CH, Richter WR, Carlborg FW. Evaluation of the dose response and *in utero* exposure to saccharin in the rat. *Food Chem Toxicol* 1985;23:475–490.
3. Clayson DB, Cooper EH. Cancer of the urinary tract. *Adv Cancer Res* 1970;13:271–381.
4. Price JM. Etiology of bladder cancer. In: Moltry E, ed. *Benign and malignant tumors of the urinary bladder*. New York: Medical Examination Publishing; 1971:189–251.
5. Cohen SM, Friedell GH. Neoplasms of the urinary system. In: Foster HL, Small JD, Fox JG, eds. *The mouse in biomedical research*. Vol IV. *Experimental biology and oncology*. New York: Academic Press; 1982:439–463.
6. Staffa JA, Mehlman MA. Innovations in cancer risk assessment (ED_{01} study). Proceedings of a symposium sponsored by the National Center for Toxicological Research, U.S. Food and Drug Administration and the American College of Toxicology. *J Environ Pathol Toxicol* 1980[Special Issue];3:1–250.

7. Nakanowatari J, Fukushima S, Imaida K, Ito N, Nagase S. Strain differences in *N*-butyl-*N*-(4-hydroxybutyl)nitrosamine bladder carcinogenesis in rats. *Jpn J Cancer Res* 1988;79:453–459.
8. Jackson CD, Frith CH, West RW, Stanley JW. Effects of 4-ethylsulfonylnaphthelene-1-sulfonamide, acetazolamide and oxamide on the mouse urinary tract. In: *Toxicology and occupational medicine*. New York: Elsevier; 1979:233–242.
9. Frith CH, Ayres PH, Shinohara Y, West R. Scanning and transmission electron microscopic observations of the acute morphological response of the mouse urinary bladder to 4-ethylsufonylnaphthalene-1-sulfonamide. *Toxicol Pathol* 1986;14:299–306.
10. Melnick RL, Boorman GA, Haseman JK, Montali RJ, Huff J. Urolithiasis and bladder carcinogenicity of melamine in rodents. *Toxicol Appl Pharmacol* 1984;72:292–303.
11. Haley TJ, Schieferstein G, Jaques WE, Farmer J, Frith CH, Sprowls RW. Time to development of urinary bladder hyperplasia in BALB/c mice fed *N*-2-fluorenylacetamide. *J Pharm Sci* 1974;63:1946–1947.
12. Frith CH, Ayres PH, Shinohara Y. A scanning and transmission electron microscopic study of normal and 2-acetylaminofluorene-treated mouse urinary bladder. *Invest Urol* 1981;19:17–19.
13. Jacobs JB, Arai M, Cohen SM, Friedell GH. Light and scanning electron microscopy of exfoliated bladder epithelial cells in rats fed *N*-[4-(5-nitro-2-furyl)-2-thiazolyl]formamide. *J Natl Cancer Inst* 1976;57:63–66.
14. Anderstrom C, Johansson SL, Von-Schultz L. The influence of phenacetin or mechanical perforation on the development of renal pelvic and urinary bladder tumors in FANFT-induced urinary tract carcinogenesis. *Acta Pathol Microbiol Immunol Scand* 1983;91:373–380.
15. Frith CH. Report of a workshop on urothelial lesions in mice. *J Environ Pathol Toxicol* 1978;1:617–626.
16. Frith CH, Townsend JW, Ayres PH. Histology, ultrastructure, urinary tract, mouse. In: Jones TC, Mohr U, Hunt RD, eds. *Monographs on pathology of laboratory animals: urinary system*. Berlin: Springer-Verlag; 1986:331–337.
17. Richter WR, Moize SM. Electron microscopic observations on the collapsed and distended mammalian urinary bladder (transitional epithelium). *J Ultrastruct Res* 1963;9:1–10.
18. Ayres PH, Shinohara Y, Frith CH. Morphological observations on the epithelium of the developing urinary bladder of the mouse and rat. *J Urol* 1985;133:506–512.
19. Cohen SM, Cano M, Sakata T, Johansson SL. Ultrastructural characteristics of the fetal and neonatal rat urinary bladder. *Scanning Microsc* 1988;2:2091–2104.
20. Frith CH, Greenman DL. Value of serial sections of the mouse urinary bladder in the determination of the incidence of bladder carcinoma. *Toxicol Lett* 1978;2:351–354.
21. Shinohara Y, Frith CH. Comparison of experimental and spontaneous urothelial hyperplasias occurring in BALB/c mice. *Invest Urol* 1981;18:235–238.
22. Cohen SM. Toxic and nontoxic changes induced in the urothelium of xenobiotics. *Toxicol Appl Pharmacol* 1989;101:484–498.
23. Frith CH, Ward JM. *A color atlas of neoplastic and nonneoplastic lesions in aging mice*. Amsterdam: Elsevier; 1988:67–70.
24. Stula EF. Adenocarcinoma, urinary bladder, mouse. In: Jones TC, Mohr U, Hunt RD, eds. *Monographs on pathology of laboratory animals: urinary system*. Berlin: Springer-Verlag; 1986:346–351.
25. Frith CH, Highman B, Burger G, Sheldon WD. Spontaneous lesions in virgin and retired breeder BALB/c and C57BL/6 mice. *Lab Anim Sci* 1983;33:273–286.
26. Gaylor DW, Greenman DL, Frith CH. Urinary bladder neoplasms induced in BALB/c female mice with low doses of 2-acetylaminofluorene. *J Environ Pathol Toxicol Oncol* 1985,6:127–136.
27. Cohen SM. Pathology of experimental bladder cancer in rodents. In: Bryan GT, Cohen SM, eds. *The pathology of bladder cancer*. Vol II. Boca Raton, FL: CRC Press; 1983:1–40.
28. Kunze E, Shauer A. Morphology, classification and histogenesis of bladder cancer. *Z Krebsforsch* 1977;75:273–289.
29. Frith CH, West RW, Stanley JW, Jackson CD. Urothelial lesions in mice given 4-ethylsulfonapthalene-1-sulfonamide, acetazolamide and oxamide. *J Exp Pathol Toxicol Oncol* 1984;5:25–38.
30. West RW, Frith CH, Stanley JW, Jackson CD. The role of urinary physiological changes in the genesis of urothelial lesions in mice given 4-ethylsulfonyl naphthalene-1-sulfonamide, acetazolamide and oxamide. *J Environ Pathol Toxicol Oncol* 1984;4/5:39–50.
31. Littlefield NA, Greeman DL, Farmer JH, Sheldon WG. Effects of continuous and discontinued exposure to 2-AAF on urinary bladder hyperplasia and neoplasia. *J Environ Pathol Toxicol* 1980;3:35–54.

32. Greenman DL, Boothe A, Kodell R. Age-dependent responses to 2-acetylaminofluorene in BALB/c female mice. *J Toxicol Environ Health* 1987;22:113–129.
33. Frith CH, Rule JE. The effects of discontinuing administration of high levels of 2-acetylaminofluorene on the mouse urinary bladder. *J Environ Pathol Toxicol* 1978;1:581–585.
34. Fukushima S, Arai M, Cohen SM, Jacobs JB, Friedell GM. Scanning electron microscopy of cyclophosphamide-induced hyperplasia of the rat urinary bladder. *Lab Invest* 1981;44:89–96.
35. Fukushima S, Cohen SM, Arai M, Jacobs JB, Friedell GH. Examination of reversible hyperplasia of the rat urinary bladder. *Am J Pathol* 1981;102:373–380.
36. Shirai T, Fukushima S, Tagawa Y, Okamura M, Ito N. Cell proliferation induced by uracil-calculi and subsequent development reversible papillomatosis in the rat urinary bladder. *Cancer Res* 1989; 49:378–383.
37. Frith CH, Farmer JH, Greenman DL, Shaw GW. Biologic and morphologic characteristics of urinary bladder neoplasms induced in BALB/c female mice with 2-acetylaminofluorene. *J Environ Pathol Toxicol* 1980;3:103–119.
38. Ito N, Shirai T. Papilloma, urinary bladder, rat. In: Jones TC, Mohr U, Hunt RD, eds. *Monographs on pathology of laboratory animals: urinary system.* Berlin: Springer-Verlag; 1986:337–341.
39. Sakata T, Masui T, St John M, Cohen SM. Uracil-induced calculi and proliferative lesions of the mouse urinary bladder. *Carcinogenesis* 1988;9:1271–1276.
40. Frith CH. Transitional cell carcinoma, urinary tract, mouse. In: Jones TC, Mohr U, Hunt RD, eds. *Monographs on pathology of laboratory animals: urinary system.* Berlin: Springer-Verlag; 1986: 331–337.
41. Frith CH, Wiley LD, Shinohara Y. Sequential morphogenesis of bladder tumors in BALB/c female mice fed 2-acetylaminofluorene. *Invest Urol* 1983;28:1071–1076.
42. Ito N, Hirose M. Squamous cell carcinoma, urinary bladder, rat. In: Jones TC, Mohr U, Hunt RD, eds. *Monographs on pathology of laboratory animals: urinary system.* Berlin: Springer-Verlag; 1986:341–346.
43. Jacobs JB, Cohen SM, Arai M, Friedell GH, Bulay O, Urman HK. Chemically induced smooth muscle tumors of the mouse urinary bladder. *Cancer Res* 1976;36:2396–2398.
44. Chandra M, Frith CH. Spontaneous occurring leiomyosarcomas of the mouse urinary bladder. *Toxicol Pathol* 1991;19:164–167.
45. Squire RA. Classification and differential diagnosis of neoplasms, urinary bladder, rat. In: Jones TC, Mohr U, Hunt RD, eds. *Monographs on pathology of laboratory animals: urinary system.* Berlin: Springer-Verlag; 1986:311–317.
46. Kunze E, Chowaniec J. Tumours of the urinary bladder. In: Turusov VS, Mohr U, eds. *Pathology of tumours in laboratory animals.* Vol 1. *Tumours of the rat.* Lyon, France: International Agency for Research on Cancer; 1990:345–397.
47. Frith CH, Baetcke KP, Nelson CJ, Schieferrstein G. Importance of the mouse liver tumor in carcinogenesis bioassay studies using benzidine dihydrochloride as a model. *Toxicol Lett* 1979;4:507–518.
48. Cohen SM, Ellwein LB. Proliferative and genotoxic cellular effects in 2-acetylaminofluorene bladder and liver carcinogenesis: Biological modeling of the ED_{01} study. *Toxicol Appl Pharmacol* 1990; 104:79–83.
49. Miller EC, Miller JA. Searches for ultimate chemical carcinogens and their reactions with cellular macromolecules. *Cancer* 1981;47:2327–2345.
50. Lai CC, Miller EC, Miller JA, Liem A. The essential role of microsomal deacetylase activity in the metabolic activation, DNA-(deoxyguanosin-8-yl)-2-aminofluorene adduct formation and initiation of liver tumors by N-hydroxy-2-acetylaminofluorene in the livers of infant male $B6C3F_1$ mice. *Carcinogenesis* 1988;9:1295–1302.
51. Lai CC, Miller EC, Miller JA, Liem A. Initiation of hepatocarcinogenesis in infant male $B6C3F_1$ mice by N-hydroxy-2-aminofluorene or N-hydroxy-2-acetylaminofluorene and formation of DNA-(deoxyguanosin-8-yl)-2-aminofluorene adducts. *Carcinogenesis* 1987;8:471–478.
52. Poirier MC, Fullerton NF, Kinouchi T, Smith BA, Beland FA. Comparison between DNA adduct formation and tumorigenesis in livers and bladders of mice chronically fed 2-acetylaminofluorene. *Carcinogenesis* 1991;12:895–900.
53. Clayson DB. Bladder carcinogenesis in rats and mice: possibility of artifacts. *J Natl Cancer Inst* 1974;52:1685–1689.
54. Jull JW. The effect of time on the incidence of carcinomas obtained by the implantation of paraffin wax pellets in mouse bladder. *Cancer Lett* 1979;6:21–25.
55. Gold LS, Bernstein L, Magaaw R, Slone TH. Interspecies extrapolation in carcinogenesis: prediction between rats and mice. *Environ Health Perspect* 1989,81:211–219.

56. Gold LS, Slone TH, Manley LB. Target organs in chronic bioassays of 533 chemical carcinogens. *Environ Health Perspect* 1991;93:233–246.
57. Huff J, Cirvello J, Haseman J, Bucher J. Chemicals associated with site-specific neoplasia in 1394 long-term carcinogenesis experiments in laboratory rodents. *Environ Health Perspect* 1991;93:247–271.
58. Lijinsky W. Species differences in nitrosoamine carcinogenesis. *J Cancer Res Clin Oncol* 1984;108:46–55.
59. Littlefield NA, Cueto C, Davis AK, Medlock K. Chronic dose-response studies in mice fed 2-AAF. *J Toxicol Environ Health* 1975;1:25–37.
60. Fullerton FR, Greenman DL, McCarty CC, Bucci TJ. Increased incidence of spontaneous and 2-acetylaminofluorene-induced liver and bladder tumors in B6C3F$_1$ mice fed AIN-76A diet versus NIH-07. *Fundam Appl Toxicol* 1991;16:51–60.
61. Fullerton FR, Greenman DL, Bucci TJ. Effects of diet type on incidence of spontaneous and 2-acetylaminofluorene-induced liver and bladder tumors in BALB/c mice fed AIN-76A diet versus NIH-07. *Fundam Appl Toxicol* 1992;18:193–199.
62. Oyasu R, Battifora HA, Eisenstein R, McDonald JH, Hass GM. Enhancement of tumorigenesis in the urinary bladder of rats by neonatal administration of 2-acetylaminofluorene. *J Natl Cancer Inst* 1968;40:377–388.
63. Cohen SM, Ellwein LB. Cell proliferation in carcinogenesis. *Science* 1990;249:1007–1911.
64. Cohen SM. Analysis of modifying factors in chemical carcinogenesis. In: Ito N, Sugano H, eds. *Progress in Experimental Tumor Research: modification of tumor development in rodents.* New York: S Karger; 1991:21–40.
65. Fukushima S. Modification of tumor development in the urinary bladder. *Prog Exp Tumor Res* 1991;33:154–174.
66. *IARC monographs on the evaluation of the carcinogenic risk of chemicals to humans.* Vol 22. *Some non-nutritive sweetening agents.* Lyon, France: International Agency for Research on Cancer, 1980.
67. Hicks R, Wakefield JStJ, Chowaniec J. Evaluation of a new model to detect bladder carcinogen or co-carcinogens; results obtained with saccharin, cyclamate and cyclophosphamine. *Chem Biol Interact* 1975;11:225–233.
68. Cohen SM, Arai M, Jacobs JB, et al. Promoting effects of saccharin and DL-tryptophan in urinary bladder carcinogenesis. *Cancer Res* 1979;39:1207–1217.
69. Boorman GA. High incidence of spontaneous urinary bladder and ureter tumors in the brown Norway rat. *J Natl Cancer Inst* 1975;52:1005–1008.
70. Shirai T, Tagawa Y, Fukushima S, et al. Strong promoting activity of reversible uracil-induced urolithiasis on urinary bladder carcinogenesis in rats initiated with *N*-butyl-*N*-(4-hydroxybutyl)nitrosamine. *Cancer Res* 1987;47:6726–6730.
71. Okumura M, Shirai T, Tamano S, Ito N, Yamada S, Fukushima S. Uracil-induced calculi and carcinogenesis in the urinary bladder of rats treated simultaneously with *N*-butyl-*N*-(4-hydroxybutyl)nitrosamine. *Carcinogenesis* 1991;12:35–41.
72. Ohtani T, Fukushima S, Okamura T, et al. Effects of intravesical instillation of antitumor chemotherapeutic agents on bladder carcinogenesis in rats treated with *N*-butyl-*N*-(4-hydroxybutyl)nitrosamine. *Cancer* 1984;54:1525–1529.
73. Frith CH, Norvell MJ, Umholtz R, Knapka JJ. Effect of dietary protein and fat levels on liver and urinary bladder neoplasia in mice fed 2-acetylaminofluorene. *J Food Safety* 1980;2:183–189.
74. Cameron E, Pauling L, Leibovitz B. Ascorbic acid and cancer: a review. *Cancer Res* 1979;39:663–681.
75. Wattenberg LW. Inhibition of chemical carcinogenesis. *J Natl Cancer Inst* 1978;60:11–18.
76. Toth B, Patil K. Enhancing effect of vitamin E on murine intestinal tumorigenesis by 1,2-dimethylhydrazine dihydrochloride. *J Natl Cancer Inst* 1983;70:1107–1111.
77. Kunze E. Hyperplasia, urinary bladder, rat. In: Jones TC, Mohr U, Hunt RD, eds. *Monographs on pathology of laboratory animals: urinary system.* Berlin: Springer-Verlag; 1986:291–310.
78. Fukushima S, Hirose M, Tsuda H, Shirai T, Hirao K, Arai M, Ito N. Histological classification or urinary bladder cancers in rats by *N*-butyl-*N*-(4-hydroxybutyl)nitrosamine. *Gann* 1976;67:81–90.
79. Ito N, Hiasa Y, Tamia A, Okajima E, Kitamura H. Histogenesis of urinary bladder tumors induced by *N*-butyl-*N*-(4-hydroxybutyl)nitrosamine in rats. *Gann* 1969;60:401–410.
80. Lijinsky W, Saavedra JE, Reuber MD. Induction of carcinogenesis in Fischer rats by methylalkylnitrosamine. *Cancer Res* 1981;41:1288–1292.
81. Pamukcu AM, Ertürk E, Yalciner S, Bryan GT. Histogenesis of urinary bladder cancer induced in rats by bracken fern. *Invest Urol* 1976;14:213–218.

82. Pamukcu AM, Yalciner S, Hatcher JF, Bryan GT. Quercetin, a rat intestinal and bladder carcinogen present in bracken fern (*Pteridium aquilinum*). *Cancer Res* 40;3648–3472.
83. Hirono I, Aiso S, Hosaka S, Yamaji T, Haga M. Induction of mammary cancer in CD rats fed bracken fern diet. *Carcinogenesis* 1983;4:885–887.
84. Ertürk E, Cohen SM, Price JM, Bryan GT. Pathogenesis, histology, and transplantability of urinary bladder carcinomas induced in albino rats by oral administration of N-[4-(5-nitro-2-furyl)-thiazolyl]formamide. *Cancer Res* 1969;29:2219–2228.
85. Hicks RM, Wright R, Wakefield JStJ. The induction of rat bladder cancer by 2-naphthylamine. *Br J Cancer* 1982;46:646–661.
86. *Bioassay of p-quinone dioxime for possible carcinogenicity.* NIH publication 79-1735. Bethesda, MD: National Cancer Institute; 1979.
87. *Bioassay of o-anisidine hydrochloride for possible carcinogenicity.* NIH publication 78-1339. Bethesda, MD: National Cancer Institute; 1978.
88. *Bioassay of nitrilotriacetic acid and nitrilotriacetic, trisodium salt, monohydrate for possible carcinogenicity.* NIH publication 77-806. Bethesda, MD: National Cancer Institute; 1979.
89. *Bioassay of o-toluidine for possible carcinogenicity.* NIH publication 79-1709. Bethesda, MD: National Cancer Institute; 1979.
90. *Bioassay of 4-amino-2-nitrophenol for possible carcinogenicity.* NIH publication 78-1344. Bethesda, MD: National Cancer Institute; 1978.
91. *Bioassay of N-nitrosodiphenylamine for possible carcinogenicity.* NIH publication 79-1720. Bethesda, MD: National Cancer Institute; 1979.
92. *Carcinogenesis bioassay of allyl isothiocyanate in F-344/N rats and B6C3F1 mice (gavage study).* NIH publication 83-1790. Research Triangle Park, NC: National Toxicology Program; 1983.
93. *Carcinogenesis bioassay of melamine in F344/N rats and B6C3F1 mice (feed study).* NIH publication 83-2501. Research Triangle Park, NC: National Toxicology Program; 1983.
94. Alden C, Frith CH. Urinary system. In: Haschek-Hock WM, Rousseau CG, eds. *Fundamentals of toxicologic pathology.* Orlando, FL: Academic Press; 1991;316–387.
95. Frith CH, Dooley K. Brief communication: hepatic cytologic and neoplastic changes in mice given benzidine dihydrochloride. *J Natl Cancer Inst* 1976;56:679–682.
96. Highman B, Frith CH, Littlefield NA. Alkaline phosphatase activity in hyperplastic and neoplastic epithelium of mice fed 2-acetylaminofluorene. *J Natl Cancer Inst* 1975;54:257–261.
97. Hinderer RK, Lankas GR, Knezevich AL, Auletta CS. The effects of long-term dietary administration of the rubber accelerator, N-oxydiethylene thiocarbamyl-n-oxydiethylene sulfenamide, to rats. *Toxicol Appl Pharmacol* 1986;82:521–531.

7

Chemically Associated Respiratory Carcinogenesis in Rodents and in Humans

James Huff

Environmental Carcinogenesis Program, National Institute of Environmental Health Sciences, Research Triangle Park, North Carolina 27709

> [T]he lung is one of the preferred target organs for those agents and complex exposures that have been established as carcinogenic to humans.   (L. Tomatis, 1990)

Diseases collectively grouped under the term *cancer* remain a leading and devastating cause of morbidity and mortality throughout the world (1,2). In the United States alone, more than 1,170,000 cases of cancer will be diagnosed in 1993, and another 515,000 persons will die from the disease (3). Cancer kills more children aged 1 to 14 than does any other disease, and almost 85,000,000 Americans now living will eventually get cancer. Obviously, these numbers are in reality probably higher, because not every case of cancer is diagnosed and not every death from cancer is so attributed (4). Unfortunately, trends in certain common tumor sites, including lung and respiratory tract, are upward (5,6).

Lung cancers are the most rapidly increasing cancers in Western Europe and North America (2). In the United States, cancer of the lung and bronchus will be diagnosed in 170,000 people in 1993 (nearly twice as many males as females) (3). The 1989 lung cancer incidence rate of 80.1 per 100,000 is second only to prostate among males, and the rate of 39.3 per 100,000 among females is in second place behind breast cancer (7). Lung cancer is the chief cause of cancer death in both sexes. In 1993, nearly 93,000 men and 53,000 women will die from cancer (3). Due to the poor relative survival rates for lung cancer, there is a very close correspondence between incidence and mortality rates and trends. Between the years 1973 and 1989, incidence increased 33.4% (males, 10.5%; females 108.4%) and mortality increased 38.4% (males, 18.3%; females, 118.3%) (7).

Estimates of lung cancers from non-tobacco-smoking causes remain unclear, yet some claim as high a figure as 15% (see Ref. 8). Whether these cancers originate uniquely from environmental sources such as chemicals is also still unknown. Nonetheless, the influence of cofactors on the incidence of lung cancers from tobacco cannot be ignored; these include asbestos, other fibers, and particulates; radon and decay products; air pollution; chemical exposures in the environment, home, and workplace; over-the-counter drugs and pharmaceuticals; and airborne chemicals and pesticides. Shopland et al. (9) propose that 90% of the 92,000 male and 78.5% of the 51,000 female lung cancer deaths in the United States are attributable to smoking. Axelson et al. (10) suggest that for men in industrial nations (except Japan) at least 85% of lung cancer is attributable to smoking, as is about 75% in women. This high frequency of an association of tobacco smoking and lung cancer tends to obscure other potentially significant causative attributions. Nonetheless, sizable numbers of lung cancers are probably due to factors or cofactors other than smoking, or synergistic with smoking; as trends in the numbers of people stopping tobacco smoking continue, together with fewer new smokers, the other factors causing lung cancer may become clearer.

Considering air pollution as an example generically, and controlling for differences in smoking behavior, Tomatis et al. (11) estimate that excess relative risks of lung cancer in urban areas are generally on the order of 50% or less. Of this excess lung cancer risk, up to 20% may be attributed to air pollution exposure. As another example, consider populations at risk residing in communities that have not met air quality standards, estimated as ranging from 74,000 children aged 5 years or under to 31 million preadolescent children aged 13 years and under (12). If these figures are even close to reality, reducing the potential adverse impact of air pollution on public health must be considered a national priority.

Exposures to natural and synthetic environmental agents can and do contribute to the development of cancers (13–17) (see the chapter, "Chemicals Causally Associated with Cancers in Humans and Laboratory Animals, by Huff). Strategies to reduce, eliminate, and prevent the incidence and mortality of cancer attributed both directly and indirectly to environmental factors rely primarily on (a) identifying and preventing the causes of these diseases; (b) educating the public on cancer risks; (c) preventing, reducing, and eliminating exposures to environmental agents; (d) intervention into the processes of carcinogenesis; (e) identifying biological indicators (biomarkers) of the organ-specific diseases; (f) via use of animal surrogates, determining those chemicals and exposure circumstances most likely to represent cancer risks; and (g) developing better, innovative, and more directed treatment regimens for particular identified cancers.

PURPOSE

In this chapter we concentrate on those chemicals and exposure circumstances identified as causing lung/respiratory tract cancers in humans and compare these findings with those from experimental animals exposed to the same agents. We further endorse the value and usefulness of animal model systems to identify potential human carcinogens, centering on those chemicals that have been studied and evaluated for carcinogenesis predominantly by inhalation exposure. We have selected this major subgroup of agents because inhalation is the cardinal route of exposure to environmental chemicals. However, one should remain cognizant that inhalational exposures often result in cancers at sites distant to the lung: for instance, cancers of the urinary bladder and pancreas, and possibly liver and kidney, due to tobacco smoke (18,19). Similarly, this is not uncommon in chemical carcinogenesis experiments (20,21).

Table 1 lists the target organs for 450 chemicals evaluated to date in our program. Cancers of the lung were induced by 44 chemicals (9.8%), and cancers of the nasal cavity were caused by 11 chemicals (2.4%). Certain empirical data are given for

TABLE 1. Numbers of chemicals associated with site-specific tumor induction in experimental carcinogenesis studies[a]

Organ, tissue, or system	Number of chemicals
Adrenal gland	33
Bone	3
Brain	12
Circulatory system	17
Clitoral gland	14
Epididymis	1
Esophagus[b]	3
Forestomach[b]	39
Glandular stomach	2
Harderian gland	12
Heart	4
Hematopoietic syst (leuk./lymp.)	53
Intestines	19
Kidney	48
Liver	141
Lung	44
Mammary gland	37
Mesothelium (abd. cav./tun. vag.)	12
Nasal cavity	11
Oral cavity[b]	11
Ovary	9
Pancreas	15
Parathyroid gland	1
Pituitary gland	7
Preputial gland	18
Seminal vesicle	1
Skin[b]	23
Spleen	12
Subcutaneous tissue	17
Thyroid gland	33
Ureter	2
Urinary bladder	19
Uterus/cervix	18
Zymbal's gland	24
No carcinogenic response	131

[a]Overall number of chemicals evaluated in long-term carcinogenesis experiments, 425.
[b]Other target sites for inhalation carcinogenesis.

these respiratory carcinogens (Table 2). Few of these chemicals are single-site carcinogens; most chemicals in this data set did not associate with cancer induction in both organs. Dibromoethane, for example, caused lung tumors by three routes of exposure (inhalation, gavage, dermal), but nasal cavity tumors only by inhalation exposure. In fact, the inhalation exposure route seems to correlate better for cancers of the nasal cavity than for the lung. Mice appear to respond more readily to lung carcinogens than do rats, whereas the opposite is true for nasal cavity carcinogens. Several were evaluated more than once (butadiene, dibromochloropropane, dibromoethane, dichloromethane) and the evidence of carcinogenicity was confirmed. In a companion report (see the chapter, "Chemicals Causally Associated with Cancer in Humans and Laboratory Animals," by Huff) we expand on the correspondence between identified animals and human carcinogens without dependence on route of exposure, and the usefulness and value of long-term chemical carcinogenesis experiments in laboratory animals (4,22–24).

BACKGROUND AND METHODS

Major and historical foundations for our knowledge on environmentally associated cancers center largely on the International Agency for Research on Cancer, in particular the IARC Monographs Series (15). Their objective evaluations of epidemiological and experimental evidence as to the carcinogenicity (and other relevant information) of chemicals, mixtures of chemicals, industrial processes, occupations, lifestyles and cultural habits, and varied exposure circumstances establishes a foundation for other organizations and governments to use in the protection of public health. IARC has identified approximately 110 environmental agents or conditions recognized as causing cancer in humans (13,25–29). The major and primary route of exposure for most human carcinogens is inhalation.

The National Toxicology Program (and prior to that the National Cancer Institute) strengthened and "standardized" the experimental protocols for identifying chemicals causing cancer in laboratory animals, and using a strength-of-the-evidence approach (4,23,30), attempts to identify those chemicals considered most likely to present carcinogenic hazards to humans (31). To date, 450 long-term chemical carcinogenesis studies in two species of laboratory animals have been reported (18,22,32–34). Thus from these major sources of international information, we compared those chemicals considered to cause lung (and other site-specific) cancer in humans by inhalation with the same chemicals studied in animals. Lewtas (35) compiled and compared experimental and human evidence for the carcinogenicity of air pollutants, based largely on the IARC Monographs (volumes 1–46) and the bioassay database of the U.S. Environmental Protection Agency.

Additionally, we have identified a sizable number of agents for which evidence for cancer was first discovered in animal model systems and only subsequently associated with cancers in humans (36,37) and have compared and summarized the target-organ sites for those chemicals through experimental and epidemiological

TABLE 2. Summary data of chemicals causing lung and/or nasal cavity tumors in 450 NCI/NTP carcinogenesis bioassays

Site	Number of chemicals	Rodent, sex-species[a]				Exposure route[b]						Only[c]
		MR	FR	MM	FM	G	F	I	W	SP	IJ	
Lung	44 (9.8%)	10	10	25	27	15	13	11	2	2	1	4
Nasal cavity	11 (2.4%)	11	9	3	4	2	2	5	1	1	0	2

Empirical observations:
1. Comparatively, mice seem more responsive to lung cancer, whereas rats develop nasal cavity cancer.
2. Male rat was responsive to all 11 nasal cavity carcinogens.
3. Most chemicals causing lung cancer (but not nasal cavity) did so by routes other than inhalation.
4. Four chemicals (3 single-sex, single species; 2 were equivocal) affected only the lung, and two (trans-sex, trans-species) for the nasal cavity.
5. Two single-site carcinogens caused cancer in all four sex-species experiments: tetranitromethane and lung cancer at all exposure levels, propylene oxide and nasal cavity at highest exposure groups only.
6. Four chemicals caused tumors at both sites: dibromochloropropane, dibromoethane, dibromopropanol, epoxybutane.
7. Nearly 75% of lung carcinogens were mutagenic to Salmonella, only one nasal cavity carcinogen was nonmutagenic: 1,4-dioxane.
8. Correspondence between sexes of a species for lung was 21 of 44 and for nasal cavity was 10 of 11.

[a]MR, male rat; FR, female rat; MM, male mice; FM, female mice.
[b]G, gavage; F, feed; I, inhalation; W, drinking water; SP, skin paint; IJ, injection.
[c]Only, no other organ sites of cancer.

studies. Based on the knowledge gained from these animal studies, alternative approaches to identifying environmental cancer agents are suggested.

The IARC has identified approximately 60 agents [group 1: "The agent (mixture) is carcinogenic to humans. The exposure circumstance entails exposures that are carcinogenic to humans"] that are recognized as causing cancers in humans, and these chemicals or processes have been determined to be carcinogenic to humans based on epidemiological data. Further, IARC has identified an additional 51 chemicals, groups of chemicals, or industrial processes that are probably carcinogenic to humans [group 2A: "The agent (mixture) is probably carcinogenic to humans. The exposure circumstance entails exposures that are probably carcinogenic to humans"], based on human epidemiological studies and/or on experimental results from animal studies (13,15,28,29).

The group 1 and 2A chemicals for which animal inhalation studies are available are reviewed and the results of target-organ lesions are compared to those in humans (Tables 3 and 4). The IARC Monographs (15) as well as the available literature, the DHHS/NTP Annual Reports on Carcinogens (16,31), and the NTP Carcinogenesis bioassay database and Technical Reports Series (32,34) have been reviewed to identify those agents for which the animal studies were the initial basis for identifying

TABLE 3. *IARC Group 1 chemicals causing lung/respiratory cancers in humans and lung/respiratory cancers in animals*

Group 1 chemicals	Species	Target organs in humans and in animals (suspect)
Aflatoxins	Human	Liver (lung)
	Rat	Liver, kidney, colon, local
	Mouse	Liver, lung
	Hamster	Liver
	Monkey	Liver, pancreas
Arsenic and As compounds	Human	Lung, skin (liver, GIT, kidney, hematopoietic)
	Mouse	Lung and respiratory tract
	Hamster	Lung and respiratory tract
Asbestos	Human	Lung, pleura, peritoneum (larynx, GIT)
	Rat	Lung, pleura, peritoneum
	Mouse	Peritoneum
	Hamster	Pleura, peritoneum
Benzene	Humans	Leukemia, lung (multiple myeloma, malignant lymphoma, liver)
	Rat	Zymbal gland, nasal and oral cavity, skin (ovary, uterus, lung, mammary)
	Mouse	Lung, Zymbal gland, lymphoma, mammary gland, ovary
Beryllium and Be compounds	Human	Lung
	Rat	Lung
Bis(chloromethyl)ether and chloromethylmethyl ether	Human	Lung
	Rat	Lung, nasal cavity,
	Mouse	Lung, local, skin
	Hamster	(Respiratory tract)
Cadmium and Cd compounds	Human	Lung, stomach, (prostate gland)
	Rat	Lung, prostate gland, leukemia, testes, local
	Mouse	Lung
Chromium (VI) compounds	Human	Lung, nasal cavity (GIT)
	Rat	Lung, local
	Mouse	Lung, (nasal cavity), local
Coal-tars	Human	Lung, skin, (urinary bladder)
	Rat	Lung
	Mouse	Lung, skin, local
Mustard gas (sulfur mustard)	Human	Lung, larynx, pharynx
	Mouse	(Lung, local)
Nickel and Ni compounds	Human	Lung, nasal cavity
	Rat	Lung, local
	Mouse	Lung, local
	Hamster	Local
Radon and decay products	Human	Lung
	Dog	Lung
	Rat	Lung
Soots	Human	Lung, skin
	Rat	Lung
	Mouse	Skin, local
Talc containing asbestiform fibers	Human	Lung (pleura)
	Rat (pure)	Lung, adrenal gland
Tobacco smoke	Human	Lung, urinary bladder, oral cavity, pharynx, larynx, kidney, plus
	Rat	Respiratory system
	Hamster	Respiratory system
Vinyl chloride	Human	Liver, blood vessels brain, lung (breast, GIT)
	Rat	Lung, liver, blood vessels, mammary gland, skin, Zymbal gland
	Mouse	
	Hamster	

Mixtures causing lung cancers in humans that have not been studied at all or inadequately in experimental animals include: coal-tar pitches (lung, skin urinary bladder), mineral oils (skin [lung, respiratory tract, GIT]).

Exposure circumstances causing lung cancers in humans that are unlikely to be studied in experimental animals include: aluminum production (lung, urinary bladder [lymphatic system]), boot and shoe manufacture and repair (nasal cavity, hematopoietic system, [lung, pharynx, others]), coal gasification (lung, skin, urinary bladder), coke production (lung, skin, urinary bladder), furniture and cabinet making (nasal cavity), iron and steel founding (lung [GIT, genitourinay and hematopoietic systems]), isopropyl alcohol manufacturing (strong acid process) (nasal cavity [larynx]), painter (occupation) (lung), rubber industry (urinary bladder, hematopoietic system. [lung, GIT, skin]) underground hematite mining and exposure to radon (lung).

TABLE 4. IARC Group 2A chemicals causing lung cancers in humans and respiratory cancers in animals

Group 2A chemical	Subject	Results of animal inhalation studies and epidemiology studies
Acryolnitrile	Rats	Neoplasms of the central nervous system, mammary gland, Zymbal's gland, forestomach
	Humans	Lung, CNS, and other sites
Benzo[a]pyrene	Rats	Lung tumors
	Hamsters	Negative
	Humans	No data
1,3-Butadiene	Rats	Multiple sites, including pancreas, uterus, testes, mammary gland, Zymbal's gland, brain, thyroid
	Mice	Multiple sites, including lung, heart, lymphoma, liver, kidney, Harderian gland, preputial gland
	Humans	Leukemia, lymphoma
Dimethylcarbamoyl chloride	Rats	Nasal tract carcinomas
	Hamsters	Nasal tract carcinomas
	Humans	No data
Dimethyl sulfate	Rats	Lung tumors
	Humans	Bronchial carcinomas
Epichlorohydrin	Rats	Nasal cavity tumors; equivocal evidence for lung tumors
	Humans	Equivocal evidence of lung neoplasms
Ethylene oxide	Rats	Mononuclear cell leukemia, brain tumors, peritoneal mesotheliomas
	Mice	Lung tumors, Harderian gland, uterine, mammary carcinomas, malignant lymphomas
	Humans	Limited evidence of leukemia
Formaldehyde	Rats	Squamous cell carcinomas of the nasal cavity
	Mice	Uncertain findings
	Humans	Limited evidence
Propylene oxide	Rats	Papillary adenomas of the nasal turbinates
	Mice	Hemangiomas and hemangiosarcomas of the nasal submucosa
	Humans	Inadequate data
Silica crystalline	Rats	Adenocarcinomas and squamous cell carcinomas, lung
	Humans	Lung
Vinyl bromide	Rats	Liver, Zymbal's gland
	Humans	No data

carcinogenic risks and only later were discovered to be associated with cancer in humans (see, e.g., refs. 36,37).

COMPARATIVE CARCINOGENESIS RESULTS

For the IARC group 1 chemicals (Table 3), there are adequate experimental inhalation studies in animals for 11: asbestos; benzene; beryllium and beryllium compounds; bis(chloromethyl) ether (BCME) and bis(chloromethylethyl) ether (BCMEE); cadmium and cadmium compounds; mustard gas (sulfur mustard); nickel and nickel compounds; radon and decay products; shale oil; tobacco smoke; and vinyl chloride. For the group 2A chemicals (Table 4) there are 11: acrylonitrile; benzo[a]pyrene; 1,3-butadiene; dimethylcarbamoyl chloride; dimethylsulfate; epichlorohydrin; ethylene oxide; formaldehyde; propylene oxide; silica crystalline; and vinyl bromide. Experimental studies using the inhalation route of exposure for these 22 IARC chemicals have shown consistently that when the respiratory system was a primary organ site for cancer in humans, the respiratory system was also a target site for cancer in rodents. Importantly, there were typically, albeit not always (e.g., propylene oxide), additional organ sites of chemically induced carcinogenesis in the rodent (Table 2).

Except for the consistency of carcinogenesis of the respiratory tract (lung in particular) for these chemicals, there seems to be a general lack of commonality in other target-site tumorigenesis in either humans or animals. Obviously, this reflects the specificity of the particular chemical or exposure circumstance. In humans, an added factor may be the comparatively incomplete search for other tumor sites once a chemical–cancer association has been established. For example, benzene has long been known to cause leukemia in humans, yet only recently have other causative cancers been substantiated, although these were predicted years ago.

DISCUSSION

Current and internationally accepted methods for identifying a carcinogenic potential for chemicals relies primarily on epidemiological investigations or on experimental studies in laboratory animals (33,38–41). We can reduce the national and international cancer disease burden only by identifying environmental causes and synergistic influences with more certainty. This would be particularly beneficial in ascertaining the primary causes for the major human cancers, which include cancers of the lung, stomach, breast, colon–rectum, and cervix. The task is formidable, of course, and has been pursued for more than 200 years. For most of these target organs none or only a few agents have been identified. Some have proposed that the environment is responsible for more than 90% of the cancer burden (42), others have placed considerable emphasis on diet as the major cause of cancers (43); still others debate the latter assignment (13,14,44).

Our review of the more than 110 agents designated with IARC groups 1 and 2A shows that experimental studies have been most effective in identifying chemicals that also cause cancer in humans; and in particular for identifying chemicals that may contribute to the burden of lung cancer, a leading cause of cancer morbidity and mortality in the world. [Obviously, a large proportion (but not all) of these cases are related to tobacco smoking (18).] Inhalation studies in rodents have been reported for 20 of the chemicals that the IARC has designated as being carcinogenic to humans. Of these, 19 were studied in rats, 8 in mice, and 6 in hamsters. All 19 human carcinogens studied in the rat gave positive carcinogenic responses in this species. When the respiratory system was a target-organ site in humans, the respiratory system was also a target site in rats, although there often were additional organ or tissue sites of carcinogenesis in the rat.

The mouse and hamster have in some cases been less responsive than the rat to inhalation chemical carcinogenesis (for some of these agents). For example, whereas cadmium exposure produced tumors of the respiratory tract in the rat, exposure to cadmium gave no or minimal evidence for respiratory tract tumors in hamsters and mice (45–49). Formaldehyde caused respiratory tract (nasal cavity) tumors in rats but not in mice (50). Studies with bis(chloromethyl) ether showed that at 0.1 ppm the incidence of tumors of the nasal cavity and lung was much higher in rats than in hamsters (51). Both rats and hamsters developed nasal cavity tumors after exposure to dimethylcarbamoyl chloride, but in rats the percentage of tumor yield was almost double that in hamsters and the tumors appeared earlier (52). Furst and Schlauder (53) reviewed studies of metals in hamsters by a variety of routes of administration and indicate that hamsters develop fewer tumors than rats do in response to heavy metals.

For the chemicals evaluated in our research program, however, the mouse seems to be more sensitive to lung carcinogens, with the rat identifying more carcinogens for the nasal cavity (Tables 2 and 3). As strains of rodents do sometimes differ in response to the same chemical, one needs to consider this in evaluating chemicals for toxicologic endpoints. Most often, one observes consistency in carcinogenic responses, yet one also finds differences in target-organ responses and potency (20,54). Obviously, these differences may be due to, among others, differences in metabolism or to metabolic activation. Varying experimental conditions are often discovered to explain differences in response to the same chemical among species or strains; these are frequently due to experimental limitations (e.g., few animals, short duration of exposure, low exposures, scanty pathology, etc.).

Some of the differences in carcinogenic responsiveness among rodent species may be due in part to differences in respiratory anatomy, genetic differences, species peculiarities in metabolism (55,56), or simply that one need not insist that results must necessarily be identical in all species (54). After all, the range of responses in humans stretches from none to blatant carcinogenicity: witness the fact that not all humans get cancer from smoking tobacco (18). Granted that laboratory animals are more homogeneous and have been likened to "test tubes," the range of responses does vary among and between sexes, strains, and species (20,54).

A variable often overlooked concerns the relatively short duration of these experiments; another comes from the observation that one sex responds stochastically later than the other; kidney carcinogens in Fischer rats are predominantly seen in males, yet for those chemicals that do affect both sexes, females are less responsive, with typically longer latency periods (57,58). Perhaps some chemicals seen to induce kidney cancer only in males might have been seen in females as well if the studies had been conducted for a longer period or for their entire life span.

Certain human diseases have been traced to exposure to environmental and occupational chemicals (see, e.g., refs. 13,14,44). In many instances the first evidence of potential adverse effects came from experimental studies and were subsequently discovered in humans. Associations of human cancers, as a diverse group of diseases, and chemicals have been made since the mid-eighteenth century. Since then, more than 100 chemicals, mixtures of chemicals, or exposure circumstances have been recognized as being carcinogenic to humans or strongly implicated in human carcinogenicity. Of the fewer than 1,000 agents evaluated adequately for carcinogenicity in laboratory animals (23), a varying spectrum of data from studies on humans is available for only about 20% to 25%. So far, more than 60 agents are linked unequivocally as causing cancer in humans, and another 50 or so are strongly suspected of being carcinogenic to humans. Not all of these have been or can be evaluated in animals because some are industrial processes or occupations, some are environmental and cultural risk factors, and some are mixtures of agents. For those that can be studied experimentally, the qualitative concordance between humans and animals approaches unity (see the chapter, "Chemicals Causally Associated with Cancer in Humans and Laboratory Animals," by Huff) and in every case there is at least one common organ site of cancer in both species (13,14,25–28).

An important fact of which most people are unaware is that evidence of carcinogenicity in experimental animals preceded that observed in humans for nearly 30 agents (36,37). The historical data show that nearly 25% to 30% of those agents, substances, or chemicals that have been causally or strongly associated with cancer in humans were first identified as being carcinogenic in experimental animals. One wonders whether some suffering and death could have been avoided had more attention been given to these findings. Similarly, for those chemicals shown unequivocally to cause cancer in laboratory animals that have not yet been studied epidemiologically, all unnecessary exposures should probably be reduced or eliminated. Meanwhile, cohorts being exposed to these agents should be identified and evaluated (23). To ignore or compromise experimental chemical carcinogenesis data for reasons of confounding or uncertainty factors or until we decipher the mechanism of activity must not be permitted to delay preventive public health measures (4,40).

Regarding the identity of "new" carcinogens for humans, Tomatis et al. (13) make the stringent observation that "it has been the rule rather than the exception that it takes a very long time before a 'new' carcinogenic hazard is recognized and fully appreciated: about 100 years elapsed from the time cigarette smoking became a widespread habit before the carcinogenic hazard was fully recognized and accepted." (Even today, many still insist that tobacco smoking or side-stream exposures are not carcinogenic.) Clemmesen (59) presents a historical perspective about the delays and attitudes regarding tobacco smoking and cancer causality, "The final epidemiologic proof of carcinogenicity is when reduction or elimation of exposure to the suspect agent results, in due course, in reduction in prevalence of the associated neoplasms. Alternative proofs are indirect, complicated, and involve studies extending over decades." Yet what we must deal with in protecting public health cannot await this "final proof"; in fact, most often no human data are available to confirm identification of carcinogenic hazards from experimental research. Thus one must intervene to preserve health using the totality of the information currently existing; typically, one must devise appropriate prevention strategies using carcinogenesis findings from long-term studies in laboratory rodents.

Several chemicals from our historical collection of 450 long-term carcinogenesis experiments have been selected to illustrate some particularly potent inhalational carcinogens: 1,3-butadiene (1,3-B), dibromochloropropane (DBCP), dibromoethane (EDB), ethylene oxide (EtOx), and tetranitromethane (TNM). These have been chosen from among the 26 chemicals (37 additional studies are ongoing) that we have studied by the inhalation route for potential human health hazard. For each of these five chemicals (Table 5) the carcinogenic responses were observed at every exposure level in all exposure groups. Thus we would expect carcinogenic effects below these concentrations. The exposure levels ranged from a low of 0.5 ppm (TNM) to a high of 50 ppm (EtOx). 1,3-B has been evaluated with the largest exposure range: 6.5 to 1,250 ppm (210-fold; others used an 8,000-ppm exposure, a 1,230-fold spread). Further, in all but one case (TNM) the organ/tissue sites of carcinogenesis included not only the lung, but numerous distant-site cancers as well: from 5 (DBCP) to 16 (1,3-B). Two chemicals (1,3-B and EtOx) have evidence of carcinogenicity in humans. From a public health perspective, an expanded effort should be directed toward identifying exposed cohorts to investigate for possible carcinogenic effects from the other chemicals as well.

TABLE 5. Chemicals and inhalation carcinogenesis (some NTP examples)

Chemical[a]	Exposure concentration (ppm)	Routes of exposure	Tumor sites
1,3-Butadiene	6.25–1250	Inhalation[b]	12 [+4]
Dibromochloropropane (DBCP)	0.6–3.0	Inhalation (and by gavage)	5
1.2-Dibromoethane (EDB)	10–40	Inhalation (and by gavage)	6
Ethylene oxide	50–100	Inhalation[c]	5 [+4]
Tetranitromethane (TNM)	0.5–5.0	Inhalation[d]	1

[a]These chemicals have been selected on a comparative basis from the 450 chemical NTP database largely on the low exposure levels used, the number of organs showing induced cancers, and/or on the uniqueness and consistency of the carcinogenic responses.
[b]Mice only; a study in rats has been reported by others showing four other tumor sites.
[c]Mice only; studies in rats showed four other tumor sites.
[d]This one organ-site carcinogen is included because the exposures are very low and the magnitude of the responses was overwhelming.

Results of *in vivo* carcinogenesis studies in laboratory animals for the human/animal chemicals can now be used to develop renewed strategies for predicting whether a chemical will be a carcinogen based on:

1. *Salmonella* test results (60)
2. Structural alerts (61), structure–activity, or induction-based paradigms (62)
3. Other short- or midterm *in vitro/in vivo* tests (30,38,63,64)
4. Modified experimental protocols (4,23,65)
5. Mechanistic information (4,28,66–76)

A key question needing considerable involvement centers on which chemicals, mixtures of chemicals, exposure circumstances, or lifestyles and personal habits we should then subject to long-term rodent studies:

1. Those with the highest probability of being carcinogenic (or noncarcinogenic)?
2. Those with the highest production volume and exposure circumstances (77)?
3. Those about which we are uncertain of the presumed outcome?
4. Those with the highest probability of extending our knowledge of mechanisms of carcinogenicity?
5. Those agents already shown to cause cancer in humans not yet evaluated at all or studied inadequately in experimental animals?
6. Those showing equivocal or marginal results in previous experiments?
7. Those mixtures composed of "typical" concoctions to which various segments of society (e.g., high-fluoride areas) or occupations (e.g., farmers, migrant workers, sprayers exposed to multiple pesticides) or ethnic groups (e.g., diets) are exposed?

SUMMARY AND CONCLUSIONS

Exposure to environmental agents occurs most often via inhalation, and this is the predominant route of exposure for the chemicals and exposure circumstances identified by the International Agency for Research on Cancer as being carcinogenic or probably carcinogenic to humans (13,15,26). For somewhat more than one-half of these 110 exposures, there are sufficient epidemiological data to determine carcinogenic causality in humans. For the remaining chemicals the evidence is not considered sufficient for determining definitive causality, and these are designated as being "probably carcinogenic to humans." Experimental data from long-term inhalation chemical carcinogenesis studies are available that allow comparisons of results from humans and animals for 15 of these chemicals. Cancers of the respiratory tract in humans have been associated with inhalation exposure to 14 of these 15 chemicals, and cancers of the respiratory tract have also been found in the rat after exposure to 13 of these 14 chemicals.

Review of available experimental inhalation studies for these chemicals, including those done by the National Toxicology Program (NTP), reveals that when a carcinogenic response occurs in the respiratory system in rats and/or in humans, results from inhalation studies in other animal species (e.g., mice or hamsters) might give inconsistent responses or carcinogenic effects in other target organs. Thus in this limited data set, the correlation between positive responses in humans and rats as well as for target-organ (respiratory system) specificity approaches unity.

1. Experimental inhalation carcinogenesis studies in animals were available for 20 of the approximately 100 chemicals identified by the IARC as human carcinogens.
2. A positive carcinogenic response was observed in inhalation studies in rats for 19 of these IARC chemicals.
3. The respiratory system was a common site for carcinogenesis in rats and humans, but a carcinogenic response in rats was often observed at other sites as well.
4. Available information on carcinogenic concordance between chemical exposure in humans and the mouse and/or hamster was more limited than for the rat.
5. In the NTP series of chemicals generated as vapors, there were excellent agreement between carcinogenesis in rats and mice; carcinogenic chemicals were also identified as mutagens in the *Salmonella* test.
6. Species differences were observed with some chemicals, including cadmium and other metals, formaldehyde, and bis(chloromethyl) ether.
7. Carcinogenesis findings from experiments in laboratory animals are relevant for identifying carcinogenic hazards in humans.

ACKNOWLEDGMENTS

The author thanks Dr. Michael Waalkes and Dr. Jerrold Ward, National Cancer Institute, for inviting him to prepare this chapter and for offering critical comments on the manuscript. Dr. John Bucher and Dr. Michael Elwell, National Institute of Environmental Health Sciences, reviewed the manuscript and made valuable suggestions.

REFERENCES

1. Miller BA, Ries LAG, Hankey BF, Kosary CL, Edwards BK, eds. *Cancer statistics review: 1973–1989*. Bethesda, MD: National Cancer Institute; 1992.
2. Parkin DM, Muir CS, Whelan SL, Gao Y-T, Ferlay J, Powell J, eds. *Cancer incidence on five continents*. Vol VI. IARC scientific publication 120. Lyon, France: International Agency for Research on Cancer; 1992.
3. ACS. *Cancer facts and figures—1993*. Atlanta, GA: American Cancer Society; 1993. 30pp.
4. Huff JE. Issues and controversies surrounding qualitative strategies for identifying and forecasting cancer causing agents in the human environment. *Pharmacol Toxicol* 1993;72[Suppl 1]:12–27.
5. Bailer JC III, Smith EM. Progress against cancer. *N Engl J Med* 1986;314:1226–1232.
6. Davis DL, Hoel DG. Trends in cancer mortality in industrial countries. *Ann NY Acad Sci* 1990;609:1–347.
7. Kessler LG. Lung and bronchus. Section XV. In: Miller BA, Ries LAG, Hankey BF, Kosary CL, Edwards BK, eds. *Cancer statistics review: 1973–1989*. Bethesda, MD: National Cancer Institute; 1992:1–13.

8. Castonguay A. Methods and strategies in lung cancer control. *Cancer Res* 1992;52:2641s-2651s.
9. Shopland DR, Eyre HJ, Pechacek TF. Smoking-attributable cancer mortality in 1991: is lung cancer now the leading cause of death among smokers in the United States? *J Natl Cancer Inst* 1991; 83:1142-1148.
10. Axelson O, Davis DL, Forestiere F, Schneiderman M, Wagener D. Lung cancer not attributable to smoking. *Ann NY Acad Sci* 1990;609:165-178.
11. Tomatis L, Fishbein L, Hemminki K, Lewitas J, Pershagen G, Simonato L, Graham JD. Concluding remarks. In: Tomatis L, ed. *Air pollution and human cancer*. New York: Springer-Verlag, 1990:85-86. 86pp.
12. MMWR. Populations at risk from air pollution—United States, 1991. *Morbid Mortal Weekly Rep* 1993;42:301-303 (Apr 30). Reprinted in *JAMA* 1993;269:2493.
13. Tomatis L, Aitio A, Wilbourn J, Shuker L. Human carcinogens so far identified. *Jpn J Cancer Res* 1989;80:795-807.
14. Huff JE, Rall DP. [1992]. Relevance to humans of carcinogenesis results from laboratory animal toxicology studies. In: Last JM, Wallace RB, eds. *Maxcy-Rosenau-Last's Public Health and Preventive Medicine*. 13th ed. Norwalk, CT: Appleton & Lange; 1992:433-440, 453-457. 1257 pp.
15. IARC. *IARC monographs on the carcinogenic risks to humans*. Vols 1-58. Lyon, France: International Agency for Research on Cancer; 1972-1993.
16. DHHS/NTP. *Annual reports on carcinogens*. Research Triangle Park, NC: National Toxicology Program, Department of Health and Human Services; 1978-1993.
17. Dunnick JK, Huff JE. Respiratory carcinogenicity in humans and in animals from inhalation exposure to chemicals. *Proc Am Assoc Cancer Res* 1992;33:178 (abstr no 1066).
18. IARC. *IARC monographs on the evaluation of carcinogenic risks to humans*. Vol 38. *Tobacco smoking*. Lyon, France: International Agency for Research on Cancer; 1986. 421pp.
19. Tomatis L. Air pollution and cancer: an old and new problem. In: Tomatis L, ed. *Air pollution and human cancer*. New York: Springer-Verlag; 1990:1-7. 86pp.
20. Huff JE, Cirvello J, Haseman JK, Bucher JR. Chemicals associated with site-specific neoplasia in 1394 long-term carcinogenesis experiments in laboratory rodents. *Environ Health Perspect* 1991; 93:247-271.
21. Huff JE, Bucher JR, Cirvello J, Melnick RL, Fung V. Chemicals inducing site-specific neoplasia in 1394 carcinogenesis experiments in rodents. *Proc Am Assoc Cancer Res* 1993;34:174 (abstr no 1038).
22. Huff JE, Haseman JK. Long-term chemical carcinogenesis experiments for identifying potential human cancer hazards. Collective data base of the National Cancer Institute and National Toxicology Program (1976-1991). *Environ Health Perspect* 1991;96:23-31.
23. Huff JE, Haseman JK, Rall DP. Scientific concepts, value, and significance of chemical carcinogenesis studies. *Annu Rev Pharmacol Toxicol* 1991;31:621-652.
24. Huff JE, Hoel DG. (1992). Perspective and overview of the concepts and value of hazard identification as the initial phase of the risk assessment for cancer and human health. *Scand J Work Environ Health* 1992;18[Suppl 1]:83-89.
25. Wilbourn J, Haroun L, Heseltine E, Kaldor J, Partensky C, Vainio H. Response of experimental animals to human carcinogens: an analysis based upon the IARC monographs programme. *Carcinogenesis* 1986;7:1853-1863.
26. IARC. *IARC monographs on the evaluation of carcinogenic risks to humans: overall evaluations of carcinogenicity: an updating of IARC monographs volumes 1 to 42*. Suppl 7. Lyon, France: International Agency for Research on Cancer; 1987. 440pp.
27. Vainio H, Coleman M, Wilbourn J. Carcinogenicity evaluations and ongoing studies: the IARC databases. *Environ Health Perspect* 1991;96:5-9.
28. Vainio H, Wilbourn J. Identification of carcinogens within the IARC monograph program. *Scand J Environ Health* (1992);18[Suppl 1]:64-73.
29. IARC. Lists of IARC evaluations. *IARC monographs on the evaluation of carcinogenic risks to humans*. Lyon, France: International Agency for Research on Cancer; May 1993. 35pp.
30. Huff JE. A historical perspective of the classification developed and used for chemical carcinogens by the National Toxicology Program: 1983-1992. *Scand J Work Environ Health* 1992;18[Suppl 1]:74-82.
31. DHHS/NTP. *Seventh annual report on carcinogens*. Research Triangle Park, NC: National Toxicology Program, Department of Health and Human Services; 1994. 745pp.
32. NCI. *NCI bioassay of "chemical" for possible carcinogenicity*. Carcinogenesis technical report series 2-100, 202-205. Bethesda, MD: National Cancer Institute; 1976-1980.

33. Huff JE. Design strategies, results, and evaluations of long-term chemical carcinogenesis studies. *Scand J Work Environ Health* 1992;18[Suppl 1]:31–37.
34. NTP. *NTP toxicology and carcinogenesis studies of "chemical" ("CAS no") in F344/N rats and B6C3F1 mice ("exposure route")*. Technical report series 201, 206–443. Research Triangle Park, NC: National Toxicology Program; 1980–1993.
35. Lewtas L. Experimental evidence for the carcinogenicity of air pollutants. In: Tomatis L, ed. *Air pollution and human cancer*. New York: Springer-Verlag; 1990:49–61. 86pp.
36. Tomatis L. The predictive value of rodent carcinogenicity tests in the evaluation of human risks. *Annu Rev Pharmacol Toxicol* 1979;19:511–530.
37. Huff JE. Chemicals and cancer in humans: first evidence in experimental animals. *Environ Health Perspect* 1993;100:201–210.
38. Montesano R, Bartsch H, Vainio H, Wilbourn J, Yamasaki H. *Long-term and short-term assays for carcinogens: a critical appraisal*. IARC scientific publication 83. Lyon, France: International Agency for Research on Cancer; 1986. 564pp.
39. Rall DP, Hogan MD, Huff JE, Schwetz BA, Tennant TW. Alternatives to using human experience in assessing health risks. *Annu Rev Public Health* 1987;8:355–385.
40. Huff JE, McConnell EE, Haseman JK, Boorman GA, Eustis SL, Schwetz BA, Rao GN, Jameson CW, Hart LG, Rall DP. Carcinogenesis studies: results from 398 experiments on 104 chemicals from the U.S. National Toxicology Program. *Ann NY Acad Sci* 1988;534:1–30.
41. Chabra RS, Huff JE, Schwetz, BS, Selkirk J. An overview of prechronic and chronic toxicity/carcinogenicity experimental study designs and criteria used by the National Toxicology Program. *Environ Health Perspect* 1990;86:313–321.
42. Boyland E. A chemist's view of cancer prevention. *Proc Roy Soc Med* 1967;60:93–99.
43. Doll R, Peto R. The causes of cancer. *J Natl Cancer Inst* 1981;66:1191–1308. Also. *The causes of cancer* Oxford: Oxford Medical Publications, Oxford University Press;1981:1191–1312.
44. Schmahl D, Preussmann R, Berger MR. Causes of cancer: an alternative view to Doll and Peto (1981). *Klin Wochenschr* 1989; 67:1169–1173.
45. Thiedemann KU, Luthe N, Paulini I, Kreft A, Heinrich U, Glaser U. Ultrastructure observations in hamster and rat lungs after chronic inhalation of cadmium compounds. *Exp Pathol* 1989;37:264–268.
46. Heinrich U, Peters L, Ernst H, Rittinghausen S, Dasenbrock C, Konih H. Investigation on the carcinogenic effects of various cadmium compounds after inhalation exposure in hamsters and mice. *Exp Pathol* 1989;37:253–258.
47. Nordberg GF, Herber RFM, Alessio L, eds. *Cadmium in the human environment: toxicity and carcinogenicity*. IARC scientific publication 118. Lyon, France: International Agency for Research on Cancer; 1993:1–469.
48. Heinrich U. Pulmonary carcinogenicity of cadmium by inhalation in animals. In: Nordberg GF, Herber RFM, Alessio L, eds. *Cadmium in the human environment: toxicity and carcinogenicity*. IARC scientific publication 118. Lyon, France: International Agency for Research on Cancer; 1993:405–413. 469pp.
49. IARC. *IARC monographs on the evaluation of carcinogenic risks to humans. Vol. 58. Beryllium, cadmium, mercury, and exposures in the glass manufacturing industry*. Lyon, France: International Agency for Research on Cancer; 1994.
50. Kerns WD, Pavkov KL, Donofrio DJ, Gralla EJ, Swenberg JA. Carcinogenicity of formaldehyde in rats and mice after long-term inhalation exposure. *Cancer Res* 1983;43:4382–4392.
51. Kuschner M, Laskin S, Drew RT, Cappiello V, Nelson N. Inhalation carcinogenicity of alpha halo ethers. II. Lifetime and limited period inhalation studies with bis(chloromethyl) ether at 0.1 ppm. *Arch Environ Health* 1975;30:73–77.
52. Sellakumar AR, Laskin S, Kuschner M, Rusch G, Katz GV, Snyder CA, Albert RE. Inhalation carcinogenesis by dimethylcarbamoyl chloride in Syrian golden hamsters. *J Environ Pathol Toxicol* 1980;4:107–115.
53. Furst A, Schlauder MC. The hamster as a model for metal carcinogenesis. *Proc West Pharmacol Soc* 1971;14:68–71.
54. Lijinsky W. Species differences in carcinogenesis. *In Vivo* 1993;7:65–72.
55. Gross EA, Swenberg JA, Fields S, Popp JA. Comparative morphometry of the nasal cavity in rats and mice. *J Anat* 1982;135:83–88.
56. Procter DF, Alternative methods to evaluate species differences in upper airway structure–function. In: *Extrapolation of dosimetric relationships for inhaled particles and gases*. New York: Academic Press; 1989:35–43.
57. Barrett JC, Huff JE. Cellular and molecular mechanisms of chemically induced renal carcinogen-

esis. In: Bach PH, Gregg NJ, Wiks MF, Delacruz L, eds. *Nephrotoxicity: mechanisms, early diagnosis, and therapeutic management*. New York: Marcel Dekker; 1991:287-306. 585pp. Reprinted as updated: *Renal Failure* 1991;13:211-225.
58. Huff JE. Carcinogenicity of ochratoxin A in experimental animals. In: Castegnaro M, Plestina R, Dirheimer G, Chernozemsky IN, Bartsch H, eds. *Mycotoxins, endemic nephropathy, and urinary tract tumours*. IARC scientific publication 115. Lyon, France: International Agency for Research on Cancer; 1991:229-244. 340pp.
59. Clemmesen J. Lung cancer from smoking: delays and attitudes, 1912-1965. *Am J Ind Med* 1993;23:941-953.
60. Tennant R, Margolin B, Shelby M, Zeiger E, Haseman J, Spalding J, Caspary W, Resnick M, Stasiewicz S, Anderson B, Minor R. Prediction of chemical carcinogenicity in rodents from *in vitro* genetic toxicity assays. *Science* 1987;236:933-941.
61. Ashby J, Tennant RW. Definitive relationships among chemical structure, carcinogenicity and mutagenicity for 301 chemicals tested by the U.S. NTP. *Mutat Res* 1991;257:229-306.
62. Bahler D, Bristol DW. The induction of rules for predicting chemical carcinogenesis in rodents. In: Hunter L, Shavlik J, Searls D, eds. *Intelligent systems for molecular biology*. Menlo Park, CA: American Association for Artificial Intelligence/MIT Press, 1993;29-37.
63. Ward JM, Ito N. Development of new medium-term bioassays for carcinogens. *Cancer Res* 1988;48: 48:5051-5054.
64. Ito N, Shirai T, Hasegawa R. Medium-term bioassays for carcinogens. In: Vainio H, Magee P, McGregor D, McMichael A, eds. *Mechanisms of carcinogenesis in risk identification*. IARC scientific publication 116. Lyon, France: International Agency for Research on Cancer 1992:353-388. 615pp.
65. Huff JE. Modified protocols and possible alternatives for long-term chemical carcinogenicity studies ("bioassays") in rodents. 1993 [*submitted*].
66. Boyd JA, Barrett JC. Genetic and cellular basis of multistep carcinogenesis. *Pharmacol Ther* 1990;46:469-486.
67. Barrett JC. Mechanism of action of known human carcinogens. In: Vainio H, Magee P, McGregor D, McMichael A, eds. *Mechanisms of carcinogenesis in risk identification*. IARC scientific publication 116. Lyon, France: International Agency for Research on Cancer; 1992:115-134. 615pp.
68. Barrett JC. Mechanisms of multistep carcinogenesis and risk assessment. *Environ Health Perspect* 1993;100:9-20.
69. Lucier GW. Receptor-mediated carcinogenesis. In: Vainio H, Magee P, McGregor D, McMichael A, eds. *Mechanisms of carcinogenesis in risk identification*. IARC scientific publication 116. Lyon, France: International Agency for Research on Cancer; 1992:87-112. 615pp.
70. Melnick RL. Does chemically induced hepatocyte proliferation predict liver carcinogenesis? *FASEB J* 1992;6:2698-2706.
71. Melnick RL. An alternative hypothesis on the role of chemically induced protein droplet (a2m-globulin) nephropathy in renal carcinogenesis. *Regul Toxicol Pharmacol* 1992;16:111-125.
72. Melnick RL, Huff JE. Liver carcinogenesis is not a predicted outcome of chemically induced hepatocyte proliferation. In: Mehlman MA, Upton A, eds. *Identification and public health control of environmental and occupational diseases*. Princeton, NJ: Princeton Scientific Publishing; 1994 [*in press*].
73. Huff JE. Chemical toxicity and chemical carcinogenesis. Is there a causal connection? A comparative morphological evaluation of 1500 experiments. In: Vainio H, Magee P, McGregor D, McMichael A, eds. *Mechanisms of carcinogenesis in risk identification*. IARC scientific publication 116. Lyon, France: International Agency for Research on Cancer; 1992:437-475. 615pp.
74. Huff JE. Mechanisms, chemical carcinogenesis, and risk assessment: cell proliferation and cancer. *Amer J Indust Med* 1993 [*in press*].
75. Huff JE. Absence of morphologic correlation between chemical toxicity and chemical carcinogenesis. *Environ Health Perspect* 1993;101[Suppl 4] 73-82.
76. Barrett JC, Wiseman RW. Molecular carcinogenesis in humans and rodents. In: Klein-Szanto A, Anderson M, Barrett JC, Slaga TJ, eds. *Comparative molecular carcinogenesis*. Vol 376. New York: Wiley, 1992:1-30.
77. Fung VA, Huff JE, Weisburger E, Hoel DG. Predictive strategies for selecting 379 NCI/NTP chemicals evaluated for carcinogenic potential: scientific and public health impact. *Fundam Appl Toxicol* 1993;20:413-436.

Carcinogenesis, edited by
M.P. Waalkes and J.M. Ward.
Raven Press, Ltd., New York © 1994.

8

Upper Respiratory Tract Carcinogenesis in Experimental Animals and in Humans

R. A. Woutersen, A. van Garderen-Hoetmer,
*P. J. Slootweg, and Victor J. Feron

*Department of Biological Toxicology, TNO-Toxicology and Nutrition Institute, 3704 HE, Zeist, The Netherlands; *Department of Pathology, University Hospital, 3508 GA, Utrecht, The Netherlands*

Epidemiological studies have demonstrated an increased risk of upper respiratory tract cancer, primarily nasal tumors, in several occupations, such as nickel refinery workers and workers engaged in the manufacture of wooden furniture or leather boots and shoes (1). In addition, nasopharyngeal cancer in southeastern China and Hong Kong has been associated with the consumption of salted fish, which appeared to contain high concentrations of volatile nitrosamines capable of inducing nasal tumors in experimental animals (2). Tobacco smoking and alcohol drinking are important causes of laryngeal cancer in humans (3,4). There are some indications for an increased risk of laryngeal cancer among workers who manufactured furniture, mustard gas, isopropyl alcohol, or sulfuric acid (5).

An increasing number of chemicals are capable of inducing upper respiratory tract tumors in rodents. Nasal tumors are encountered most frequently; laryngeal tumors are relatively rare (6–9). A great number of nitrosamines are capable of inducing nasal tumors in rats and hamsters (2,10–12). Furthermore, tumors of the nose develop in experimental animals after exposure to a variety of important industrial chemicals (Table 1), such as ethylene dibromide (13), dimethyl sulfate (14), acetaldehyde (15), bis(chloromethyl) ether (16), hexamethylphosphoramide (17), propylene oxide (18), phenylglycidyl ether (19), dimethylcarbamoyl chloride (20), epichlorohydrin (21), and vinyl chloride (22). There are no epidemiological data indicating an increased risk of nasal cancer in workers exposed to any of these industrial compounds. Clearly, this may be due to a lack of powerful epidemiological studies or to the absence of an association between nasal cancer in humans and exposure to these chemicals. However, another factor involved may be the striking differences in size and internal shapes of the nose and the possible differences in physiology of the nose between humans and rodents. Moreover, in contrast to humans, rodents are obligatory nose breathers. Therefore, it seems not illogical to

TABLE 1. Chemicals that induce nasal tumors in laboratory rodents

Compound	Species	Ref.
Acetaldehyde	Rat, hamster	15
Acrylonitrile	Rat	168
Benzene	Rat	168
Bis(chloromethyl) ether	Rat	16
p-Cresidine	Rat	168
Diallylnitrosamine	Rat, hamster	168
1,2-Dibromo-3-chloropropane	Rat, mouse	168
1,2-Dibromoethane	Rat, mouse	168
2,3-Dibromo-1-propanol	Rat	90
Dimethylcarbamoyl chloride	Hamster	20
Dimethylsulfate	Rat	14
Dimethylvinyl chloride	Rat	168
Dinitrosophomopiperazine	Rat	168
1,4-Dioxane	Rat	168
Epichlorohydrin	Rat	21
1,2-Epoxybutane	Rat	169
2-Ethyl-O,N,N-azoxyethane	Rat	168
Ethylene dibromide	Rat	13
Ethylnitrosocyanamide	Rat	168
Formaldehyde	Rat, mouse	168
Hexamethyl phosphoramide	Rat	17
Hydrazine	Rat, hamster	168
Nitrosaminoketone	Rat	90
Nitroso-2,6-dimethylmorpholine	Hamster	168
N-Nitroso-N-methyldecylamine	Rat	168
Di(N-nitroso)perhydropyrimidine	Rat	168
N-Nitroso(2,2,2-trifluoroethyl)ethylamine	Rat	168
1-Nitroso-3,4,5-trimethylpiperazine	Rat	168
N-Nitrosoallyl-2,3-dihydroxypropylamine	Rat	168
N-Nitrosoallyl-2-hydroxypropylamine	Rat	168
N-Nitrosoallyl-2-oxopropylamine	Hamster	168
N-Nitrosoallylethanolamine	Rat	168
N-Nitrosobis(2-hydroxypropyl)amine	Rat	168
N-Nitrosobis(2-oxopropyl)amine	Rat	168
N-Nitrosodiethanolamine	Rat	168
N-Nitrosodipropylamine	Rat	168
N-Nitrosomethyl-2,3-dihydroxypropylamine	Rat, hamster	168
N-Nitrosomethyl-2-hydroxypropylamine	Rat	168
N-Nitrosomorpholine	Hamster	168
N'-Nitrosonornicotine	Hamster	168
N'-Nitrosonornicotine-1-N-oxide	Rat	168
N-Nitrosopiperidine	Hamster	168
Phenacetin	Rat	168
Phenylglycidylether	Rat	19
Procarbazine	Rat, mouse	90
Propylene oxide	Rat, mouse	18
Tris(aziridinyl)phosphine sulfide	Rat	90
Vinyl chloride	Rat	22
2,6-Xylidine	Rat	169

assume that changes found in the noses of rodents after inhalation exposure may be predictive of effects on more distal parts of the respiratory tract in humans. Two examples are epichlorohydrin and bis(chloromethyl) ether, which produce nasal carcinomas in rats and lung cancer in humans (23). Laryngeal cancer has been encountered in Syrian golden hamsters after exposure by inhalation to whole smoke (4,24,25) or to acetaldehyde vapor (26), and after intratracheal instillation of benzo[a]pyrene or administration of nitrosamines in various ways (27). In this chapter we review upper airway carcinogenesis in rodents and humans.

HISTOLOGY OF THE UPPER RESPIRATORY TRACT

Histology of the Nasal Passages and Larynx of Rodents

Nose

The normal histology of the nasal cavity of rodents has been described in detail by Young (28) and Uraih and Maronpot (29). This section deals with the location of the lining epithelium, which is particularly relevant to the subject of the present chapter. There is considerable variation among animal species in the distribution of the nasal epithelial populations and the types of cells within these defined populations. All commonly used laboratory animals have four specifically defined epithelial regions: (a) stratified squamous epithelium in the nasal vestibule; (b) ciliated, pseudostratified respiratory epithelium, mainly located anteriorly in the nose; (c) nonciliated cuboidal transitional epithelium in the region between the squamous and respiratory epithelium; and (d) olfactory epithelium, mainly located more posteriorly in the nose. In rats, the transitional epithelium is restricted to the anterior lateral wall, whereas in humans transitional epithelium is present on both the lateral and septal walls of the anterior nasal cavity (30).

The various types of epithelium lining the nasal passages at six cross sections (levels I to VI, Fig. 1) examined routinely in our laboratory are described below.

Level I

The first cross section is located immediately anteriorly to the roots of the upper incisor teeth (Fig. 2). At this level the entire nasal cavity is lined by (keratinized) stratified squamous epithelium.

Level II

The second cross section runs down the middle of the upper incisors (Fig. 3). The roots of the teeth are seen laterally in the section. The naso- and maxilloturbinates have a hooklike shape. The nasal cavity is mainly lined by respiratory epithelium at

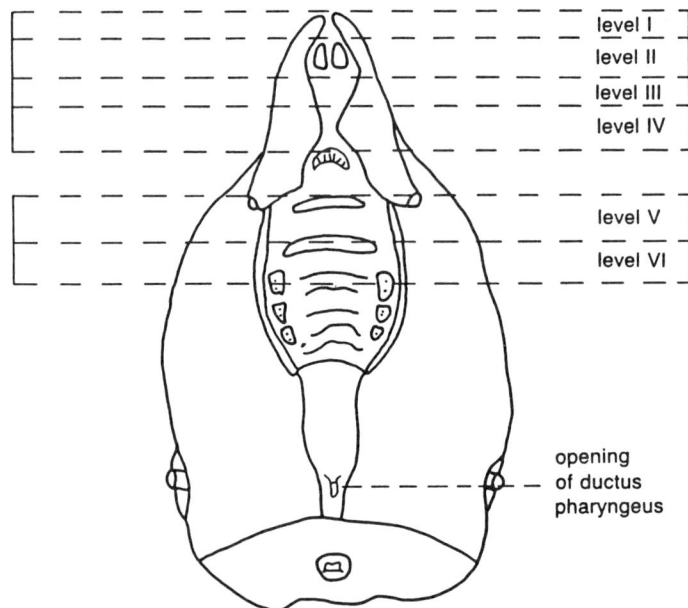

FIG. 1. Ventral view of the rat hard palate region with the lower jaw removed, indicating the six standard cross sections through the nose (I to VI).

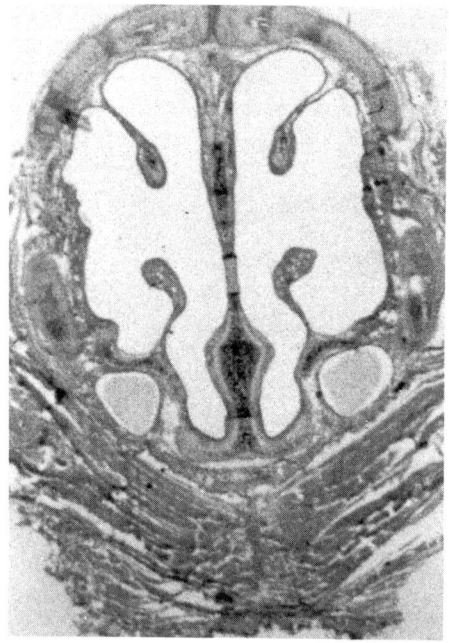

FIG. 2. Cross section at level I of the rat nasal cavity just anterior to the roots of the upper incisor teeth. H&E, ×7.1.

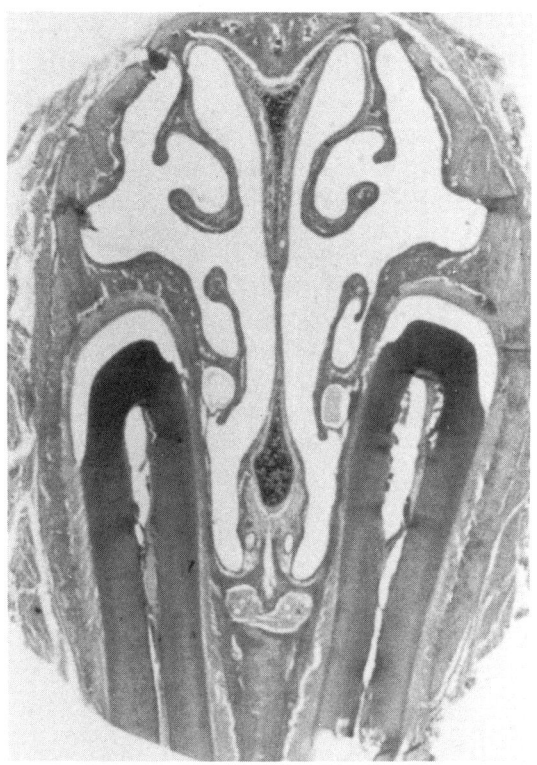

FIG. 3. Cross section at level II of the rat nasal cavity just through the middle of the upper incisor teeth. The roots of the teeth are seen laterally in the section. H&E, ×7.1.

this level. Slightly keratinized stratified squamous epithelium lines the vestibule and ventral meatus.

Six different types of cells can be distinguished in the respiratory epithelium. The nasal septum is lined by ciliated, columnar cells, goblet cells, and basal cells. The lateral aspects of the maxillo- and nasoturbinates show nonciliated columnar cells with a microvillous border, cuboidal cells, and brush cells. We have found brush cells also on the nasal septum. The function of these slender, pear-shaped cells showing dense microvilli is still unknown, but the morphological similarities between brush cells and intestinal M-cells are remarkable enough to suggest a role of brush cells in the immunological defense system, but this needs further elucidation (31). At this cross section the early effects of irritating compounds that are easily soluble in water can be observed. It has been found that transitional cell epithelium which covers the lateral wall at this cross section is highly sensitive to irritating substances. These early effects are characterized by disarrangement, hyperplasia, and occasionally, stratified squamous metaplasia of the respiratory and transitional epithelium. Rats exposed to 0.4 ppm ozone exhibited disarrangement and hyper-

and metaplasia of the transitional epithelium lining the maxillary and nasal turbinates and the lateral wall at this cross section, whereas the nasal septum was not visibly affected (32).

Level III

Level III is located immediately posterior to the upper incisor teeth (Fig. 4). At this cross section the paired vomeronasal organ (organ of Jacobson), nasolachrymal ducts, and septal glands are encountered. At this level the septum, maxillo- and nasoturbinates, and the lateral wall are covered by respiratory epithelium. The vestibule and ventral meatus is lined by slightly keratinized stratified squamous epithelium. Dorsomedially olfactory epithelium can be found, but a transition zone between respiratory and olfactory epithelium is often visible. Care should be taken not to misinterpret the presence of respiratory epithelium as replacement of olfactory epithelium.

The paired vomeronasal organ is lined by ciliated columnar epithelium on the one side and by olfactory neurons and sustentacular cells on the opposite side. Stratified squamous epithelium is normally found both at the origin and the end of the na-

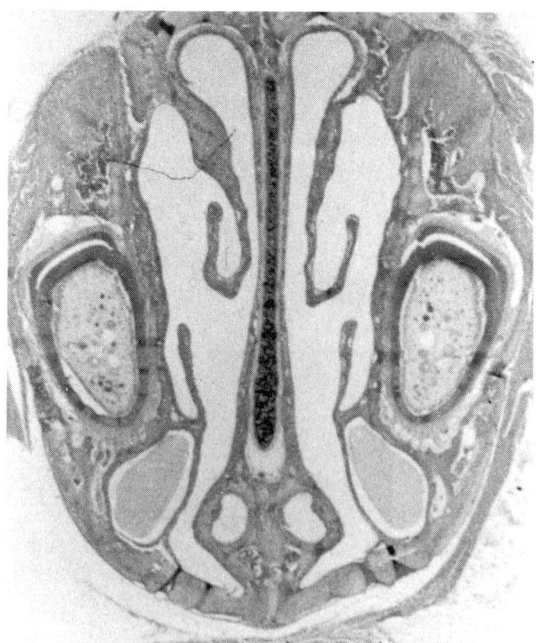

FIG. 4. Cross section at level III of the rat nasal cavity immediately posterior to the upper incisor teeth. At this cross section the vomeronasal organ, nasolachrymal ducts, and septal glands are encountered. H&E, ×7.1.

solachrymal ducts, which are further lined by pseudostratified nonciliated columnar epithelium, frequently showing squamous metaplasia.

Level IV

At level IV (Fig. 5), the upper incisor roots are still prominent and the nasolachrymal ducts are now lateral to the teeth. The maxilloturbinates are reduced to small projections from the lateral wall. The lumina of the vomeronasal organ are no longer visible at this cross section. At this level bilateral communication with the oral cavity via the incisive ducts can be seen. The ducts are lined by stratified squamous epithelium, and occlusion by inflammatory exudate or foreign bodies such as hair shafts may be seen occasionally. The dorsal meatus is lined by olfactory epithelium and there is a sharp demarcation between the respiratory and the olfactory epithelium on the septum. At this cross section, the organ of Masera may be present (septal olfactory organ of Rodolfo Masera), which is a small islet of olfactory epithelium surrounded by respiratory epithelium. In rats exposed to acetaldehyde, this septal olfactory epithelium exhibited severe hyperplasia and keratinizing squamous metaplasia (Fig. 6).

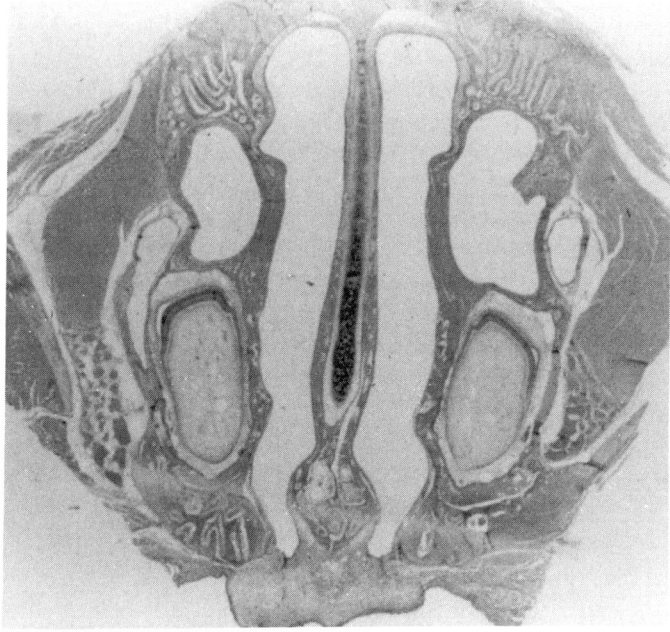

FIG. 5. Cross section at level IV of the rat nasal cavity. The maxilloturbinates are seen as small projections from the lateral wall. At this cross section the septal olfactory organ of Rodolfo Masera may be present (see Fig. 6). H&E, ×7.1.

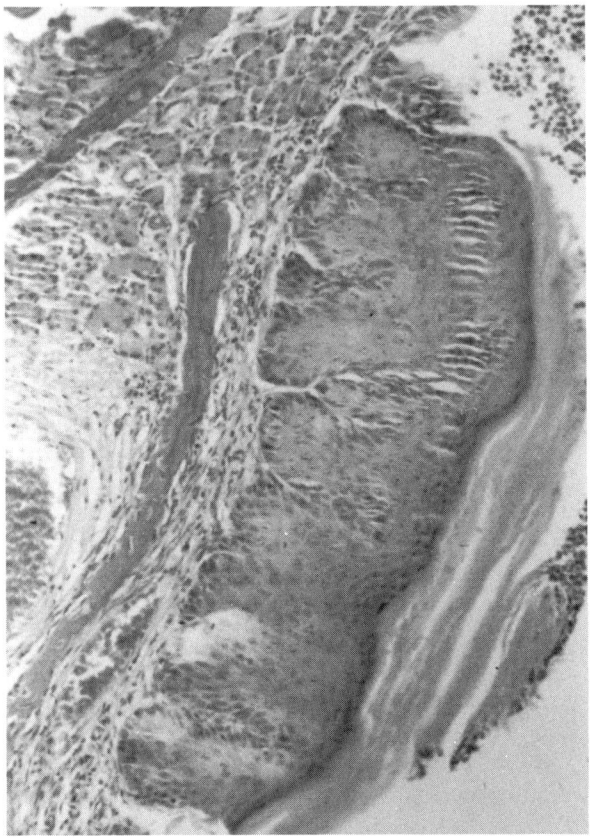

FIG. 6. Hyperplasia and keratinized squamous metaplasia of the organ of Masera, a small islet of olfactory epithelium surrounded by respiratory epithelium. Male rat exposed to 1,500 ppm acetaldehyde for 28 months. H&E, ×280.

Level V

The fifth cross section runs down the second palatal ridge (Fig. 7). The septal window is found at this level. Although the septum in most mammals, including humans, effectively divides the chamber into two symmetrical compartments, the septum of rats, mice, hamsters, and guinea pigs has a septal window, which is distinctly present at this cross section. Further, the paired maxillary sinus, the dorsolachrymal duct, and the beginning of the nasopharyngeal duct can be found. The mucosa at this cross section is lined primarily by olfactory epithelium, whereas the maxillary sinus is covered with respiratory epithelium. The olfactory epithelium is composed of three cell types: sustentacular (supporting) cells, sensory cells (olfactory neurons), and basal cells. Since the basal cells are the stem cells for the sensory

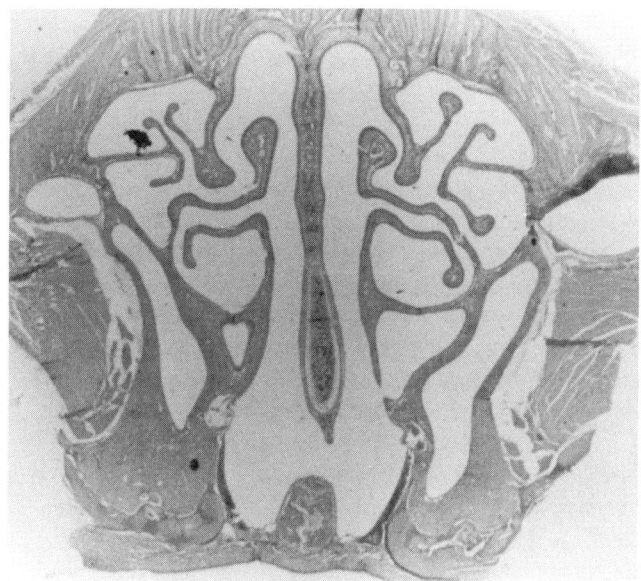

FIG. 7. Cross section at level V of the rat nasal cavity just down the second palatal ridge. The septal window is present at this level. H&E, ×7.1.

cells and the rat neuroepithelium exhibits a certain turnover (approximately 30 days), some areas may have multiple layers of basal cells associated with a decrease in numbers of mature sensory cells—olfactory neurons (33,34).

Level VI

At the sixth cross section (just posterior to the first upper molar tooth), the pharyngeal duct is fully formed in the ventral part of the section and lined by respiratory epithelium (Fig. 8). At levels IV, V, and VI an area of lymphoid tissue is present at the entrance and around the pharyngeal canal. This lymphoid tissue has been shown to contain T- and B-cell areas and to possess the same characteristics as gut- and bronchus-associated lymphoid tissue (GALT and BALT). Spit et al. (31) suggested designating this tissue as nose-associated lymphoid tissue (NALT). Except for small areas of respiratory epithelium on the lateral aspects of some ectoturbinates and the lateral wall, the lining epithelium at this cross section is entirely olfactory. Dorsally in this cross section the olfactory lobes of the brain can be seen and the Harderian glands are present laterally in the orbita.

Larynx

In rodents, the larynx is lined by stratified squamous epithelium and pseudostratified ciliated columnar epithelium. The dorsal part of the lateral walls of the

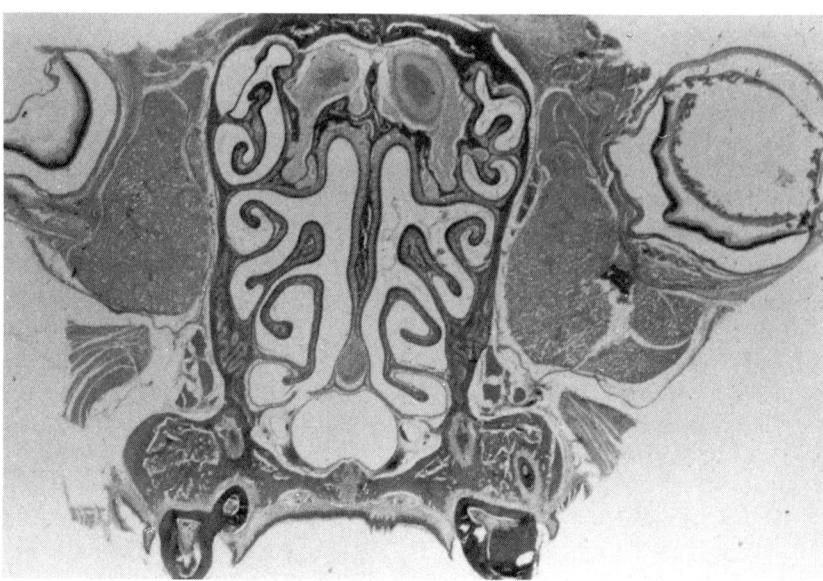

FIG. 8. Cross section at level VI of the rat nasal cavity just posterior to the first upper molar teeth. H&E, ×7.1.

vestibule of the larynx is covered with stratified squamous epithelium, whereas its ventral surface is lined by pseudostratified ciliated columnar epithelium. The vocal cords are lined by stratified squamous epithelium. Caudally to the vocal cords, ciliated columnar to cuboidal epithelium is found which extends to the trachea.

Histology of the Upper Respiratory Tract in Humans

The upper respiratory tract extends from the nostrils to the subglottic area of the larynx and includes the nose and paranasal sinuses, naso-, oro-, and hypopharynx, and larynx. For obvious reasons in humans standard (cross) sections are rarely used for histopathological examination of the upper respiratory tract. Therefore, other than in experimental animals, in the following paragraphs the histology of the various epithelia lining the different parts of the upper respiratory tract is discussed. These epithelia, each of which is more or less restricted to specific areas (35), comprise:

1. *Keratinized stratified squamous epithelium*, which covers the most external area of the nostrils. It can be considered as an intranasal extension of the adjacent epidermis of the outer surface of the nose. Just as epidermis elsewhere, it consists of a basal layer that through a sequence of prickle cells and cells with keratohyalin granules matures into a cornified surface consisting of anuclear dead cells composed merely of keratin. In the underlying dermis, sebaceous and sweat glands are found, and hair follicles are present that give rise to short stiff hairs, the so-called vibrissae.

2. *Nonkeratinized stratified squamous epithelium*, which is found at a variety of locations. It is the lining of the posterior one-third of the nasal vestibule, the major part of the anterior and posterior surface of the nasopharynx, and minor parts of its lateral walls. Moreover, it covers the tonsillar area, the anterior epiglottic surface, the cranial part of the dorsal epiglottic surface, the hypopharynx, the ary-epiglottic fold, and the true vocal cord. Nonkeratinized stratified squamous epithelium is similar to keratinized stratified squamous epithelium, except that the upper cell layers do not keratinize but exhibit hydropic swelling with shrinkage of their nuclei. The most superficial cell layer consists of flattened cells with clear cytoplasm and still-visible small dark nuclei.

3. *Respiratory epithelium*, which covers the nasal cavity, the paranasal sinuses, and parts of the anterior, posterior, and lateral walls of the nasopharynx and the inner surface of the larynx, except for the areas covered with nonkeratinized stratified squamous epithelium as outlined above. Respiratory epithelium is a pseudostratified columnar ciliated epithelium with goblet cells scattered among ciliated cells. There are some minor differences in the number of goblet cells relative to ciliated cells. In the mucosal lining of the paranasal sinuses, goblet cells are fewer in number (Fig. 9). Underneath nonkeratinized squamous epithelium as well as respiratory epithelium, numerous mucosal glands are found comprising mucous-secretory cells and serous-secretory units. The only area where these glands are absent is the vocal cords.

4. *Olfactory epithelium*, which is present at the superoposterior portion of each

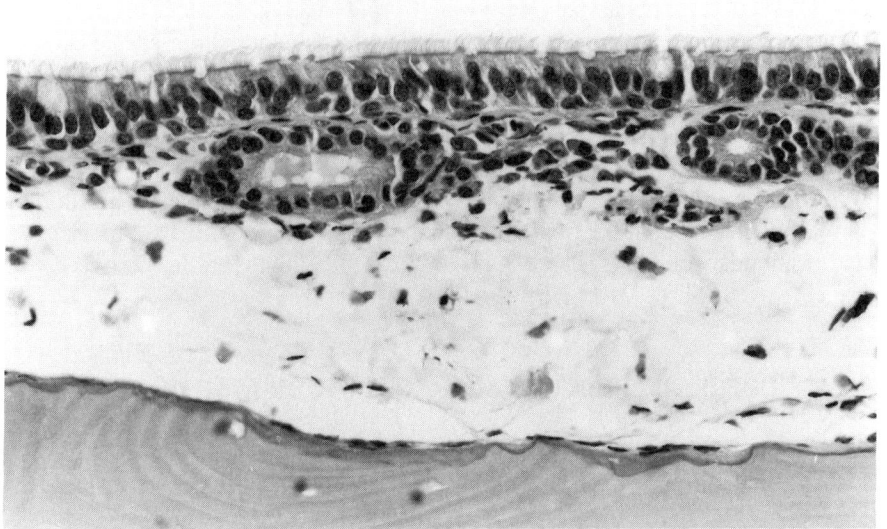

FIG. 9. Respiratory epithelium. Single-layered pseudostratified epithelium consisting of cylindrical cells rests on a loosely textured stromal tissue that contains some mucoserous glands. H&E, ×340.

nasal cavity, involving the upper part of the nasal septum, the posterior part of the roof of the nasal cavity, and the upper and medial area of the superior conchae. It is a single-layered epithelium consisting of three different cell types: basal cells, sustentacular cells, and olfactory cells (Figs. 10 and 11). The basal cells are reserve cells for the sustentacular cells as well as the olfactory cells; they lay between the basal portions of the sustentacular cells, and the sustentacular cells bear microvilli on their surface. The olfactory cells are bipolar spindle-shaped receptor neurons with a distal and a proximal process. The distal process passes between the sustentacular cells toward the mucosal surface and forms the olfactory rod with some cilia and olfactory vesicles. The proximal cytoplasmic extension, the filum olfactorium, perforates the skull base to make connection with the olfactory bulb. Olfactory cells are the only neurons that may renew themselves during one's lifetime, and this may explain why tumors originating in these cells occur much later in life than do other neuronal neoplasms. Underneath the olfactory epithelium are the glands of Bowman, which produce a watery fluid that bathes the olfactory area.

5. *Intermediate epithelium*, occasionally called *transitional epithelium* because of its resemblance to the urothelium covering the urinary tract (36), which is stratified, five or six cell layers thick, and devoid of cilia. The basal cells are cuboidal or low columnar, the upper cells form a surface of rounded cells, and polyhedral cells are interposed between the basal and superficial cell layers. Sometimes a single cell can be shown to contain mucus or keratohyaline granules (Fig. 12). However, whether intermediate epithelium really exists is questionable. This epithelium is located at areas were respiratory and stratified squamous epithelium meet: the lateral nasopharyngeal wall, the posterior wall of the pharyngeal tonsils, and other areas in oral and nasopharynx. Moreover, from a cytological point of view intermediate epithelium shows characteristics of squamous epithelium and respiratory epithelium by containing mucus as well as keratohyalin granules. Finally, epithelium resembling intermediate epithelium has been observed as a transient stage in metaplasia of respiratory epithelium to squamous epithelium (37). It is probable that intermediate epithelium is, in fact, respiratory epithelium that has not yet completed its transformation to stratified squamous epithelium. This metaplastic transformation plays a great role in the final distribution of the various epithelial linings in the upper respiratory tract, as the area of respiratory epithelium is strongly reduced with advancing age (36).

UPPER RESPIRATORY TRACT CANCER IN HUMANS

Epidemiology

Nasal Cancer

Malignant tumors of the interior of the human nose and accessory air sinuses are rare. The frequency of these tumors is placed in perspective when it is considered that the incidence in both sexes is about one-hundredth that of the most common

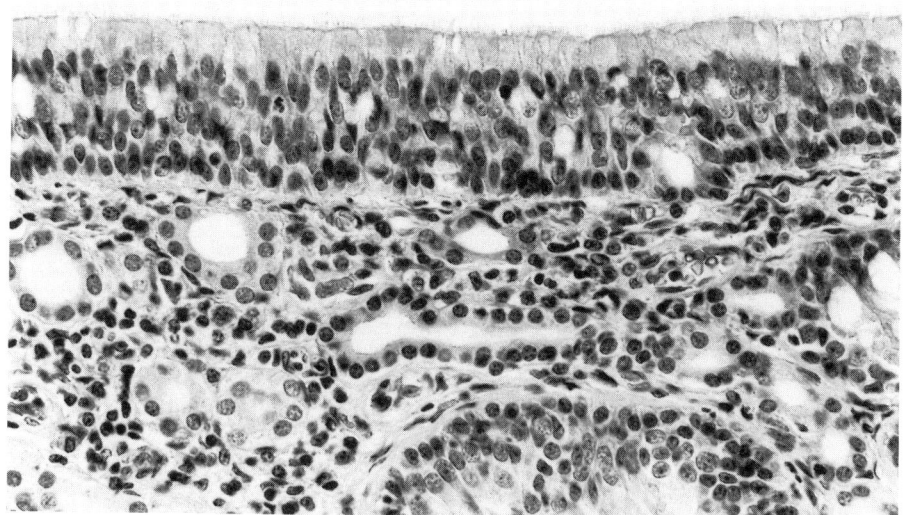

FIG. 10. Olfactory epithelium. Although the epithelium is cylindrical, just as respiratory epithelium, the cells are taller and the nuclei are arranged in several layers. The underlaying stroma contains numerous serous glands. H&E, ×340.

malignant tumors in most developed countries: that is, carcinoma of the bronchus in men and carcinoma of the breast in women. However, six occupational groups have an unequivocal association with nasal cancer (1): chromate workers, nickel refiners and workers, makers of isopropyl alcohol (by the strong-acid process), mustard gas manufacturers, makers of wooden furniture and certain other woodworkers, and boot and shoe workers exposed to leather dust. In the nose, squamous cell tumors account for more than three-fourths of all malignant tumors. Adenocarcinomas and anaplastic tumors account for about 10% each.

Chromium

Workers in the chromate production industry and the chromate pigment industry, who experience an increased risk of lung cancer, also experience an increased risk of cancer of the accessory nasal sinuses (38,39). An important consumer of chromium has been the tanning industry. Epidemiologic studies imply that hexavalent chromium compounds are the main cause of respiratory tract cancers in chromate workers (40). Animal work incriminates certain hexavalent chromium compounds as definite carcinogens (41).

Nickel

Striking increases in risk for both nasal and lung cancer have been described in nickel refiners in several countries. The majority of nasal cancer cases (mainly

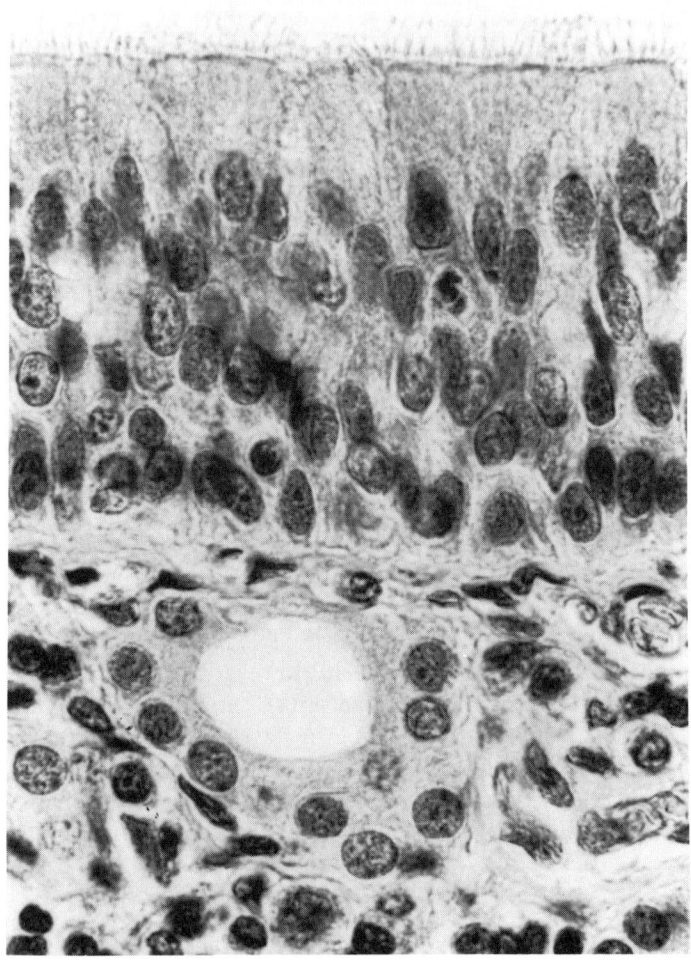

FIG. 11. Olfactory epithelium. Higher magnification from Fig. 10. Nuclei from sustentacular and olfactory cells lay higher in the epithelium than the nuclei of the basal cells. H&E, ×1,000.

squamous cell carcinomas) can be related to dust exposure during the process of roasting and leaching, suggesting a link with exposure to nickel sulfides or nickel oxides (42). No cases of nasal cancer have been observed within 15 years of first exposure; thereafter the risk rises rapidly and is still increasing 40 years following first exposure (42). Kaldor et al. (43) also demonstrated an increasing risk with increasing age at first exposure and a strong relationship with duration of employment in high-risk areas. In the Report of the International Committee on Nickel Carcinogenesis in Man (44), a review is given of past epidemiologic studies of nickel-exposed populations. The primary conclusion reached is that more than one form of nickel gives rise to lung and nasal cancer. In nickel refinery workers, expo-

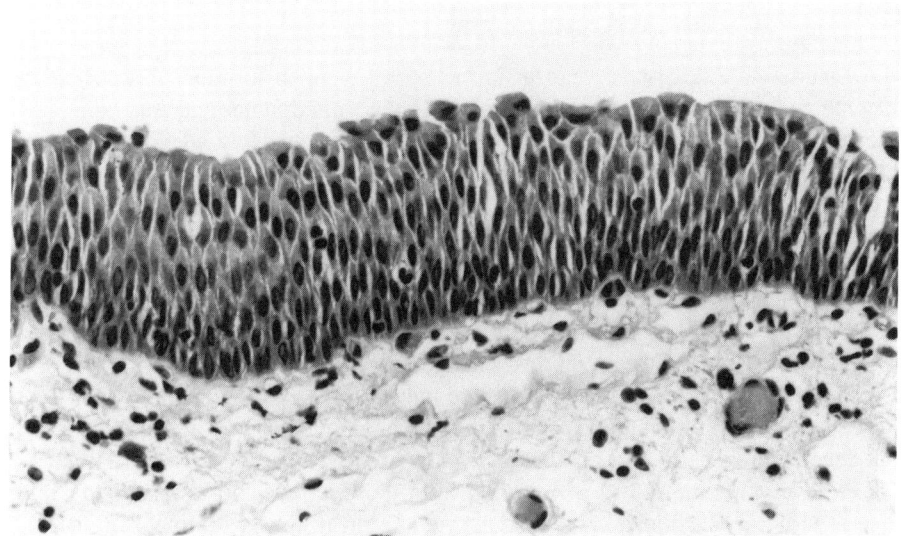

FIG. 12. Intermediate epithelium. A multilayered epithelium with a superficial layer of cells of the umbrella-type similar to those seen in the lining of the urinary tract. H&E, ×340.

sure to mixtures of oxidic and sulfidic nickel turned out to be the major risk factor. It was also evident that exposure to soluble nickel increased the risk. There was, however, no evidence that metallic nickel was associated with increased cancer risks. There is at present a need for more long-term inhalation experiments in laboratory animals to determine the relative carcinogenic potency of the various nickel compounds. On the positive side, it seems clear that outside the refineries, exposure to nickel compounds is such that no measurable risk (at least for nasal sinus cancer) is involved.

Isopropyl Alcohol

An excess risk of nasal cancer (and possibly of laryngeal cancer) has been found in three factories in which isopropyl alcohol was manufactured by the strong-acid process (45). The nature of the carcinogen is unknown. Alderson and Rattan (46) described a historical prospective study of workers in an isopropyl alcohol plant. Specific examination was carried out of observed and expected nasal sinus cancer. Although only one observed (not further specified) cancer occurred, the expected figure was so low that the difference was statistically significant.

Mustard Gas

In a group of Japanese workers who manufactured mustard gas before and during World War II, a high incidence of nasal (laryngeal and lung) cancer (47) was observed.

Wood Dust

An increased risk of nasal cancer in makers of wooden furniture has now been documented in most European countries and in the United States and Australia (48). The tumors that occur in these workers are almost exclusively adenocarcinomas. According to Hadfield (49), the inhalation of wood dust in the furniture industry over an extended period of time depressed mucociliary clearance. This phenomenon, which may be due to loss of cilia, leads to stasis and retention of wood dusts at the anterior end of the middle turbinate. This, in turn, may lead to penetration of the mucous glands by a carcinogen and to the occurrence of adenocarcinomas. Other work has shown that the prevalence of mucociliary stasis in woodworkers is related to the concentration of the wood dust inhaled (50).

Acheson (51) suggested that the factors inducing the nasal tumors were at least present in the furniture industry in the United Kingdom between 1920 and 1940 and that beech almost certainly, and oak probably, are associated with the disease. The risk of developing nasal cancer was highest for those in jobs with exposure to wood dust as turners, machinists, and sanders rather than in jobs with exposure to polishes, varnishes, and the like. On the basis of occurrences of nasal cancer in various types of woodworkers, Acheson believed that wood dust itself, rather than any of the other extraneous chemicals that might be met by a worker in the furniture industry, is the factor related to the workplace that contributes to the development of malignant neoplasms. The substance may be a naturally occurring agent or an agent produced by pyrolysis during the action of high-speed grinding and cutting machines. There are many complex compounds in wood dust (e.g., condensed tannins) but also a number of complex aldehydes. This is of particular interest in view of the carcinogenic action of formaldehyde and acetaldehyde in rats. However, in the United Kingdom, formaldehyde was not used prior to World War II in the furniture industry. IARC (48) concluded that there was sufficient evidence that nasal adenocarcinomas had been caused by employment in the furniture-making industry. The excess risk occurred mainly among those exposed to wood dust. From 1981 onward there are some reports indicating that softwood dust exposure appears to be associated with squamous cell carcinomas (51–55). Hayes et al. (56) presented a case-control study in the Netherlands, examining the relationships between type of woodworking (and extent of wood-dust exposure) and the risk for specific histologic types of sinonasal cancer. They found that the risk for nasal adenocarcinomas was elevated. The association between wood-dust exposure and adenocarcinoma was strongest for those employed in wood-dust-related occupations between 1930 and 1941. The risk of adenocarcinoma in the sinonasal area did not appear to decrease for at least 15 years after termination of wood-dust exposure. No cases of adenocarcinoma were observed in men whose first exposure to wood dust had occurred after 1941.

Miller et al. (57) investigated cause-specific mortality among U.S. members of a national furniture workers' union first employed between 1946 and 1962. Nasal cancer was not found to be significantly raised in this cohort, although the average follow-up period (21 years) may not have been long enough to detect an excess risk for this uncommon type of tumor. The mean latency for occupationally related nasal adenocarcinoma has been reported to be about 40 years, with a minimum observed latency of 27 years (58). Most cases of nasal cancer among furniture workers have been identified among workers first employed before World War II. It has been suggested that this may be due either to an insufficient latency period for detecting cases among more recently exposed workers or to some change in workplace exposures (e.g., introduction of mechanical production techniques with high dust exposures in the 1930s, followed by the introduction of improved hygiene measures in the 1940s).

Viren and Imbus (59) reviewed the literature dealing with the association between nasal and sinus cancers and wood dust. They presented the results of a case-control study of nasal cancer deaths in four American states and concluded that "there seems to be no association between nasal cancer and industry/occupation normally identified with wood dust." Finkelstein (60), however, showed that the data of Viren and Imbus are compatible with an interpretation opposite to theirs: namely, that there is, indeed, an association between the risk of nasal cancers and occupational exposure to wood dust.

Kleinsasser and Schroeder (61) studied the epidemiology, clinical behavior, and histopathology of nasal adenocarcinomas collected in the former Federal Republic of Germany. Of the patients with intestinal v-type adenocarcinoma, 79 had been exposed intensively to wood dust. Each year approximately 10 to 15 new cases of this disease are diagnosed in the former Federal Republic of Germany. The authors hypothesized that the rare cases of intestinal v-type adenocarcinomas of the nose published before 1960 indicate that this occupational disease has become more frequent within the last 20 years, perhaps by some still unknown change in the woodworking processes.

Boot and Shoe Workers

Nasal cancer has been described and accepted as an occupational risk in makers and repairers of leather boots and shoes both in England and Italy (62–64). In people working in this industry it is possible to demonstrate increased risks of adenocarcinoma and of other histological types of nasal tumors. The occurrence of these tumors is concentrated in two small areas in the factories: the areas where dusty work is done with leather used to make heels and soles. It is important to point out that the hard, durable leather used for soles and heels is tanned exclusively by vegetable extracts and not by chrome.

Formaldehyde

In recent years the carcinogenic effects of formaldehyde have been widely discussed, since it was shown that it is a potent nasal carcinogen in rats exposed to high concentrations. Exposure to formaldehyde is very common in both industrial and domestic environments. However, epidemiological studies conducted to date have not provided unequivocal evidence that exposure can induce nasal or other types of cancer (65,66).

Halperin et al. (67) reported a case of squamous cell carcinoma of the nasal cavity of a man who had 25 years of occupational exposure to low concentrations of formaldehyde in the textile-finishing industry. Holmström and Lund (68) described three cases of malignant mucosal melanoma of the nasal cavity in patients who had been occupationally exposed to formaldehyde. Holmström et al. (69) also investigated the histological effects on the human nasal mucosa of long-term exposure to formaldehyde alone and in combination with wood dust. Significant changes (e.g., epithelial dysplasia) were found in the formaldehyde group but not in the group exposed to both formaldehyde and wood dust. No correlation was found between histological changes and duration of exposure, doses of exposure, or smoking habits.

Boysen et al. (70) studied the histological changes in the nasal mucosa of workers exposed to formaldehyde (for more than 5 years) and found a higher degree of metaplastic alterations compared with age-matched referents. These results indicate that formaldehyde might be carcinogenic to humans. Combining this finding with the inconclusive epidemiological studies suggests that formaldehyde may be a weak carcinogen, but that occupational exposure to formaldehyde alone is insufficient to induce nasal cancer.

It is worth considering whether formaldehyde can be held responsible for the occurrence of nasal cancer in the furniture, boot, and shoe industries. At the present time it is used extensively in both, principally in adhesives. However in the United Kingdom formaldehyde was not used prior to World War II in either industry, yet it is known that a number of workers who subsequently developed the disease had left the industry prior to 1930 in the furniture industry (71) and before 1920 in the boot and shoe industry (64,72). It therefore seems very unlikely that formaldehyde can be incriminated in these industries.

Laryngeal Cancer

Tobacco smoking is an important cause of laryngeal cancer. Pipe and/or cigar smoking appear to increase the risk to about the same extent as cigarette smoking (4). Drinking of alcoholic beverages is another major cause of laryngeal cancer. There is no indication that the effect is dependent on type of beverage (73). A combination of tobacco smoking and high doses of alcohol leads to an additional risk, although there are indications that this is more valid for pharyngeal cancer than for laryngeal cancer (74). A number of occupational exposures, such as exposure to asbestos, nickel, mustard gas, isopropyl alcohol, sulfuric acid, and wood dust have been associated with increased risk of laryngeal cancer, but the results are often conflicting (5). However, recent cohort and case-control studies clearly demonstrate an increased risk of laryngeal cancer in workers exposed to strong inorganic-acid mists containing sulfuric acid (75–78). In a case-control study, low dietary vitamin A levels appeared to be associated with increased risk of cancer of the larynx (79).

Histopathology

Neoplasms of the upper respiratory tract include a variety of benign and malignant tumors. The majority of these are epithelial, approximately 70% versus 30% that are from a diversity of other tissues (80). Malignant epithelial tumors may be derived from the surface epithelium or from the underlying salivary glands. They are broadly divided into tumors showing squamous or glandular differentiation (81,82), these accounting for 50% and 20%, the remaining carcinomas being classified as undifferentiated. Within the nonepithelial malignancies, malignant lymphoma, malignant melanoma, and olfactory neuroblastoma together make up 50% of this group, the other 50% being formed by an immense diversity of malignancies that each account for less than 1% (80). Our discussion of upper respiratory tract cancers is restricted to the more common lesions.

Squamous cell carcinoma is the most common malignancy in the human upper respiratory tract. The characteristic element in this tumor is the polygonal spinous cell (keratinocyte, prickle cell) that forms intercellular bridges. In well-differentiated cases, these cells are abundant, and differentiation proceeds toward the formation of clusters of cells compounded almost exclusively of keratin lamellae, the so-called *keratin pearls*. Loss of differentiation parallels loss of spinous cells, and when these are entirely absent, the squamous nature of an individual tumor may become difficult to ascertain. Squamous cell carcinomas are classified as well, moderately, or poorly differentiated, depending on the amount of prickle cells and keratin pearls. The tumor occurs anywhere in the upper respiratory tract, including the paranasal sinuses and nasopharynx. Invasively growing squamous cell carcinoma may be preceded by a noninvasive precursor lesion. These lesions show changes as cellular and nuclear pleomorphism, increased number of mitoses, and hyperchromasia. Moreover, the normal maturation sequence from basal cells to spinous cells and subsequently to superficial flattened cells may be disturbed; cells being found at levels abnormal for their stage of maturation. Depending on the severity of these by definition intraepithelial alterations, the lesion may be classified as showing mild, moderate, or severe dysplasia, or carcinoma *in situ*.

Verrucous carcinoma is a variant of squamous cell carcinoma that is characterized by an extremely well-differentiated nature that contrasts with its locally destructive nature. The tumor consists of broad bulbs of well-differentiated epithelium that infiltrate into the underlying tissue by pushing them away.

Another variant of squamous cell carcinoma is *spindle cell carcinoma*. In this tumor, the epithelial cells have transformed into poorly differentiated spindle cells sometimes exhibiting a whorling arrangement. Epithelial features may become so rudimentary that they are visible only at the ultrastructural level. The squamous nature of this neoplasm is further substantiated by the simultaneous occurrence of spindle cell areas and ordinary squamous cell carcinoma in the same lesion and by the observation that spindle cell carcinoma may recur as conventional squamous cell carcinoma, or vice versa (83).

The next variant of squamous cell carcinoma consists of ribbons of stratified epithelium exhibiting flattening of the surface cells. They exhibit no keratinization, but ultrastructurally, squamous differentiation is shown. The epithelial strands are usually sharply demarcated from the adjacent stroma (Fig. 13). Because of a resem-

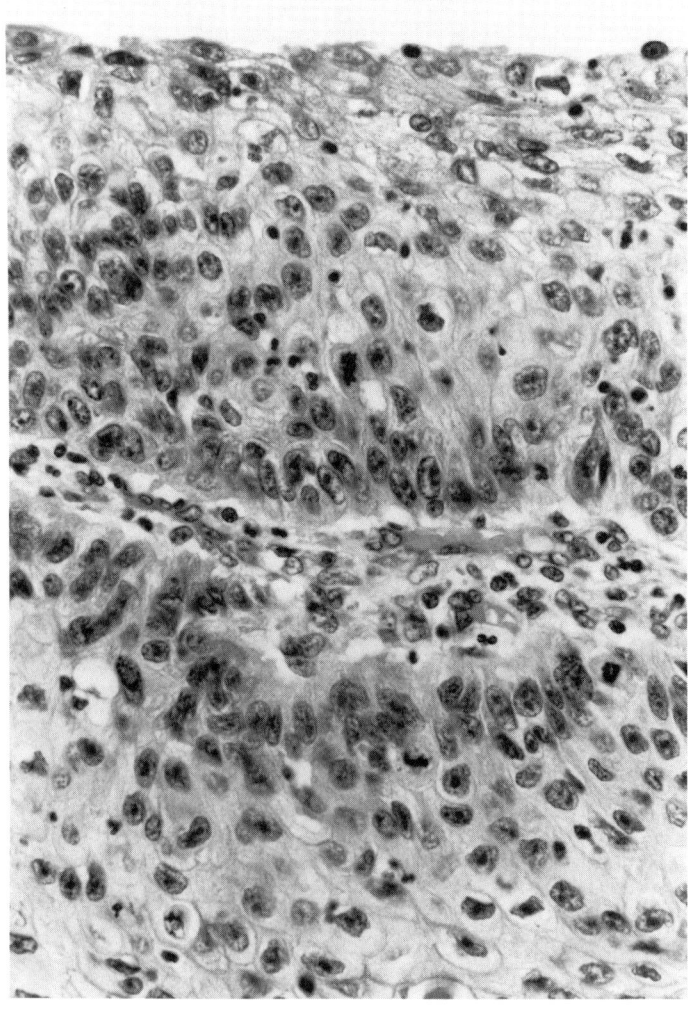

FIG. 13. Transitional squamous cell carcinoma. A multilayered epithelium exhibiting cellular and nuclear atypia is sharply demarcated from the underlying stroma. H&E, ×400.

blance to the transitional epithelium that lines the urinary bladder, these tumors are labeled *transitional* or *transitional cell carcinoma*. Sometimes these tumors also contain many cylindrical cells; in that event the designation *cylindrical cell carcinoma* is employed. Also, mucus located either intra- or intercellularly may be present, probably due to preexistent goblet cells being overgrown by tumor. This type of squamous cell carcinoma preferably occurs in the sinonasal tract and also in the nasopharynx, where it is designated as *nonkeratinizing nasopharyngeal carcinoma* (82). Other nasopharyngeal carcinomas are the conventional squamous cell carcinoma exhibiting keratin pearls and prickle cells and the so-called *undifferentiated carcinoma of nasopharyngeal type*. Undifferentiated carcinoma of nasopharyngeal type is essentially a very poorly differentiated squamous cell carcinoma (82). It consists of tumor cells with oval or round vesicular nuclei, prominent nucleoli, and a syncytial appearance. Sometimes the tumor nests are surrounded by a dense lymphocytic infiltrate, which in the past has given origin to the erroneous designation "lymphoepithelioma."

Tumors exhibiting *glandular differentiation* may be divided into those originating from salivary gland epithelium and those originating from surface epithelium. The former are the conventional salivary gland adenocarcinomas, such as adenoid cystic carcinomas, mucoepidermoid carcinomas, and others. The reader is referred to monographs on this topic (84). The cancers from surface epithelium with glandular differentiation are very interesting from a toxicological point of view, since they were the first to be related to certain occupations (61,85,86). Because of their resemblance to gastrointestinal carcinomas, these cancers are collectively labeled *intestinal-type adenocarcinoma*. These tumors may be well or poorly differentiated and are composed of single- or multilayered columnar epithelium that may arrange to form cysts, tubules, or papillary structures (Fig. 14). Cellular differentiation may include goblet cell or signet cell formation. Occasionally, the tumor cells lay dispersed in large pools of mucus. According to Kleinsasser and Schroeder (61,86), this type of nasal cancer has become more frequent among woodworkers in Germany during the last few decades.

Olfactory neuroblastoma originates from the olfactory epithelium situated in the upper roof of the nose. The tumor is characterized by the presence of well-demarcated lobules of uniform tumor cells laying in a highly vascular stroma. The distinct lobular architecture is retained even when there is progression from lower to higher grades of malignancy (87). These grades of malignancy are defined as follows. Grade 1 tumors consist of large lobules in which cells with round to ovoid nuclei lay dispersed in a neurofibrillary background. Mitoses are not present (Fig. 15). In grade 2 tumors, the lobuli are smaller, the nuclei show more pleomorphism, mitoses may be observed, and neurofibrillar material is scarce and usually present as dots surrounded by tumor cells, giving origin to so-called *pseudorosettes* or *Homer Wright rosettes* (Fig. 16). Grade 3 tumors show still more anaplasia at the cellular and nuclear levels. Their histologic hallmark are the *Flexner–Wintersteiner rosettes*: radially orientated cylindrical cells surrounding an empty space; similar structures are seen in ocular retinoblastomas (Fig. 17). Grade 4 tumors lack any

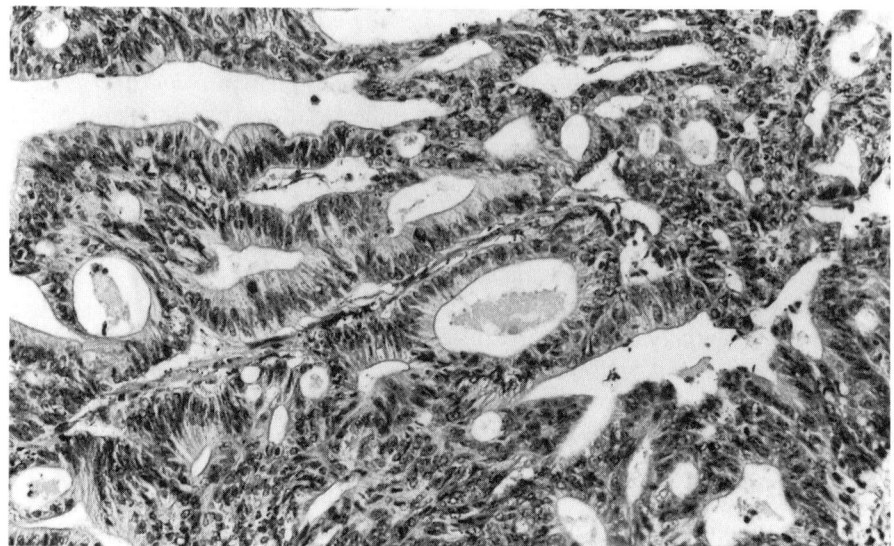

FIG. 14. Adenocarcinoma of the gastrointestinal type occurring in the sinonasal cavities. The arrangement of atypical cylindrical cells in strands and lining ductlike spaces is clearly displayed. H&E, ×170.

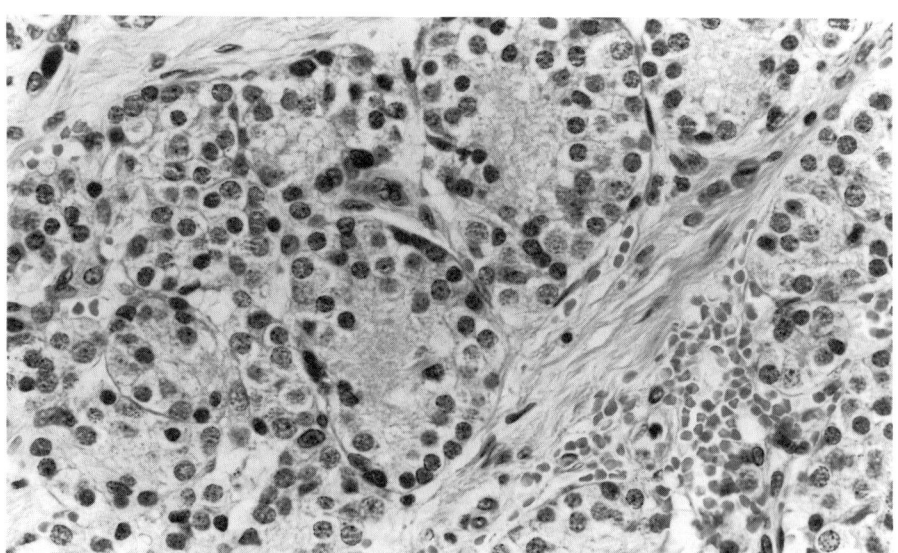

FIG. 15. Olfactory neuroblastoma grade I. Cells with monotonous vesicular nuclei and ample cytoplasm are arranged in lobuli. Neurofibrillary material occupies the center of some lobuli. H&E, ×340.

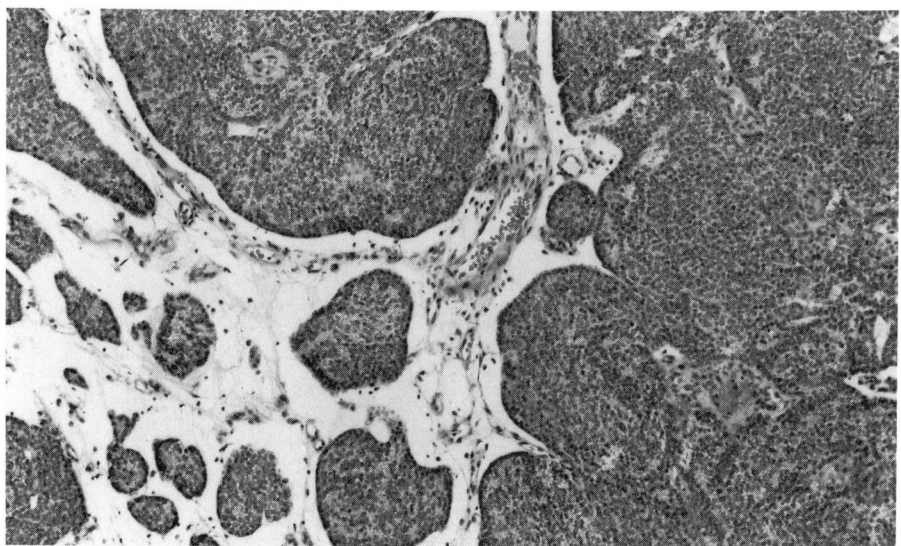

FIG. 16. Olfactory neuroblastoma grade II. The cells are darker and the lobular architecture is less pronounced than in grade I tumors. H&E, ×85.

evidence of differentiation at the light microscopical level. This diagnosis is suggested by the lobular architecture and the vascular stroma but needs support from ultrastructural demonstration of neurosecretory granules. Olfactory neuroblastomas grade 1 and 2 were formerly called *esthesioneurocytomas*, *esthesioneuroepithelioma* and *esthesioneuroblastoma* being the designations employed for grade 3 and grade 4 tumor, respectively. These diagnostic labels are, however, no longer in use (82).

Sometimes olfactory neuroblastomas contain glandlike structures (Fig. 18). This observation has led to the proposition of an entity called *neuroendocrine carcinoma*. However, these glandlike structures are often combined with more classical features such as neurofibrillary matrix or rosettes. Moreover, olfactory neuroblastomas seem to be derived from the basal cells of the olfactory membrane (83; our own observation, Figs. 18 and 19) and as these cells give origin to sensory neurons as well as sustentacular cells (88), the presence of cylindrical cells investing ductlike spaces should be considered as an additional differentiation of the neoplastically altered basal cells. Thus there seems to be no need for creating a separate category of neuroendocrine carcinoma. In summary, olfactory neuroblastomas show cell-rich lobuli lying in a highly vascular stroma, neurofibrillary matrix, and rosettes or pseudorosettes, glandlike spaces being optional and ultrastructurally demonstrable neurosecretory granules being obligate.

Malignant lymphoma in the upper respiratory tract is mainly one of the types of non-Hodgkin's malignant lymphoma. B- as well as T-cell lymphomas may occur

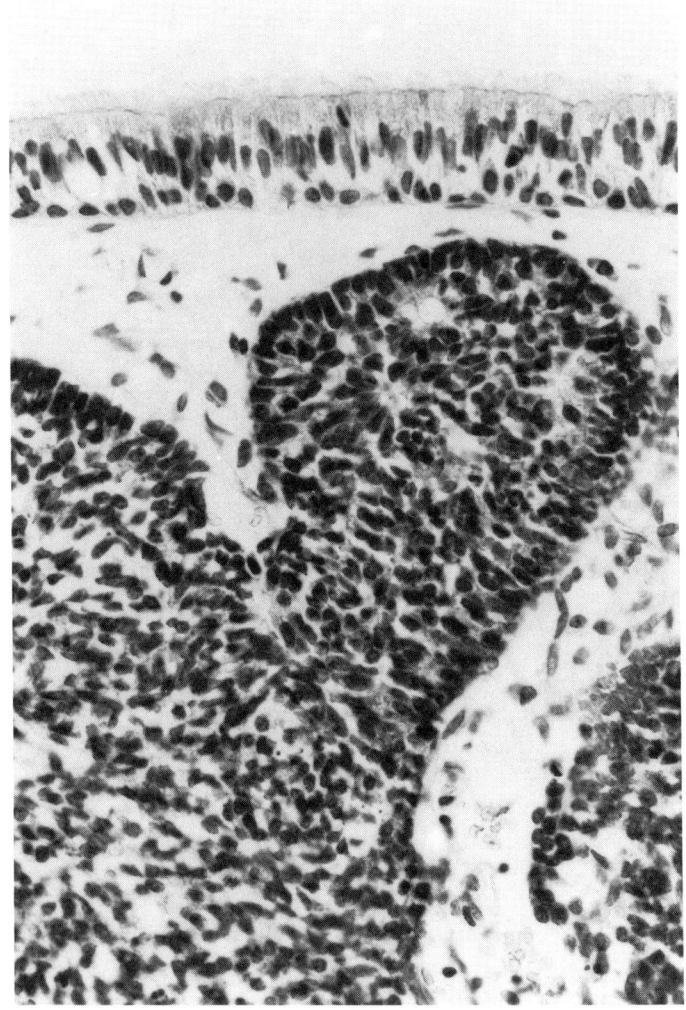

FIG. 17. Olfactory neuroblastoma grade III. The cells are small with dark nuclei. Flexner–Wintersteiner rosettes are present. H&E, ×400.

and their presence may be hidden behind signs suggesting an ordinary inflammation clinically as well as histologically (89).

Malignant melanoma occurs predominantly in the nose and paranasal sinuses. If well differentiated, the tumor is readily recognized by the presence of large cells with highly pleomorphic nuclei, large nucleoli, and melanin pigment. They may,

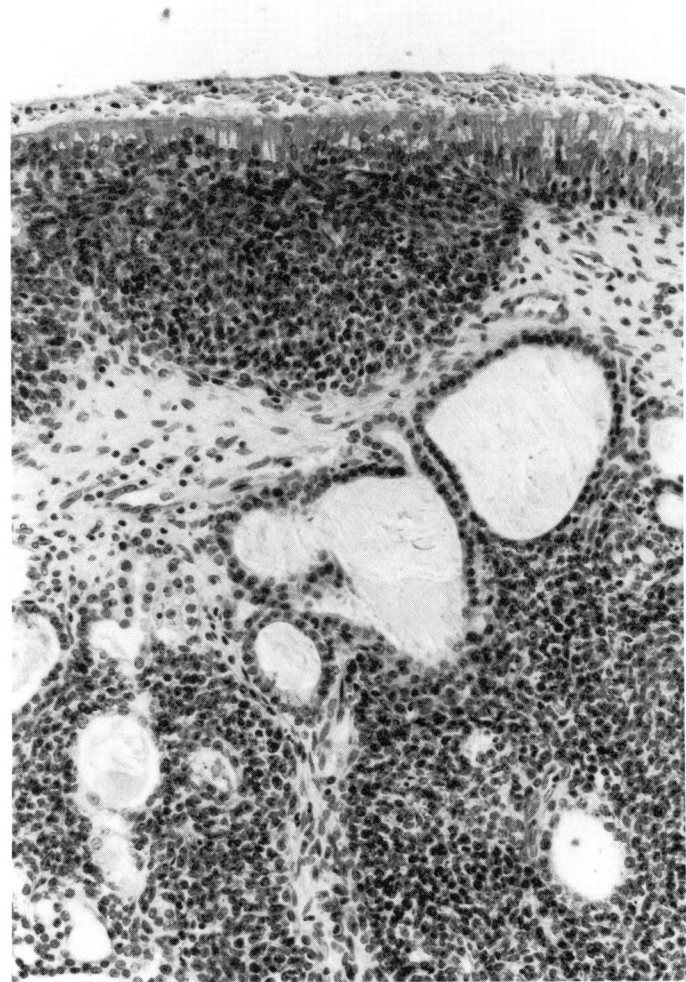

FIG. 18. Derivation of olfactory neuroblastoma from the basal layer of the olfactory epithelium (**right**). The tumor engulfs preexistent glands of Bowman (**left**). H&E, ×200.

however, also be less differentiated, with a predominant spindle cell morphology, or even entirely undifferentiated at the light microscopic level. It is obvious that the upper respiratory tract is a very significant organ system from an oncologic point of view. A plethora of tumors does occur in this region, and ideas on their etiology are only beginning to emanate.

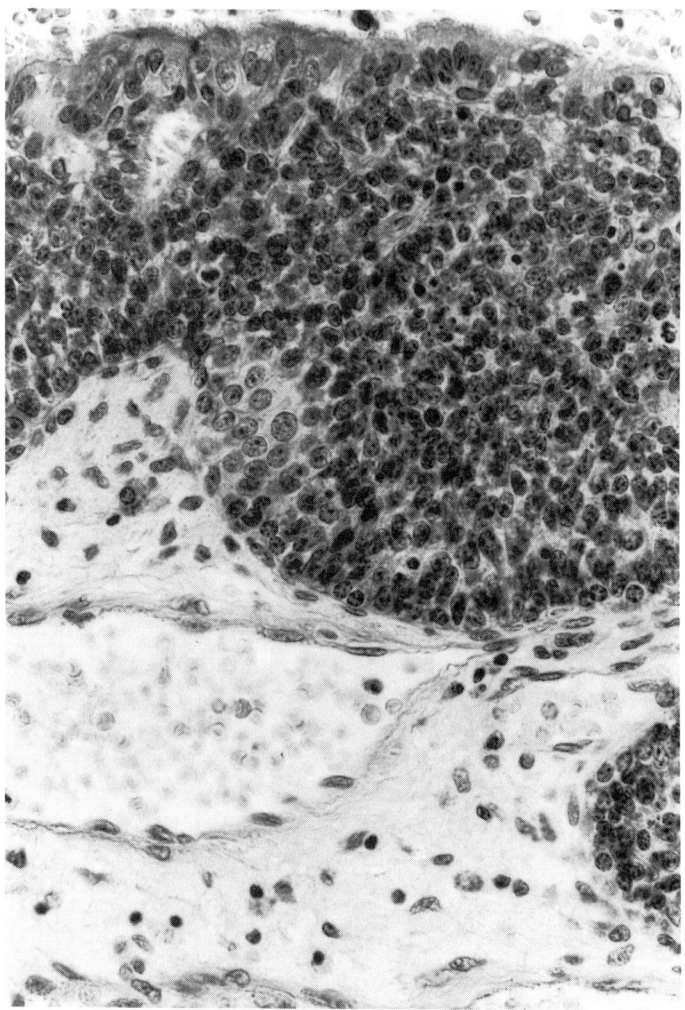

FIG. 19. Higher magnification from Fig. 18 in which the relationship of the tumor with a disorganized olfactory epithelium is exhibited. H&E, ×400.

UPPER RESPIRATORY TRACT CANCER IN RODENTS

Spontaneous Nasal and Laryngeal Tumors

In a previous paper (9) we have given a survey of upper respiratory tract tumors in Cpb:WU (Wistar random) rats, including those found in untreated controls. It appeared that 7 out of 661 untreated male control animals (1.1%) developed a nasal tumor, whereas none of the 492 untreated female control rats were found to bear a nasal tumor. The nasal tumors observed in those seven male controls were invariably squamous cell carcinomas. Six tumors were large, unilateral, well-differentiated keratinizing squamous cell carcinomas located in the anterior half of the nose. These tumors had destroyed turbinates and bones and extended into the subcutis. Three of these tumors were associated with odontodystrophy, severe necrotizing (peri)odontitis, and rhinitis. One small infiltrating squamous cell carcinoma was seen in an inflamed nasolachrymal duct. The site of origin of large nasal tumors is generally uncertain, although they are probably derived from (metaplastic) respiratory epithelium lining the anterior sinonasal structures. Other types of (spontaneous) nasal tumors detected in chemically treated animals, but considered unrelated to treatment, included one carcinoma *in situ*, one osteosarcoma, one fibrosarcoma, and four odontogenic tumors (see below) in males and one papilloma in a female. In none of the 420 untreated male control rats and in only one female of the 422 untreated female controls (0.2%) was a laryngeal tumor found. The latter tumor was an adenoma (9).

The incidence of spontaneous tumors of the upper respiratory tract in the National Toxicology Program (NTP) archives was less than 0.5% for any tumor type in any location. The most common type of spontaneous tumor seen in the upper respiratory tract of rats was squamous cell carcinoma (90). In hamsters and mice, spontaneous tumors of the upper respiratory tract are rare. In mice, Stewart et al. (91) reported a polypoid tumor covered by stratified squamous epithelium. Pour et al. (92,93) found upper respiratory tract tumors in up to 3% of the hamsters. Many of these tumors were located in the nasal cavity and larynx/trachea and included polyps lined by stratified squamous or cuboidal epithelium and clear cell carcinomas of unknown cellular origin in the larynx. These authors also found a carcinoma of the nasoturbinates with formation of rosettes and production of mucus.

Spontaneous Tumors Extending into the Nasal Cavity

Nasal tumors must be discriminated from tumors arising in the oral cavity or skin, or, for example, from Zymbal's glands and expanding into the nasal cavity. Spontaneously occurring odontogenic tumors in rats are extremely rare (94). Recently, we presented a case of a spontaneous odontogenic tumor in the maxilla of a male Wistar rat (95). This tumor was classified as an adenomatoid odontogenic tumorlike epithelioma and consisted of epithelial islands of varying size composed of densely packed spindle-shaped cells with large oval nuclei with finely dispersed chromatin and weakly eosinophilic cytoplasm.

Spontaneous tumors, apparently arising from the periodontal ligament and sometimes extending into the nasal cavity, have also been described by others (9,96). The rat incisor teeth develop from cells that are derived from a continuously proliferating elliptical sheath, the enamel epithelium, which is located at the base of the tooth and which encloses the connective tissue of the primitive pulp. An adult incisor tooth undergoes functional attrition as a normal wearing process. When, by reason of accident, one of the incisors is broken or when a malocclusion occurs, the nonattrition of the opposing incisor and its continuous growth results in an elongation or overgrowth; the term "overgrowth" is misleading, as in reality, this elongation is not related to the rate of growth of the tooth but is result of the lack of wear (97). In three of seven untreated Cpb:WU, Wistar random rats with a nasal squamous cell carcinoma (9), the tumor was seen to be associated with severe necrotizing (peri)odontitis and rhinitis which involved the entire area of the incisor tooth, the maxillary turbinate, and the maxillary sinus. Since such inflammatory reactions are accompanied by sustained tissue damage, which is known to predispose to tumor formation in other locations (e.g., liver, colon, skin, lungs), it seems reasonable to assume that the malocclusion syndrome may enhance the risk of the development of squamous cell carcinoma or ameloblastoma, originating from metaplastic respiratory or odontogenic epithelium, respectively. It is possible that in rats a certain percentage of nasal squamous cell carcinomas could be considered part of the malocclusion syndrome.

Brown (90) described several tumors observed in the NTP database having a distinct morphology but an uncertain origin. These tumors were termed "poorly differentiated spindle-cell tumors of dental or nasolachrymal duct origin." Such tumors occur anterior to the root of the incisor teeth at the level where the nasolachrymal duct lies immediately lateral to the tooth. The neoplasm appears to be centered around the tooth but involves the nasolachrymal duct extensively. Typically, the ductal epithelium is characterized by papillary folding of squamous epithelium that is six to eight cell layers thick. Mitotic activity is quite high in the lower one-third of the epithelium, and there is a variable degree of subacute inflammation and inflammatory exudate associated with the epithelium. Beneath the epithelium and around the tooth is a population of spindle cells that appeared to be fairly uniform in a given tumor but somewhat pleomorphic when comparing different tumors. Nuclei varied from being elongated and hyperchromatic to being more vesicular and rounded with a marginated chromatin pattern and a prominent nucleolus. Cellular morphology was either elliptical, indistinct and tightly compacted, or more loosely arranged as polygonal, individual cells with more abundant eosinophilic cytoplasm. Both types often appeared to merge with the adjacent nasolachrymal duct epithelium to a variable extent. The pattern of growth was basically in sheets that had no distinctive features. The incisor tooth involved was distorted.

Chemically Induced Upper Respiratory Tract Tumors

Tumors of Squamous Epithelium and Respiratory Mucosa of the Nose

Antecedent to tumors of the respiratory epithelium, different types of hyperplasia (simple, papillary, nodular, or pseudoepitheliomatous) and stratified squamous metaplasia with keratinization have been found in experimental animals following oral or subcutaneous administration of various nitrosamines or other compounds (Table 2) (98–102). Takano et al. (103) studied the sequential changes in the development of preneoplastic and neoplastic lesions in the nasal respiratory epithelium of rats given 1,4-dinitrosopiperazine in their drinking water. With respect to the nonneoplastic lesions, they distinguished simple hyperplasia, papillary hyperplasia, and nodular hyperplasia. Simple hyperplasia was defined as focal thickening of the mucosa with slightly irregular cells; papillary hyperplasia consisted of exophytic protrusions with a thin fibrovascular stalk; and nodular hyperplasia was seen as downward growth into the submucosa, which occasionally showed glandular structures containing periodic acid–Schiff-positive material. There was evidence that the papillary hyperplasia progressed to papillomas and the nodular hyperplasia to adenocarcinomas. Rats exposed to phenylglycidyl ether developed hyperplastic and metaplastic respiratory epithelium, occasionally showing dysplastic glandular acini with hyperplastic goblet cells (19).

In our chronic inhalation study with acetaldehyde in rats, squamous cell carcinomas were found primarily in the top-concentration group (3,000 ppm decreased to 1,000 ppm after 52 weeks), in which a nearly 100% incidence of keratinized stratified squamous metaplasia of large areas of the nasal respiratory epithelium occurred (104). A similar response of the nasal respiratory epithelium has been reported in rats exposed to 15 ppm formaldehyde for life (105,106). Acetaldehyde-induced squamous cell carcinomas varied from large tumors, filling one or both sides of the nasal cavity, destroying turbinates and bones, and extending into the subcutis and brain, to small neoplasms invading the submucosa of the nasal epithelium (104). The large tumors often showed extensive keratinization, and their origin could not be determined with certainty.

Most small squamous cell carcinomas were seen to originate from metaplastic, keratinized, stratified squamous respiratory epithelium, and they occurred in the anterior part of the nose. A few squamous cell carcinomas appeared to be derived from metaplastic, keratinized, squamous olfactory epithelium located in the dorsomedial and posterior part of the nasal cavity (15). Formaldehyde-induced squa-

TABLE 2. Nasal tumors originating from the respiratory mucosa in rodents

Papilloma
  Exophytic
  Endophytic (inverted)
Adenoma (of submucosal glands)
Polypoid adenoma (exophytic)
Squamous cell papilloma
Squamous cell carcinoma
Adenocarcinoma
Adenosquamous carcinoma
Anaplastic carcinoma

mous cell carcinomas were relatively large keratinizing or nonkeratinizing tumors originating from the naso- and maxilloturbinates or from the lateral wall at the level of these turbinates; they invariably invaded bones and/or the subcutis (107). Squamous cell carcinomas of the respiratory epithelium were also found in Cpb:WU (Wistar random) rats with their respiratory mucosa severely damaged by electrocoagulation and exposed to 10 ppm formaldehyde for 28 months (108). Chronic exposure of hamsters to a high concentration of acetaldehyde (2,500 ppm decreased to 1,650 ppm after 45 weeks) resulted in only a few nasal tumors (one adenoma, one adenocarcinoma, and one anaplastic carcinoma in a total of 53 animals), despite severe and extensive keratinized squamous metaplasia of the respiratory epithelium (26). Also, hamsters exposed to 10 ppm formaldehyde gas for life showed hyper- and metaplasia of the respiratory tract but developed no nasal tumors (109). Apparently, the nasal respiratory epithelium of hamsters is less susceptible to the carcinogenic activity of these aldehydes than is that of rats.

The squamous cell carcinomas seen in our studies with formaldehyde (107,108) were seen to originate from the same region in the nasal cavity as described earlier by Morgan et al. (110). They reported that most squamous cell neoplasms occurred on the lateral side of the nasoturbinate and adjacent lateral wall at cross section II. Other tumors were located on the midventral nasal septum (cross sections II and III) and on the dorsal septum and the roof of the dorsal meatus (cross sections II and III). Only a small number was found on the maxilloturbinate at cross sections II and III (Figs. 1 to 4). In several rats exposed to high concentrations of acetaldehyde (1,500 or 3,000 ppm) carcinomas *in situ* developed in metaplastic stratified squamous respiratory epithelium (15). Clearly, these tumors were part of the neoplastic response of the nasal respiratory epithelium to acetaldehyde and may be considered precursors of the frequently found squamous cell carcinomas. A total of four polypoid adenomas were observed in the Cpb:WU (Wistar random) rat used in our laboratory, namely two in male rats exposed to 20 ppm formaldehyde for 4 or 8 weeks, respectively, followed by an observation period of over 2 years (107,111), one in a male rat exposed to 10 ppm formaldehyde for 3 months, followed by an observation period of 25 months (107), and one in a male rat exposed to 1.5/2.0 ppm trichlorobutene for 83 weeks (112). Those seen after exposure to 20 ppm formaldehyde are considered compound induced, while those seen in the other studies may or may not be treatment related. We never found a polypoid adenoma in an untreated control rat. One of the formaldehyde-related polypoid adenomas was derived from the epithelium lining the maxilloturbinate and the adjacent lateral wall (Figs. 20 and 21); it was an exophytic sessile tumor protruding into the nasal cavity. The other formaldehyde-induced tumor was a small pedunculated adenoma, originating from the lateral wall at the level of the nasoturbinate. In addition to solid sheets of epithelial cells and microcysts, the latter neoplasm contained one large cystic structure partially lined by keratinized stratified squamous epithelium. A third polypoid adenoma, possibly related to formaldehyde exposure, was a small pedunculated adenoma, derived from the ventral margin of the nasoturbinate. The polypoid adenoma found in the trichlorobutene-exposed rat was an exophytic sessile

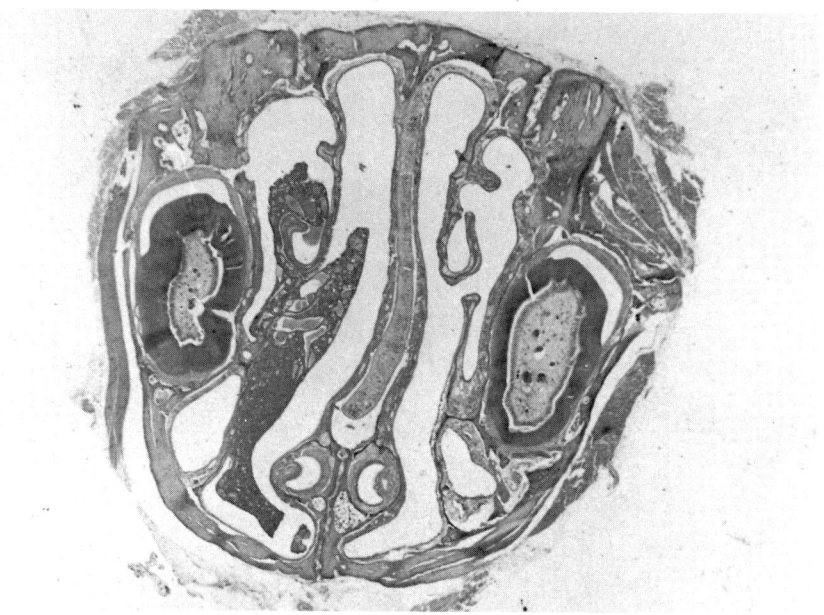

FIG. 20. Sessile polypoid adenoma originating from the maxilloturbinate and lateral wall. Male rat exposed to 20 ppm formaldehyde for 4 weeks. H&E, ×10.

adenoma, arising from the respiratory epithelium lining the lateral aspect of the nasoturbinate and lateral wall. The diagnosis of polypoid adenoma was based on the criteria described by Kerns (113), who reported a number of polypoid adenomas in rats exposed to formaldehyde vapor. In view of the tumors' localization, histology, and cytology, there seems to be little doubt that polypoid adenomas originate from respiratory epithelium. Ultrastructural studies demonstrate that these tumors have the characteristics of respiratory epithelium (114).

In hamsters, tumors of the nasal cavity were observed after oral and intratracheal application of nitrosodiethylamine (NDE) (95,115–117). Herrold (118) also reported that intratracheal instillation in Syrian hamsters of *N*-nitroso-*N*-methylurea induced squamous cell carcinomas of the nasopharyngeal tube, pharynx, larynx, trachea, and bronchi. Mohr et al. (119) repeatedly injected NDE subcutaneously into the common European hamster (*Cricetus cricetus* L.) for life and induced tumors at many sites in the respiratory tract, with the main target organ being the nose. Furthermore, adenomas, squamous cell carcinomas, adenocarcinomas, and anaplastic carcinomas have been found in the nose of hamsters exposed to acetaldehyde, either alone or in combination with benzo[*a*]pyrene or diethylnitrosamine (26). Thyssen et al. (120) induced nasal cavity, larynx, and trachea tumors in hamsters with benzo[*a*]pyrene condensed on sodium chloride prior to inhalation. Dimethylcarbamoyl chloride is another compound known to induce squamous cell carcinomas in the nasal cavity of Syrian golden hamsters (121).

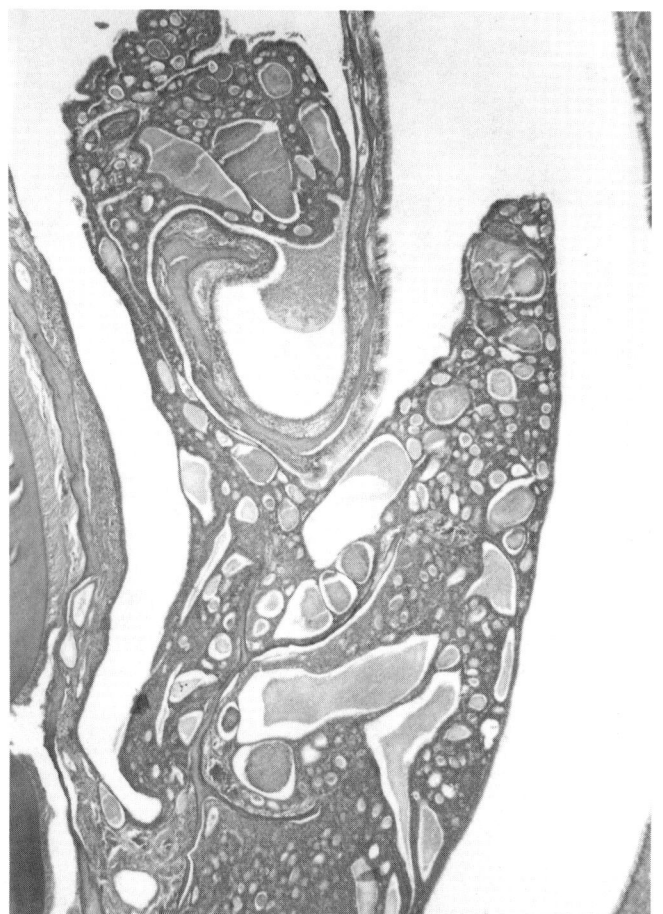

FIG. 21. Polypoid adenoma; higher magnification of tumor depicted in Fig. 20. H&E, ×40.

The mouse has been used much less than the hamster and the rat for upper respiratory tract carcinogenesis studies. Hemangiomas and hemangiosarcomas of the nasal submucosa have been found in mice exposed to 400 ppm propylene oxide by inhalation for up to 103 weeks (18). In mice, squamous cell carcinomas and adenoacanthomas in the anterior portion of the nasal cavity can be induced easily by diethylnitrosamine (122). Several of these carcinomas invaded the nasal bones and infiltrated the submucosa of the septum.

Tumors of the Olfactory Mucosa of the Nose

Focal atrophy with or without hyperplasia of olfactory epithelium and Bowman's glands has been found to accompany the development of tumors of the olfactory epithelium in rats exposed to quinoxaline-1,4-dioxide (123), to 1,2-dibromo-3-chloropropane (124), or to vinyl chloride (22) (Table 3). Atrophy of the olfactory epithelium accompanied by loss of nerve bundles and a thickened submucosa has been observed in mice and rats after prolonged exposure to high concentrations of formaldehyde (6 or 15 ppm) (125) and in Syrian hamsters and rats exposed to acetaldehyde at concentrations of 1,500 ppm and above (26,104,126). Proliferation of (most probably) basal cells was seen occasionally in rats exposed to lower concentrations of acetaldehyde (750 or 1,500 ppm). In the 3,000/1,000 ppm acetaldehyde exposure groups, 40 of 101 (19 of 48 males and 21 of 53 females) had developed an adenocarcinoma. For the mid- and low-concentration groups these figures are 55 of 105 (28 of 52 males and 27 of 53 females) and 20 of 96 (14 of 48 males and 6 of 48 females). For 66 of 115 (57%) adenocarcinomas, it was possible to establish the cross section where the tumor originated with high accuracy (127). The majority of the adenocarcinomas had developed from olfactory epithelium lining the ecto- and endoturbinates at standard cross section VI, and 18% probably originated from olfactory epithelium at cross section V. Six adenocarcinomas probably originated from cross section III and 13 from cross section IV. The adenocarcinomas found at cross section III seem to originate from glandular epithelium present in the submucosa beneath the respiratory epithelium.

There were no obvious differences in the gross and microscopic appearance between adenocarcinomas induced by vinyl chloride (22), trichlorobutene (112), or acetaldehyde (15). These adenocarcinomas varied in size from small groups of atypical cells to large tumors. Small atypical foci were located in the lamina propria of the olfactory epithelium, grew endophytically along the structures of the nasal passages, and invaded nerve bundles. Large osteolytic exophytic tumors with areas of necrosis grew outside the nasal cavity into the subcutis and the cerebrum via the olfactory lobe. The tumors consisted of compact sheets and cords of cells separated by strands of fibrous tissue varying widely in thickness. Tumor cells were pleomorphic, and bizarre mitotic figures were often observed. Tumors often contained both

TABLE 3. Nasal tumors originating from the olfactory mucosa in rodents

Adenocarcinoma/neuroepithelial carcinoma
  Basal cell differentiation or neuroblastoma-like rosettes (Flexner–Wintersteiner or
    Homer Wright rosettes)
  Glands of Bowman
  Sustentacular cell differentiation
    (Flexner–Wintersteiner, Homer Wright, or vascular rosettes)
  Solid pattern
  Neuroendocrine differentiation
  Mixed
  Undifferentiated
Adenosquamous carcinoma
Squamous cell carcinoma
Inverted papilloma

dark and light cells with big hyperchromatic round-to-oval nuclei (Fig. 22). Dark cells were small with scanty cytoplasm, sharp nuclear membranes, a fine nuclear chromatin pattern, and small, distinct nucleoli. Several tumors exhibited rosettes, pseudorosettes, and palisading and glandular formations, suggestive of a neurogenic origin (Fig. 23). A male rate exposed to 5,000 ppm vinyl chloride for 52 weeks (22) was found to have a nasal tumor consisting almost entirely of columnar cells arranged in rosettes. The spaces lined by the tall cells often contained eosinophilic material. This histological appearance is highly suggestive of an olfactory neuroblastoma. Metastases were seen in three cases; two tumors had metastasized to cervical lymph nodes, and one tumor, to the lungs (15).

From electron microscopic studies performed on acetaldehyde-induced adenocarcinomas, it was found that the cytoplasm of the tumor cells contained small mitochondria, a few cisternae of rough endoplasmic reticulum, and many free polyribosomes, but they contained no unique structures. Nuclei were big and indented and had large compact nucleoli. Desmosomelike structures occurred between adjacent cells. Neurofibrils could not be identified. The overall picture pointed to the basal cells of the olfactory epithelium as the cells of origin. This cell type has been

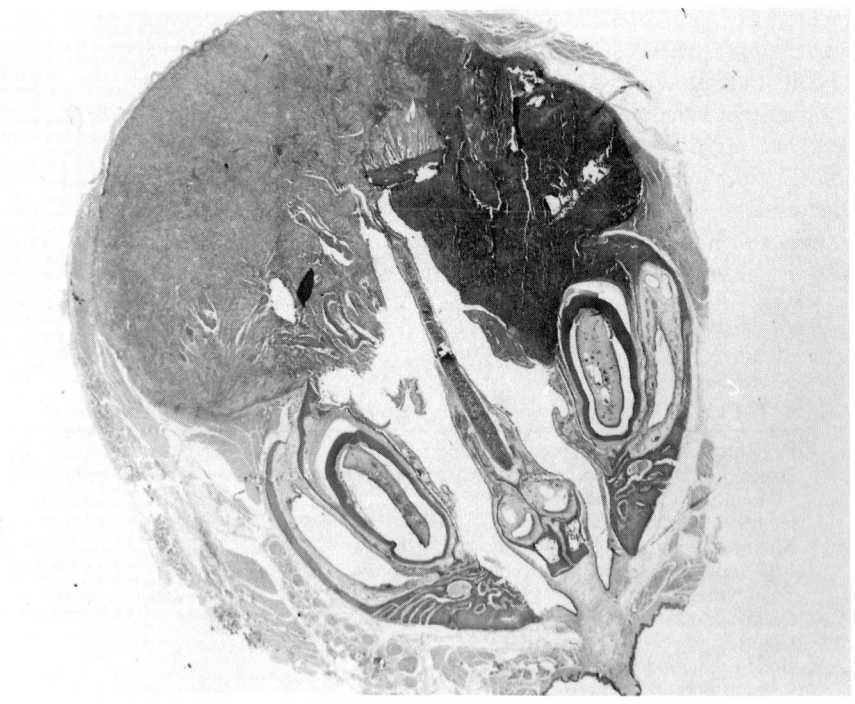

FIG. 22. Adenocarcinoma of the olfactory epithelium exhibiting areas of dark and light cells. Male rat exposed to 750 ppm acetaldehyde for 28 months. H&E, ×10.

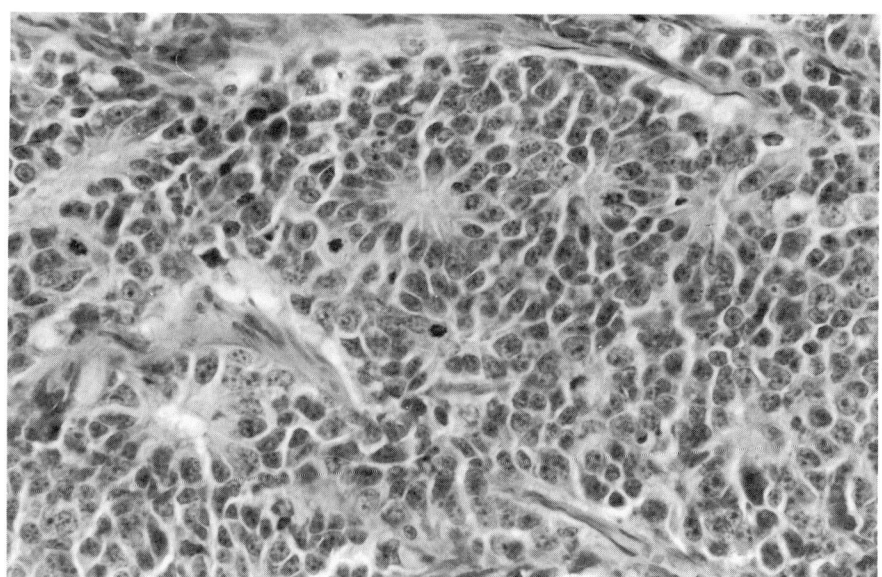

FIG. 23. Adenocarcinoma of olfactory epithelium showing rosettes and "owl eye" nuclei. Female rat exposed to 1,000/3,000 ppm acetaldehyde for 88 weeks. H&E, ×320.

suggested as the stem cell from which both olfactory sustentacular cells and sensory cells develop (88). In view of their localization, prevailing histologic pattern, and cytology, the nasal adenocarcinomas are considered to be derived from olfactory stem cells or sustentacular cells.

A number of investigators have reported neuroepitheliomas, esthesioneuroepitheliomas, (esthesio)neuroblastomas, esthesioneuromas, or esthesioneurocytomas of the nasal olfactory epithelium in experimental animals treated with carcinogens (8,128). The neurogenic origin of this lesion, termed preferably *olfactory neuroblastoma*, should appear from the unequivocal presence of neurotubules, neurosecretory granules, or neuritic processes of tumor cells (98,124,129,130). Neuroblasts are supposedly the precursor cells from which olfactory sensory cells differentiate during embryonic development (33,34). Atrophy and toxic degeneration of olfactory sensory cells could create a stimulus for stem cells to proliferate. In addition, tumors classified as poorly differentiated adenocarcinomas may originate from neuroblasts that have lost their characteristic morphological markers (e.g., neurotubules, axons), and in this case, they are probably of neurogenic origin and should be classified as olfactory neuroblastomas. On the other hand, poorly differentiated adenocarcinomas exhibiting ductlike spaces resembling rosettes and pseudorosettes may have been misdiagnosed as olfactory neuroblastomas. Relevant to a discussion on classification and nomenclature of tumors of the olfactory epithelium may be an observation that we made in a study into the recovery of severe acetaldehyde-induced damage to the olfactory epithelium of rats (131). After termination of the exposure to acetaldehyde, the dorsomedial part of the nose normally lined by olfactory epithelium was seen to be covered by uni- or multilayered basal cells. During the recovery period these undifferentiated cells were seen to differentiate into groups of sensory cells accompanied by the formation of nerve bundles. This striking finding supports the view of Graziadei and Monti Graziadei (33,34) that basal cells may be the stem cells of the sensory neurons, and it also supports Rivenson et al.'s suggestion (132) that all types of tumors derived from the olfactory epithelium be classified as olfactory neuroblastomas. Further subclassification of nasal olfactory neuroblastomas could then be based on the prevailing type of tumor cells (90).

Tumors of the Larynx

In rats, laryngeal tumors have been described in animals exposed to acetaldehyde or propylene oxide. These tumors included a carcinoma *in situ* in a female rat exposed to 1,500 ppm acetaldehyde (Fig. 24), a squamous cell carcinoma in one male exposed to 300 ppm propylene oxide and in one female exposed to 1,500 ppm acetaldehyde, and an adenocarcinoma in a male exposed to 300 ppm propylene oxide. These tumors were all considered to be related to treatment.

In hamsters, tumors of the larynx were found after inhalation of cigarette smoke for more than 24 months (24,25,133,134). Furthermore, papillomas, carcinomas (*in situ*), and squamous cell carcinomas were found in the larynx of hamsters exposed to acetaldehyde vapor alone or simultaneously to benzo[a]pyrene or diethylnitrosamine (26). Intratracheal instillation of benzo[a]pyrene or administration of carcinogenic nitrosamines via various routes leads to laryngeal tumors in Syrian golden hamsters (27).

ROLE OF TISSUE DAMAGE IN UPPER RESPIRATORY TRACT CARCINOGENESIS

Sustained Hyperplasia and Cancer Formation

There is substantial evidence that persistent tissue damage in humans and experimental animals may act as a precursor of tumor formation (135). In humans liver cancer is 10 times more likely in patients with cirrhotic than with noncirrhotic livers (136); colon cancer is frequently seen in persons with chronic colitis (137); squamous cell carcinoma may develop in the hyperplastic epithelium around chronic skin ulcers (138); lung cancer grows in areas of scarring (139). In experimental animals subcutaneous sarcomas develop at the site of repeated injection of compounds such as common salt or glucose (140); liver cancer in rats often occurs in enlarged livers (135); urinary bladder cancer develops in rats following implantation of solid objects into the bladder (141). Taken collectively, an overall picture

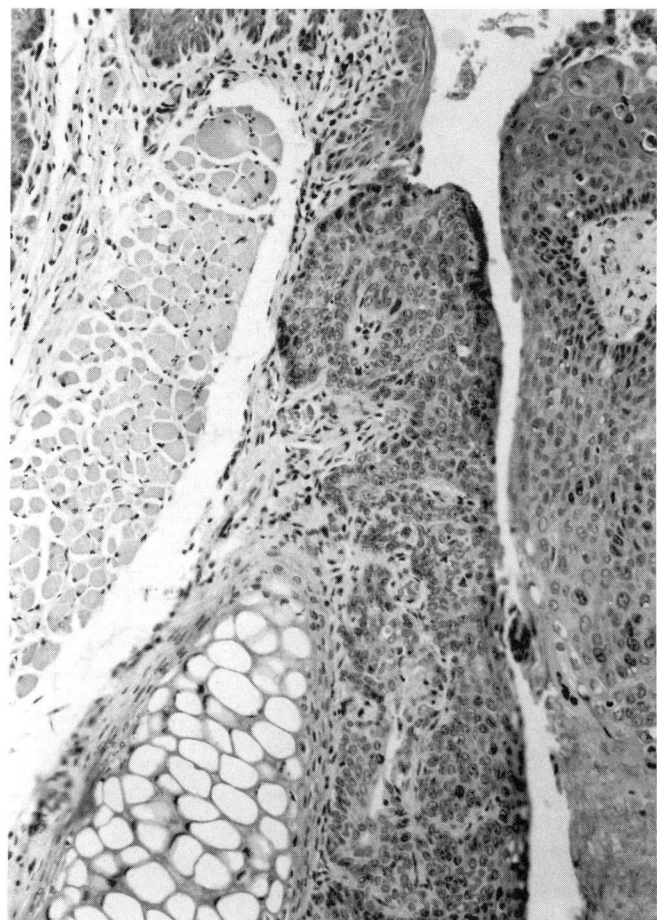

FIG. 24. Carcinoma *in situ* of the larynx. Female rat exposed to 1,500 ppm acetaldehyde for 122 weeks. H&E, ×400.

emerges that sustained hyperplasia renders various sites in the rodent (135) and in humans vulnerable to tumor development.

Wood-Dust Carcinogenesis in Humans

Epidemiological studies have convincingly shown an association between nasal cancer and occupational exposure to wood dust (142). Irritation of the nasal mucosa leading to reduction in mucociliary transport, epithelial hyperplasia, metaplasia, and dysplasia are considered etiological factors in the development of nasal cancer associated with exposure to wood dust (143–146). Chemicals introduced in wood or wood's natural constituents, and mechanical irritation of the nasal mucosa by wood-dust particles, have been suggested as causative or enhancing agents (143,144).

Chronic Rhinitis and Sinusitis and Nasal Cancer in Humans

The nose is subjected to a huge number of environmental insults. Many people have inflammatory and metaplastic lesions and even papillomas in their nose. It is striking, however, how rarely cancer follows these lesions. Thus despite the suggestion by Sato (147), simple damage to the nasal mucosa and chronic sinusitis are not predisposing factors for cancer of the nasal passages or paranasal sinuses in humans (148). Clearly, not all sustained hyper- and metaplasia are necessarily preneoplastic. It is not yet clear how preneoplastic potential of (nasal) hyper- and metaplastic lesions can be distinguished from nonpreneoplastic counterparts.

Malocclusion Syndrome in Rats

As discussed in an earlier paragraph, a portion of nasal squamous cell carcinomas and odontogenic tumors in rats may be part of the malocclusion syndrome. Madsen (149) reported a high incidence of nasal, oral, and pharyngeal carcinomas in rats suffering from chronic irritation and inflammation in mouth, pharynx, and nose caused by chaff from oat and barley in the feed squeezed between molars and gingiva. Obviously, in animals other than humans, sustained tissue damage and hyperproliferation of nasooral tissue renders this site vulnerable to cancer formation.

Formaldehyde Carcinogenesis

Formaldehyde is a highly irritating, genotoxic carcinogen capable of inducing malignant tumors in the nose of rats after long-term inhalation exposure (106). There is substantial experimental evidence to suggest a crucial role for tissue damage and persistent hyper- and metaplasia of the nasal respiratory epithelium in formaldehyde carcinogenesis (110,150). A very important piece of evidence originates from a long-term inhalation study in which male rats with a severely damaged or an undamaged nasal mucosa were exposed to 0, 0.1, 1.0, or 10.0 ppm formaldehyde for 6 hours/day, 5 days/week, for either 28 months or for 3 months followed by an observation period of 25 months (108). The damage to the nasal mucosa was induced by bilateral intranasal electrocoagulation. Treatment-related nasal tumors occurred only in the 10 ppm group of rats with a damaged nose exposed to formaldehyde for the full 28 months. Evidently, "drastic" conditions were required for tumor formation: severe damage plus a high concentration of formaldehyde.

Acetaldehyde Carcinogenesis

Just like formaldehyde, acetaldehyde is a highly irritating genotoxic nasal carcinogen in rats (15). With both formaldehyde and with acetaldehyde, nasal tumors were seen to arise from epithelium that had been damaged by acetaldehyde, indicating a significant role for the cytotoxicity of acetaldehyde in its carcinogenicity. However, the lowest exposure level of acetaldehyde tested in a long-term study (750 ppm) induced both cytotoxic and neoplastic changes. Therefore, it cannot be excluded that noncytotoxic levels of acetaldehyde are capable of inducing nasal tumors in rats. Consequently, for the time being, the role of tissue damage in acetaldehyde carcinogenesis is much less convincing than in formaldehyde carcinogenesis (151).

Irritating Nasal Noncarcinogens in Rodents

Acrolein, a very irritating unsaturated aldehyde, induced rhinitis and hyperplasia and metaplasia of the nasal respiratory and olfactory epithelium in Syrian hamsters, but no (nasal) tumors (152). Chronic exposure of Syrian hamsters to *furfural*, a heterocyclic aldehyde, resulted in highly characteristic alterations of the olfactory epithelium but did not lead to tumors (153). Two-year exposure of rats to *dimethylamine* led to concentration-dependent lesions of the nasal olfactory mucosa, including destruction of sensory cell and nerve bundles; no nasal tumors occurred (154). In a 2-year inhalation study with *ethyl acrylate* in rats, the compound did not induce nasal tumors, but the olfactory epithelium was severely damaged, showing atrophy of sensory cells, basal cell hyperplasia, and intraepithelial glandular structures (155). Despite marked damage to the nasal mucosa, no nasal tumors were found in Syrian hamsters after chronic exposure to *formaldehyde* vapor (109). The aforementioned examples clearly demonstrate that the local tissue conditions created by these nasal irritants apparently did not meet the requirements for tumor development.

Generalization Not Possible

Undoubtedly, chronic tissue damage, often accompanied by hyperproliferation, may play a role in the formation of cancer in both humans and experimental animals. Although many factors may be involved (deposition, clearance, metabolism, DNA repair), sustained hyperproliferation as such seems to be a key factor. Therefore, in humans, recurrent chronic tissue injury should be avoided where possible. In experimental carcinogenesis, one should be aware of the impact that tissue damage and hyperproliferation may have on the different steps of the process of carcinogenesis (135,156). Moreover, the occurrence of tissue damage and hyperproliferation should be taken into account in interpreting the results of carcinogenicity studies, particularly in predicting low-dose effects from high-dose findings, and in estimating human health risk (151).

As far as the nose is concerned, in humans chronic inflammation is not considered a predisposing factor for cancer of the maxillary sinus (148). However, chronic necrotizing (peri)odontitis, rhinitis, and sinusitis may be involved in the development of nasal squamous cell carcinomas in untreated control rats (149,150). Moreover, rats suffering from such chronic inflammatory changes may be more susceptible than normal rats to nasal carcinogens. Chemical and mechanical irritation may contribute to the induction of nasal cancer in furniture industry workers (143,144). Studies in animals to elucidate the role of irritation in wood-dust carcinogenesis are needed. A working hypothesis could be that wood-dust levels not leading to irritation are low enough to avoid substantial risk of nasal cancer (151).

The crucial role of tissue damage followed by hyperplasia and metaplasia of the nasal respiratory epithelium in formaldehyde carcinogenesis has now been widely recognized and should be included in human cancer risk assessment. Despite differences in anatomy and physiology of the nose between rats and humans, the respiratory tract defense systems are similar in both species. It is therefore reasonable to conclude that the response of the respiratory tract to formaldehyde will be qualitatively similar in rats and humans. If in humans exposure to formaldehyde were to be accompanied by recurrent tissue damage and repair at the site of contact, formaldehyde in cytotoxic concentrations may be assumed to have carcinogenic potential in humans. It has been shown that in rats such recurrent tissue damage must be accompanied by exposure to *high*, cytotoxic concentrations of formaldehyde in order that nasal tumors will be formed (108,157). Correspondingly, if the respiratory tract tissue is not recurrently injured, exposure of humans to relatively low, noncytotoxic levels of formaldehyde can be assumed to represent a negligible cancer risk. Human exposure to formaldehyde should be minimized for its potency to damage tissue. In humans, formaldehyde exposure should be controlled to levels below that likely to produce a significant irritant effect. This threshold is about 1 ppm. Thus an exposure limit of 1 ppm would be likely to virtually eliminate any carcinogenic risk that might have existed at higher exposure concentrations in the past (150).

The role of tissue damage and hyperproliferation is clear in formaldehyde carcinogenesis; its role in acetaldehyde carcinogenesis seems similar but needs further study to justify inclusion in risk estimation. Compounds such as acrolein, furfural, dimethylamine, and ethyl acrylate are very cytotoxic to the nasal mucosa and induced hyperproliferative changes but did not cause nasal tumors. Apparently, the local tissue conditions created by these compounds did not meet the requirements for tumor initiation, promotion, and progression. However, ethyl acrylate, being a nasal noncarcinogen, did cause carcinomas in the forestomach of rats and mice after administration by gavage (158). Such differences in response between organs may be due to differences in local tissue dose and/or tissue-specific differences in sensitivity. Such differences can, for example, result in metabolic overload and the production of genotoxic metabolites in one tissue but not in another tissue (J. J. Clary, I. C. Munro, and J. Orr, personal communication), or with one parent compound and not with another parent compound, or in one species and not in another species. Even if genotoxic metabolites are not involved, it is conceivable that hyperproliferation induced by one compound will lead to tumors on the basis of a certain epigenetic mechanism, whereas hyperproliferation induced by another substance will not lead to tumor formation. For instance, differences in toxifying or detoxifying mechanisms, or in time available for DNA repair, ultimately determine whether or not "background" initiators and promoters will get hold of the tissue and eventually will result in neoplastic transformation. In brief, as far as neoplastic transformation is concerned, hyperproliferative nasal tissue may easily behave differently from hyperproliferative forestomach tissue induced, for example, by the same agent; also, hyperproliferative nasal epithelium induced by ethyl acrylate may behave very differently from hyperproliferative nasal epithelium induced by, for example, furfural (153) or electrocoagulation (108). Thus species-, tissue-, and compound-specific factors largely if not entirely determine the role of tissue injury in (nasal) carcinogenesis. Consequently, a status of sustained hyperplasia may, but does not necessarily, lead to (nasal) neoplasia. On the other hand, for a compound causing (nasal) neoplasia *only* at concentrations also causing tissue injury followed by hyperplasia, induction of injury plus hyperproliferation probably, but not necessarily, is a prerequisite for the manifestation of the compound's carcinogenic potential (151).

DISCUSSION AND CONCLUSIONS

From a comparative viewpoint, humans have relatively simple noses with primary function for breathing, while other mammals have more complex nasal cavities with primary function for olfaction. Consequently, the anatomy of the nasal cavity in relation to the oral cavity is arranged in such a way that humans can breathe both orally and oronasally, whereas rodents are obligatory nose breathers (159). Despite the differences in complexity and the variations in shape, the noses of most rodents have characteristics similar to those of humans. On the other hand, there are major structural differences between humans and rodents in the nasal cavities that can modify the course of the air currents. When compared among species, the mouse has more respiratory epithelium available for filtering air per unit volume of the nasal cavity than does the rat. The surface area values are useful for calculating the theoretical dose of a chemical or particulate that is likely to be disposed upon the nasal surface.

The nature and site of damage in the respiratory tract are influenced by a series of factors relating to the airborne substance (solubility, polarity, diffusion rate, particle size, shape, and density), the exposure pattern (e.g., continuous, interrupted, peak loads), or the subject (e.g., anatomy of the respiratory tract, respiration rate, detoxification systems, pathological conditions such as distortions, occlusions, impaired lung, or other functions). Obviously, the combined action of a large number of factors determines the site(s) and type of biological response. For example, a polar, highly soluble gas inhaled through the nose will affect the nasal mucosa but will not reach the pulmonary tissue, whereas an apolar poorly soluble gas inhaled through the mouth penetrates the lungs and may damage the pulmonary tissue. In view of the increasing significance of inhalation toxicity testing, analyses of airborne substances in the different segments of the respiratory system are becoming increasingly important, particularly with respect to their relevance to humans. Acetaldehyde and formaldehyde, for example, show similarities but also considerable differences in site and type of the lesions induced in the upper respiratory tract. Both aldehydes appeared capable of damaging the nasal mucosa and inducing squamous cell carcinomas. Adenocarcinomas of the olfactory epithelium, however, occurred only after exposure to acetaldehyde (7,104,125).

Low effective concentrations of acetaldehyde (400 to 1,000 ppm) affected only the olfactory epithelium, while low effective concentrations of formaldehyde (2 to 3 ppm) damaged only the respiratory epithelium (125), indicating that the impact of acetaldehyde occurred more than that of formaldehyde in the posterior part of the nose. That impact, rather than susceptibility of the two types of epithelium to the cytotoxic action of these aldehydes, determines initially the site of damage is also supported by the observation that alterations of the respiratory epithelium induced by formaldehyde were restricted to the anterior part of the nasal septum and the nasomaxillary turbinates and, as the study progressed, extended to the posterior segments of the nose.

Druckrey et al. (160) found that dinitrosopiperazine and N-nitrosopiperidine given subcutaneously and N-nitrosomorpholine and N-nitrosomethylallylamine given intraveneously produced olfactory neuroblastomas in the nose of rats. When the rats were subjected to exposure by inhalation to nitrosodimethylamine, they also developed olfactory neuroblastomas, but rats exposed to N-nitrosomethylvinylamine by inhalation developed squamous cell carcinomas of the nasal cavity similar to those induced in mice by cutaneous applications of nitrosodiethylamine. Thus tumor induction in the upper respiratory tract may be influenced by the route of administration and the type of carcinogen. Species differences also play an important role in the effects of chemicals on the upper respiratory tract. Formaldehyde-induced nasal carcinomas were observed in numerous rats, in only a few mice, and not at all in hamsters exposed to similar concentrations for comparable periods of time (101,105,161). Exposure of rats to acetaldehyde at concentrations of 750 ppm and higher resulted in nasal carcinomas (104), whereas in hamsters only a few nasal tumors were found following prolonged exposure to the "maximum tolerated concentration" of acetaldehyde (2,500 ppm gradually decreased to 1,650 ppm). Similar species differences were observed with bis(chloromethyl) ether (BCME). Although BCME produced some pulmonary adenomas and adenocarcinomas in mice and one nasal olfactory neuroblastoma in Syrian golden hamsters, the rat appeared much more sensitive to the carcinogenic effect of this chemical. In 86.5% of the rats exposed to 100 ppb BCME for 6 months, Leong et al. (16) found olfactory neuroblastomas.

However, such differences in sensitivity between species should be interpreted with circumspection. For example, we concluded that rats are more sensitive than mice to the cytotoxic and carcinogenic activity of formaldehyde. However, it has been shown that mice are able to minimize the inhalation of irritating concentrations of formaldehyde more effectively than rats (162). Taking into account minute volumes and surface area of the nasal mucosa, it was calculated that the dose of formaldehyde per square centimeter of nasal mucosa during a 6-h exposure to 15 ppm formaldehyde is about 40% lower in mice than in rats (163). This finding is consistent with the lower incidence of nasal tumors in mice than in rats at 15 ppm (164) and also indicates that the nasal mucosa of rats and mice differ much less in sensitivity to formaldehyde than would appear from the results of the long-term inhalation studies. This example also demonstrates that certain differences in response between species may be concentration specific. With subirritating concentrations of formaldehyde, mice are unlikely to reduce their inhalation of the compound.

Humans are more likely than rodents to inhale through the mouth, because rodents are obligatory nose breathers. Mouth breathing means bypassing filtration by the nasal passages (165). Rodents have highly developed tortuous nasal turbinates, whereas humans have relatively simple noses containing less complex turbinates (159,166). The implication of these physiological and anatomical differences between rodents and humans may be that the effects of chemicals on the nose of rodents have a predictive value for effects in humans on more distal parts of the respiratory tract, such as larynx, bronchi, and lungs (7).

Active inhalation of cigarette smoke is an illustrative example of mouth breathing. The gas phase of cigarette smoke contains high concentrations of aldehydes discussed in this paper (167). It is therefore conceivable that smokers who actively inhale cigarette smoke expose their larynx and bronchi to high concentrations of these compounds. Consequently, these chemicals may contribute significantly to the induction of laryngeal and bronchial cancer by cigarette smoke.

REFERENCES

1. Acheson ED. Epidemiology of nasal cancer. In: Barrow CS, ed. *Toxicology of the nasal passages*. Washington, DC: Hemisphere; 1986:135–141.
2. Tricker AR, Preussmann R. Carcinogenic *N*-nitrosamines in the diet: occurrence, formation, mechanisms and carcinogenic potential. *Mutat Res* 1991;259:277–289.
3. Burch JD, Howe GR, Miller AB, Semenciw R. Tobacco, alcohol, asbestos, and nickel in the etiology of cancer of the larynx: a case-control study. *J Natl Cancer Inst* 1981;67:1219–1224.
4. IARC. *IARC monographs on the evaluation of the carcinogenic risk of chemicals to humans*. Vol 38. *Tobacco smoking*. Lyon, France: International Agency for Research on Cancer, WHO; 1986.
5. Schouten LJ, Knipschild PG. Epidemiologie van het larynxcarcinoom, een overzicht van de literatuur. *Tijdschr Soc Gezondheidszorg* 1985;63:375–378.
6. Reznik G, Stinson SF. *Nasal tumors in animals and man*. Vol 3. *Experimental nasal carcinogenesis*. Boca Raton, FL: CRC Press; 1983.
7. Feron VJ, Woutersen RA, Appelman LM. Epithelial damage and tumours of the nose after exposure to four different aldehydes by inhalation. In: Grosdanoff P, Bass R, Hackenberg U, Henschler D, Müller D, Klimisch HJ, eds. *Problems of inhalatory toxicity studies*. Munich: MMV Medizin Verlag; 1984:587–609.
8. Feron VJ, Woutersen RA, Spit BJ. Pathology of chronic nasal toxic responses including cancer. In: Barrow CS, ed. *Toxicology of the nasal passages*. Washington, DC: Hemisphere; 1986:67–89.

9. Feron VJ, Woutersen RA, van Garderen-Hoetmer A, Dreef-van der Meulen HC. Upper respiratory tract tumors in Cpb:WU (Wistar random) rats. *Environ Health Perspect* 1990;85:305-315.
10. Reznik-Schüller HM. Nitrosamine-induced nasal cavity carcinogenesis. In: Reznik G, Stinson SF, eds. *Nasal tumours in animals and man.* vol 3. *Experimental nasal carcinogenesis.* Boca Raton, FL: CRC Press; 1983:47-78.
11. Lijinsky W, Reuber MD. Transnitrosation by nitrosamines *in vivo*. *IARC Sci Publ* 1987;41: 625-631.
12. Klein RG, Janowsky I, Pool-Zobel BL, et al. Long-term inhalation of low-dose N-nitrosodimethylamine (NDMA) in rats. *Proc Am Assoc Cancer Res* 1990;31:87.
13. NCI. Carcinogenesis bioassay of 1,2-dibromomethane (inhalation study), TR-210 (CAS no 106-93-4). *Carcinogenesis testing program.* DHHS publication no (NIH) 81-1766. Bethesda, MD: National Cancer Institute: 1981.
14. Schlögel FA, Bannasch P. Toxicity and cancerogenic properties of inhaled dimethyl sulfate. *Arch Pharmacol* 1970;266:441.
15. Woutersen RA, Appelman LM, van Garderen-Hoetmer A, Feron VJ. Inhalation toxicity of acetaldehyde in rats. III. Carcinogenicity study. *Toxicology* 1986;41:213-231.
16. Leong BKJ, Kociba RJ, Jersey GC. A lifetime study of rats and mice exposed to vapours of bis(chloromethyl) ether. *Toxicol Appl Pharmacol* 1981;58:269-281.
17. Lee KP, Trochimowicz HJ. Metaplastic changes of nasal respiratory epithelium in rats exposed to hexamethylphosphoramide (HMPA) by inhalation. *Am J Pathol* 1982;106:8-19.
18. Renne RA, Giddens WE, Boorman GA, Kovatch R, Haseman JE, Clarke WJ. Nasal cavity neoplasia in F344/N rats and (C57BL/6xC3H)F1 mice inhaling propylene oxide for up to two years. *J Natl Cancer Inst* 1986;77:573-582.
19. Lee KP, Schneider PW, Trochimowicz HJ. Morphological expression of glandular differentiation in the epidermoid nasal carcinomas induced by phenylglycidylether inhalation. *Am J Pathol* 1983; 111:140-148.
20. Sellakumar A, Snyder C, Patil G, Burns F. Inhalation carcinogenesis of dimethylcarbamoyl chloride. A dose response effect and induction of naso-pharyngeal and nasal cavity tumors in rats. *Proc Am Assoc Cancer Res* 1989;30:140.
21. Laskin S, Sellakumar AR, Kuschner M, et al. Inhalation carcinogenicity of epichlorohydrin in noninbred Sprague-Dawley rats. *J Natl Cancer Inst* 1980;65:751-757.
22. Feron VJ, Kroes R. One year time-sequence inhalation toxicity study of vinyl chloride in rats. II. Morphological changes in the respiratory tract, ceruminous glands, brain, kidneys, heart and spleen. *Toxicology* 1979;13:131-141.
23. IARC. *IARC monographs on the evaluation of carcinogenic risks to humans.* Suppl 7. *Overall evaluations of carcinogenicity: an updating of IARC monographs vols 1 to 42.* Lyon, France: International Agency for Research on Cancer, WHO; 1987.
24. Dontenwill W, Chevalier HJ, Harke HP, Lafrenz U, Reckzeh G, Schneider B. Investigations on the effects of chronic cigarette smoke inhalation in Syrian golden hamsters. *J Natl Cancer Inst* 1973;51:1781-1832.
25. Bernfeld P, Homburger F, Russfield AB. Strain differences in the response of inbred Syrian hamsters to cigarette smoke inhalation. *J Natl Cancer Inst* 1974;53:1141-1157.
26. Feron VJ, Kruysse A, Woutersen RA. Respiratory tract tumours in hamsters exposed to acetaldehyde vapour alone or simultaneously to benzo(*a*)pyrene or diethylnitrosamine. *Eur J Cancer Clin Oncol* 1982;18:13-31.
27. Saffiotti U, Stinson SF, Keenan KP, McDowell EM. Tumor enhancement factors and mechanisms in the hamster respiratory tract carcinogenesis model. *Carcinogenesis* 1985;8:63-92.
28. Young JT. Light microscopic examination of the rat nasal passages: preparation and morphologic features. In: Barrow CS, ed. *Toxicology of the nasal passages.* Washington, DC: Hemisphere; 1986:27-36.
29. Uraih LC, Maronpot RR. Normal histology of the nasal cavity and application of special techniques. *Environ Health Perspect* 1990;85:187-208.
30. Harkema JR. Comparative pathology of the nasal mucosa in laboratory animals exposed to inhaled irritants. *Environ Health Perspect* 1990;85:231-238.
31. Spit BJ, Hendriksen EGJ, Bruijntjes JP, Kuper CF. Electron microscopy of nasal brush cells and nose-associated lymphoid tissue (NALT). *Toxicol Tribune* 1988;3:3.
32. Reuzel PGJ, Wilmer JWGM, Woutersen RA, Zwart A, Rombouts PJA, Feron VJ. Interactive effects of ozone and formaldehyde on the nasal respiratory lining epithelium in rats. *J Toxicol Environ Health* 1990;29:279-292.

33. Graziadei PPC, Monti Graziadei GA. Neurogenesis and neuron regeneration in the olfactory system of mammals. I. Morphological aspects of differentiation and structural organization of the olfactory sensory neurons. *J Neurocytol* 1979;8:1–18.
34. Monti Graziadei GA, Graziadei PPC. Neurogenesis and neuron regeneration in the olfactory system of mammals. II. Degeneration and reconstitution of the olfactory sensory neurons after axotomy. *J Neurocytol* 1979;8:197–213.
35. Friedmann I. Nose, throat and ears. In: Symmers WSC, ed. *Systemic pathology*. Vol 1. Edinburgh: Churchill Livingstone; 1986.
36. Batsakis JG, Solomon AR, Rice DH. The pathology of head and neck tumors: carcinoma of the nasopharynx, part 11. *Head Neck Surg* 1981;3:511–524.
37. Boysen M. The surface of the human nasal mucosa. I. Ciliated and metaplastic epithelium in normal individuals. A correlated study by scanning/transmission electron and light microscopy. *Virchows Arch B Cell Pathol* 1982;40:279–294.
38. Bidsrup PL, Case RAM. Carcinoma of the lung in workmen in the biochromates-producing industry in Great Britain. *Br J Ind Med* 1956;13:260–264.
39. Enterline PE. Respiratory cancer amongst chromate workers. *J Occup Med* 1974;16:523–526.
40. Sunderman FW Jr. A review of the carcinogenicities of nickel, chromium and arsenic compounds in man and animals. *Prev Med* 1976;5:279.
41. IARC. *IARC monographs on the evaluation of the carcinogenic risk of chemicals to humans*. vol 23. *Some metals and metallic compounds*. Lyon, France: International Agency for Research on Cancer, WHO; 1980.
42. Easton DF. Epidemiology of nasal cancer in nickel workers. In: Feron VJ, Bosland MC, eds. *Nasal carcinogenesis in rodents: relevance to human health risk*. Wageningen, The Netherlands: Pudoc; 1989:85–90.
43. Kaldor J, Peto J, Easton D, Doll R, Hermon C, Morgan L. Models for respiratory cancer in nickel refinery workers. *J Natl Cancer Inst* 1986;77:841–848.
44. Anonymous. Report of the International Committee on Nickel Carcinogenesis in Man. *Scand J Work Environ Health* 1990;16:1–82.
45. Hueper WC. Occupational and environmental cancer of the respiratory system. *Recent Results Cancer Res* 1966;3:105–107.
46. Alderson MR, Rattan NS. Mortality of workers on an isopropyl alcohol plant and two MEK dewaxing plants. *Br J Ind Med* 1980;37:85–89.
47. Yamada A. On the late injuries following occupational inhalation of mustard gas, with special reference to carcinoma of the respiratory tract. *Acta Pathol Jpn* 1963;13:131–155.
48. IARC. *IARC monographs on the evaluation of the carcinogenic risk of chemicals to humans*. vol 25. *Wood, leather and some associated industries*. Lyon, France: International Agency for Research on Cancer, WHO; 1981.
49. Hadfield EH. A study of adenocarcinoma of the paranasal sinuses in woodworkers in the furniture industry. *Ann R Coll Surg Engl* 1970;46:301–319.
50. Boysen M, Solberg LA. Changes in the nasal mucosa of furniture workers: a pilot study. *Scand J Work Environ Health* 1982;8:273–282.
51. Acheson ED. Nasal cancer in the furniture and boot and shoe manufacturing industries. *Prev Med* 1976;5:295–315.
52. Elwood JM. Wood exposure and smoking: association with cancer of the nasal cavity and paranasal sinuses in British Columbia. *Can Med Assoc J* 1981;124:1573–1577.
53. Hernberg S, Westerholm P, Schultz-Larsen K, et al. Nasal and sinonasal cancer: connection with occupational exposures in Denmark, Finland and Sweden. *Scand J Work Environ Health* 1983;9:315–326.
54. Voss R, Stenersen T, Roald Oppedal B, Boysen M. Sinonasal cancer and exposure to softwood. *Acta Otolaryngol* 1985;99:172–178.
55. Vaughan TL, Davis S. Wood dust exposure and squamous cell cancers of the upper respiratory tract. *Am J Epidemiol* 1991;133:560–564.
56. Hayes RB, Gerin M, Raatgever JW, de Bruyn A. Wood-related occupations, wood dust exposure, and sinonasal cancer. *Am J Epidemiol* 1986;124:569–577.
57. Miller BA, Blair AE, Raynor HL, Stewart PA, Hoar Zahm S, Fraumeni JF Jr. Cancer and other mortality patterns among United States furniture workers. *Br J Ind Med* 1989;46:508–515.
58. Acheson ED. Nasal cancer in furniture workers: the problem. *The carcinogenicity and mutagenicity of wood dust*, Scientific report 1. Southampton, Hampshire, England: Medical Research Council; 1982.

59. Viren JR, Imbus HR. Case-control study of nasal cancer in workers employed in wood-related industries. *J Occup Med* 1989;31:35–40.
60. Finkelstein MM. Nasal cancer among North American woodworkers: another look. *J Occup Med* 1989;31:899–901.
61. Kleinsasser O, Schroeder HG. Adenocarcinomas arising after exposure to wood dust. *Pathol Res Pract* 1989;184:554–558.
62. Acheson ED, Cowdell RH, Jolles B. Nasal cancer in the Northamptonshire boot and shoe industry. *Br Med J* 1970;1:385–393.
63. Cecchi F, Buiatti E, Kriebel D, Nastasi L, Santucci M. Adenocarcinoma of the nose and paranasal sinuses in shoe makers and wood workers in the province of Florence, Italy (1963–1977). *Br J Ind Med* 1980;37:222–225.
64. Acheson ED, Pippard EC, Winter PD. Nasal cancer in the Northamptonshire boot and shoe industry: is it declining? *Br J Cancer* 1982;46:940–946.
65. Blair A, Walrath J, Malker H. Review of epidemiologic evidence regarding cancer and exposure to formaldehyde. *Adv Chem Ser* 1985;210:263–273.
66. Nelson N, Levine RJ, Albert RE, et al. Contribution of formaldehyde to respiratory cancer. *Environ Health Perspect* 1986;70:23–35.
67. Halperin WE, Goodman M, Stayner L, Elliott LJ, Keenlyside RA, Landrigan PJ. Nasal cancer in a worker exposed to formaldehyde. *JAMA* 1983;249:510–512.
68. Holmström M, Lund VJ. Malignant melanomas of the nasal cavity after occupational exposure to formaldehyde. *Br J Ind Med* 1991;48:9–11.
69. Holmström M, Wilhelmsson B, Hellquist H, Rosén G. Histological changes in the nasal mucosa in persons occupationally exposed to formaldehyde alone and in combination with wood dust. *Acta Otolaryngol* 1989;107:120–129.
70. Boysen M, Zadig E, Digernes V, Abeler V, Reith A. Nasal mucosa in workers exposed to formaldehyde: a pilot study. *Br J Ind Med* 1990;47:116–121.
71. Acheson ED, Cowdell RH, Hadfield E, Macbeth RG. Nasal cancer in woodworkers in the furniture industry. *Br Med J* 1968;2:587–596.
72. Acheson ED, Cowdell RH, Rang E. Adenocarcinoma of the nasal cavity and sinuses in England and Wales. *Br J Ind Med* 1972;29:21–30.
73. IARC. *IARC monographs on the evaluation of carcinogenic risks to humans.* vol 44. *Alcohol drinking.* Lyon, France: International Agency for Research on Cancer, WHO; 1988.
74. Hirayama T. Prospective studies on cancer epidemiology based on census population in Japan. In: Nieburgs HE, ed. *Prevention and detection of cancer.* vol 1. *Etiology.* New York: Marcel Dekker; 1978:1139–1147.
75. Forastiere F, Valesini S, Salimei E, Magliola ME, Perucci CA. Respiratory cancer among soap production workers. *Scand J Work Environ Health* 1987;13:258–260.
76. Soskolne CL, Zeighami EA, Hanis NM, Kupper LL, Herrmann N, Amsel J, Mausner JS, Stellman JM. Laryngeal cancer and occupational exposure to sulfuric acid. *Am J Epidemiol* 1984;120:358–369.
77. Soskolne C, Jhangri G, Checkoway H, Risch H, Siemiatycki J, Lakhani R, Burch D, Howe G, Miller A. Sulfuric acid exposure in laryngeal cancer: induction and latency estimates from a lagged exposure window analysis (Abstract). In: *Proceedings of the 12th scientific meeting of the International Epidemiological Association,* Los Angeles, Aug 5–9, 1990.
78. Steenland K, Schnorr T, Beaumont J, Halperin W, Bloom T. Incidence of laryngeal cancer and exposure to acid mists. *Br J Ind Med* 1988;45:766–776.
79. Graham S, Mettlin C, Marshall J, et al. Dietary factors in the epidemiology of cancer of the larynx. *Am J Epidemiol* 1981;113:675–680.
80. Weber AL, Stanton AC. Malignant tumours of the paranasal sinuses; radiologic, clinical and histopathologic evaluation. *Head Neck Surg* 1984;6:761–766.
81. Heffner DK. Classification of human upper respiratory tract tumours. *Environ Health Perspect* 1990;85:219–229.
82. Hyams VJ, Batsakis JG, Michaels L. *Tumours of the upper respiratory tract and ear.* Washington, DC: Armed Forces Institute of Pathology; 1988.
83. Slootweg PJ, Roholl PJM, Müller H, Lubsen H. Spindle cell carcinoma of the oral cavity and larynx. Immunohistochemical aspects. *J Craniomaxillofac Surg* 1989;17:234–236.
84. Ellis GL, Gnepp DR. Unusual salivary gland tumours. In: Gnepp DR, ed. *Pathology of the head and neck.* New York: Churchill Livingstone; 1988:585–661.

85. Barnes L. Intestinal type adenocarcinoma of the nasal cavity and paranasal sinuses. *Am J Surg Pathol* 1986;10:192–202.
86. Kleinsasser O, Schroeder HG. Adenocarcinomas of the inner nose after exposure of wood dust. *Arch Otolaryngol* 1988;245:1–15.
87. Michaels L. *Ear, nose and throat histopathology.* Berlin: Springer-Verlag; 1987:194–199.
88. Jafek BW. Ultrastructure of human nasal mucosa. *Laryngoscope* 1983;93:1576–1599.
89. Ho CS, Choy D, Loke SL, et al. Polymorphic reticulosis and conventional lymphomas of the nose and upper aerodigestive tract. *Hum Pathol* 1990;21:1041–1050.
90. Brown HR. Neoplastic and potentially prenoplastic changes in the upper respiratory tract of rats and mice. *Environ Health Perspect* 1990;85:291–304.
91. Stewart HL, Dunn TB, Snell KC, Deringer MK. Tumours of the respiratory tract. In: Turusov VS, ed. *Pathology of tumours in laboratory animals.* Vol II. *Tumours of the mouse.* Lyon, France: WHO; 1979:251–288.
92. Pour P, Mohr U, Cardesa A, Althoff J, Kmoch N. Spontaneous tumours and common diseases in two colonies of Syrian golden hamsters. II. Respiratory tract and digestive system tumours. *J Natl Cancer Inst* 1976;56:937–948.
93. Pour P, Althoff J, Salmasi SZ, Stepan K. Spontaneous tumors and common diseases in three types of hamsters. *J Natl Cancer Inst* 1979;63:797–811.
94. Gorlin RJ. Odontogenic tumors in mammals and fish. *Oral Surg* 1972;33:86–90.
95. Slootweg PJ, Woutersen RA, Feron VJ. Odontogenic epithelioma in a male Wistar rat. *J Oral Pathol Med* 1992;21:138–140.
96. Cullen JM, Ruebner BH, Hsieh DPH, Burkes EJ Jr. Odontogenic tumours in Fischer rats. *J Oral Pathol Med* 1987;16:469–473.
97. Schour I, Massler M. The teeth. In: Griffith JQ, Farris EJ, eds. *The rat in laboratory investigation.* Philadelphia: JB Lippincott; 1942:102–163.
98. Reznik G, Reznik-Schüller HM, Hayden DW, Russfield A, Krishna Murthy AS. Morphology of nasal cavity neoplasms in F-344 rats after chronic feeding of *p*-cresidine, an intermediate of dyes and pigments. *Anticancer Res* 1981;1:279–286.
99. Herrold K. Epithelial papillomas of the nasal cavity. Experimental induction in Syrian hamsters. *Arch Pathol* 1964;78:189–195.
100. Pour P, Krüger FW, Cardesa A, Althoff J, Mohr U. Carcinogenic effect of di-*n*-propylnitrosamine in Syrian golden hamsters. *J Natl Cancer Inst* 1973;51:1019–1027.
101. Pour P, Gingell R, Langenbach R, Nagal D, Grandjean C, Lawson T, Salmasi S. Carcinogenicity of *N*-nitrosomethyl(2-oxopropyl)amine in Syrian hamsters. *Cancer Res* 1980;40:3585–3590.
102. Reznik-Schüller HM, Mohr U. Ultrastructure of *N*-nitrosodibutylamine-induced tumours of the nasal cavity in the European hamster. *J Natl Cancer Inst* 1976;57:401–407.
103. Takano T, Shirai T, Ogiso T, Tsuda H, Baba S, Ito N. Sequential changes in tumour development induced by 1,4-dinitrosopiperazine in the nasal cavity of F-344 rats. *Cancer Res* 1982;42:4236–4240.
104. Woutersen RA, Appelman LM, Feron VJ, van der Heijden CA. Inhalation toxicity of acetaldehyde in rats. II. Carcinogenicity study: interim results after 15 months. *Toxicology* 1984;31:123–133.
105. Albert RE, Sellakumar AR, Laskin S, Kuschner M, Nelson N, Snyder CA. Gaseous formaldehyde and hydrogen chloride induction of nasal cancer in the rat. *J Natl Cancer Inst* 1982;68:597–603.
106. Kerns WD, Pavkov KL, Donofrio DJ, Gralla EJ, Swenberg JA. Carcinogenicity of formaldehyde in rats and mice after long-term inhalation exposure. *Cancer Res* 1983;43:4382–4392.
107. Feron VJ, Bruijntjes JP, Woutersen RA, Immel HR, Appelman LM. Nasal tumours in rats after short-term exposure to a cytotoxic concentration of formaldehyde. *Cancer Lett* 1988;39:101–111.
108. Woutersen RA, van Garderen-Hoetmer A, Bruijntjes JP, Zwart A, Feron VJ. Nasal tumours in rats after severe injury to the nasal mucosa and prolonged exposure to 10 ppm formaldehyde. *J Appl Toxicol* 1989;9:39–46.
109. Dalbey WE. Formaldehyde and tumours in hamster respiratory tract. *Toxicology* 1982;24:9–14.
110. Morgan KT, Jiang X-Z, Starr JB, Kerns WD. More precise localization of nasal tumours associated with chronic exposure of F-344 rats to formaldehyde gas. *Toxicol Appl Pharmacol* 1986;82:264–271.
111. Feron VJ, Immel HR, Wilmer JWGM, Woutersen RA, Zwart A. Nasal tumours in rats after severe injury to the nasal mucosa and exposure to formaldehyde vapour: preliminary results. In: Tyiak E, Gullner G, eds. *The role of formaldehyde in biological systems.* Budapest: Sote Press; 1987:73–77.

112. Reuzel PGJ, Feron VJ, Immel HR, Dreef-van der Meulen HC. *Chronic (25-month) inhalation toxicity/carcinogenicity study with 2,3,4-trichlorobutene-1 in rats.* CIVO/TNO report V81.133/ 267399. Zeist, The Netherlands: CIVO; 1981.
113. Kerns WD. Polypoid adenoma of the nasal cavity in the laboratory rat. In: Jones TC, Mohr U, Hunt RD, eds. *Monographs on pathology of laboratory animals: respiratory system.* New York: Springer-Verlag; 1985:41–47.
114. Monteiro-Riviere NA, Popp JA. Ultrastructural characterization of the nasal respiratory epithelium in the rat. *Am J Anat* 1984;169:31–43.
115. Herrold KM. Induction of olfactory neuroepithelial tumors in Syrian hamsters by diethylnitrosamine. *Cancer* 1964;17:114–121.
116. Herrold KM. Effect of the route of administration on the carcinogenic action of diethylnitrosamine. *Br J Cancer* 1964;18:763–767.
117. Herrold KM, Dunham LJ. Induction of tumors in the Syrian hamster with diethylnitrosamine (N-nitrosodiethylamine). *Cancer Res* 1963;23:773–777.
118. Herrold KM. Upper respiratory tract tumors induced in Syrian hamsters by N-methyl-N-nitrosourea. *Int J Cancer* 1970;6:217–222.
119. Mohr U, Althoff J, Page N. Tumors of the respiratory system induced in the common European hamster by N-diethylnitrosamine. *J Natl Cancer Inst* 1972;49:595–597.
120. Thyssen J, Althoff J, Kimmerle G, Mohr U. Inhalation studies with benzo(a)pyrene in Syrian golden hamsters. *J Natl Cancer Inst* 1981;66:575–577.
121. Sellakumar AR, Laskin S, Kuschner M, Rusch G, Katz GV, Snyder CA, Albert RE. Inhalation carcinogenesis by dimethylcarbamoyl chloride in Syrian golden hamsters. *J Environ Pathol Toxicol* 1980;4:107–115.
122. Hoffman F von, Graffi A. Nasenhöhlentumoren bei Mäusen nach percutaner Diäthylnitrosaminapplikation. *Arch Geschwulstforsch* 1964;23:274–288.
123. Tucker MJ. Carcinogenic action of quinoxaline 1,4-dioxide in rats. *J Natl Cancer Inst* 1975;55: 137–146.
124. Reznik G, Reznik-Schüller HM, Ward JM, Stinson SF. Morphology of nasal cavity tumours in rats after chronic inhalation of 1,2-dibromo-3-chloropropane. *Br J Cancer* 1980;42:772–781.
125. Battelle. *A chronic inhalation toxicology study in rats and mice exposed to formaldehyde.* Final report, CIIT, Dec 31, 1981. Columbus, OH: Battelle Columbus Laboratories; 1981:173.
126. Feron VJ. Effects of exposure to acetaldehyde in Syrian hamsters simultaneously treated with benzo(a)pyrene or diethylnitrosamine. *Prog Exp Tumor Res* 1979;24:162–176.
127. Woutersen RA, Feron VJ. Localization of nasal tumours in rats exposed to acetaldehyde or formaldehyde. In: Feron VJ, Bosland MC, eds. *Nasal carcinogenesis in rodents: relevance to human health risk.* Wageningen, The Netherlands: Pudoc; 1989:70–75.
128. Pepelko WE. Experimental respiratory carcinogenesis in small laboratory animals. *Environ Res* 1984;33:144–188.
129. Cardesa A, Pour P, Haas H, Althoff J, Mohr U. Histogenesis of tumours from the nasal cavities induced by diethylnitrosamine. *Cancer* 1976;37:346–358.
130. Reznik-Schüller HM. Pathogenesis of tumours induced with N-nitrosomethylpiperazine in the olfactory region of the rat nasal cavity. *J Natl Cancer Inst* 1983;71:165–172.
131. Woutersen RA, Feron VJ. Inhalation toxicity of acetaldehyde in rats. IV. Progression and regression of nasal lesions after discontinuation of exposure. *Toxicology* 1987;47:295–305.
132. Rivenson A, Furuya K, Hecht SS, Hoffmann D. Experimental nasal cavity tumours induced by tobacco-specific nitrosamines (TSNA). In: Reznik G, Stinson SF, eds. *Nasal tumours in animals and man.* Vol 3. *Experimental nasal carcinogenesis.* Boca Raton, FL: CRC Press; 1983:79–114.
133. Dontenwill W. Experimental investigations on the effect of cigarette smoke on laboratory animals. In: Hanna MG Jr, Netteshein P, Gilbert JR, eds. *Inhalation carcinogenesis.* Oak Ridge, TN: US AEC Division of Technical Information; 1970:389–409.
134. Wehner AP, Olson RJ, Busch RH. Increased life span and decreased weight in hamsters exposed to cigarette smoke. *Arch Environ Health* 1976;31:146–153.
135. Grasso P, Sharratt M, Cohen AJ. Role of persistent, non-genotoxic tissue damage in rodent cancer and relevance to humans. *Annu Rev Pharmacol Toxicol* 1991;31:253–287.
136. Johnson P, Williams R. Cirrhosis and the aetiology of hepatocellular carcinoma. *J Hepatol* 1987; 4:140–147.
137. Laroye GJ. How efficient is immunological surveillance against cancer and why does it fail? *Lancet* 1974;1:1097–1100.

138. Haber H, Milne JA, Symmers WSC. The skin. In: Symmers WSC, ed. *Systemic pathology.* Vol 6, 2nd ed. London: Churchill Livingstone; 1980:2575–2604.
139. Bennett DE, Sasser WF, Ferguson TB. Adenocarcinoma of the lung in men. *Cancer* 1969;23: 431–439.
140. Grasso P. Persistent organ damage and cancer production in rats and mice. Mechanisms and models in toxicology. *Arch Toxicol Suppl* 1987;11:75–83.
141. Roe FJC. An illustrated classification of the proliferative and neoplastic changes in mouse bladder epithelium in response to prolonged irritation. *Br J Urol* 1964;36:253–328.
142. Scheidt R, Ehrhardt HP, Bartsch R. Gehäuftes Auftreten von bösartigen Tumoren im Bereich der Nase und ihrer Nebenhöhlen bei Werktätigen der Holzindustrie und anderen Industriezweigen. *Arch Geschwulstforsch* 1987;57:393–399.
143. Mohtashamipur E, Norpoth K. Zur Frage beruflich bedingter Tumoren in der holzverarbeitenden Industrie. *Arbeitsmed Sozialmed Praeventivmed* 1983;18:49–52.
144. Boysen M. Histopathology of the nasal mucosa in furniture workers. *Rhinology* 1985;23:109–113.
145. Boysen M, Voss R, Solberg LA, The nasal mucosa in softwood exposed furniture workers. *Acta Otolaryngol* 1986;101:501–508.
146. Wilhelmsson B, Hellquist H, Olofsson J, Klintenberg C. Nasal cuboidal metaplasia with dysplasia. *Acta Otolaryngol* 1985;99:641–648.
147. Sato T. High-risk factors in the development of head and neck cancers. *Gan To Kagaku Ryoko* 1987;14:2626–2631.
148. Higginson J, Bolt HM, Bosland MC. Concluding remarks. In: Feron VJ, Bosland MC, eds. *Nasal carcinogenesis in rodents: relevance to human health risk.* Wageningen, The Netherlands: Pudoc; 1989:205–209.
149. Madsen C. Squamous-cell carcinoma and oral, pharyngeal and nasal lesions caused by foreign bodies in feed. Cases from a long-term study in rats. *Lab Anim* 1989;23:241–247.
150. Feron VJ, Wilmer JWGM, Woutersen RA, Zwart A. Inhalation toxicity and carcinogenicity of formaldehyde in animals: significance for assessment of human health risk. In: Mohr U, Bates DV, Dungworth DL, et al, eds. *Assessment of inhalation hazards.* ILSI monographs. Berlin: Springer-Verlag; 1989:131–138.
151. Feron VJ, Woutersen RA. Role of tissue damage in nasal carcinogenesis. In: Feron VJ, Bosland MC, eds. *Nasal carcinogenesis in rodents: relevance to human health risk.* Wageningen, The Netherlands: Pudoc; 1989:76–84.
152. Feron VJ, Kruysse A. Effects of exposure to acrolein vapour in hamsters simultaneously treated with benzo(a)pyrene or diethylnitrosamine. *J Toxicol Environ Health* 1977;3:379–394.
153. Feron VJ, Kruysse A. Effects of exposure to furfural vapour in hamsters simultaneously treated with benzo(a)pyrene or diethylnitrosamine. *Toxicology* 1978;11:127–144.
154. Swenberg JA. Twenty four month final report inhalation toxicity of dimethylamine in F-344 rats and B6C3F1 mice. Research Triangle Park, NC: Chemical Industry Institute of Toxicology; 1990 (Docket 11957).
155. Miller RR, Young JT, Kociba RJ, Keyes DG, Bodner KM, Calhoun LL, Ayres JA. Chronic toxicity and oncogenicity bioassay of inhaled ethyl acrylate in Fischer 344 rats and B6C3F1 mice. *Drug Chem Toxicol* 1985;8:1–42.
156. Roe FJC. Non-genotoxic carcinogenesis: implications for testing and extrapolation to man. *Mutagenesis* 1989;4:407–411.
157. Feron VJ. Recent inhalation and chronic oral studies with formaldehyde in rats. In: *The toxicology forum, Given Institute of Pathobiology.* Washington, DC: Toxicology Forum; 1988:116–139.
158. Maronpot RR. NTP technical report on the carcinogenesis bioassay of ethyl acrylate in rats and mice. NTP technical report 259. Research Triangle Park, NC: *National Toxicology Program*; 1983.
159. Reznik GK. Comparative anatomy, physiology, and function of the upper respiratory tract. *Environ Health Perspect* 1990;85:171–176.
160. Druckrey H, Ivankovic S, Mennel HD, Preussman R. Selektive Erzeugung von Carcinomen der Nasenhöhle bei Ratten durch N,N'-Dinitrosopiperazin, Nitrosopiperidin und Methyl-vinyl-nitrosamin. *Z Krebsforsch* 1964;66:138–150.
161. Swenberg JA, Kerns WD, Mitchell RI, Gralla EJ, Pavkov KL. Induction of squamous cell carcinomas of the rat nasal cavity by inhalation exposure to formaldehyde vapour. *Cancer Res* 1980; 40:3398–3402.

162. Chang JCF, Steinhagen WH, Barrow CS. Effect of single or repeated formaldehyde exposure on minute volume of B6C9F1 mice and F-344 rats. *Toxicol Appl Pharmacol* 1981;61:451–459.
163. Chang JCF, Gross EA, Swenberg JA, Barrow CS. Nasal cavity deposition, histopathology, and cell proliferation after single or repeated formaldehyde exposures in B6C9F1 mice and F-344 rats. *Toxicol Appl Pharmacol* 1983;68:161–176.
164. Heck H d'A, Casanova-Schmitz M. Biochemical toxicology of formaldehyde. *Rev Biochem Toxicol* 1984;6:155–189.
165. Page NP. Concepts of a bioassay program in environmental carcinogenesis. In: Kraybill H, Mehlman H, eds. *Environmental carcinogenesis*. Washington, DC: Hemisphere; 1977:87–171.
166. WHO. *Principles and methods for evaluating the toxicity of chemicals*. Part I. *Environmental health criteria 6*. Geneva: World Health Organization; 1978.
167. Groenen PJ. *Bestanddelen van tabaksrook. Aard en hoeveelheid, potentiële invloed op de gezondheid*. CIVO/TNO report 5787. Zeist, The Netherlands: CIVO; 1978.
168. Gold LS, Slone TH, Manley NB, Bernstein L. Target organs in chronic bioassays of 533 chemical carcinogens. *Environ Health Perspect* 1991;93:233–246.
169. Huff J, Cirvello J, Haseman J, Bucher J. Chemicals associated with site-specific neoplasia in 1394 long-term carcinogenesis experiments in laboratory rodents. *Environ Health Perspect* 1991;93:247–270.

9
Multistage Skin Carcinogenesis in Mice

John DiGiovanni

Department of Carcinogenesis, University of Texas, M.D. Anderson Cancer Center, Smithville, Texas 78957

Skin carcinogenesis in mice can be accomplished using either multistage or complete protocols (1,2). Complete carcinogenesis experimental protocols involve the administration of a single dose or repeated applications of smaller doses of a carcinogen to an experimental animal. In the mouse skin tumorigenesis system, multiple papillomas and carcinomas can be produced on the backs of mice following a single application of as little as 600 to 800 nmol of a pure polycyclic aromatic hydrocarbon (PAH) such as 7,12-dimethylbenz[a]anthracene (DMBA) (3,4). The induction of mouse skin tumors can also be accomplished by using a multistage model that involves the processes defined operationally and mechanistically as initiation and promotion (1,2,5). Initiation is generally accomplished by topical application of a single subcarcinogenic dose of a skin carcinogen, such as DMBA. An initiating dose of a carcinogen, per se, will not lead to the development of visible tumors. Visible tumors will result only following prolonged and repeated topical applications of a tumor promoter, such as croton oil or its most active constituent, 12-O-tetradecanoylphorbol-13-acetate (TPA), to the initiated skin (1,2). It is generally assumed that both the initiating and promoting components are present during complete carcinogenesis experimental protocols.

A schematic representation of multistage carcinogenesis in mouse skin is depicted in Fig. 1. As noted above, the initiation stage of mouse skin tumorigenesis is effected by a single application or exposure to a subcarcinogenic dose of a skin carcinogen. Initiation is a rapid process that produces no apparent morphological alterations in the epidermis (reviewed in refs. 1,2,6,7). The initiation event occurs as a result of interaction of a reactive form of a skin carcinogen with the DNA of an epidermal target cell (5,8,9). As a result of interaction of a reactive carcinogenic intermediate with DNA, one can usually measure a transient dose-dependent inhibition of epidermal DNA synthesis (10,11). One of the hallmarks of tumor initiation in mouse skin is that it persists for the lifetime of the animal (12–15) despite the fact that the epidermis renews itself approximately once every 6 to 8 days (16). Thus some important characteristics of skin tumor initiators can be summarized as fol-

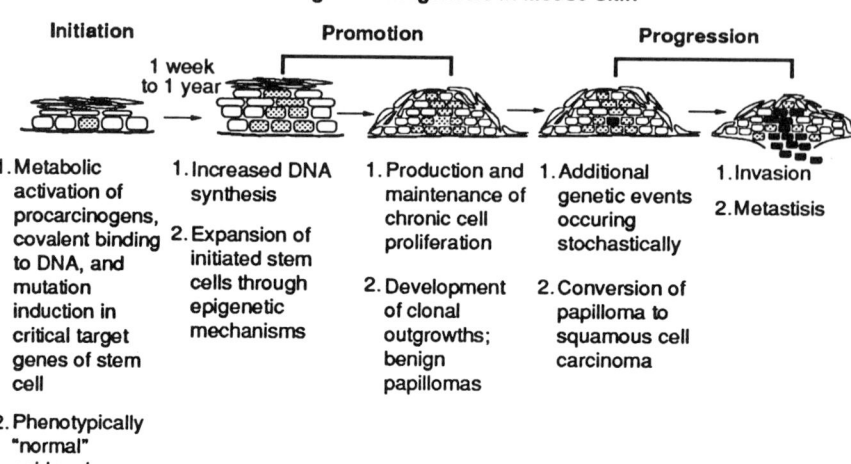

FIG. 1. Overview of multistage carcinogenesis in mouse skin. Carcinogenesis in mouse skin can be divided into three main stages: initiation, promotion, and progression. The promotion and progression stages are further clarified by indicating early versus later events associated with these stages. Major events and/or changes associated with each stage are summarized below the sketches representing the physical appearance of the skin or major lesion at the particular stage.

lows (reviewed in refs. 5,9,17): (a) initiators react covalently with or indirectly modify cellular macromolecules such as DNA, RNA, and protein; (b) initiators produce an essentially irreversible event after a single application or exposure; and (c) initiators are mutagenic in bacterial and mammalian cells.

In contrast to the initiation stage, treatment of mouse skin with a tumor-promoting agent produces dramatic morphological and biochemical effects that are reversible in the absence of continued treatment (2,6,18–21), although some effects may persist for longer periods of time after discontinuation of promoter treatment (20–23). Thus tumor promoters must be given at an optimal frequency and duration to effect tumor development. The process of tumor promotion in mouse skin is believed to involve the selective clonal expansion of initiated cells into visible clonal outgrowths (papillomas) by one or a combination of several mechanisms (reviewed in 5,9,24). While genetic mechanisms have been postulated to play a role in the tumor promotion stage (25–29), the eventual reversibility of promoter-induced effects (21,23,30) argues that this is accomplished primarily through epigenetic mechanisms as originally postulated by Boutwell (2,6) and others. Since the early studies of Boutwell (1), several laboratories have extended the observation that the tumor promotion stage of mouse skin tumorigenesis can be subdivided into two distinct stages (31–33). However, this concept has been challenged by recent studies demonstrating that the first or "conversion" stage can, in fact, be effected for a limited time, prior to application of the initiator (23,30,34,35).

The first tumors that appear during a two-stage mouse skin tumorigenesis protocol using DMBA and TPA as the initiator and promoter, respectively, are premalignant lesions called papillomas (reviewed in ref. 36). The papillomas that initially develop during mouse skin initiation–promotion procotols have long been considered heterogeneous in that some will persist, some will disappear or regress, and only a small proportion will "progress" to an invasive squamous cell carcinoma (SCC) during the time frame of most experiments (37–42). This information has led to the hypothesis that different subclasses of papillomas exist with different probabilities of malignant progression and, indeed, to the hypothesis that some papillomas (referred to as "terminally benign") (38,39,41,43) are not at risk for progression to SCC. On the other hand, other studies (44) have suggested, based on a sequential cytogenetic and histopathological study, that skin papillomas generated during an initiation–promotion regimen progress to SCC at different rates and that many of the papillomas generated during initiation–promotion have the potential to become SCC. Furthermore, recent studies (45–47) have demonstrated that many factors (e.g., tumor burden) can dramatically influence the apparent growth potential of papillomas and hence influence final carcinoma yields. Studies such as these have provided additional support for the hypothesis that a significant proportion of papillomas generated by initiation–promotion protocols in sensitive mouse strains should be considered premalignant lesions (48).

Tumor progression in the classical mouse skin initiation–promotion model involves the conversion of papillomas to SCC. Based on the available evidence (reviewed in refs. 36,48,49), most, if not all, SCCs arise from preexisting papillomas. The process of tumor progression appears to involve the accumulation of additional genetic changes in cells comprising skin papillomas (44,50–55). These genetic changes appear to occur stochastically in that once a maximum papilloma yield is obtained on a given mouse, further promoter treatment is not necessary to produce a maximum SCC yield (39,40,45,50).

As noted above, the major types of tumors produced in mouse skin using initiation–promotion regimens with PAH initiators and phorbol ester promoters are squamous papillomas and SCCs. However, other tumor types have been noted to various extents such as keratoacanthomas, melanomas, and adnexal tumors (36,56–60). The appearance of these tumor types may be highly dependent on the type of initiator and/or promoter used and on the genetic background of mouse stock or strain utilized (36,56–60).

TUMOR INITIATION

The initiation stage of mouse skin carcinogenesis can be effected by a variety of both direct- and indirect-acting chemical carcinogens (61,62). In general, where appropriately tested, complete carcinogens for mouse skin possess at least some tumor-initiating activity (17,62). However, several compounds, including urethane, diol-epoxide derivatives of benzo[a]pyrene (BaP) and benz[a]anthracene, and possibly several other compounds, have been suggested to possess only skin tumor–initiating activity (17,62). PAHs are one of the major chemical classes of carcinogens that possess both tumor-initiating and complete carcinogenic activity on mouse skin (17,62,63). These compounds are widely utilized and studied for their mechanism(s) of skin tumor initiation. In addition to PAH, many other chemical classes of compounds possess, albeit in some cases low activity, the ability to initiate skin tumors in mice. Comprehensive listings of known chemical carcinogens and tumor initiators on mouse skin can be found elsewhere (17,61,62,64,65).

Many chemical carcinogens and skin tumor initiators, including the widely studied PAH, require metabolic activation in order to express their carcinogenic and tumor-initiating properties in mouse skin (reviewed in refs. 63,66–68). PAHs are metabolized by cytochrome P450-dependent monooxygenase enzymes to a wide variety of primary metabolites, including epoxides, dihydrodiols, quinones, and phenols (reviewed in refs. 69–72). Some of these primary oxidation products can serve as substrates for conversion to water-soluble glutathione, glucuronide and sulfate conjugates (69,70,72). A number of the products of initial oxidation (i.e., phenols and diols) can be reoxidized and recycled through these same metabolic pathways (69–72). Of particular interest is the formation of the highly reactive PAH diol-epoxides. Studies in a variety of tissues and species of the ubiquitous PAH, BaP, for example, have shown that it is activated to mutagenic and carcinogenic derivatives by a two-step mechanism leading to the formation of a "bay-region" diol-epoxide (71,72) and that the various isomers of this diol-epoxide bind covalently to different extents at various positions on DNA bases, particularly on deoxyguanosine (dGuo) residues (71–73). This two-step oxidation mechanism appears to be a major pathway of metabolic activation of BaP and other PAH for tumor initiation in mouse skin (reviewed in refs. 73,74).

Skin tumor initiators have been shown to bind covalently to a wide variety of cellular macromolecules, including DNA, RNA, and protein (8,66,75). However, it is the interaction with DNA that correlates most closely with skin tumor–initiating activity (8,17,76). Considerable effort has been expended in characterizing covalent interactions between activated carcinogen metabolites (primarily PAH) and the DNA of epidermal cells, the target cells for tumor initiation in mouse skin. Following topical application of the prototypic PAH, BaP, to mouse skin *in vivo*, the major DNA adduct formed is (+) *anti*-BaP-diol-epoxide bound through *trans* addition of the exocyclic amino (N^2) group of dGuo [(+)-*anti*-BPDE-N^2-dGuo] (Fig. 2 and reviewed in (refs. 71,74). Although much attention has focused on (+)-*anti*-BPDE-N^2-dGuo, a number of studies in various tissues, including mouse epidermis (71–73,77–82), have found DNA adducts arising from reaction of the anti BaP-diol-epoxides with deoxyadenosine (dAdo). In addition, at least one dGuo adduct with a *syn*-BaP-diol-epoxide has been identified in mouse epidermal DNA following topical application of BaP to mouse skin (80,81). Furthermore, studies of BaP-diol-epoxide DNA binding *in vitro* have indicated the formation of O^6- and N^7-dGuo and N^4-deoxycytidine (dCyto) derivatives (83–87); however, less is known about their formation in mouse skin or other target tissues *in vivo*.

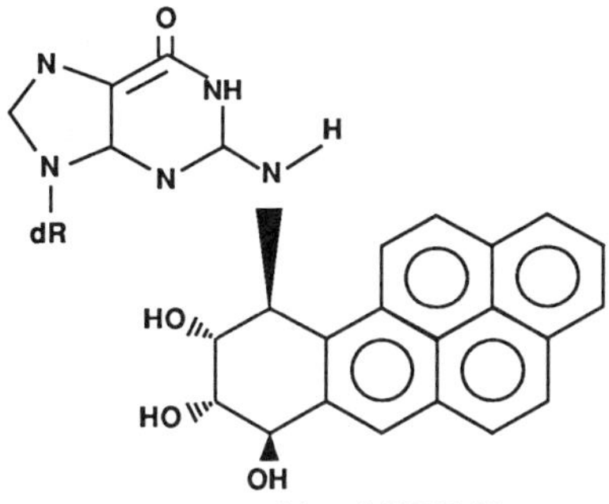

FIG. 2. Chemical structure of the major BaP–DNA adduct in most target tissues, including mouse epidermis; (+)-*anti*-BPDE-*trans*-dGuo.

Less is known about the total spectrum of DNA adducts formed in mouse epidermis from other PAH skin tumor initiators. DMBA, another widely studied PAH, is metabolized to a variety of reactive intermediates that bind extensively to epidermal DNA, including both *syn* and *anti* diol-epoxides (71). Interestingly, these diol-epoxide metabolites of DMBA bind much more extensively to dAdo residues in epidermal DNA than BaP and it has been hypothesized that this preference for dAdo residues could account, in part, for the difference in biological potency between BaP and DMBA (71,88). The reader is referred to several extensive reviews on the subject of PAH DNA adduct formation in various cellular systems, including mouse skin (71,73).

GENES AND GENETIC CHANGES ASSOCIATED WITH SKIN TUMOR INITIATION

The capacity of many carcinogens to cause point mutations in DNA (89,90), together with the irreversible nature of skin tumor initiation (reviewed in refs. 1,9, 76,89) led to the hypothesis that initiation involves the induction of point mutations in a gene(s) that confers some selective growth advantage to the target epidermal cell(s). A number of genes have frequently been found to be altered by translocation or mutation in human or animal tumors (reviewed in refs. 91–96). Most genes in this category are members of the *ras* family, comprising Harvey-(Ha-), Kirsten-(Ki-), and N-*ras*, although several other genes have also been identified (93, 94). Balmain et al. (97) demonstrated that a high percentage of DMBA-induced mouse skin carcinomas and papillomas had an activated c-Ha-*ras*. In addition, the fact that this gene was activated in papillomas led to the conclusion that this alteration must have occurred at a relatively early stage in the carcinogenic process. Further support for a role of Ha-*ras* activation in the process of skin tumor initiation comes from studies where an activated Ha-*ras* gene (i.e., v-Ha-*ras*) has been introduced directly into epidermal cells in culture, allowing them to form papillomas in growth chambers on nude mice (98) or *in vivo* followed by treatment with TPA (99). In the latter study, although introduction of v-Ha-*ras* alone did not lead to the development of skin tumors, subsequent promoter treatment led to the formation of both papillomas and SCC. Finally, the importance of activated *ras* in mouse skin tumor initiation has been demonstrated by the development of skin tumors, primarily at sites of wounding in transgenic mice harboring an activated *ras* under the control of an epidermal keratin promoter (100). These studies as well as others (reviewed in ref. 101) strongly implicate *ras* gene involvement in mouse skin tumor initiation.

Evidence has also been emerging that point mutations in the mouse c-Ha-*ras* gene obtained from skin papillomas and carcinomas can be highly dependent on the initiator (94–96,102–104). Whereas tumors from mice initiated with DMBA, dibenz[*c,h*]acridine, and urethane produced almost exclusively $A^{182} \rightarrow T$ transversions at codon 61 of the second exon of c-Ha-*ras*, methylnitrosourea (MNU)-, or *N*-methyl-*N*'-nitro-*N*-nitrosoguanidine (MNNG)-induced papillomas and carcinomas did not have this point mutation in their DNA (102–106). In fact, MNU- or MNNG-induced papillomas contained primarily $G^{35} \rightarrow A$ transition mutations in codon 12 of c-Ha-*ras* (106). These observations are similar to those of Barbacid and co-workers (94,107,108), in whose work DNA from rat mammary carcinomas induced by MNU contained an activated c-Ha-*ras* gene with a point mutation in codon 12, whereas with DMBA the same $A^{182} \rightarrow T$ transversion in codon 61 was observed. Recent studies from our laboratory have characterized the DNA adducts found in mouse epidermal DNA (109,110) and the c-Ha-*ras* mutations in skin tumors resulting from topical application of dibenz[*a,j*]anthracene (DB[a,j]A) (110, 111). This compound is interesting in that in mouse epidermis *in vivo*, considerable binding occurs at both dGuo and dAdo residues (110). A high percentage (80%) of skin papillomas initiated by this compound possessed $A^{182} \rightarrow T$ transversion mutations in codon 61 of c-Ha-*ras* (Table 1). In addition, papillomas induced by initiation with the putative ultimate tumor-initiating diol-epoxide of DB[a,j]A (*anti*-DB[*a,j*]A-3,4-diol-1,2-epoxide) possessed the same mutation as those found in tumors initiated with the parent hydrocarbon (i.e., $A^{182} \rightarrow T$ transversions in condon 61). These mutations in c-Ha-*ras* are consistent with the presence of specific dAdo adducts from the *anti*-diol-epoxide formed in mouse epidermal cells following exposure to the parent hydrocarbon, DB[a,j]A (109,110). The reason why the majority of the Ha-*ras* mutations observed with this compound were at dAdo residues despite the distribution of DNA adducts at both dGuo as well as dAdo residues remains unknown at present. We have also analyzed skin tumors from SENCAR mice initiated with 7-methylbenz[*a*]anthracene (7-MBA). This compound has not been studied as extensively for its DNA binding *in vivo*, although studies with the (±)*anti*-diol-epoxide of 7-MBA have been conducted *in vitro* (112). This diol-epoxide binds extensively to dGuo residues upon reaction with calf thymus DNA, and the mutation spectrum using the supF gene in Ad 293 cells is predominated by mutations at G·C base pairs (113). Interestingly, a preliminary analysis of six papillomas initiated by 7-MBA indicated that five of them possessed $A^{182} \rightarrow T$ transver-

TABLE 1. Analysis of point mutations ($A^{182} \to T$ transversions) in codon 61 of c-Ha-Ras from skin papillomas initiated by several PAH[a]

PAH initiator	Promoter	Number positive/ number tested
—[b]	—	0/5
DMBA	TPA	9/10
DB[a,j]A[c]	TPA	8/10
(±)anti-DB[a,j]A-DE[c]	TPA	5/5
7-MBA	TPA	5/6

[a]Papillomas were generated during standard initiation–promotion protocols using 10 nmol DMBA, 400 nmol of DB[a,j]A or (±)anti-DB[a,j]A-DE, or 400 nmol of 7-MBA at initiation, followed 2 weeks later by twice-weekly applications of 3.4 nmol of TPA. All tumors were harvested between weeks 20 and 34 of promotion.
[b]DNA from control epidermis.
[c]Data regarding DB[a,j]A and (±)anti-DB[a,j]A-DE from Gill et al. (111).

sion mutations in the sixty-first codon of c-Ha-*ras* (Table 1). Therefore, 7-MBA appears to be very similar to DB[a,j]A and further raises a question regarding the relationship between DNA adducts and mutations in the c-Ha-*ras*. One possible interpretation is that dAdo adducts from both of these PAH are responsible for the mutations observed. It should be noted that skin papillomas and carcinomas induced by promoter treatment alone have been reported to contain an activated c-Ha-*ras* (sixty-first codon $A^{182} \to T$ mutation) (114). Based on these and other data (114–116) it has been hypothesized that certain mutations in c-Ha-*ras* can occur spontaneously. Further work will be necessary to determine if some Ha-*ras* mutations in mouse epidermis may occur by mechanism(s) other than as a result of the presence of a DNA adduct.

TUMOR PROMOTION

As noted earlier in this chapter, the phorbol esters are the most widely studied skin tumor promoters. These compounds are derivatives of the tetracyclic diterpene phorbol, esterified in the 12 and 13 positions (see Fig. 3). The tumor-promoting activity of the phorbol esters appears to be related to a delicate hydrophobic–hydrophilic balance determined by positions 12-O, 13-O, and 20. TPA is the most potent of the phorbol ester series (117,118). The structure–activity relationships of phorbol esters, as well as other diterpene esters, have been reported in detail by Hecker (117,118). Although the phorbol esters have been the most widely studied skin tumor promoters to date, many other chemical compounds have been shown to possess skin tumor–promoting properties (Table 2). In addition to chemical promoting agents, a number of other types of stimuli can act as promoters of skin tumors in this model system. Ultraviolet light has a strong promoting action in mouse skin (57,119,120). Physical trauma of sufficient magnitude has long been known to promote skin tumor formation in previously initiated mice (121–126). In this regard,

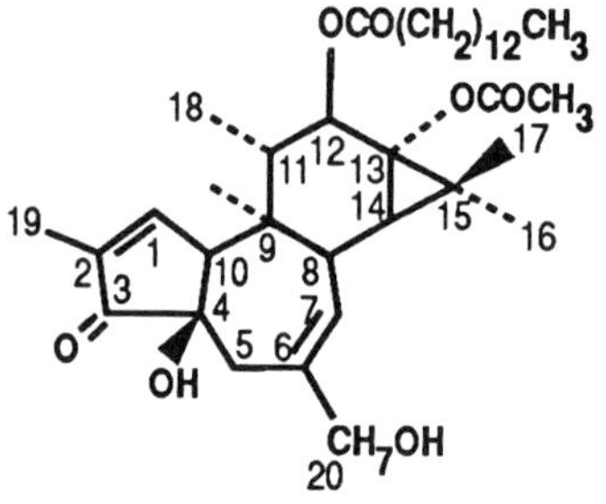

TPA

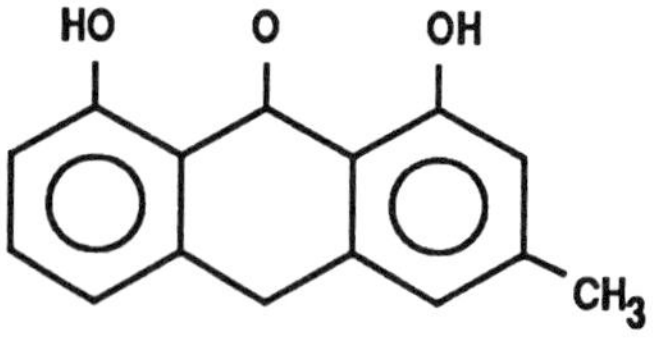

1,8-dihydroxy-3-methyl-9-anthrone (Chrysarobin)

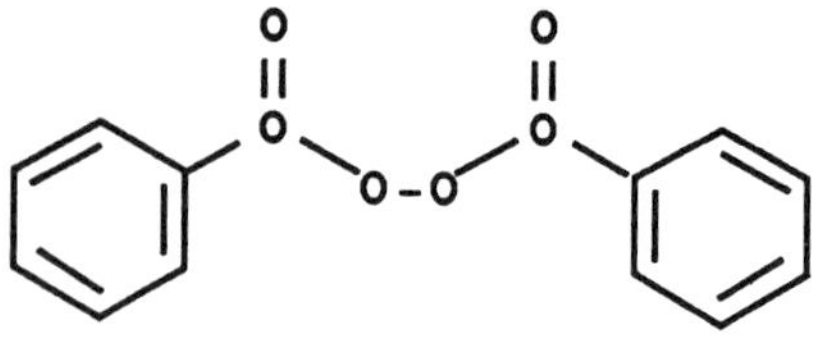

Benzoyl peroxide

FIG. 3. Chemical structures of representative skin tumor promoters, including TPA.

repeated physical abrasion can promote skin tumors (124–126). Finally, full-thickness skin wounding is a very strong promoting stimulus for epidermal tumorigenesis (122,123). Recently, another type of physical skin tumor–promoting agent has been identified: biogenic silica fibers (127). These fibers, obtained from the grain of *Phalaris canariensis*, are effective skin tumor promoters when rubbed on the backs of previously initiated mice (127). Interestingly, recent evidence suggests that these biogenic silica fibers work by a mechanism distinctly different from physical abrasion (128). One has to marvel at the diversity of stimuli that possess skin tumor–promoting activity and whether there are some common effects at the biochemical and molecular level responsible for tumor promotion by all these different agents (see Table 2).

Tumor–promoting agents produce substantial cellular changes when topically applied to mouse epidermis. Within a few hours after application of a single effective

TABLE 2. *Diversity of mouse skin tumor promoting stimuli*

Promoter stimuli	Relative activity
Chemicals	
Croton oil	Strong
Certain phorbol esters found in croton oil	Strong
Some synthetic phorbol esters	Strong
Certain euphorbia latices	Strong
Teleocidins	Strong
Polyacetates (e.g., aplysiatoxin)	Strong
Okadaic acid	Strong
Calyculin A	Strong
Palytoxin	Strong
Thapsigargin	Strong
Anthrones (e.g., anthralin, chrysarobin)	Moderate
Extracts of unburned tobacco	Moderate
Tobacco smoke condensate	Moderate
1-Fluoro-2,4-dinitrobenzene	Moderate
7-Bromomethylbenz[a]anthracene	Moderate
Benzo[e]pyrene	Moderate
Benzoyl peroxide	Moderate
Certain fatty acids and fatty acid methyl esters	Weak
Certain long-chain alkanes	Weak
A number of phenolic compounds	Weak
Surface-active agents (sodium lauryl sulfate, Tween 60)	Weak
Citrus oils	Weak
Iodoacetic acid	Weak
Others	
Full-thickness wounding	Strong
Abrasion	Moderate
UV light	Moderate
Biogenic silica fibers	Moderate

dose of the phorbol ester, TPA, to mouse skin, localized edema and erythema characteristic of inflammation and irritation are evident, and by 24 h, there is leukocytic infiltration of the dermis (7,129). At that time there is also a 5- to 10-fold increase in the percentage of DCs in the interfollicular epidermis (130–132). These DCs are characterized by their strong basophilia, dense chromatin, and large numbers of free ribosomes. They increase in number in TPA-induced hyperplasia to a greater extent than in hyperplasia induced by mezerein or more weakly promoting hyperplastic agents (131,133). These observations have led to the hypothesis that an increase in their number may be an important component of the promotion stage of skin carcinogenesis (132,134,135). Several investigators have reported the presence of both viable and nonviable DCs in promoter-treated epidermis (20,136–144). The importance of any or all of these types of DCs in the process of tumor promotion remains an open question at present.

Within 1 to 2 days after a single promoter treatment, stimulation of mitotic activity in the basal cell layer of the epidermis continues for several days and results in an increased number of nucleated cell layers (130). This is followed by a phase of increased keratinization of the upper layers of the epidermis (130,145,146). Without additional promoter treatments, all these responses to the promoter gradually subside and the epidermis regains its normal appearance within approximately 2 to 3 weeks of treatment (147). Repeated promoter treatment, however, prevents this decrease in response, and the skin appears to be in a chronic state of irritation and regenerative hyperplasia (21). In fact, repeated treatment with TPA leads to a potentiation of the hyperplasia response in species and mouse strains that are susceptible to skin tumor promotion by phorbol esters (148,149). Table 3 illustrates the potentiated hyperplasia that occurs after four or more topical applications of TPA, chrysarobin, or benzoyl peroxide to a promotion-responsive mouse stock (i.e, SENCAR) compared to a single application. Note that where adequately tested, all tumor promoters produce such a potentiated hyperplasia, although the magnitude and kinetics of this response can differ with each type of promoting agent (125,126,150). The ability to produce a potentiated hyperplasia after multiple treatments and the magnitude of this response appear to correlate most closely with the tumor-promoting ability of various compounds (125,126,150,151).

It has been argued for many years that the induction of cell proliferation and hyperplasia was a necessary but not sufficient condition for tumor promotion in the mouse skin model (2,6,7). This argument was based on the observations that certain chemicals could produce dramatic epidermal hyperplasia after a single application [e.g., acetic acid, mezerein, ethyl phenyl propiolate (EPP)] and yet these compounds exhibited only poor papilloma-promoting ability (133,152–154). However, careful examination of these compounds revealed that they are unable to maintain a potentiated epidermal hyperplasia and cell proliferation when given repeatedly, due, in part, to severe epidermal toxicity (151,155–157). Epidermal toxicity appears to be an important limiting factor in the promoting activity of both the an-

TABLE 3. Comparison of epidermal hyperplasia induced by TPA and chrysarobin following single and multiple treatments[a]

Compound (dose)	Treatment protocol	Epidermal thickness (μm)
Acetone (0.2 mL)	Single	15.8 ± 1.0
	Multiple	15.0 ± 1.0
TPA (3.4 nmol)[b]	Single	42.8 ± 2
	Multiple	71.5 ± 4.9[c]
Chrysarobin (220 nmol)[b]	Single	20.8 ± 1.2
	Multiple	54.2 ± 3.2[c]
Benzoyl peroxide (20 mg)	Single	17.2 ± 0.9
	Multiple	22.3 ± 1.2[c]

[a]Three female SENCAR mice were used for each experimental group. TPA (3.4 nmol) was applied either as a single application or as five applications given twice weekly over a 2½-week period. Chrysarobin (220 nmol) was applied either as a single application or as five applications given once weekly over 5 weeks. BzPo (20 mg) was applied either as a single application or as five applications given twice weekly over a 2½-week period. Animals were sacrificed 48 h after the last application.
[b]Data for TPA and chrysarobin are from Kruszewski et al. (150).
[c]Significantly greater ($p<0.05$) than the value after a single application.

thrones (158) as well as EPP (159). These observations, as well as the fact that regenerative hyperplasia alone can promote skin tumors (124,125), supports the hypothesis that epidermal hyperplasia and cell proliferation of a specific type, magnitude, and duration is sufficient for skin tumor promotion in susceptible mouse strains and stocks (125,126).

BIOCHEMICAL AND MOLECULAR MECHANISMS OF TUMOR PROMOTION

Phorbol diesters with promoting activity produce an initial inhibition of tritiated thymidine incorporation into epidermal DNA (130,160,161). This is soon followed by greatly increased rates of nucleic acid and protein synthesis (122,160,161). Promoter-treated skin shows an increase in phospholipid turnover (162–164) and prostaglandin accumulation (165,166), a decreased responsiveness to epidermal chalones (167,168) and β-adrenergic agonists (167–172), a decrease in the basal activities of epidermal superoxide dismutase (SOD) and catalase (173,174), a decrease in the glucocorticoid receptor (175–177), and an increase in the activity of xanthine oxidase (174). Tumor promoter treatments also lead to a decrease in epidermal histidase (178) and histidine decarboxylase (179), modification of epidermal keratins and keratin expression (146,180–182), increased synthesis and phosphorylation of histones (183–185), and a large induction of ornithine decarboxylase (ODC) (186,187), the rate-limiting enzyme in polyamine biosynthesis. As a result of the induction of epidermal ODC, the levels of putrescine, and especially spermidine, in the epidermis become elevated (188–191). The elevated spermidine/spermine ratio that occurs after TPA treatment is linked tightly to the DNA synthesis response induced by this promoter (190,191).

Phorbol esters and several other classes of tumor promoters, including the teleocidins and the aplysiatoxins, appear to exert some of their effects by initially binding to high-affinity sites on individual PKC isozymes, with a resultant increase in membrane-associated kinase activity and subsequent changes in the phosphorylation of cellular proteins (192–194). By activating PKC, phorbol esters such as TPA are believed to bypass a normal cellular mechanism(s) for regulating cell proliferation (195–197). In keratinocytes of mouse skin, an important mechanism presumably involves the interaction of growth factors with their receptors [e.g., the epidermal growth factor receptor (EGFr)] (198). In this regard, tumor-promoting phorbol esters are able to modulate the transcription of a number of cellular and viral genes (199–213). Some of these genes, including c-*myc* and c-*fos*, whose transcription is induced by phorbol esters in cultured cells (199,200) and mouse skin *in vivo* (206), are the same competence genes induced by activation of the EGFr and other growth factor receptors (reviewed in refs. 214,215). In many of these cases, activation of PKC by TPA has been implicated in the mechanism of altered transcription and presumably mitogenesis.

Evidence is emerging that the generation of free radicals may be involved in the skin tumor–promoting actions of several classes of promoting agents (27,28), including the phorbol esters. For example, TPA stimulates production of O_2^- and possibly other free radicals by polymorphonuclear leukocytes (PMNs) (216–218), probably by activating the ubiquitous membrane-bound NADPH oxidase system (219,220). Fischer et al. (221) demonstrated the production of O_2^- in isolated epidermal cells by active, but not inactive, phorbol ester analogs using a chemiluminescence assay and its suppression by antipromoters (222). More direct evidence for the involvement of free radicals in tumor promotion comes from studies with free-radical-generating compounds such as the organic peroxides and anthrones. Benzoyl peroxide and other organic peroxides are effective skin tumor promoters in sensitive mouse stocks and strains (223,224). In addition, structure–activity studies for tumor-promoting activity with anthrone derivatives strongly suggest that oxidation at C_{10} of the molecule, with subsequent generation of free-radical intermediates, is crucial for their tumor-promoting actions (225,226). A number of additional studies have also demonstrated that free-radical-generating systems such as xanthine/xanthine oxidase can mimic the effects of phorbol esters on enhancing cell transformation in cultured C3H10T 1/2 (227) and mouse epidermal JB6 cells (228). Antioxidants are effective inhibitors of chemical carcinogenesis and skin tumor promotion, which further supports a role for free radicals in tumor promotion (reviewed in refs. 28,229). TPA, benzoyl peroxide, and anthralin have also been shown to decrease the activities of SOD and catalase in mouse epidermis, shortly after their application (173,174,224). Perchellet et al. (230) have demonstrated that a wide variety of tumor promoters decrease the reduced (GSH)/oxidized (GSSG) glutathione ratio in mouse epidermal cells treated with a variety of promoting agents. TPA was also found to stimulate a rapid, transient increase in GSH-peroxidase followed by a prolonged depression in the activity of this enzyme (230). These changes presumably reflect the induction of a prooxidant state in the epidermal cells by TPA and other types of tumor promoters. More recent studies by Perchellet and co-workers (231,232) have demonstrated that tumor promoters can induce the production of hydroperoxides in mouse epidermal homogenates. Taken together, all these studies support a role for free radicals in tumor promotion by certain types of compounds.

The exact biochemical and molecular mechanism(s) whereby certain free-radical intermediates might lead to the process of tumor promotion remain unknown. Both genetic and epigenetic mechanisms have been postulated (reviewed in refs. 27–29, 233). Cerutti (27,233) has proposed that the induction of a prooxidant state leads to altered gene expression through activation of poly(ADP-ribose) synthetase and subsequent ADP ribosylation of chromosomal proteins. The activation of poly (ADP-ribose) synthetase is proposed to result from oxidant-induced DNA strand breaks and increased levels of oxidized pyridine nucleotides. Because of the reactivity of unsaturated and sulfur-containing molecules with free radicals, proteins containing such functional groups will be susceptible to free-radical-mediated amino acid modification (28,234). A variety of cellular proteins and/or enzymatic pathways could thus be changed, leading to altered phenotypic characteristics of a cell (reviewed in refs. 28,223,235). In this regard, anthralin is known to inhibit glucose-6-phosphate dehydrogenase (G6PDH) *in vitro* as well as in epidermal preparations of human skin (236,237). The ability of anthralin to inhibit G6PDH *in vitro* correlates with its ability to undergo oxidation to 1,8-dihydroxyanthraquinone and the anthralin dimer (237). PKC may be regulated to a certain extent by direct oxidation. In this regard, mild oxidation of the regulatory domain of PKC may eliminate the requirement for Ca^{2+} and phospholipid for its activation (238). Furthermore, H_2O_2 has been reported to alter the distribution of PKC in JB6 cells (239) and benzoyl peroxide to alter PKC distribution in mouse epidermis (240). The activities of other proteins may also be regulated to a certain extent directly by redox reactions, including c-*fos* (241); c-*jun* (241); a tyrosine kinase located in the endoplasmic reticulum (242); GSSG reductase and Mg^{2+}-dependent, Na^+,K^+ stimulated ATPase (243); and possibly many others.

During oxidative stress, most cells suffer from compromised energy homeostasis due to uncoupling of oxidative phosphorylation, decreased levels of GSH, and decreased levels of NADPH as a result of its utilization by the GSH-peroxidase redox cycle leading to subsequent release of intracellular Ca^{2+} stores (244–246). The resulting increase in intracellular Ca^{2+} concentrations could lead to the activation of a cascade of biochemical pathways (reviewed in refs. 244,246). It is interesting to note that PKC and Ca^{2+} are believed to act synergistically in stimulating various cellular responses (295,247). In addition, release of intracellular Ca^{2+} has been postulated to account for phosphorylation of the ribosomal protein, S6, in cells treated with H_2O_2 (248) through an intermediate Ca^{2+}/-calmodulin-sensitive kinase (233,248). The reported downregulation of epidermal PKC by anthrone tumor promoters (249) could result from the activation of Ca^{2+}-dependent proteases (250) through a similar mechanism.

Despite the fact that tumor promoters are not mutagenic in different test systems (251,252) and do not bind covalently to DNA, there is cumulative evidence that TPA induces alterations at the genetic level that could result in toxicity and/or alterations in gene expression. It has been shown that TPA induces replication of endogeneous and integrated viral genomes (199,200,253,254), enhances sister chromatid exchanges in hamster fibroblasts (255), and induces DNA single-strand breaks in human leukocytes (256) and mouse keratinocytes (257,258). Moreover, TPA treatment induces and/or enhances numerical and structural chromosomal aberrations in different systems, such as yeast (259), human leukocytes (260,261), and mouse keratinocytes (262–264). It has been reported that TPA also induced cytogenetic changes in cultures of primary mouse keratinocytes (25).

Chemicals such as okadaic acid, calyculin A, and similar compounds appear to be relatively specific inhibitors of cellular serine/threonine protein phosphatases [primarily PP-1 and PP-2A (265)], which may mediate, in part, their skin tumor–promoting activities (266–269). The sesquiterpene lactone thapsigargin promotes tumorigenesis in mouse skin but does not activate PKC and is classified as a nonphorbol ester type of tumor promoter (270,271). Thapsigargin has been demonstrated to release Ca^{2+} specifically from the inositol triphosphate–sensitive intracellular pool in parotid acinar cells (272). Studies in rat hepatocytes suggest that the mechanism of action of thapsigargin involves inhibition of the Ca^{2+}-activated endoplasmic reticulum ATPase, the presumptive intracellular Ca^{2+} pump (273). Thapsigargin elevates intracellular Ca^{2+} in a dose-dependent manner, providing a unique tool to study the effect of intracellular Ca^{2+} concentration on gene transcription and tumor promotion. The biochemical and molecular mechanism(s) by which the many other nonphorbol ester skin tumor promoters work remain(s) to be determined. However, it should be stressed again that all known skin tumor promoters that have been studied adequately to date induce a sustained and potentiated hyperplasia and cell proliferation response following multiple treatments (125,126,151), and it is the latter response that appears to be the most universal among the different types of promoting stimuli.

ROLE OF EGFr AND TGF-α IN SKIN TUMOR PROMOTION AND PROGRESSION IN MOUSE SKIN

Phorbol ester tumor promoters have been shown in a variety of studies to alter the binding of EGF to its cellular receptor (274–277). This change is apparently due to the loss of high-affinity binding of EGF; however, the exact mechanism for this alteration is currently unknown. TPA activation of PKC induces phosphorylation of Thr-654, which may lead to reduced affinity of the receptor for its ligand (278–280). However, TPA also alters receptor affinity in cells transfected with an Ala-654-containing EGFr, in addition to altering affinity of the wild-type EGFr (278), suggesting that alternative pathway(s) (other than PKC activation) may also mediate alterations in EGFr affinity (281). Recently, several nonphorbol ester skin tumor promoters, such as thapsigargin (282), okadaic acid (283), palytoxin (284), and chrysarobin (277), have been shown to inhibit the binding of EGF to its receptor through a protein kinase C–independent pathway(s). In addition, ultraviolet-B (UVB) irradiation (285) as well as phenobarbital (286) have been shown to inhibit EGF binding to its receptor on specific cell types. Thus many known skin tumor promoters appear to inhibit EGF binding initially, especially using cultured cells. These relatively short-term effects of various tumor promoters on the EGFr appear, on the surface, unrelated to their ability to induce rather marked proliferative responses in mouse skin *in vivo* and various cells in culture, including keratinocytes (2,6,24,287–289). However, Imamoto et al. (249) reported that topical application of both TPA and chrysarobin led to the loss of epidermal PKC and ultimately, elevation of [^{125}I]EGF binding to its membrane receptor. In addition, these authors reported that both types of tumor promoters increased the levels of TGF-α mRNA and protein, suggesting a possible role for the EGFr in tumor promoter–induced cell proliferation and a possible common mechanism among some tumor promoters for induction of cell proliferation in mouse epidermis (249). Both TPA and 2,3,7,8-TCDD have been shown to induce TGF-α mRNA and protein synthesis in human keratinocytes (211,290). In addition, UVB-radiation leads to increased expression of TGF-α protein in cultured human melanocytes (291). All of these studies support a possible role of both the EGFr and TGF-α in the process of skin tumor promotion.

The ability of tumor promoters to modulate the expression of growth factors (both positive and negative) in mouse epidermis is becoming increasingly apparent (292). In addition to TGF-α (249), several laboratories (208,293) have demonstrated that promoter treatment of mouse skin leads to increased production of TGF-β mRNA and presumably, TGF-β protein. TGF-β has been shown to inhibit DNA synthesis in human and mouse keratinocytes (292–298). However, many transformed epithelial cell lines are resistant to this effect (299,300). It has also been postulated that initiated cells respond differently to growth inhibitory signals (9,24,292) such as those mediated by TGF-β or other growth regulatory molecules and that this may play a role in the selection process that takes place during tumor promotion (24, 292). Recently, combined intradermal injections of both TGF-α and TGF-β were reported to substitute for TPA in the first stage of a two-stage promotion protocol, supporting this hypothesis (297).

We have recently found in preliminary experiments that topical treatment of SENCAR mouse epidermis with TPA leads to elevated EGFr protein as shown in Fig. 4. This observation may help explain, in part, the elevated binding of [^{125}I]EGF to its membrane receptor in mouse epidermal preparations observed after

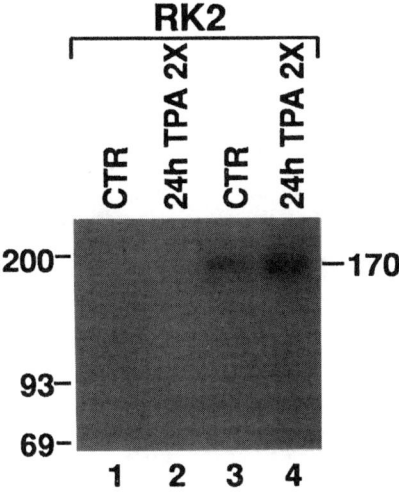

FIG. 4. Changes in EGFr levels as a result of TPA treatment *in vivo*. Groups of mice were treated with either acetone (0.2 mL) or TPA 3.4 nmol twice (Monday and Thursday) and then sacrificed 24 h later (Friday). Epidermal preparations from groups of four SENCAR mice were prepared as described previously (194) and adjusted to equal protein concentrations. Equal amounts of protein were then incubated 2 h (4°C) with protein A–Sepharose beads precoated with either *anti*-EGFr antibody (RK2) or normal rabbit serum (NRS). After incubation, the beads were washed and then 30 µL of Laemmli buffer was added to the pelleted beads followed by boiling for 4 min. Ten microliters of the denatured samples were then loaded onto 7.5% acrylamide SDS-PAGE gels. After electrophoresis, proteins were transferred to either PVDF membranes for immunoblotting. Immunoblotting was then performed using *anti*-EGFr antibodies (RK2) followed by protein B–biotin conjugate (Zymed) and then [^{125}I]streptavidin (Amersham). Immunoblots were then developed by autoradiography. Lanes 1 and 2 were from samples immunoprecipitated with NRS; lanes 3 and 4 were from samples immunoprecipitated with RK2. Lanes 1 to 4 were immunoblotted with RK2. CTR, samples from control animals treated with acetone.

several topical treatments with TPA (249). An alternative mechanism, currently being explored, involves decreased phosphorylation (especially at Thr-654) of the EGFr as a result of TPA-induced downregulation of PKC (249).

We have also obtained recent preliminary evidence suggesting that alterations in the levels of mRNA for both TGF-α and EGFr may play a role in the growth and progression of skin tumors in the mouse skin model of multistage tumorigenesis (301). In this regard, virtually all papillomas and SCCs examined to date have elevated TGF-α mRNA (see Fig. 5). The earliest papillomas examined to date were collected at 20 weeks of promotion. These data suggest that overexpression of TGF-α may be an early event in the development of autonomous growth in skin papillomas generated by initiation–promotion regimens. Examination of the levels of EGFr mRNA in papillomas and carcinomas revealed that very few of the papillomas examined to date (<25%) displayed elevated transcripts for the growth factor receptor (two positive papillomas are shown in Fig. 6). Interestingly, however, a high percentage of SCCs had elevated transcripts (>75%) for the EGFr receptor (six positive carcinomas are shown in Fig. 6). These data suggest the possibility that changes in expression of the EGFr may be associated with malignant

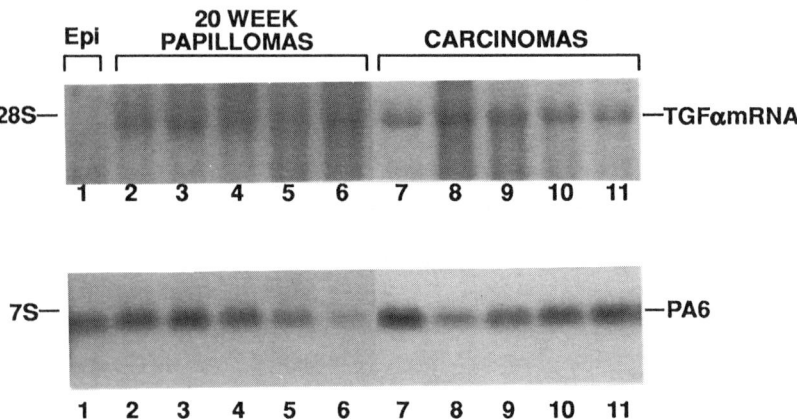

FIG. 5. TGF-α mRNA levels in normal epidermis (Epi), papillomas (20 weeks of promotion), and squamous cell carcinomas (30 to 33 weeks of promotion) generated in SENCAR mice using DMBA initiation followed by TPA (3.4 nmol) promotion. Papillomas were harvested after 20 weeks of promotion, whereas carcinomas were harvested between weeks 30 and 33 as they appeared. Total RNA (20 μg/lane) isolated as described (194) was electrophoresed in a 1% agarose–6% formaldehyde gel. The gel was soaked in 50 mM NaOH and 10 × SCC and transferred to a cationized nylon membrane. The oligonucleotide probe for human TGF-α was 5′ end-labeled with γ-[^{32}P]ATP and T4 polynucleotide kinase. The membrane was hybridized with the probe in 1.0 M NaCl, 50 mM Tris, pH 7.5, 10% dextran sulfate, 1% SDS, 100 μg/mL denatured salmon sperm DNA at 50°C for 16 h. The probe for 7S cytoplasmic RNA (PA6) was labeled using a random primed DNA labeling kit (USB). After stripping off the TGF-α probe the membrane was rehybridized with labeled PA6. After washing, the membranes were autoradiographed at −70°C. The position of transcripts for the 4.8-kb TGF-α mRNA or the 7S cytoplasmic RNA is indicated on the right-hand side of the figure.

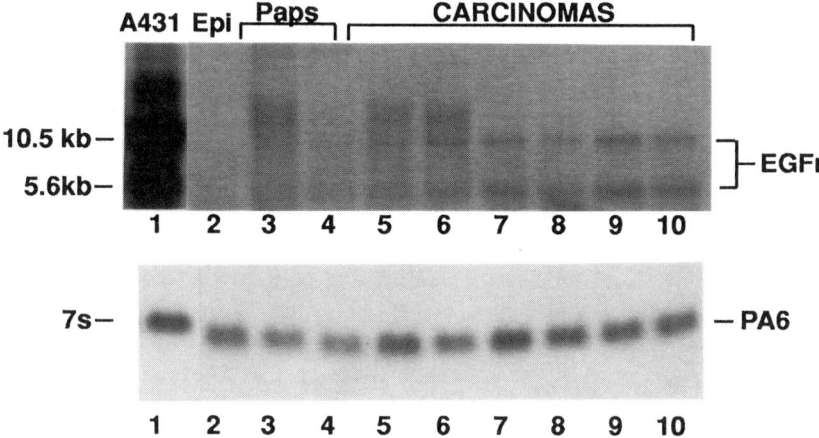

FIG. 6. EGFr mRNA levels in normal epidermis (Epi), and papillomas (20 to 22 weeks) and squamous cell carcinomas (33 and 60 weeks) generated in SENCAR mice by initiation with DMBA or BaP and promotion with either TPA or chrysarobin. Total RNA (20 μg/lane) was electrophoresed in a 1% agarose–6% formaldehyde gel. The RNA was transferred to a nitrocellulose membrane. The EGFr (PE7, ATCC) probe was random prime labeled using klenow. The membrane was hybridized with the probe in 50% formamide, 5 × Denhardt's, 5 × SSPE, 0.1% SDS, and 100 μg/mL salmon sperm DNA at 43°C for 16 h. The probe for 7S cytoplasmic RNA (PA6) was labeled as described in Fig. 5. The positions of the transcripts for the 10.5 kb and the 5.6-kb EGFr mRNA or the 7S cytoplasmic RNA are indicated on the right-hand side of the figure. Total RNA (5 μg) from A431 cells was loaded in lane 1 as a positive control.

progression in the mouse skin initiation–promotion model system. Preliminary data also indicate that at least some of the tumors that have elevated EGFr transcripts also have elevated amounts of EGFr protein. Changes in the levels (mRNA and protein) or function of TGF-α and/or the EGFr have been found in a variety of human tumors, including SCCs of the skin (302–306). The latter studies have led to the hypothesis that autocrine/paracrine stimulation plays an important role in malignant transformation. Such an autocrine/paracrine mechanism may also occur in the mouse skin model system, which is ideally suited to study its role during both the premalignant and malignant stages of carcinogenesis.

GENETIC FACTORS REGULATING SUSCEPTIBILITY TO SKIN CARCINOGENESIS

Mouse skin is generally considered most sensitive to epidermal carcinogenesis by application of either the complete carcinogenesis protocol or the initiation–promotion protocol (reviewed in refs. 17,149). Other species, such as the rat, hamster, and rabbit, are less sensitive, and the guinea pig is very resistant (reviewed in refs. 17,149). In addition to these species differences, there are marked strain differences with respect to epidermal two-stage carcinogenesis (reviewed in ref. 149). A number of studies have demonstrated that a major determinant of susceptibility to multistage skin carcinogenesis among mouse strains and between species is their susceptibility to the tumor promotion stage (17,149). Nevertheless, numerous studies have suggested a positive correlation between the level of AHH (both basal and induced) and susceptibility to tumorigenesis by PAH in several tissues and within the same tissue when comparing different mouse strains (307–313). Nebert and Gelboin (314) found that certain strains of mice could be classified as being "responsive" to induction of AHH activity in liver by PAH, whereas others were "nonresponsive." This variation in enzyme induction has been studied extensively in the mouse and has been linked to the expression of a cytosolic protein, MW 95 kDa (i.e., the Ah receptor), which is capable of binding PAH within the cell (315,316), an event postulated to result in its translocation to the nucleus, ultimately leading to the expression of a number of genes encoding cytochrome P450 (primarily the P450I family) and other enzyme activities (317,318). It was hypothesized that "responsive" strains would demonstrate increased susceptibility to PAH-induced tumorigenesis compared with equivalent "nonresponsive" animals. In general, this has been found to be the case when using complete carcinogenic regimens, but the correlation is not necessarily a strict one (319). For instance, which PAH is used as the carcinogen (307,317), the route of its administration (320), or the tissue being examined (314,321,322) may all be important determining factors. Again, there are particular strains (321) and species (323) that may be defined as being "responsive," yet they are resistant to hydrocarbon-induced tumorigenesis. In theory, such differences could have a dramatic influence on susceptibility to skin tumor initiation in mice. Legraverend et al. (320) have reported a correlation between the relative amounts of induced BaP metabolism in mouse skin microsomes and BaP-induced complete carcinogenesis in mouse skin using three inbred mouse strains. However, to date it has not been possible to establish a clear correlation between levels of tissue monooxygenase activity (basal or induced) and tumor initiation by PAH in mouse skin (324–331). This could be due to the fact that mouse epidermis constituitively expresses the major cytochrome P450 specie(s) (e.g., P450IA1) responsible for metabolic activation of PAH carcinogens to reactive diol-epoxides at levels sufficient for tumor initiation under most experimental conditions (74).

Although it is known that genetic differences exist in the enzyme systems responsible for metabolism of PAH and other skin carcinogens, the available data suggest that certain aspects of skin tumor initiation with PAH are qualitatively and quantitatively similar in mouse strains that differ in their sensitivity to epidermal carcinogenesis as noted above (reviewed in refs. 149,330,331). Additional data have led to the conclusion that the primary determinant in strain differences to epidermal chemical carcinogenesis is at the level of responsiveness to the tumor promoter (reviewed in refs. 149, 330, 331). A tentative genetic model has been developed using inbred mouse strains that are relatively sensitive (DBA/2, C3H/He) and relatively resistant (C57BL/6) to phorbol ester skin tumor promotion (143,329,332,333). This model has the following characteristics: (a) susceptibility to TPA promotion in B6D2F$_1$ and B6C3F$_1$ hybrid mice is inherited as an incomplete dominant trait; (b) neither cytoplasmic genetic determinants nor the X chromosome appear to play a major role in susceptibility of mice to phorbol ester promotion; (c) the degrees of sustained epidermal hyperplasia and DC induction after multiple TPA treatments show excellent correlation with inherited susceptibility to promotion; (d) the incidence of tumors in backcrosses between F_1 mice and TPA-resistant C57BL/6 mice, in $B6D2F_2$ and $B6C3F_2$ mice, and in BXD and BXH recombinant inbred mice can be explained by a model with a minimum of three loci (two dominant and one recessive locus) controlling TPA promotion sensitivity.

It is interesting to note that C57BL/6 mice, although relatively refractory to two-stage carcinogenesis and skin tumor promotion by TPA, are quite sensitive to complete carcinogenesis protocols with both BaP and DMBA. Bock and Burns (334) presented earlier data suggesting that C57/st mice were less sensitive to anthralin than Swiss mice initiated with the same dose of DMBA, although small numbers of animals were used in the experimental groups of this study. In further studies, CD-1 mice appeared to be less sensitive than SENCAR mice to the promoting effects of 7-bromomethylbenz[a]anthracene (41) and UV light (335). More detailed studies (336) have clearly shown that when tested under appropriate conditions, mouse stocks and strains generally show similar strain distribution patterns for sensitivity to several different classes of promoting agents. In addition, C57BL/6 mice are highly refractory to wounding as a promoting stimulus (DiGiovanni et al., submitted for publication). In contrast to these studies, Reiners et al. (329) reported that C57BL/6 mice were highly sensitive to benzoyl peroxide tumor promotion. Despite the latter inconsistency, the current body of data suggest that there may be some common genetic factors controlling responsiveness to tumor-promoting agents and by inference some common biochemical and molecular events in tumor promotion by diverse chemical and physical stimuli.

SUMMARY AND CONCLUSIONS

The mouse skin model of multistage carcinogenesis continues to serve as a major *in vivo* model for studying the sequential and stepwise evolution of the cancer process by chemical and physical carcinogens. The initiation stage of mouse skin carcinogenesis involves genetic damage in the form of DNA adducts or initiator-induced DNA base changes. These changes ultimately lead to mutations in critical target genes of epidermal stem cells. The Ha-*ras*, and to a limited extent, N-*ras* genes have been identified as target genes for certain tumor initiators in this model system. While some data exist showing the correlation between specific DNA adduct formation and mutations in the Ha-*ras* gene, sufficient data exist for only a few compounds. Further work establishing the relationship between the type of DNA damage and the point mutations observed in *ras* genes should help further substantiate this relationship. The report that tumors induced by TPA treatment alone possessed sixty-first codon Ha-*ras* mutations (114) raises questions about the mechanism(s) of mutation induction in this gene *in vivo* which must be addressed.

The promotion stage of mouse skin carcinogenesis involves the production and maintenance of a chronic state of hyperplasia and cell proliferation and ultimately, the selective clonal expansion of initiated cells. The hallmark of all tumor promoters that have been adequately tested is their ability to induce a potentiated hyperplasia after several treatments that is greater than that observed after a single application. Tumor promoters produce many effects when applied topically to mouse skin. Many of the effects that occur after a single application of phorbol esters such as TPA appear to be mediated by its interaction with PKC (194). An important question is whether the activation of PKC, *per se*, is responsible for tumor promotion by TPA. Since repetitive treatments with TPA lead to a sustained loss of PKC, it is possible that other effects, not mediated by PKC but produced by phorbol esters and related compounds, may play an important role in the production and maintenance of chronic hyperplasia and cell proliferation in the skin and for skin tumor promotion. In addition, more attention should be placed on studying the promoting actions of other compounds outside the most commonly studied phorbol esters. Investigations of some of these compounds already have and will continue to provide important clues regarding possible common pathways shared by diverse promoting agents. One such pathway may involve the EGFr and its ligand TGF-α. As discussed in this review, it is now evident that many different types of promoting agents increase production of TGF-α (211,249,290,291). Although many tumor promoters initially decrease the binding of [^{125}I]EGF to the EGFr in specific cell types, including mouse epidermal cells, the long-term effects of tumor promoters, especially after repetitive treatments, may be considerably different. Tumor promoters may ultimately lead to a sensitization of this receptor pathway (194,249) as well as other pathways regulated by PKC. Further studies to determine the role of the EGFr and possibly other growth factor–mediated pathways in tumor promoter–induced hyperplasia and cell proliferation will probably yield important insights into the overall promotion process.

Other evidence supporting some common mechanism(s) shared by diverse tumor-promoting agents comes from studies of genetic differences in response to diverse promoting stimuli. The available evidence suggests that, in general, mice less sensitive to phorbol esters are also less sensitive to other chemical classes of promoters (330,331,336). Furthermore, C57BL/6 mice, which are very resistant to phorbol ester promotion, are also very resistant to tumor promotion by full-thickness skin wounding (J. DiGiovanni, submitted for publication). Collectively, these studies support the hypothesis that tumor promotion by diverse chemical agents may mimic events occurring during the process of wound healing (24,125,126,292). Thus a major emphasis should be placed on studying the nature and mechanism(s) of wounding-induced tumor promotion in mouse skin and its similarities and differences to the mechanisms of chemical and physical promoting stimuli.

In conclusion, although no rodent carcinogenesis model system can define mechanisms for all types of cancer and cancer-causing agents, further understanding of the process in this specific epithelial model system will probably continue making significant contributions to our understanding of multistage carcinogenesis in humans.

REFERENCES

1. Boutwell RK. Some biological aspects of skin carcinogenesis. *Prog Exp Tumor Res* 1964;4: 207–250.
2. Boutwell RK. The function and mechanism of promoters of carcinogenesis. *CRC Crit Rev Toxicol* 1974;2:419–443.
3. Terracini B, Shubik P, Della Porta G. A study of skin carcinogenesis in the mouse with single applications of 910-dimethyl-12-benzathracene at different dosages. *Cancer Res* 1960;20:1538–1542.
4. Turusov V, Day N, Andrianov L, Jain D. Influence of dose on skin tumor induced in mice by single application of 7,12-dimethylbenz(a)-anthracene. *J Natl Cancer Inst* 1971;47:105–111.
5. Slaga TJ. Cellular and molecular mechanisms involved in multistage skin carcinogenesis. In: Conti CJ, Slaga TJ, Klein-Szanto AJP, eds. *Carcinogenesis*. Vol 11. *Skin tumors: experimental and clinical aspects*. New York: Raven Press; 1989:1–18.
6. Boutwell RK. The biochemistry of preneoplasia in mouse skin. *Cancer Res* 1976;36:2631–2635.
7. Scribner JD, Suss R. Tumor initiation and promotion. In: Richter GW, Epstein MA, eds. *International review of experimental pathology*. Vol 18. New York: Academic Press; 1978:137–198.
8. Brookes P, Lawley PD. Evidence for the binding of polynuclear aromatic hydrocarbons to the nucleic acids of mouse skin: relation between carcinogenic power of hydrocarbons and their binding to DNA. *Nature* 1964;202:781–784.
9. Yuspa SH, Poirier MC. Chemical carcinogenesis: from animal models to molecular models in one decade. *Adv Cancer Res* 1988;50:25–70.
10. Slaga TJ, Bowden GT, Shapas BG, Boutwell RK. Macromolecular synthesis following a single application of alkylating agents used as initiators of mouse skin tumorigenesis. *Cancer Res* 1973; 33:769–776.
11. Slaga TJ, Bowden GT, Shapas BG, Boutwell RK. Macromolecular synthesis following a single application of polycyclic hydrocarbons used as initiators of mouse skin tumorigenesis. *Cancer Res* 1974;34:771–777.
12. Berenblum I, Shubik P. The persistence of latent tumor cells induced the mouse's skin by a single application of 910-dimethyl-12-benzanthracene. *Br J Cancer* 1949;3:384–386.
13. Roe FJC, Carter RL, Mitchley BCV, Peto R, Hecker E. On the persistence of tumour initiation and the acceleration of tumour progression in mouse skin tumorigenesis. *J Cancer* 1972;9:264–273.
14. Van Duuren BL, Sivak A, Katz C, Seidman I, Melchionne S. The effect of aging and interval between primary and secondary treatment in two-stage carcinogenesis on mouse skin. *Cancer Res* 1975;35:502–505.
15. Loehrke H, Schweizer J, Dederer E, Hess B, Rosenkranz G, Goerttler K. On the persistence of tumor initiation in two-stage carcinogenesis on mouse skin. *Carcinogenesis* 1983;6:771–775.
16. Potten CS. Stem cells in epidermis from the back of the mouse. In: Potten CS, ed. *Stem cells: their identification and characterization*. New York: Churchill Livingstone; 1983:200–232.
17. Slaga TJ, Fischer SM. Strain differences and solvent effects in mouse skin carcinogenesis experiments using carcinogens tumor initiators and promoters. *Prog Exp Tumor Res* 1983;26:85–109.
18. Argyris TS. Epidermal growth following a single application of 12-O-tetradecanoylphorbol-13-acetate in mice. *Am J Pathol* 1980;639–646.
19. Argyris TS. The regulation of epidermal hyperplastic growth. *CRC Crit Rev Toxicol* 1981;19:151–200.
20. Klein-Szanto AJP. Morphological evaluation of tumor promoter effects on mammalian skin. In: Slaga TJ, ed. *Mechanisms of tumor promotion*. Vol 2. *Tumor promotion and skin carcinogenesis*. Boca Raton, FL: CRC Press; 1984:42–72.
21. Aldaz CM, Conti CJ, Gimenez IB, Slaga TJ, Klein-Szanto AJP. Cutaneous changes during prolonged application of 12-O-tetradecanoylphorbol-13-acetate on mouse skin and residual effects after cessation of treatment. *Cancer Res* 1985;45:2753–2759.
22. Fürstenberger G, Sorg B, Marks F. Tumor promotion by phorbol esters in skin: evidence for a memory effect. *Science* 1983;220:89–91.
23. Fürstenberger G, Kinzel V, Schwarz M, Marks F. Partial inversion of the initiation-promotion sequence of multistage tumorigenesis in the skin of NMRI mice. *Science* 1985;230:76–78.
24. Parkinson EK. Defective responses of transformed keratinocytes to terminal differentiation stimuli. Their role in epidermal tumour promotion by phorbol esters and by deep skin wounding. *Br J Cancer* 1985;52:479–493.

25. Petrusevska RT, Fürstenberger G, Marks F, Fusenig NE. Cytogenetic effects caused by phorbol ester tumor promoters in primary mouse keratinocytes: correlation with the convertogenic activity of TPA in multistage skin carcinogenesis. *Carcinogenesis* 1988;9:1207–1215.
26. Fürstenberger G, Schurich B, Kaina B, Petrusevska RT, Fusenig NE, Marks F. Tumor induction in initiated mouse skin by phorbol esters and methyl methane sulfonate: correlation between chromosomal damage and conversion stage I of tumor promotion *in vivo*. *Carcinogenesis* 1989;10:749–752.
27. Cerutti PA. Prooxidant states and tumor promotion. *Science* 1985;227:375–381.
28. Kensler TW, Taffe BG. Free radicals in tumor promotion. *Adv Free Radical Biol Med* 1986;2:347–387.
29. Perchellet J-P, Perchellet EM. Phorbol ester tumor promoters and multistage skin carcinogenesis In: *Atlas of science pharmacology*. Philadelphia: ISI; 1988:325–333.
30. Ewing MW, Crysup SE, Phillips JL, Slaga TJ, DiGiovanni J. Enhancement of mezerein-promoted papilloma formation by treatment with 12-*O*-tetradecanoylphorbol-13-acetate or mezerein prior to initiation. *Carcinogenesis* 1989;405–410.
31. Slaga TJ, Fischer SM, Nelson K, Gleason GL. Studies on the mechanism of skin tumor promotion: evidence for several stages in promotion. *Proc Natl Acad Sci USA* 1980;77:3659–3663.
32. Slaga TJ, Klein-Szanto AJP, Fischer SM, Weeks CE, Nelson K, Major S. Studies on mechanism of action of *anti*-tumor-promoting agents: their specificity in two-stage promotion. *Proc Natl Acad Sci USA* 1980;77:2251–2254.
33. Fürstenberger G, Berry DL, Sorg B, Marks F. Skin tumor promotion by phorbol esters is a two-stage process. *Proc Natl Acad Sci USA* 1981;78:7722–7726.
34. Ordman AB, Cleaveland JS, Boutwell RK. Tetradecanoyl-phorbol-13-acetate promotes tumors prior to initiation in two-stage promotion. *Cancer Lett* 1985;29:79–84.
35. Marks F, Fürstenberger G. The conversion stage of skin carcinogenesis. *Carcinogenesis* 1990;11:2085–2092.
36. Klein-Szanto AJP. Pathology of human and experimental skin tumors. In: Conti CJ, Slaga TJ, Klein-Szanto AJP, eds. *Carcinogenesis*. Vol II. *Skin tumors: experimental and clinical aspects*. New York: Raven Press; 1989:19–53.
37. Shubik P, Baserga R, Ritchie AC. The life and progression of induced skin tumors in mice. *Br J Cancer* 1953;7:342–351.
38. Burns FJ, Vanderlaan M, Sivak A, Albert RE. Regression kinetics of mouse skin papillomas. *Cancer Res* 1976;36:1422–1427.
39. Burns FJ, Vanderlaan M, Snyder B, Albert RE. Induction and progression kinetics of mouse skin papillomas In: Slaga TJ, Sivak A, Boutwell RK, eds. *Carcinogenesis*. Vol 2. *Mechanisms of tumor promotion and cocarcinogenesis*. New York: Raven Press; 1978:91–96.
40. Verma AK, Boutwell RK. Effects of dose and duration of treatment with the tumor-promoting agent 12-*O*-tetradecanoylphorbol-13-acetate on mouse skin carcinogenesis. *Carcinogenesis* 1980;1:271–276.
41. Scribner JD, Scribner NK, McKnight B, Mottet NK. Evidence for a new model of tumor progression from carcinogenesis and tumor promotion studies with 7-bromomethylbenz(*a*)anthracene. *Cancer Res* 1983;43:2034–2041.
42. Hennings H, Shores R, Mitchell P, Spangler EF, Yuspa SH. Induction of papillomas with a high probability of conversion to malignancy. *Carcinogenesis* 1985;6:1607–1610.
43. Reddy AL, Caldwell M, Fialkow PJ. Studies of skin tumorigenesis in PGK mosaic mice: many promoter-independent papillomas and carcinomas do not develop from pre-existing promoter-dependent papillomas. *Int J Cancer* 1987;39:261–265.
44. Aldaz CM, Conti CJ, Klein-Szanto AJP, Slaga TJ. Progressive dysplasia and aneuploidy are hallmarks of mouse skin papillomas: relevance to malignancy. *Proc Natl Acad Sci USA* 1987;84:2029–2032.
45. Ewing MW, Conti CJ, Kruszewski FH, Slaga TJ, DiGiovanni J. Tumor progression in SENCAR mouse skin as a function of initiator dose and promoter dose duration and type. *Cancer Res* 1988;48:7048–7054.
46. Ewing MW, Conti CJ, Phillips JL, Slaga TJ, DiGiovanni J. Further characterization of skin tumor promotion and progression by mezerin in SENCAR mice. *J Natl Cancer Inst* 1989;81:676–682.
47. Aldaz CM, Conti CJ, Chen A, Bianchi A, Walker SB, DiGiovanni J. Promoter independence as a feature of most skin papillomas in SENCAR mice. *Cancer Res* 1991;51:1045–1050.
48. Aldaz CM, Conti CJ. The premalignant nature of mouse skin papillomas: Histopathologic cytogenetic and biochemical evidence. In: Conti CJ, Slaga TJ, Klein-Szanto AJP, eds. *Carcinogen-*

esis. Vol II. *Skin tumors: experimental and clinical aspects.* New York: Raven Press; 1989:227–242.
49. Burns FJ, Albert RE, Altschuler B. Cancer progression in mouse skin. In: Slaga TJ, ed. *Mechanisms of tumor promotion.* Vol 2. *Tumor promotion and skin carcinogenesis.* Boca Raton, FL: CRC Press; 1984:17–29.
50. Hennings H, Shores R, Wenk ML, Spangler EF, Tarone ML, Yuspa SH. Malignant conversion of mouse skin tumors is increased by tumor initiators and unaffected by tumor promoters. *Nature* 1983;304:67–69.
51. O'Connell JF, Klein-Szanto AJP, DiGiovanni DM, Fries JW, Slaga TJ. Malignant progression of mouse skin papillomas treated with ethylnitrosourea N-methyl-N'-nitro-N-soguanidine or 12-O-tetradecanoylphorbol-13-acetate. *Cancer Lett* 1986;30:269–274.
52. Aldaz CM, Trono D, Larcher F, Slaga TJ, Conti CJ. Sequential trisomization of chromosomes 6 and 7 in mouse skin premalignant lesions. *Mol Carcinog* 1989;2:22–26.
53. Brenner R, Balmain A. Genetic changes in skin tumor progression: correlation between presence of a mutant *ras* gene and loss of heterozygosity on mouse chromosome 7. *Cell* 1990;61:407–417.
54. Bianchi AB, Aldaz CM, Conti CJ. Nonrandom duplication of the chromosome bearing a mutated Ha-*ras*-1 allele in mouse skin tumors *Proc Natl Acad Sci USA* 1990;87:6902–6906.
55. Bianchi AB, Navone NM, Aldaz CM, Conti CJ. Overlapping loss of heterozygosity by mitotic recombination on mouse chromosome 7F1-ter in skin carcinogenesis. *Proc Natl Acad Sci USA* 1991;88:7590–7594.
56. Berkelhammer J, Oxenhandler RW. Evaluation of premalignant and malignant lesions during the induction of mouse melanomas. *Cancer Res* 1987;47:1251–1254.
57. Husain Z, Pathak MA, Flotte T, Wick MM. Role of ultraviolet radiation in the induction of melanocytic tumors in hairless mice following 7,12-dimethylbenz[a]anthracene application and ultraviolet irradiation. *Cancer Res* 1991;51:4964–4970.
58. Jaffe D, Bowden GT. Ionizing radiation as an initiator: effects of proliferation and promotion time on tumor incidence in mice. *Cancer Res* 1987;47:6692–6696.
59. Monks TJ, Walker SE, Flynn LM, Conti CJ, DiGiovanni J. Epidermal ornithine decarboxylase induction and mouse skin tumor promotion by quinones. *Carcinogenesis* 1990;11:1795–1801.
60. O'Connell JF, Klein-Szanto AJP, DiGiovanni DM, Fries JW, Slaga TJ. Enhanced malignant progression of mouse skin tumors by the free-radical generator benzoyl peroxide. *Cancer Res* 1986; 46:2863–2865.
61. Pereira MA. Skin tumorigenesis research data base. *J Am Coll Toxicol* 1982;1:47–82.
62. Slaga TJ, Nesnow S. SENCAR mouse skin tumorigenesis. In: Milman HA, Weisburger EK, eds. *Handbook of carcinogen testing.* Park Ridge, NJ: Noyes Publications; 1985:230–250.
63. Gelboin HV, Ts'o POP, eds. *Polycyclic aromatic hydrocarbons and cancer.* Vols 1 and 2. New York: Academic Press; 1978.
64. Nesnow S, Triplett LL, Slaga TJ. Tumorigenesis of diesel exhaust gasoline exhaust and related emission extracts on SENCAR mouse skin. In: Waters MD, Sandhu SS, Huisingh JL, Claxton L, Nesnow S, eds. *Short-term bioassays in the analysis of complex environmental mixtures II.* New York: Plenum Press; 1981:277–297.
65. Slaga TJ, Fischer SM, Triplet LL, Nesnow S. Comparison of complete carcinogenesis and tumor initiation and promotion in mouse skin: the induction of papillomas by tumor initiation–promotion a reliable short term assay. *J Am Coll Toxicol* 1982;1:83–100.
66. Miller EC. Some current perspectives on chemical carcinogenesis in humans and experimental animals: presidential address. *Cancer Res* 1978;38:1479–1496.
67. Beland FA, Poirier MC. DNA adducts and carcinogenesis. In: Sirica AE, ed. *The pathobiology of neoplasia.* New York: Plenum Press; 1989:57–80.
68. Cooper CS, Grover PL, eds. *Handbook of experimental pharmacology.* Vol 94/I. *Chemical carcinogenesis and mutagenesis.* Berlin: Springer-Verlag, 1990.
69. Gelboin HV. Benzo[a]pyrene metabolism activation and carcinogenesis: role and regulation of mixed-function oxidases and related enzymes. *Physiol Rev* 1980;60:1107–1165.
70. Pelkonen O, Nebert DW. Metabolism of polycyclic aromatic hydrocarbons: etiologic role in carcinogenesis. *Pharmacol Rev* 1982;34:189–222.
71. Dipple A, Moschel RC, Bigger CAH. Polynuclear aromatic carcinogens. In: Searle CE, ed. *Chemical carcinogens,* 2nd ed, vol 1. Washington, DC: American Chemical Society; 1984:41–163.
72. Hall M, Grover PL. Polycyclic aromatic hydrocarbons: metabolism activation and tumour initiation. In: Cooper CS, Grover PL, eds. *Handbook of experimental pharmacology.* Vol 94/I. *Chemical carcinogenesis and mutagenesis.* Berlin: Springer-Verlag; 1990:327–372.

73. Baird WM, Pruess-Schwartz D. Polycyclic aromatic hydrocarbon-DNA adducts and their analysis: a powerful technique for characterization of pathways of metabolic activation of hydrocarbons to ultimate carcinogenic metabolites. In: Yang SK, Silverman BD, eds. *Polycyclic aromatic hydrocarbon carcinogenesis: Structure–activity relationships.* Vol II. Boca Raton, FL: CRC Press; 1988:141–179.
74. DiGiovanni J. Metabolism of polycyclic aromatic hydrocarbons and phorbol esters by mouse skin: relevance to mechanism of action and trans-species/strain carcinogenesis In: Slaga TJ, Klein-Szanto AJP, Boutwell RK, Stevenson DE, Spitzer HL, D'Motto B, eds. *Progress in clinical and biological research.* Vol 298. *Skin carcinogenesis: mechanisms and human relevance.* New York: Alan R Liss; 1989:167–199.
75. Heidelberger C. Chemical carcinogenesis. *Annu Rev Biochem* 1975;44:79–121.
76. Slaga TJ, Fischer SM, Weeks CE, Klein-Szanto AJP, Reiners J. Studies on the mechanisms involved in multistage carcinogenesis in mouse skin. *J Cell Biol* 1982;18:99–119.
77. Ivanovic V, Geacintov NE, Yamasaki H, Weinstein IB. DNA and RNA adducts formed in hamster embryo cell cultures exposed to benzo[a]pyrene. *Biochemistry* 1978;17:1597–1603.
78. Ashurst SW, Cohen GM. *In vivo* formation of benzo[a]pyrene diol-epoxide deoxyadenosine adducts in the skin of mice susceptible to benzo[a]pyrene-induced carcinogenesis. *Int J Cancer* 1981;27:357–364.
79. Ashurst SW, Cohen GM. The formation and persistence of benzo[a]pyrene metabolite-deoxyribonucleoside adducts in rat skin *in vivo. Int J Cancer* 1981;28:387–392.
80. Ashurst SW, Cohen GM, Nesnow S, DiGiovanni J, Slaga TJ. Formation of benzo[a]pyrene/DNA adducts and their relationship to tumor initiation in mouse epidermis. *Cancer Res* 1983;43:1024–1029.
81. DiGiovanni J, Decina PC, Prichett WP, Fisher EP, Aalfs KK. Formation and disappearance of benzo[a]pyrene DNA-adducts in mouse epidermis. *Carcinogenesis* 1985;6:741–747.
82. Sims P. Chemical carcinogenesis. *Br Med Bull* 1980;36:11–18.
83. Straub KM, Meehan T, Burlingname AL, Calvin M. Identification of the major adducts formed by reaction of benzo[a]pyrene diolepoxide with DNA *in vitro. Proc Natl Acad Sci USA* 1977;74:5285–5289.
84. Osborne MR, Harvey RG, Brookes P. The reaction of *trans*-7,8-dihydroxy-*anti*-9,10-epoxy-7,8,9,10-tetrahydrobenzo[a]pyrene with DNA involves attack at the N^7-position of guanine moieties. *Chem Biol Interact* 1978;20:123–130.
85. Meehan T, Straub K, Calvin M. Benzo[a]pyrene diol-epoxide covalently binds deoxyguanosine and deoxyadenosine in DNA. *Nature* 1977;269:725–727.
86. Meehan T, Straub K. Double-stranded DNA stereoselectively binds benzo[a]pyrene diol-epoxides. *Nature* 1979;277:410–412.
87. Osborne MR, Jacobs S, Harvey RG, Brookes P. Minor products from the reaction of + and − benzo[a]pyrene-*anti*-diolepoxide with DNA. *Carcinogenesis* 1981;2:553–558.
88. DiGiovanni J, Sawyer TW, Fisher EP. Correlation between formation of a specific hydrocarbon-deoxyribonucleoside adduct and tumor-initiating activity of 7,12-dimethylbenz[a]anthracene and its 9- and 10-monofluoroderivatives in mice. *Cancer Res* 1986;46:4336–4341.
89. Huberman E, Barr SH, eds. *The role of chemicals and radiation in the etiology of cancer carcinogenesis: a comprehensive survey.* Vol 10. New York: Raven Press; 1985.
90. Cooper CS, Grover PL, eds. *Handbook of experimental pharmacology.* Vol 94/II. *Chemical carcinogenesis and mutagenesis.* Berlin: Springer-Verlag; 1990.
91. Klein G, Klein E. Oncogene activation and tumor progression. *Carcinogenesis* 1984;5:429–435.
92. Balmain A. Transforming *ras* oncogenes and multistage carcinogenesis *Br J Cancer* 1985;51:1–7.
93. Weinberg RA. The action of oncogenes in the cytoplasm and nucleus. *Science* 1985;230:770–776.
94. Barbacid M. *Ras* genes. *Annu Rev Biochem* 1987;56:779–827.
95. Guerrero I, Pellicer A. Mutational activation of oncogenes in animal model systems of carcinogenesis. *Mutat Res* 1987;185:293–308.
96. Balmain A, Brown K. Oncogene activation in chemical carcinogenesis. *Adv Cancer Res* 1988;51:147–182.
97. Balmain A, Ramsden M, Bowden GT, Smith J. Stages of carcinogenesis: activation of the mouse cellular Harvey-*ras* gene in chemically induced benign skin papillomas. *Nature* 1984;307:658–660.
98. Roop DR, Lowy DR, Tambourin PE, et al. An activated Harvey *ras* oncogene produces benign tumours on mouse epidermal tissue. *Nature* 1986;323:822–824.
99. Brown K, Quintanilla M, Ramsden M, Kerr IB, Young S, Balmain A. V-*ras* genes from Harvey

and BALB murine sarcoma viruses can act as initiators of two-stage mouse skin carcinogenesis. *Cell* 1986;46:447–456.
100. Bailleul B, Surani MA, White S, et al. Skin hyperkeratosis and papilloma formation in transgenic mice expressing a *ras* oncogene from a suprabasal keratin promoter. *Cell* 1990;62:697–708.
101. Balmain A. Molecular events associated with tumor initiation promotion and progression in mouse skin. In: Graf T, Kahn P, eds. *Oncogenes and growth control*. Heidelberg: Springer-Verlag; 1986:115–135.
102. Quintanilla M, Brown K, Ramsden M, Balmain A. Carcinogen-specific mutation and amplification of Ha-*ras* during mouse skin carcinogenesis. *Nature* 1986;322:78–80.
103. Bizub D, Wood AW, Skalka AM. Mutagenesis of the Ha-*ras* oncogene in mouse skin tumor induced by polyclic aromatic hydrocarbons. *Proc Natl Acad Sci USA* 1986;83:6048–6052.
104. Cooper CS. The role of oncogene activation in chemical carcinogenesis. In: Cooper CS, Grover PL, eds. *Handbook of experimental pharmacology*. Vol 94/II. *Chemical Carcinogenesis and Mutagenesis*. Berlin: Springer-Verlag; 1990:319–352.
105. Bonham K, Embry T, Gibson D, Jaffe DR, Roberts RA, Cress AE, Bowden GT. Activation of the cellular Harvey *ras* gene in mouse skin tumors initiated with urethane. *Mol Carcinog* 1989;2:34–39.
106. Brown K, Buchmann A, Balmain A. Carcinogen-induced mutations in the mouse c-Ha-*ras* gene provide evidence of multiple pathways for tumor progression. *Proc Natl Acad Sci USA* 1990;87:538–542.
107. Zarbl H, Sukumar S, Arthur AV, Martin-Zanca D, Barbacid M. Direct mutagenesis of Ha-*ras*-1 oncogene by *N*-nitroso-*N*-methylurea during initiation of mammary carcinogenesis in rats. *Nature* 1985;315:382–385.
108. Barbacid M. Oncogenes mutagens and cancer. *Proc Am Assoc Cancer Res* 1986;27:435.
109. Nair RV, Gill RD, Nettikumara AN, Baer-Dubowska W, Cortez C, Harvey RG, DiGiovanni J. Characterization of covalently modified deoxyribonucleosides formed from dibenz[*aj*]anthracene in primary cultures of mouse keratinocytes. *Chem Res Toxicol* 1991;4:115–122.
110. DiGiovanni J, Gill RD, Nettikumara AN, Koostra A. Analysis of point mutations in Ha-*ras* of skin papillomas produced by initiation with dibenz[*aj*]anthracene DB[*aj*]A and its 714-dimethyl-derivative. *Proc Am Assoc Cancer Res* 1991;32:135.
111. Gill RD, Beltrán L, Nettikumara AN, Harvey RG, Kootstra A, DiGiovanni J. Analysis of point mutations in murine c-Ha-*ras* of skin tumors initiated with dibenz[*aj*]anthracene and derivatives. *Mol Carcinog* 1992;6:53–59.
112. Peltonen K, Cheng SC, Hilton BD. Effect of bay region methyl group on reactions of *anti*-benz[*a*]anthracene-3,4-dihydrodiol 1,2-epoxides with DNA. *J Org Chem* 1991;56:4181–4188.
113. Bigger CAH, Flickinger DJ, St John J, Harvey RG, Dipple A. Preferential mutagenesis at G-C base pairs by the *anti* 3,4-dihydrodiol 1,2-epoxide of 7-methylbenz[*a*]anthracene. *Mol Carcinog* 1991;4:176–179.
114. Pelling JC, Neades R, Strawhecker J. Epidermal papillomas and carcinomas induced in uninitiated mouse skin by tumor promoters alone contain a point mutation in the 61st codon of the Ha-*ras* oncogene. *Carcinogenesis* 1988;9:665–667.
115. Greenhalgh DA, Welty DJ, Srickland JE, Yuspa SH. Spontaneous Ha-*ras* gene activation in cultured primary murine keratinocytes: consequences of Ha-*ras* gene activation in malignant conversion progression. *Mol Carcinog* 1989;2:199–207.
116. Quintanilla M, Haddow S, Jonas D, Jaffe D, Bowden GT, Balmain A. Comparison of *ras* activation during epidermal carcinogenesis *in vitro* and *in vivo*. *Carcinogenesis* 1991;12:1875–1881.
117. Hecker E. Isolation and characterization of the cocarcinogenic principles from croton oil. In: Busch H, ed. *Methods in Cancer Research*. Vol 6. New York: Academic Press; 1971:439–484.
118. Hecker E. Structure–activity relationships in diterpene esters irritant and cocarcinogenic to mouse skin. In: Slaga TJ, Sivak A, Boutwell RK, eds. *Carcinogenesis*. Vol 2. *Mechanisms of tumor promotion and cocarcinogenesis*. New York: Raven Press; 1978:11–18.
119. Verma AK, Lowe NJ, Boutwell RK. Induction of mouse epidermal ornithine decarboxylase activity and DNA synthesis by ultraviolet light. *Cancer Res* 1979;39:1035–1040.
120. Lowe N, Verma AK, Boutwell RK. Ultraviolet light induces epidermal ornithine decarboxylase activity. *J Invest Dermatol* 1978;71:417–418.
121. Pullinger BD. A measure of the stimulating effect of simple injury combined with carcinogenic chemicals on tumor formation in mice. *J Pathol Bacteriol* 1945;57:477–481.
122. Hennings H, Boutwell RK. Studies on the mechanism of skin tumor promotion. *Cancer Res* 1970;30:312–320.

123. Clark-Lewis I, Murray AW. Tumor promotion and the induction of epidermal ornithine decarboxylase activity in mechanically stimulated mouse skin. *Cancer Res* 1978;38:494–497.
124. Argyris TS. Tumor promotion by abrasion induced epidermal hyperplasia in the skin of mice. *J Invest Dermatol* 1980;75:360–362.
125. Argyris TS. Regeneration and the mechanism of epidermal tumor promotion. *CRC Crit Rev Toxicol* 1985;14:211–258.
126. Argyris TS. Epidermal tumor promotion by damage in the skin of mice. In: Slaga TJ, Klein-Szanto AJP, Boutwell RK, Stevenson DE, Spitzer HL, D'Motto B, eds. *Progress in clinical and biological research*. Vol 298. *Skin carcinogenesis. Mechanisms and human relevance*. New York: Alan R Liss; 1989:63–80.
127. Bhatt TS, Coombs M, O'Neil C. Biogenic silica fibre promotes carcinogenesis in mouse skin. *Int J Cancer* 1984;4:519-528.
128. Bhatt TS, Beltran LM, Walker SE, DiGiovanni J. Induction of epidermal ornithine decarboxylase activity in mouse skin exposed to biogenic silica fibers. *Carcinogenesis* 1992;13:617–620.
129. Stenback F, Garcia H, Shubik P. Present status of the concept of promoting action of cocarcinogenesis in skin. In: Shubik P, ed. *The physiopathology of cancer biology and biochemistry*. Basel: S Karger; 1974:155–225.
130. Raick AN. Ultrastructural histological and biochemical alterations produced by 12-O-tetradecanoylphorbol-13-acetate on mouse epidermis and their relevance to skin tumor promotion. *Cancer Res* 1973;33:269–286.
131. Klein-Szanto AJP, Major SK, Slaga TJ. Induction of dark keratinocytes by 12-O-tetradecanolyphorbol-13-acetate and mezerein as an indicator of tumor-promoting efficiency. *Carcinogenesis* 1980;1:399–406.
132. Klein-Szanto AJP, Slaga TJ. Numerical variation of dark cells in normal and chemically induced hyperplastic epidermis with age of animal and efficiency of tumor promoter. *Cancer Res* 1981;41:4437–4440.
133. Raick AN, Burdzy K. Ultrastructural and biochemical changes induced in mouse epidermis by a hyperplastic agent ethylphenylpropiolate. *Cancer Res* 1973;3:2221–2230.
134. Slaga TJ, Klein-Szanto AJP. Initiation–promotion versus complete skin carcinogenesis in mice: importance of dark basal keratinocytes stem cells. *Cancer Invest* 1983;5:425–436.
135. Slaga TJ. Mechanisms involved in multistage skin tumorigenesis. In: Huberman E, Barr SH, eds. *Carcinogenesis*. Vol 10. *The role of chemicals and radiation in the etiology of cancer*. New York: Raven Press; 1985:189–199.
136. Parsons DF, Marko M, Bruan SJ, Wansor KJ. "Dark cells" in normal hyperplastic and promoter-treated mouse epidermis studied by conventional and high-voltage electron microscopy. *J Invest Dermatol* 1983;81:62–67.
137. Glaso M, Ree K, Iversen OH, Hovig T. The influence of different fixatives and a tumor promoter 12-O-tetradecanoyl-phorbol-13-acetate TPA on the induction of so-called dark cells in mouse epidermis. A light microscopical study. *Virchows Arch B Cell Pathol*. 1986;50:355–372.
138. Glaso M, Iversen OH, Hovig T. The influence of fixation on the relative amount of cytoplasmic ribosomes in mouse epidermal basal keratinocytes. A morphometric study of so-called "dark cells" and their putative role in epidermal carcinogenesis. *Virchows Arch B Cell Pathol* 1989;56:221–235.
139. Glaso M, Hovig T. The influence of fixation on the morphology of mouse epidermis. A light and electron microscopical study with special reference to "dark cells" and epidermal carcinogenesis. *Virchows Arch B Cell Pathol* 1987;54:73–88.
140. Glaso M, Haskjold E. The morphology of the denuded epidermal basal cell layer of the hairless mouse after different preparation methods a scanning and transmission electron microscopical study. *Virchows Arch B Cell Pathol* 1989;57:181–194.
141. Glaso M, Wetteland P. Morphometric evaluation of the changes affecting the basal keratinocytes in hairless mouse epidermis during early 2-stage chemical carcinogenesis and after two different fixation methods. *APMIS* 1990;98:695–712.
142. Murakami Y, Hibino T, Arai M, Kuroki T. Appearance of dark keratinocytes following intracutaneous injection of cholera toxin in mouse skin. *J Invest Dermatol* 1985;85:115–117.
143. Naito M, Chenicek KJ, Naito Y, DiGiovanni J. Susceptibility to phorbol ester skin tumor promotion in C57BL/6 x DBA/2 F1 mice is inherited as an incomplete dominant trait: evidence for multilocus involvement. *Carcinogenesis* 1988;4:639–645.
144. Chiba M, Slaga TJ, Klein-Szanto AJP. A morphometric study of dedifferentiated and involutional dark keratinocytes in 12-O-tetradecanolyphorbol-13-acetate-treated mouse epidermis. *Cancer Res* 1984;44:2711–2717.

145. Bach H, Goerttler K. Morphologische Untersuchungen zur hyper-plasiogenen Wirkung des biologisch aktiven Phorbol Esters $_A$1. *Virchows Arch* 1971;8:196–205.
146. Balmain A. The synthesis of specific proteins in adult mouse epidermis during phases of proliferation and differentiation induced by the tumor promoter TPA and in basal and differentiating layers of neonatal mouse epidermis. *J Invest Dermatol* 1976;67:243–253.
147. Raick AN. Late ultractructural changes induced by 12-O-tetradecanoylphorbol-13-acetate in mouse epidermis and their reversal. *Cancer Res* 1973;33:1096–1103.
148. Sisskin EE, Gray T, Barret JC. Correlation between sensitivity to tumor promotion and sustained epidermal hyperplasia of mice and rats treated with 12-O-tetradecanoylphorbol-13-acetate. *Carcinogenesis* 1982;3:403–407.
149. Naito M, DiGiovanni J. Genetic background and development of skin tumors. In: Conti CJ, Slaga TJ, Klein-Szanto AJP, eds. *Carcinogenesis*. Vol III. *Skin tumors: experimental and clinical aspects*. New York: Raven Press; 1989:187–212.
150. Kruszewski FH, Naito M, Naito Y, DiGiovanni J. Histologic alterations produced by chrysarobin 18-dihydroxy-3-methyl-9-anthrone in SENCAR mouse skin: relationships to skin tumor promoting activity. *J Invest Dermatol* 1989;92:64–71.
151. Naito M, Naito Y, DiGiovanni J. Comparison of the histological changes in the skin of DBA/2 and C57BL/6 mice following exposure to various promoting agents. *Carcinogenesis* 1987;8:1807–1815.
152. Slaga TJ, Bowden GT, Boutwell RK. Acetic acid a potent stimulator of mouse epidermal macromolecular synthesis and hyperplasia but with weak tumor-promoting ability. *J Natl Cancer Inst* 1975;55:983–987.
153. Slaga TJ. Multistage skin tumor promotion and specificity of inhibition. In: Slaga TJ, ed. *Mechanisms of tumor promotion: tumor promotion and skin carcinogenesis*. Boca Raton, FL: CRC Press; 1984:189–196.
154. Mufson RA, Fischer SM, Verma AK, Gleason GL, Slaga TJ, Boutwell RK. Effects of 12-O-tetradecanoylphorbol-13-acetate and mezerein on epidermal ornithine decarboxylase activity isoproterenol-stimulated levels of cyclic adenosime 3:5-monophosphate and induction of mouse skin tumors. *Cancer Res* 1979;39:4791–4798.
155. Argyris TS. Nature of epidermal hyperplasia produced by mezerein a weak tumor promoter in initiated skin of mice. *Cancer Res* 1983;43:1768–1773.
156. Argyris TS. An analysis of the epidermal hyperplasia produced by acetic acid a weak tumor promoter in the skin of female mice initiated with dimethylbenzanthracene. *J Invest Dermatol* 1983;80:430–435.
157. Baxter CS, Andringa A, Chalfin K, Miller ML. Comparative histomorphometric changes in SENCAR mouse epidermis in response to multiple treatments with complete and stage-specific tumor promoting agents. *Carcinogenesis* 1989;10:1855–1861.
158. Kruszewski FH, Conti CJ, DiGiovanni J. Characterization of skin tumor promotion and progression by chrysarobin in SENCAR mice. *Cancer Res* 1987;47:3783–3790.
159. Cameron GS, Baldwin JK, Klann RC, Patrick KE, Fischer SM. Tumor-promoting activity of ethyl phenylpropiolate. *Cancer Res* 1991;51:5642–5648.
160. Paul D, Hecker E. On the biochemical mechanism of tumorigenesis in mouse skin. II. Early effects on the biosynthesis of nucleic acids induced by initiating doses of DMBA and by promoting doses of phorbol-1213-diester TPA. *Z Krebsforsch* 1969;73:149–163.
161. Baird WM, Sedgwick JA, Boutwell RK. Effects of phorbol and four diesters of phorbol on the incorporation of tritiated precursors into DNA RNA and protein in mouse epidermis. *Cancer Res* 1971;31:1434–1439.
162. Rohrschneider LR, O'Brien DH, Boutwell RK. The stimulation of phospholipid metabolism in mouse skin following phorbol ester treatment. *Biochim Biophys Acta* 1972;280:57–70.
163. Suss R, Kinzel V, Kreibich G. Cocarcinogeneic croton oil factor A_1 stimulates lipid synthesis in cell cultures. *Experientia* 1971;27:46–47.
164. Balmain A, Hecker E. On the biochemical mechanism of tumorigenesis in mouse skin. VI. Early effects of growth-stimulating phorbol esters on phosphate transport and phospholipid synthesis in mouse epidermis. *Biochim Biophys Acta* 1974;62:457–468.
165. Verma AK, Ashendel CL, Boutwell RK. Inhibition by protaglandin synthesis inhibitors of the induction of epidermal ornithine decarboxylase activity the accumulation of prostaglandins and tumor promotion caused by 12-O-tetradecanoylphorbol-13-acetate. *Cancer Res* 1980;40:308–315.
166. Fürstenberger G, Marks F. Early prostaglandin E synthesis is an obligatory event in the induction of cell proliferation in mouse epidermis *in vivo* by the phorbol ester TPA. *Biochem Biophys Res Commun* 1980;42:749–756.

167. Marks F, Bertsch S, Grimm W, Schweizer J. Hyperplastic transformation and tumor promotion in mouse epidermis: possible consequences of disturbances of endogenous mechanisms controlling proliferation and differentiation. In: Slaga TJ, Sivak A, Boutwell RK, eds. *Carcinogenesis*. Vol 2. *mechanisms of tumor promotion and cocarcinogenesis*. New York: Raven Press; 1978:97–116.
168. Marks F. Epidermal growth control mechanisms hyperplasia and tumor promotion in the skin. *Cancer Res* 1976;36:2636–2643.
169. Marks F, Grimm W. Diurnal fluctuation and β-adrenergic elevation of cyclic AMP in mouse epidermis *in vivo*. *Nature New Biol* 1972;240:178–179.
170. Grimm W, Marks F. Effect of tumor-promoting phorbol esters on the normal and the isoproterenol-elevated level of adenosine 3′5′-monophosphate in mouse epidermis. *Cancer Res* 1974;34:3408–3413.
171. Verma AK, Murray AW. The effect of benzo[a]pyrene on the basal and isoproterenol-stimulated levels of cyclic adenosine 3′5′-cyclic monophosphate in mouse epidermis *in vivo*. *Cancer Res* 1974;34:3128–3134.
172. Mufson RA, Simsiman RC, Boutwell RK. The effect of the phorbol ester tumor promoters on the basal and catecholamine-stimulated levels of cyclic adenosine 3′5′-monophosphate in mouse skin and epidermis *in vivo*. *Cancer Res* 1977;37:665–669.
173. Solanki V, Rana RS, Slaga TJ. Diminution of mouse epidermal superoxide dismutase and catalase activities by tumor promoters. *Carcinogenesis* 1981;2:1141–1146.
174. Reiners JJ Jr, Kodari E, Cappel RE, Gilbert HF. Assessment of the antioxidant/prooxidant status of murine skin following topical treatment with 12-O-tetradecanoylphorbol-13-acetate and throughout the ontogeny of skin cancer. II. Quantitation of glutathione and glutathione disulfide. *Carcinogenesis* 1991;12:2345–2352.
175. Davidson KA, Slaga TJ. Effects of phorbol ester tumor promoters and hyperplasiogenic agents on cytoplasmic glucocortidoid receptors in epidermis. *J Invest Dermatol* 1982;9:378–382.
176. Davidson KA, Slaga TJ. Glucocorticoid receptor levels in mouse skin after repetitive applications of 12-O-tetradecanoylphorbol-13-acetate and mezerin. *Cancer Res* 1983;43:3847–3851.
177. Warren BS, Naylor MF, Vo TK-O, Sandoval A, Davis MM, Slaga TJ. Phorbol ester tumor promoter treated epidermis papillomas carcinomas and tumor derived epidermal cell lines have decreased levels of the glucocorticoid receptor. *Proceedings AACR* 1991;32:162.
178. Colburn NH, Lau S, Head R. Decrease of epidermal histidase activity by tumor-promoting phorbol esters. *Cancer Res* 1975;35:3154–3159.
179. Watanabe T, Taguchi Y, Sasaki K, Tsuyama K, Kitamura Y. Increase in histidine decarboxylase activity in mouse skin after application of the tumor promoter tetradecanoylphorbol acetate. *Biochem Biophys Res Commun* 1981;1:427–432.
180. Schweizer J, Winter H. Changes in regional keratin polypeptide patterns during phorbol ester-mediated reversible and permanently sustained hyperplasia of mouse epidermis. *Cancer Res* 1982;42:1517–1529.
181. Nelson KG, Slaga TJ. Effect of inhibitors of tumor promotion on 12-O-tetradecanoyl-phorbol-13-acetate-induced keratin modification in mouse epidermis. *Carcinogenesis* 1982;3:1311–1315.
182. Roop DR, Hawley-Nelson P, Cheng CK, Yuspa SH. Keratin gene expression in mouse epidermis and cultured epidermal cells *Proc Natl Acad Sci USA* 1983;80:716–720.
183. Raineri R, Simsiman R, Boutwell RK. Stimulation of the phosphorylation of mouse epidermal histones by tumor-promoting agents. *Cancer Res* 1973;33:134–139.
184. Raineri R, Simsman RC, Boutwell RK. Stimulation of the synthesis of the H1 and H3 histone fractions of mouse epidermis by 12-O-tetradecanoylphorbol-13-acetate. *Cancer Lett* 1978;5:277–284.
185. Link R, Marks F. Histone phosphorylation in phorbol ester stimulated and β-adrenergically stimulated mouse epidermis *in vivo* and characterization of an epidermal protein phosphorylation system. *Biochim Biophys Acta* 1981;675:265–275.
186. O'Brien TG, Simsiman RC, Boutwell RK. Induction of the polyamine-biosynthetic enzymes in mouse epidermis by tumor-promoting agents. *Cancer Res* 1975;35:1662–1670.
187. O'Brien TG, Simsiman RC, Boutwell RK. Induction of the polyamine-biosynthetic enzymes in mouse epidermis and their specificity for tumor promotion. *Cancer Res* 1975;35:2426–2433.
188. O'Brien TG. The induction of ornithine decarboxylase as an early possibly obligatory event in mouse skin carcinogenesis. *Cancer Res* 1976;36:2644–2653.
189. Weeks CE, Slaga TJ. Inhibition of phorbol ester-induced polamine accumulation in mouse epidermis by anti-inflammatory steroid. *Biochem Biophys Res Commun* 1979;91:1488–1496.

190. Astrup EG, Paulsen JE. Changes in epidermal polyamine biosynthesis and specific activity of DNA following a single application of 12-O-tetradecanoylphorbol-13-acetate to hairless mouse skin. *Carcinogenesis* 1981;2:545–551.
191. Kruszewski FH, DiGiovanni J. Alterations in epidermal polyamine levels and DNA synthesis following topical treatment with chrysarobin in SENCAR mice. *Cancer Res* 1988;48:6390–6395.
192. Blumberg PM. Protein kinase C as the receptor for the phorbol ester tumor promoters. *Cancer Res* 1988;48:1–18.
193. Weinstein IB. The origins of human cancer: molecular mechanisms of carcinogenesis and their implications for cancer prevention and treatment. *Cancer Res* 1988;48:4135–4143.
194. Nishizuka Y. Studies and prospectives of protein kinase C family for cellular regulation. *Cancer* 1989;63:1892–1903.
195. Berridge MM, Irvine R. Inositol triphosphate a novel second messenger in cellular signal transduction. *Nature* 1984;312:315–321.
196. Nishizuka Y. Studies and prospectives of the protein kinase C family for cellular regulation. *Cancer* 1989;63:1892–1903.
197. Pandiella A, Beguinot L, Vicentini LM, Meldolesi J. Transmembrane signalling at the epidermal growth factor receptor. *Trends Pharmacol Sci* 1986;10:411–414.
198. King LE, Gates RE, Stoscheck CM, Nanney LB. The EGF/TGFα receptor in skin. *J Invest Dermatol* 1990;94:1645–1705.
199. Fisher PB, Weinstein IB, Eisenberg D, Ginsberg HS. Interactions between adenovirus a tumor promoter and chemical carcinogens in transformation of rat embryo cell cultures. *Proc Natl Acad Sci USA* 1978;75:2311–2314.
200. zur-Hausen H, O'Neill FJ, Freeze UK, Hecker E. Persisting oncogenic herpesvirus induced by tumor promoter TPA. *Nature* 1978;272:373–375.
201. Monier R, Daza-Grosjean L, Sarasin A. The effect of 12-O-tetradecanoylphorbol-13-acetate TPA on cell transformation by simian virus 40 mutants. In: Pullman B, Tso P, Gelboin H, eds. *Carcinogenesis: fundamental mechanisms and environmental effects.* Dordrecht, The Netherlands: D Reidel; 1980:371–378.
202. Amtmann E, Sauer G. Activation of non-expressed bovine papilloma virus genomes by tumor promoters. *Nature* 1982;196:675–677.
203. Cochran BJ, Zullo J, Vermain I, Stiles CD. Expression of the c-*fos* gene and of a *fos*-related gene is stimulated by platelet-derived growth factor. *Science* 1984;226:1080–1082.
204. Greenberg ME, Ziff EB. Stimulation of 3T3 cells induces transcription of the c-*fos* protooncogene. *Nature* 1984;311:433–438.
205. Lau LF, Nathans D. Identification of a set of genes expressed during the Go/G_1 transition of cultured cells. *EMBO J* 1985;4:3143–3151.
206. Angel P, Poting A, Mallick U, Rahmsdorf HJ, Schorpp M, Herrlich P. Induction of metallothionein and other mRNA species by carcinogens and tumor promoters in primary human skin fibroblasts. *Mol Cell Biol* 1986;6:1760–1766.
207. Verma AK, Erickson D, Dolnick BJ. Increased mouse epidermal ornithine decarboxylase activity by the tumor promoter 12-O-tetradecanoylphorbol 13-acetate involves increased amounts of both enzyme protein and messenger RNA. *Biochem J* 1986;237:297–300.
208. Akhurst RJ, Lee F, Balmain A. Localized production of TGFβ mRNA in tumor promoter stimulated mouse epidermis. *Nature* 1988;331:363–365.
209. Krieg P, Finch J, Fürstenberger G, Melber K, Matrisian LM, Bowden GT. Tumor promoters induce a transient expression of tumor associated genes in both basal and differentiated cells of the mouse epidermis. *Carcinogenesis* 1988;9:95–100.
210. Rose-John S, Fürstenberger G, Krieg P, Besenfelder E, Rincke G, Marks F. Differential effects of phorbol esters on c-*fos* and c-*myc* and ornithine decarboxylase gene expression in mouse skin *in vivo*. *Carcinogenesis* 1988;9:831–835.
211. Pittelkow MR, Lindquist PB, Abraham RT, Braves-Deal R, Derynck R, Coffey RJ. Induction of transforming growth factor-α expression in human keratinocytes by phorbol esters. *J Biol Chem* 1989;264:5164–5171.
212. Denhardt DT, Craig AM, Smith JH. Regulation of gene expression by the tumor promoter 12-O-tetradecanoyl-phorbol-13-acetate. In: Colburn NH, ed. *Genes and signal transduction in multistage carcinogenesis.* New York: Marcel Dekker; 1989:167–189.
213. Karin M, Herrlich P. *Cis*- and *trans*-acting genetic elements responsible for induction of specific genes by tumor promoters serum factors and stress. In: Colburn NH, ed. *Genes and signal transduction in multistage carcinogenesis.* New York: Marcel Dekker; 1989:415–440.

214. Brenner DA, Koch KS, Leffert HL. Transforming growth factor-alpha stimulates proto-oncogene c-*jun* expression and a mitogenic program in primary cultures of adult rat hepatocytes. *DNA* 1989; 8:279–285.
215. Pardee AB. G_1 events and regulation of cell proliferation. *Science* 1989;246:603–608.
216. Repine JE, White JG, Clawson CC, Holmes BM. The influence of phorbol myristate acetate on oxygen consumption by polymorphonuclear leukocytes. *J Clin Lab Med* 1974;83:911–920.
217. Kensler TW, Trush MA. Inhibition of phorbol ester stimulated chemiluminescence in human polymorphonuclear leukocytes by retinoic acid and 56-epoxyretinoic acid. *Cancer Res* 1981;41:216–222.
218. Troll W, Witz G, Goldstein B, Stone D, Sugimura T. The role of free oxygen radicals in tumor promotion and carcinogenesis. In: Hecker E, Fusenig NE, Kunz W, Marks F, Thielmann HW, eds. *Carcinogenesis*. Vol 7. *Cocarcinogenesis and biological effects of tumor promoters*. New York: Raven Press; 1982:593–597.
219. Cox JA, Jeng AY, Sharkey NA, Blumberg PM, Tauber AI. Activation of the human neutrophil nicotinamide adenine dinucleotide phosphate NADPH-oxidase by protein kinase C. *J Clin Invest* 1985;76:1932–1938.
220. Papini E, Grzeskowiak M, Bellavite P, Rossi F. Protein kinase C phosphorylates a component of NADPH oxidase of neutrophils. *FEBS Lett* 1985;190:204–208.
221. Fischer SM, Baldwin JK, Adams LM. Effects of antipromoters and mouse strain on promoter-induced oxidants in murine epidermal cells. *Carcinogenesis* 1986;7:915–918.
222. Fischer SM, Adams LM. Suppression of tumor promoter-induced chemiluminescence in mouse epidermal cells by several inhibitors of arachidonic acid metabolism. *Cancer Res* 1985;45:3130–3136.
223. Slaga TJ, Klein-Szanto AJP, Triplett LL, Yotti LP, Trosko JE. Skin tumor-promoting activity of benzoyl peroxide a widely used free radical-generating compound. *Science* 1981;213:1023–1025.
224. Slaga TJ, Solanki V, Logani M. Studies on the mechanism of action of antitumor promoting agents: suggestive evidence for the involvement of free radicals in promotion. In: Nygaard OF, Simic MG, eds. *Radioprotectors and anticarcinogens*. New York: Academic Press; 1983:471–485.
225. DiGiovanni J, Kruszewski FH, Chenicek KJ. Modulation of chrysarobin skin tumor promotion. *Carcinogenesis* 1988;9:1445–1450.
226. DiGiovanni J, Kruszewski FH, Chenick KJ. Studies on the skin tumor promoting actions of chrysarobin, G103. In: Butterworth BE, Slaga TJ, eds. *Nongenotoxic mechanisms in carcinogenesis*. Cold Spring Harbor, NY: Cold Spring Harbor Press; 1987:25–39.
227. Zimmerman R, Cerutti P. Active oxygen acts as a promoter of transformation in mouse embryo C3H/10T1/2 fibroblasts. *Proc Natl Acad Sci USA* 1984;81:2085–2087.
228. Cerutti PA. Genotoxic oxidant tumor promoters. In: Butterworth BE, Slaga TJ, eds. *Nongenotoxic mechanisms in carcinogenesis*. Cold Spring Harbor, NY: Cold Spring Harbor Laboratory; 1987:325–335.
229. Slaga TJ, DiGiovanni J. Inhibition of chemical carcinogenesis. In: Searle CE, ed. *Chemical carcinogens*. 2nd ed, vol 2. *American Chemical Society monograph* 182. Washington DC: American Chemical Society; 1984:1279–1321.
230. Perchellet J-P, Perchellet EM, Orten DK, Schneider BA. Decreased ratio of reduced/oxidized glutathione in mouse epidermal cells treated with tumor promoters. *Carcinogenesis* 1986;7:503–506.
231. Perchellet EM, Abney NL, Perchellet JP. Stimulation of hydroperoxide generation in mouse skin treated with tumor-promoting or carcinogenic agents *in vivo* and *in vitro*. *Cancer Lett* 1988;42:169–177.
232. Perchellet EM, Perchellet J-P. Characterization of the hydroperoxide response observed in mouse skin treated with tumor promoters *in vivo*. *Cancer Res* 1989;49:6193–6201.
233. Cerutti PA. Oxidant stress and carcinogenesis. *Eur J Clin Invest* 1991;21:1–5.
234. Pryor WA. The role of free radical reactions in biological systems. In: Pryor WA, ed. *Free radicals in biology*. Vol 1. New York: Academic Press; 1976:1–49.
235. Freeman BA, Crapo JD. Biology of disease: free radicals and tissue injury. *Lab Invest* 1982;47:412–426.
236. Hammar H. Glyceraldehydephosphate dehydrogenase and glucose-6-phosphate dehydrogenase activities in psoriasis and neurodermatitis and the effect of dithranol. *J Invest Dermatol* 1970;54:121–125.

237. Cavey D, Caron J-C, Shroot B. Anthralin: chemical instability and glucose-6-phosphate dehydrogenase inhibition. *J Pharm Sci* 1982;71:980–983.
238. Gopalakrishna R, Anderson W. Ca2+- and phospholipid-independent activation of protein kinase C by selective oxidative modification of the regulatory domain. *Proc Natl Acad Sci USA* 1989; 86:6758–6762.
239. Larsson R, Cerutti P. Translocation and enhancement of phosphotransferase activity of protein kinase C following exposure of mouse epidermal cells to oxidants. *Cancer Res* 1989;49:5627–5632.
240. Donnelly TE, Pelling JC, Anderson CL, Dalbey D. Benzoyl peroxide activation of protein kinase C activity in epidermal cell membranes. *Carcinogenesis* 1987;12:1871–1874.
241. Abate C, Patel L, Rauscher FJ III, Curran T. Redox regulation of *fos* and *jun* DNA-binding activity in vitro. *Science* 1990;249:1157–1161.
242. Bauskin AR, Alkalay I, Ben-Neriah Y. Redox regulation of a protein tyrosine kinase in the endoplasmic reticulum. *Cell* 1991;66:685–696.
243. Thor H, Orrenius S. The mechanism of bromobenzene-induced cytotoxicity studied with isolated hepatocytes. *Arch Toxicol* 1980;44:31–43.
244. Trump BF, Berezesky IK. Ion regulation cell injury and carcinogenesis. *Carcinogenesis* 1987;8:1027–1031.
245. Richter C, Frei B. Ca^{2+} release from mitochondria induced by prooxidants. *Free Radical Biol Med* 1988;4:365–375.
246. Reed DJ. Review of the current status of calcium and thiols in cellular injury. *Chem Res Toxicol* 1990;3:495–502.
247. Nishizuka Y. Phospholipid degradation and signal translation for protein phosphorylation. *Trends Biochem Sci* 1983;8:13–16.
248. Larsson R, Cerutti P. Oxidants induce phosphorylation of ribosomal protein S6. *J Biol Chem* 1988;263:17452–17458.
249. Imamoto A, Beltran L, DiGiovanni J. Evidence for autocrine/paracrine growth stimulation by transforming growth factor-α during the process of skin tumor promotion *Mol Carcinog* 1991;4:52–60.
250. Mellgren RL. Calcium-dependent proteases: an enzyme system active at cellular membranes. *FASEB J* 1987;1:110–115.
251. Lankas GR, Baxter CS, Christian RT. Effect of tumor promoting agents on mutation frequency in cultured V79 chinese hamster cells. *Mutat Res* 1977;45:153–156.
252. Thomson LM, Baker RM, Carrano AV, Brookman KW. Failure of phorbol ester TPA to enhance sister chromatid exchanges mitotic segregations or expression of mutations in chinese hamster cells. *Cancer Res* 1980;40:3245–3251.
253. Imbra RJ, Karin M. Phorbol ester induces the transcriptional stimulatory activity of the SV40 enhancer. *Nature* 1986;323:555–557.
254. zur-Hausen H, Bornkamm GW, Schmidt R, Hecker E. Tumor initiators and promoters in the induction of Epstein–Barr virus. *Proc Natl Acad Sci USA* 1979;76:782–785.
255. Kinsella AR, Radman M. Tumor promoter induces sister chromatid exchanges: relevance to mechanisms of carcinogenesis. *Proc Natl Acad Sci USA* 1978;75:6149–6153.
256. Birnbaim HC. DNA strand breakage in human leukocytes exposed to a tumor promoter phorbol myristate acetate. *Science* 1982;211:1247–1249.
257. Dutton DR, Bowden GT. Indirect induction of a clastogenic effect in epidermal cells by a tumor promoter. *Carcinogenesis* 1985;6:1279–1284.
258. Hartley JA, Gibson NW, Zwelling LA, Yuspa SH. The association of DNA strand breaks and terminal differentiation in mouse epidermal cells exposed to tumor promoters. *Cancer Res* 1985; 45:4864–4870.
259. Parry JM, Parry EM, Barrett JC. Tumor promoters induce mitotic aneuploidy in yeast. *Nature* 1981;294:263–265.
260. Callen DF, Ford JH. Chromosome abnormalities in chronic lymphocytic leukemia revealed by TPA as mitogen. *Cancer Genet Cytogenet* 1983;10:87–93.
261. Emerit I, Cerutti PA. Tumor promoter phorbol-12-myristate-13-acetate induces chromosomal damage via indirect action. *Nature* 1981;293:144–146.
262. Dzarlieva RT, Fusenig NE. Tumor promoter 12-O-tetradecanoylphorbol-13-acetate enhances sister chromatid exchanges and numerical and structural chromosome aberrations in primary mouse epidermal cell cultures. *Cancer Lett* 1982;16:7–17.
263. Fusenig NE, Dzarlieva RT. Phenotypic and chromosomal alterations in cell cultures are indicators

of tumor-promoting activity. In: Hecker E, Fusenig NE, Kunz W, Marks F, Thielmann HW, eds. *Carcinogenesis.* New York: Raven Press; 1982:201–216.
264. Dzarlieva-Petrusevska RT, Fusenig NE. Tumor promoter 12-*O*-tetradecanoylphorbol-13-acetate TPS-induced chromosome aberrations in mouse keratinocyte cell lines: a possible genetic mechanism of tumor promotion. *Carcinogenesis* 1985;6:1447–1456.
265. Cohen P. The structure and regulation of protein phosphatases. *Annu Rev Biochem* 1989;58:453–508.
266. Hesheler J, Mieskes G, Ruegg JC, Takai A, Trautwein W. Effects of a protein phosphatase inhibitor okadaic acid on membrane currents of isolated guinea pig cardiac myocytes. *Pflugers Arch Ges Physiol* 1988;412:248–252.
267. Haystead TAJ, Sim ATR, Carling D, Honnor RC, Tsukitani Y, Cohen P, Hardie DG. Effects of the tumor promoter okadaic acid on intracellular protein phosphorylation and metabolism. *Nature (London)* 1989;337:78–81.
268. Suganuma M, Suttajit M, Suguri H, Ohika M, Yamada K, Fujiki H. Specific binding of okadaic acid a new tumor promoter in mouse skin. *FEBS Lett* 21989;50:615–618.
269. Suganuma M, Fujiki H, Furuya-Suguri H, et al. Calyculin A an inhibitor of protein phosphatases a potent tumor promoter on CD-1 mouse skin. *Cancer Res* 1990;50:3521–3525.
270. Haikii H, Fujiki H, Suganuma M, et al. Thapsigargin a histamine secretagogue is a non-12-*O*-tetradecanoylphorbol-13-acetate TPA type tumor promoter in two-stage mouse skin carcinogenesis. *J Cancer Res Clin Oncol* 1986;111:177–181.
271. Fujiki H, Suganuma M, Suguri H, Yoshizawa S, Hirota M, Takagi K, Sugimura T. Diversity in the chemical nature and mechanism of response to tumor promoters. In: Slaga TJ, Klein-Szanto AJP, Boutwell RK, Stevenson DE, Spitzer HL, D'Motto B, eds. *Progress in clinical and biological research.* Vol 298. *Skin carcinogenesis: mechanisms and human relevance.* New York: Alan R Liss; 1989:281–291.
272. Takemura H, Hughes AR, Thastrup O, Putney JJ. Activation of calcium entry by the tumor promoter thapsigargin in parotid acinar cells. Evidence that an intracellular calcium pool and not an inositol phosphate regulates calcium fluxes at the plasma membrane. *J Biol Chem* 1989;264:12266–12271.
273. Thastrup O, Cullen PJ, Drobak BK, Hanley MR, Dawson AP. Thapsigargin a tumor promoter discharges intracellular Ca^{2+} stores by specific inhibition of the endoplasmic reticulum Ca^{2+}-ATPase. *Proc Natl Acad Sci USA* 1990;87:2466–2470.
274. Shoyab M, DeLarco JE, Todaro GJ. Biologically active phorbol esters specifically alter affinity of epidermal growth factor membrane receptors. *Nature* 21979;79:387–391.
275. Lee LS, Weinstein IB. Mechanism of tumor promoter inhibition of cellular binding of epidermal growth factor. *Proc Natl Acad Sci USA* 1979;76:5168–5172.
276. Magun BE, Bowden GT. Effects of phorbol ester tumor promoters on the binding processing and biological activity of epidermal growth factor. In: Slaga TJ, ed. *Mechanisms of tumor promotion.* Vol III. *Tumor promotion and carcinogenesis in vitro.* Boca Raton, FL: CRC Press; 1984:125–141.
277. Imamoto A, Beltran L, DiGiovanni J. Differential mechanism for the inhibition of epidermal growth factor binding to its receptor on mouse keratinocytes by anthrones and phorbol esters. *Carcinogenesis* 1990;11:1543–1549.
278. King CS, Cooper JA. Effects of protein kinase C activation after epidermal growth factor binding on epidermal growth factor receptor phosphorylation. *J Biol Chem* 1986;261:10073–10078.
279. Davis RJ. Independent mechanisms account for the regulation by protein kinase C of the epidermal growth factor receptor affinity and tyrosine–protein kinase activity. *J Biol Chem* 1988;263:9462–9469.
280. Downward J, Waterfield MD, Parker PJ. Autophosphorylation and protein kinase C phosphorylation of the epidermal growth factor receptor. Effect on tyrosine kinase activity and ligand binding affinity. *J Biol Chem* 1985;260:14538–14546.
281. Countaway JL, Northwood IC, Davis RJ. Mechanism of phosphorylation of the epidermal growth factor receptor at threonine 669. *J Biol Chem* 21989;64:10828–10835.
282. Friedman BA, Van Amsterdam J, Fujiki H, Rosner MR. Phosphorylation at threonine-654 is not required for negative regulation of the epidermal growth factor receptor by non-phorbol tumor promoters. *Proc Natl Acad Sci USA* 1989;86:812–816.
283. Hernandez-Sotomayor SMT, Mumby M, Carpenter G. Okadaic acid–induced hyperphosphorylation of the epidermal growth factor receptor. *J Biol Chem* 1991;266:21281–21286.
284. Wattenberg EV, McNeil PL, Fujiki H, Rosner MR. Palytoxin down-modulates the epidermal

growth factor receptor through a sodium-dependent pathway. *J Biol Chem* 1989;264:213–219.
285. Matsui MS, Laufer L, Scheide S, DeLeo V. Ultraviolet-B 290-320 nm-irradiation inhibits epidermal growth-factor binding to mammalian cells. *J Invest Dermatol* 1989;92:617–622.
286. Meyer SA, Gibbs TA, Jirtle RL. Independent mechanisms for tumor promoters phenobarbital and 12-O-tetradecanoylphorbol-13-acetate in reduction of epidermal growth factor binding by rat hepatocytes. *Cancer Res* 1989;49:5907–5912.
287. Yuspa SH, Lichti U, Ben T, Patterson E, Hennings H. Phorbol esters stimulate DNA synthesis and ornithine decarboxylase activity in mouse epidermal cell cultures. *Nature* 1976;262:402–404.
288. Diamond L, O'Brien TG, Giovanni R. Tumor promoters: effects on proliferation and differentiation of cells in culture. *Life Sci* 1978;23:1979–1988.
289. Diamond L. Tumor promoters and cell transformation. *Pharmacol Ther* 1982;89:89–145.
290. Choi EJ, Toscano DG, Ryan JA, Riedel N, Toscano WA Jr. Dioxin induces transforming growth factor-α in human keratinocytes. *J Biol Chem.* 1991;266:9591–9597.
291. Ellem KAO, Cullinan M, Baumann KC, Dunstan A. UVR induction of TGFα: a possible autocrine mechanism for the epidermal melanocytic response and for promotion of epidermal carcinogenesis. *Carcinogenesis* 1988;9:797–801.
292. Parkinson K, Balmain A. Chalones revisited—a possible role for transforming growth factor β in tumour promotion. *Carcinogenesis* 1990;11:195–198.
293. Krieg P, Schnapke R, Fürstenberger G, Vogt I, Marks F. TGF-β1 and skin carcinogenesis: antiproliferative effect *in vitro* and TGF-β1 mRNA expression during epidermal hyperproliferation and multistage tumorigenesis. *Mol Carcinog* 1991;4:129–137.
294. Shipley GD, Pittelkow MR, Wille JJ Jr, Scott RE, Moses HL. Reversible inhibition of normal human prokeratinocyte proliferation by type beta transforming growth factor-growth inhibitor in serum-free medium. *Cancer Res* 1986;46:2068–2071.
295. Coffey RJ, Snipes NJ, Bascom CC, Graves-Deal R, Pennington CY, Weissman BE, Moses HL. Growth modulation of mouse keratinocytes by transforming growth factors. *Cancer Res* 1988;48:1596–1602.
296. Mansbridge JN, Hanawalt PC. Role of transforming growth factor-beta in the maturation of human epidermal keratinocytes. *J Invest Dermatol* 1988;90:336–341.
297. Fürstenberger G, Rogers M, Schnapke R, Bauer G, Hofler P, Marks F. Stimulatory role of transforming growth factors in multistage skin carcinogenesis: possible explanation for the tumor-inducing effect of wounding in initiated NMRI mouse skin. *Int J Cancer* 1989;43:915–921.
298. Partridge M, Green MR, Landon JD, Feldmann M. Production of TGFα and TGFβ by cultured keratinocytes skin and oral squamous carcinomas: potential autocrine regulation of normal and malignant epithelial cell proliferation. *Br J Cancer* 1989;60:542–548.
299. Sporn MB, Roberts AB. Autocrine growth factors and cancer. *Nature* 1985;313:745–747.
300. Roberts AB, Thompson NL, Heine U, Flanders C, Sporn MB. Transforming growth factor-β: possible roles in carcinogenesis. *Br J Cancer* 1988;57:594–600.
301. Beltrán L, DiGiovanni J. Elevated expression of transforming growth factor-α (TGFα) mRNA in mouse skin papillomas and carcinomas. *Proc Am Assoc Cancer Res* 1992;33:125.
302. Derynck R, Goeddel DV, Ullrich A, Gutterman JU, Williams RD, Bringman TS, Berger WH. Synthesis of messenger RNAs for transforming growth factors α and β and the epidermal growth factor receptor by human tumors. *Cancer Res* 1987;74:707–712.
303. DiMarco E, Pierve JH, Fleming TP, Kraus MH, Molloy CJ, Aaronson SA, DiFiore PP. Autocrine interaction between TGFα and the EGF-receptor: quantitative requirements for induction of the malignant phenotype. *Oncogene* 1989;4:831–838.
304. Hendler FJ, Ozanne B. Human squamous cell lung cancers express increased epidermal growth factor receptors. *J Clin Invest* 1984;74:647–651.
305. Yamamoto T, Kamata N, Kawano H, et al. High incidence of amplification of the epidermal growth factor receptor gene in human squamous carcinoma cell lines. *Cancer Res* 1986;46:414–416.
306. Ozanne B, Richards CS, Hendler F, Burns D, Gusterson B. Over-expression of the EGF receptor is a hallmark of squamous cell carcinomas. *J Pathol* 1986;149:9–14.
307. Kouri RE, Salerno RA, Whitmore CE. Relationships between aryl hydrocarbon hydroxylase inducibility and sensitivity to chemically induced subcutaneous sarcomas in various strains of mice. *J Natl Cancer Inst* 1973;50:363–368.
308. Kouri RE, Ratrie H, Whitmore CE. Genetic control of susceptibility to 3-methylcholanthrene-induced subcutaneous sarcomas. *Int J Cancer* 1974;13:714–720.
309. Kouri RE. Relationship between levels of aryl hydrocarbon hydroxylase activity and susceptibility

to 3-methylcholanthrene and benzo[a]pyrene-induced cancers in inbred strains of mice. In: Freudenthal R, Jones P, eds. *Carcinogenesis.* Vol 1. *Polynuclear aromatic hydrocarbons: chemistry, metabolism, and carcinogenesis.* New York: Raven Press; 1976:139–141.
310. Nebert DW, Boobis AR, Yagi H, Jerina DM, Kouri RE. Genetic differences in mouse cytochrome P1-450-mediated metabolism of benzo[a]pyrene *in vitro* and carcinogenic index *in vivo*. In: Jollow DJ, Kocsis JJ, Snyder R, Vainio H, eds. *Biologically reactive intermediates.* New York: Plenum Press; 1977:125–145.
311. Nebert DW, Atlas SA, Guenthner TM, Kouri RE. The Ah locus: genetic regulation of the enzymes which metabolize polycyclic hydrocarbons and the risk for cancer. In: Gelboin HV, Tsó POP, eds. *Polycyclic hydrocarbons and cancer.* Vol 2. New York: Academic Press; 1978:346–390.
312. Kouri RE, Rude TH, Joglekar R, et al. 2378-Tetrachlorodibenzo-*p*-dioxin as cocarcinogen causing 3-methylcholanthrene-initiated subcutaneous tumors in mice genetically "nonresponsive" at Ah locus. *Cancer Res* 1978;38:2777–2783.
313. Nebert DW. Pharmacogenetics: an approach to understanding chemical and biologic aspects of cancer. *J Natl Cancer Inst* 1980;64:1279–1290.
314. Nebert DW, Gelboin HV. The *in vivo* and *in vitro* induction of aryl hydrocarbon hydroxylase in mammalian cells of different species tissues strains and developmental and hormonal states. *Arch Biochem Biophys* 1969;134:76–89.
315. Poland A, Glover E. Ca^{2+}-dependent proteolysis of the Ah receptor. *Arch Biochem Biophys* 1988;261:103–111.
316. Fernandez N, Roy M, Leska P. Binding characteristics of Ah receptors from rats and mice before and after separation from hepatic cytosols 7-Hydroxyellipticine as a competitive antagonist of cytochrome P-450 induction. *Eur J Biochem* 1988;172:585–592.
317. Nebert DW, Jensen NM. The Ah locus: genetic regulation of the metabolism of carcinogens drugs and other environmental chemicals by cytochrome P-450-mediated monooxygenases. *CRC Crit Rev Biochem* 1979;6:401–437.
318. Nebert DW, Gonzalez FJ. P-450 genes: structure evolution and regulation. *Annu Rev Biochem* 1987;56:945–993.
319. Kinoshita N, Gelboin HV. The role of aryl hydrocarbon hydroxlase in 7,12-dimethylbenz[a]anthracene skin tumorigenesis: on the mechanism of 78-benzoflavone inhibition of tumorigenesis. *Cancer Res* 1972;32:1329–1339.
320. Legraverend C, Mansour B, Nebert DW, Holland JM. Genetic differences in benzo[a]pyrene-initiated tumorigenesis in mouse skin. *Pharmacology* 1980;20:242–255.
321. Seifried HE, Birkett DJ, Levin W, Lu AYH, Conney AH, Jerina DM. Metabolism of benzo[a]pyrene. Effect of 3-methylcholanthrene pretreatment on metabolism by microsomes from lungs of genetically "responsive" and "nonresponsive" mice. *Arch Biochem Biophys* 1977;178:256–263.
322. Okey AB, Bondy GP, Mason ME, Kahl GF, Eisen HJ, Guenthner TM, Nebert DW. Regulatory gene product of the Ah locus. Characterization of the cytosolic inducer-receptor complex and evidence for its nuclear translocation. *J Biol Chem* 1979;254:11636–11648.
323. Bickers DR, Mukhtar H, Yang SK. Cutaneous metabolism of benzo[a]pyrene: comparative studies in C57BL/6N and DBA/2N mice and neonatal Sprague–Dawley rats. *Chem Biol Interact* 1983;43:263–270.
324. Nebert DW, Benedict WF, Gielen JE, Oesch F, Daly JW. Aryl hydrocarbon hydroxylase epoxide hydrase and 7,12-dimethylbenz[a]-anthracene produced skin tumorigenesis in the mouse. *Mol Pharmacol* 1972;8:374–379.
325. Benedict WG, Considine N, Nebert DW. Genetic differences in aryl hydrocarbon hydroxylase induction and benzo[a]pyrene produced tumorigenesis in the mouse. *Mol Pharmacol* 1972;9:226–277.
326. Burki K, Liebelt AG, Bresnick E. Induction of aryl hydrocarbon hydroxylase in mouse tissues from a high and low cancer strain and their F1 hybrids. *J Natl Cancer Inst* 1973;50:369–380.
327. DiGiovanni J, Slaga TJ, Juchau MR. Comparative epidermal metabolism in strains of mice with differing sensitivity to skin tumorigenesis. *Proc Am Assoc Cancer Res* 1979;20:134.
328. DiGiovanni J, Slaga TJ, Boutwell RK. Comparison of the tumor-initiating activity of 7,12-dimethylbenz[a]anthracene and benzo[a]pyrene in female SENCAR and CD-1 mice. *Carcinogenesis* 1980;1:381–389.
329. Reiners JJ Jr, Nesnow S, Slaga TJ. Murine susceptibility to two-stage skin carcinogenesis is influenced by the agent used for promotion. *Carcinogenesis* 1984;5:301–307.

330. DiGiovanni J. Genetics of susceptibility to mouse skin tumor promotion. In: Sirica AE, ed. *The pathobiology of neoplasia*. New York: Plenum Press; 1989:247–274.
331. DiGiovanni J. Genetic determinants of susceptibility to mouse skin tumor promotion in inbred mice. In: Colburn NH, ed. *Genes and signal transduction in multistage carcinogenesis*. New York: Marcel Dekker; 1989:39–67.
332. DiGiovanni J, Prichett WP, Decina PC, Diamond L. DBA/2 mice are as sensitive as SENCAR mice to skin tumor promotion by 12-O-tetradecanoylphorbol-13-acetate. *Carcinogenesis* 1984; 11:1493–1498.
333. DiGiovanni J, Walker SE, Aldaz CM, Conti CJ. Further studies on the influence of initiation dose on papilloma growth and progression during two-stage carcinogenesis in SENCAR mice. *Carcinogenesis* 1993 [*in press*].
334. Bock FG, Burns R. Tumor-promoting properties of anthralin 189-Anthratriol. *J Natl Cancer Inst* 1963;30:393–398.
335. Strickland PT. Tumor induction in SENCAR mice in response to ultraviolet radiation. *Carcinogenesis* 1982;3:1487–1489.
336. DiGiovanni J, Walker SC, Beltrán L, Naito M, Eastin WC. Evidence for a common genetic pathway controlling susceptibility to mouse skin tumor promotion by diverse classes of promoting agents. *Cancer Res* 1991;51:1398–1405.

10

Neurocarcinogenesis

Adalbert Koestner and *Keiji Marushige

Department of Veterinary Pathobiology, Ohio State University, Columbus, Ohio 43210;
*Department of Pathology, Michigan State University, East Lansing, Michigan 48824

Our knowledge about etiology and pathogenesis of primary brain tumors in humans and animals has been greatly enhanced during the past two decades. Oncogenic viruses and chemical carcinogens have been used successfully in experimental models and have revealed important new information. Advancements in molecular biology have expanded our understanding of neurocarcinogenic processes on a molecular level. It has become possible to define the interactions of chemical carcinogens with DNA molecules and assess their consequences. Methods are now available to explore the roles of oncogenes, growth factors, and supressor genes in the neurooncogenic process.

All of these advancements have naturally contributed to the understanding of neoplastic disease as a whole; however, their applicability to the central nervous system (CNS) deserves special consideration because of the uniqueness of the CNS as a target organ for carcinogenic agents. In comparison to other major target organs in cancer development (e.g., skin, lung, liver, kidney, intestine, etc.) the CNS occupies a remarkably protected location within the body. Access to the brain is further limited for bloodborne substances by the blood-brain barrier, unless these substances are nonpolar or actively transported. In addition to this specific barrier, the CNS is also unique through its lack of a lymphatic system, which makes it less accessible to immunodefense mechanisms for whatever role they may play in carcinogenesis.

Some carcinogenic substances have been demonstrated to gain access to the brain; however, several of them require transformation into active carcinogens by enzymes that mostly are not available in the brain. Finally, the major functioning cell population of the nervous system, the neurons, are unable to divide after maturation and a precursor pool is not available. Such terminally differentiated neurons are therefore unavailable for neoplastic transformation. As a consequence, tumors in the adult nervous system of human beings as well as in most animal species overwhelmingly arise from the glial element, while tumors of neuronal origin play an important role only in children. For the above and perhaps other unknown reasons, tumors of the nervous system are more easily produced by chemical carcinogens in fetuses and newborn animals than in adults. Comparably, brain tumors in adult human beings amount to only 1.2% of all autopsied deaths and 9% of all primary tumors (1), while in infants they represent 25% of all primary tumors, rated second only to leukemia (2).

In this chapter we present highlights from over two decades of research conducted in many laboratories on "resorptive" neurocarcinogens and assess the contribution of this research to an understanding of the mechanisms of neurocarcinogenesis. Morphological features of chemically induced tumors of the nervous system as well as molecular aspects of initiation of neoplastic transformation are presented with special emphasis on recent developments pertaining particularly to the later phases of neurocarcinogenesis, promotion, and progression. See also recent reviews on neurocarcinogenesis (3–5).

CARCINOGENS AND TARGET-ORGAN SPECIFICITY

The specificity of carcinogenic agents for selected organs and/or cell types of the body is well recognized. Obvious reasons for this specificity include direct access of the agent by contact (e.g., skin, eyes, and genital organs), inhalation (respiratory system), ingestion (digestive tract), excretion (digestive and urinary systems), presence of activating enzymes (e.g., liver and kidney), and inherited predisposition for tumor development (e.g., hepatic tumors in certain strains of mice, mammary and lung tumors in some strains of rats). None of the circumstances above are known to apply to the nervous system with the exception of some predisposition for brain tumor development in aging rats. Sprague–Dawley, Fischer 344, and Wistar rats have a higher prevalence of spontaneous brain tumors that other rodents, dogs, and humans at the age of 2 years and beyond. The incidence of brain tumors in these rats approaches an average of 3.0% in males and 1.6% in females (6–10). Tumor incidences of that level, although three times that of the brain tumor incidence in the adult human population (1) are still classified as rare by Environmental Protection Agency and Federal Drug Administration standards.

The rat has become the most valuable experimental animal for neurocarcinogenesis studies in the past three decades. Druckrey et al. (11), with their remarkable discovery of brain tumor production in rats with nitrosourea compounds by extraneural administration (intravenous, subcutaneous, and oral), set the stage for a new phase in experimental neurooncology. Two compounds, methylnitrosourea (MNU) and ethylnitrosourea (ENU), particularly, were shown to have a very high neurooncogenic potential. One single inoculation of 20 to 50 mg/kg ENU to a pregnant rat between days 15 and 21 of gestation resulted in 90% to 100% neurogenic tumor production in the offspring after a latency period of up to 1 year (12).

Since that discovery by Druckrey et al., over 30 chemical agents have been recognized as being capable of neurogenic tumor production by systemic inoculation. For the purpose of this chapter, dealing primarily with pathogenetic mechanisms, we selected MNU and ENU (Fig. 1) as the model neurocarcinogens, although other agents will be discussed when applicable.

The selective organ specificity of neurooncogenic agents, as with carcinogenic agents in general, are influenced by several factors, such as species, strain, age, sex, dose of the carcinogen, and method of exposure.

Species

There are remarkable species-dependent differences in susceptibility and tumor location. With repeated intravenous inoculations of MNU at optimal doses, brain tumors were produced in 77% of the rats, 50% to 70% in rabbits, 10% in mice, and 0% in hamsters. Under these experimental conditions tumors of the peripheral nervous system (PNS) occurred solely in rats among the four rodent species tested (13). On the other hand, mice and hamsters developed a high rate of stomach cancer following parenteral MNU exposure. No stomach cancer developed in rats and rabbits unless oral exposure was used. Comparable differences in tumor prevalence and location were also observed among rodent species following a single transplacental exposure to ENU (13–15). In contrast to the rat, perinatal ENU exposure to mice resulted in the development of medulloblastoma in 0.2% of the animals; this neuronal neoplasm was never encountered in the many experiments reported in rats (15). Tumors of neuronal origin were also produced by embryonal ENU induction in the opossum (16) and with the human polyoma virus in hamsters (17).

The dog deserves to be mentioned in addition to the rodents because the spontaneous brain tumors in this species show great morphological similarity to human brain tumors, and their incidence approaches that of adult human beings. While viral induction of brain tumors in dogs has been quite successful (18), chemical induction has had only limited exploration. In one experiment only four brain tumors out of 10 mixed-breed dogs developed within an average latency period of 13 months following monthly intravenous inoculations of 20 mg/kg MNU (19). In another experiment (20), using pure-bread Boxer dogs, a breed known to have a high spontaneous brain tumor incidence, brain tumors did not develop within 3 years

$$O=N-N\begin{matrix}CH_3\\ \\CO-NH_2\end{matrix} \qquad O=N-N\begin{matrix}CH_2\cdot CH_3\\ \\CO-NH_2\end{matrix}$$

Methylnitrosourea	Ethylnitrosourea

FIG. 1. Neurooncogenic *N*-nitrosoureas. The O=N·N group is the basic nitroso molecule; CH_3 or $CH_2 \cdot CH_3$ are the active alkylating radicals (methylation or ethylation), and the CO·NH$_2$ (urea) is the organ-directing radical.

following 36 weekly i.v. inoculations of 5 mg/kg MNU; however, 70% of the dogs developed neurinomas (schwannomas).

Strain or Breed

Different strains of rats express different levels of susceptibility to the neurocarcinogenic effect of *N*-nitrosourea compounds. Such differences were noticed by Jänisch and Schreiber (21) when comparing Hooded rats with Wistar rats under the same experimental conditions. Intravenous administration of 10 mg/kg MNU every 2 weeks for a total of 180 mg/kg resulted in 72% of CNS tumors in Hooded rats and only 32.7% in Wistar rats. Druckrey et al. (22) tested ENU in 10 genetically defined strains of rats, by transplacental exposure of 50 mg/kg ENU on day 15 of gestation. While the incidence of neurogenic tumors in the offspring ranged from 80% to 100% in nine of the strains and 100% in four strains it was only 55% in BD IV rats. While many rats of the more susceptible strains had more than one tumor of the nervous system, the BD IV rats did not. The latency period varied considerably among the strains. BD IX rats (among the two most susceptible) had an average latency period of 180 days while BD IV rats survived an average of 550 days. There were also differences in location. In four strains there were up to 58% of the tumors in the brain with 16% in the spinal cord, 10% in cranial nerves, and 16% in peripheral nerves. By contrast, another four groups had only 27% brain tumors, 18% tumors of the spinal cord, but 22% in cranial nerves and 33% in peripheral nerves. Similar differences exist among strains of mice, although they have been less well investigated. Some strains of mice may die early from lung and liver tumors or from leukemia before brain tumors have a chance to develop.

Age

The age of exposure has a major influence on susceptibility, location, and type of tumor. Fetuses are 50 to 100 times more susceptible than adult rats, although tumors of the nervous system cannot be induced in rats before the twelfth day of gestation. After the twelfth day the susceptibility increases with advancing pregnancy culminating toward the end of the gestation period. The susceptibility gradually declines in the newborn to day 30 postpartum when it becomes all but impossible to produce neurogenic tumors with a single dose of ENU.

There are also differences in tumor types, degree of differentiation, and location based primarily on age at exposure. If ENU is administered on day 15 of gestation, the majority of tumors will occur in the brain. Neurinomas, particularly of the trigeminal nerve, predominate when exposure occurs at the end of gestation. The brain tumors in these animals are mostly differentiated gliomas (oligodendrogliomas, astrocytomas, and mixed gliomas). The neurinomas are predominantly anaplastic. If we further compare these tumors, induced in the fetus, with those produced with multiple i.v. inoculations of MNU to adults rats, a further diversified tumor spectrum results. In contrast to the transplacentally induced tumors, MNU in adult rats produces primarily anaplastic gliomas in addition to oligodendrogliomas and astrocytomas. Gliomas usually arise in periventricular regions as monomorphous astrocytomas and in the cerebral cortex as oligodendrogliomas and as they grow larger, they become more mixed and anaplastic. Sarcomas and gliosarcomas also occur. Neurinomas in adult rats, in contrast, are much more differentiated and less numerous (Table 1).

The basis for these differences is most likely the availability of target cells and perhaps their stage of activity and proliferation. Activity in the glia and Schwann cell population may be very high during the last week of gestation, and many of these cells may still be in a precursor stage. Warkany et al. (23) preceded ENU application on day 20 of gestation with 200 rad of x-radiation in pregnant rats and expected an increase in neurogenic tumors with this combined treatment. The results revealed just the opposite. Offspring of rats treated with ENU alone developed 46 of 74 neurogenic tumors (62%) and those with x-ray + ENU only 10 of 60 (16%). The assumption is made that x-rays and ENU attack the same target population. As a consequence of x-radiation a considerable portion of the target cells may have been destroyed and was therefore not available for ENU initiation. We obtained similar results by treating pregnant rats for 5 days with NGF (nerve growth factor) and then administering 50 mg/kg of ENU i.v. (24). The prevalence of trigeminal neurinomas and early neoplastic proliferation was reduced significantly ($p<0.025$) in the NGF-pretreated group from 58% to 26% at 90 days postpartum. A possible explanation is that NGF caused differentiation in a large segment of the target cell population, thus making them less susceptible to neoplastic transformation by ENU.

TABLE 1. Classification of tumors produced in Sprague–Dawley rats with MNU (incidence of NS tumors 97%) and ENU (incidence 100% in offspring)

Tumor type	MNU 5 mg/kg i.v. weekly for 36 weeks	ENU 50 mg/kg i.v. to pregnant rats, day 20 of gestation
Astrocytoma	5	4
Oligodendroglioma	18	32
Mixed glioma	14	19
Anaplastic glioma	14	5
Gliaependymoma	0	4
Ependymoma	0	10
Gliosarcoma	7	0
Meningioma	0	1
Total CNS	58	75
Neurinoma	7	3
Anaplastic neurinoma	6	24
Total PNS	13	27
Extraneural	8	7
Total neoplasia	79	109

Reprinted with permission from Koestner (189).

Sex

Although male rats have a higher spontaneous brain tumor incidence than females just as is found in human beings, there is no statistically significant difference in susceptibility of the sexes in experimental MNU and ENU tumor induction.

Dose and Methods of Application

A striking dose-response relation can be demonstrated using single inoculations of ENU to produce tumors in the offspring; with increasing doses the tumor incidence increases and the latency period is shortened (Table 2). Tumor production in adult rats requires multiple MNU applications. Variable doses, different routes, and different regimens of exposure may be selected, depending on the objectives. The incidence of neurogenic tumors is highest with intravenous administration of MNU (95%), lower with oral (52%) and intraperitoneal (36%) routes, and lowest with subcutaneous (12%) administrations (25,26). Any route other than i.v. not only results in a decline of neurogenic tumors but also in an increased appearance of extraneural neoplasms, predominantly at the injection site. MNU and ENU do not require enzymatic activation since cleavage of the acyl residue occurs heterolytically in a neutral or slightly alkaline medium. Tumors may therefore be produced at the site of application as well as in distant organs, such as brain.

Depending on the objectives, different routes, variable doses, and different regimens of exposure may be selected. If, for instance, a high intracerebral glioma yield is desired, low weekly doses of MNU (5 mg/kg) should be applied i.v. to Sprague–Dawley rats for a total of 180 mg/kg. Over 90% glioma incidence will be achieved with this treatment (27). If tumors of the PNS are desired, male Fischer 344 rats should be exposed i.v. to 10 mg/kg MNU twice weekly for 9 weeks (28). With this regimen an 81% incidence of neurinomas (schwannomas) can be produced. Intragastric intubation of 20 mg/kg MNU twice weekly for 9 weeks, however, may result in a 100% incidence of thymic lymphomas and gastric carcinomas. The rats may not live long enough for neurogenic tumor development (29).

Single intraperitoneal administrations of 45, 90, and 180 mg/kg ENU resulted in

TABLE 2. *Transplacental tumor induction in SPF Sprague–Dawley rats by administration of ENU on day 20 of gestation*

Single dose i.v. (mg/kg)	Number of dams	Number of offspring	Number of rats with tumors	Average survival time (days)
1	4	46	13 (29%)	487 ± 119
5	3	24	14 (58%)	368 ± 149
20	2	17	16 (94%)	269 ± 77
50	2	25	25 (100%)	211 ± 70

Reprinted with permission from Koestner (189).

80% to 100% mammary carcinoma development in female and 80% in male Sprague–Dawley rats (30,31). When female BD IV rats were exposed to the same regimen, Sertoli's cell–like tumors of the ovary were produced in addition to mammary tumors (32).

Cellular and Molecular Basis for Target-Organ Specificity

The target-organ specificity is ultimately determined by the presence of a cell population susceptible to neoplastic transformation. Prospective target cells must have the capability to replicate. Terminally differentiated cells, such as mature neurons, are not susceptible to neoplastic transformation. There is convincing evidence that all chemical carcinogens produce structural alterations of cellular DNA (covalent DNA adducts). Such alterations are not restricted to target cells; however, their relative persistence or elimination distinguishes target cells from nontarget cells. Using the N-nitrosourea treatment as a model for neurogenic tumor production in rats, alkylation of guanine at the O^6-position has been considered to be a crucial alteration. It has been convincingly demonstrated that formation of O^6-methylguanine (33) or O^6-ethylguanine (34) affect target and nontarget cells alike, but their persistence is restricted to target cells. The deficiency of brain cells compared to liver cells for repair of O^6-alkylguanine from the DNA makes the nervous system a target organ for N-nitrosourea-induced neoplasia.

Chang et al. (35) studied the persistence of DNA lesions (O^6-ethylguanine) induced by different doses of ENU by comparing brain (a high target organ) with kidney (a low target organ) and liver (a nontarget organ). In addition, cellular proliferation was measured as an increment of DNA content per organ at day 7 posttreatment. They found that persistence of O^6-ethylguanine was not affected by dose levels. Comparing the three organs, the adduct persistence ranked in the order brain >kidney>liver, while the percent increase in DNA content was measured as liver >kidney>brain. When target specificity of ENU carcinogenesis in 30-day-old rats was compared to that following transplacental exposure in terms of its relationship to persistence of DNA lesions and the rate of target cell proliferation, the following conclusion could be drawn: Induction of neoplasia in target cells is not only determined by persistent DNA lesions but also by the rate of proliferation of target cells at the time of exposure. This importance of proliferative activity has been emphasized by other investigators (36,37). It is well established that partial hepatectomy leading to reparative proliferation enhances the hepatocarcinogenic effect of chemical carcinogens. Both characteristics, the high proliferative activity and an incompletely developed enzyme system responsible for DNA repair, are found in precursor cells in the developing nervous system and render them highly susceptible to neoplastic transformation.

The subependymal plate has been recognized as a predilection site for glioma development in perinatal neurocarcinogenesis studies (Fig. 2). Pilkington and Lantos carefully documented the sequential development of gliomas from the sub-

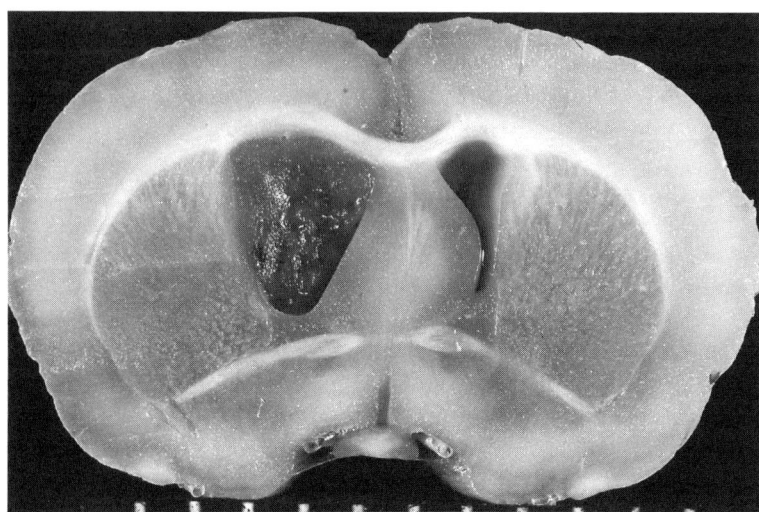

FIG. 2. Glioma arising in periventricular region of the cerebral cortex in a rat exposed to multiple i.v. inoculations of MNU.

ependymal plate following transplacental exposure to ENU (38). Kleihues et al. (39) considers the persistence of a subependymal matrix cell population a prerequisite for the development of astrocytic, ependymal, and mixed gliomas, but not for oligodendrogliomas. Using a very elegant method of fetal forebrain transplants following exposure to ENU, he and his collaborators (40) could only produce oligodendrogliomas in the transplant when the recipient rats were exposed to two additional doses of ENU. This experiment supports the hypothesis that oligodendroglioma production does not require the pluripotential precursor cells of the subependymal plate; therefore, oligodendrogliomas may arise from transformation of differentiated oligodendrocytes or precursor cells already committed to oligodendrocytic differentiation. In our studies of early stages of tumor development, packets of oligodendrocytic tumor cells were arranged in their usual satellite positions around neurons in the cerebral cortex (Fig. 3).

Tumor induction in adult animals is more difficult since it must deal with lower numbers of precursor cells and reduced cellular proliferation. Proliferation can, however, be stimulated by high (toxic) doses of carcinogens. The increased tumor burden of older people and animals might be explained by impaired cellular and molecular mechanisms responsible for repair, proliferation control, elimination of aberrant cells, and other vital cellular activities (41).

Based on these findings, a critical determinant for the risk of neoplastic transformation is the capacity of cells to repair promutagenic DNA lesions. The inability of the rat nervous system to excise O^6-alkylguanine makes it the target organ for tumor induction with alkylating alkylnitrosoureas. Although this correlation has been consistent in rat studies, it is not applicable to other species. Kleihues and Wiestler

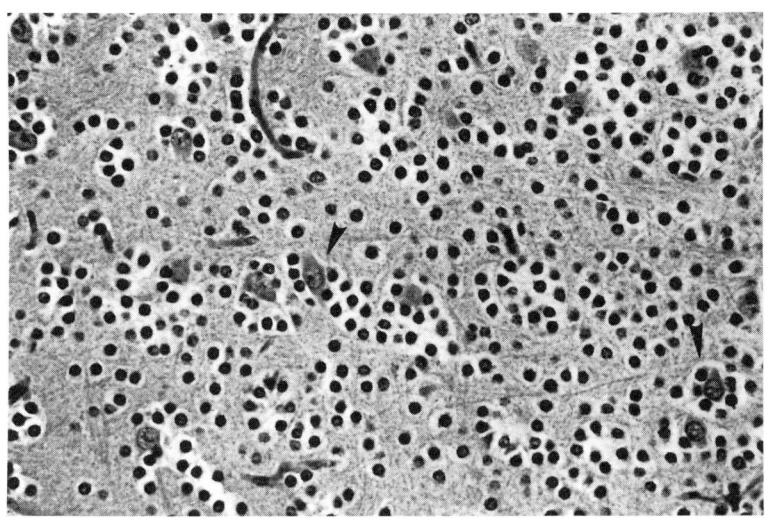

FIG. 3. Early neoplastic proliferation of oligodendrocytes in packets and in satellite position around neurons (*arrows*) in cerebral cortex. [Reprinted with permission from Koestner et al. (190).]

(42), referring to earlier studies, point out that mice (although as poor as rats in repairing O^6-alkylguanine in cerebral DNA) rarely develop nervous system tumors. Also, gerbils retained 40% of the initial concentration of O^6-ethylguanine for 6 months following a single dose of ENU, but so far, attempts to induce neurogenic tumors in this species have failed completely. The authors drew the conclusion that persistence of O^6-alkylguanine constitutes a necessary, although not a sufficient event for malignant transformation of prospective target cells.

MULTISTEP PROCESS OF CARCINOGENESIS AND ITS APPLICABILITY TO TUMORS OF THE NERVOUS SYSTEM

The concept of a multistep process of carcinogenesis has been widely tested, particularly in the hepatocarcinogenesis model. The structural alteration of DNA (adduct formation) in the target cell by the ultimate carcinogen is considered to be the primary event in the multistep process of carcinogenesis. Such DNA modifications usually result from covalent binding between nucleophilic centers (electron-rich N and O atoms) and highly reactive electrophilic derivatives of the carcinogen (4). Carcinogenic agents such as alkylating agents form 12 or more different DNA adducts. Some adducts are chemically unstable and lost from DNA, leaving an apurinic site that must be repaired. Other adducts are repaired by various DNA repair systems, including alkyltransferase, which removes O^6 lesions and the excision repair, which removes specific adducts together with some adjacent nucleotides and resynthesizes the DNA using the second DNA strand as a template. Unrepaired adducts can lead to DNA sequence changes by miscoding during DNA replication, recombinations, gene amplification, and chromosomal aberrations. Several additional steps are, however, required in the process to achieve cancer production. The reduction of the rather complicated mechanisms of carcinogenesis to three major phases has helped focusing on specific crucial events of this process and has contributed to a better understanding of cancer development. The three phases, initiation, promotion, and progression, will be treated separately with tumor induction of the nervous system in mind.

Initiation

Initiation is the primary event in the carcinogenic process. Covalent DNA adducts formed by carcinogens may result in promutagenic lesions in target cells which generate various DNA changes referred to above during DNA replication. Only cells capable of proliferation (particularly progenitor cells) are target cells for initiation. Base alkylations and resulting point mutation constitute the major DNA lesion with alkylating carcinogens, bulky DNA adducts, as derived from polycyclic aromatic hydrocarbons, aflatoxins and aromatic amines, may, in addition cause frame shifts (42). It is postulated that completed initiation prevents a stem cell from terminally differentiating (43,44). The common denominator of all mechanistic consequences of initiation is basically an interference with the genetic programs of target cells (45). The most intensive studies in the field of initiation in neurocarcinogenesis have been accomplished using alkylating agents.

Among the cytotoxic DNA adducts formed upon cell exposure to alkylating carcinogens are N^7-alkylguanine and N^3-alkyladenine, but these do not cause base mispairing. In contrast, lesions such as O^6-alkylguanine and O^4-alkylthymine frequently cause mutation owing to base mispairing. O^6-Alkylguanine, which is the most abundant mutagenic lesion, induces the GC-to-AT transition (46–48), while O^4-alkylthymine which is found at much lower levels than O^6-alkylguanine, induces transition from AT to GC (49–51). Such point mutations may activate cellular oncogenes if they occur at critical codons, and thus play a critical role in the initiation of carcinogenesis. O^6-Alkylguanine can be repaired by the ubiquitous O^6-alkylguanine DNA alkyltransferase that transfers the alkyl group to a cysteine residue within the protein itself (52–54). O^4-Alkylthymine is also known to be recognized by the eukaryotic alkyltransferase (54,55). When the coding sequence of the *Escherichia coli* O^6-alkylguanine alkyltransferase gene was transfected into Chinese hamster V79 cells that lack endogenous alkyltransferase activity, a clone expressing high levels of the bacterial alkyltransferase rapidly repaired O^6-methylguanine produced in the host genome following exposure to MNU and reduced its mutagenic effects (56). When a vector containing O^6-methylguanine or O^6-ethylguanine was introduced in parallel into a pair of Chinese hamster ovary cells, in which one was deficient in the repair enzyme O^6-alkylguanine DNA alkyltransferase and the other was proficient in this activity, a high frequency of mutations (almost exclusively G→A transitions) was observed in the cells deficient in alkyltransferase, and a low frequency of mutations was detected in the repair-proficient cells (57). These observations clearly indicate that O^6-alkylguanine adducts are indeed capable of inducing G→A mutations in mammalian cells, and that the O^6-alkylguanine DNA alkyltransferase plays a significant role in reducing such a mutation. Moreover, when O^6-ethylguanine-repair-proficient variants and repair-deficient derivatives of the 208F rat fibroblast cell line were tested for tumorigenic conversion after exposure to ENU, the frequencies of foci in monolayer culture and of anchorage-independent colonies in a semisolid agar medium in the repair-proficient variants, were as low as $1/28$ and $1/56$ of those in the repair-deficient wild type (58). The relative capacity of cells for repair of O^6-alkylguanine is therefore a critical determinant for the probability of transformation by N-nitroso carcinogens. This, in turn, further supports the notion that mutation is an event crucial to the initiation of carcinogenesis.

Induction of mammary tumors in rats by a single exposure to MNU often involves activation of c-Ha-*ras* protooncogenes by G→A transition in codon 12 (59,60). Similarly, MNU-induced mammary tumors in mice have a G→A mutation in codon 12 of the c-Ki-*ras* gene (61). Because of the highly labile nature of MNU, the binding to DNA must occur within minutes following its administration. The mutational events are therefore probably involved in the initiation of the carcinogenesis process (62). Mutations of N-*ras*, which cause substitution of position 61 of the protein product, have been reported in cell lines of human neuroblastoma (63) and human melanoma (64).

The *neu* (c-*erb*B-2) gene, which encodes a protein closely related to the epidermal growth factor (65–67), is a protooncogene that can be activated by a point mutation. The *neu* oncogene was found consistently to be activated in established cell lines derived from ENU-induced neurogenic tumors of BD IX rats by a T→A transversion in a sequence that encodes the transmembrane region of the gene product (68). The replacement of valine by glutamic acid in this region induces an aggregated state that may mimic aspects of ligand-induced receptor aggregation, and results in intrinsic activation of tyrosine kinase (69). Transfection of DNA of primary gliomas and schwannomas transplacentally induced by ENU demonstrated that the activation of *neu* oncogene was specifically associated with tumors of the PNS (70).

The establishment of a DNA nucleotide sequence alteration (mutation) induced by replication of DNA containing an adduct such as O^6-alkylguanine or O^4-alkylthymine is probably the crucial factor in the initiation process. Of course, only point mutations in critical codons of a protooncogene may result in oncogene activation (42,53,59).

Promotion

Promotion is viewed as the process whereby initiated cells develop focal proliferations such as altered hepatocellular foci in the liver or papillomas of the skin.

These focal proliferations may regress or they may progress into malignant neoplasms. In contrast to initiation and progression, promotion is a reversible process. Proposed mechanisms of promotion include alterations of gene expression (e.g., expression of an oncogene product, inhibition of intercellular communication by gap junctions, suppression of immune surveillance, receptor binding, and oxidant injury). Although promotion has been studied intensively in the liver and other nonneural organs, little is known about promotion of tumors of the nervous system. Kokunai et al. (71) tested the promoting effect of 12-O-tetradecanoylphorbol-13-acetate (TPA) using cultured cells obtained from the cerebrum of rat fetuses exposed transplacentally to ENU (50 mg/kg) on day 18 of gestation. TPA was added in various doses to the cell cultures. When compared to untreated cells, the TPA-treated cells exhibited an increased plating efficiency in agar, an increased agglutinability to concanavalin A, and a higher tumorigenicity upon intracerebral implantation into syngeneic rats with a significantly reduced latency period. The authors attributed these effects to the tumor-promoting capacity of TPA. Phenobarbital was ineffective as a neurogenic tumor promoter in both mice (72) and rats (73).

Promotion occurs sometime between initiation and progression and may determine the start of cancer development, following months or years of dormancy of initiated cells. The time between initiation and the appearance of recognizable tumors is generally referred to as the latency period. This period varies greatly among species. Using identical experimental conditions (weekly i.v. injections of 5 mg/kg MNU for a total dose of 180 mg/kg) the average latency period in rats was 8½ months, while in dogs it was 3 years. Known latency periods in humans may extend over decades, as the Hiroshima atom bomb exposure and the diethylstilbestrol-linked vaginal clear cell carcinoma (74) indicate. The latency period also varies with age of exposure, carcinogenic potential of the agent, dose, and tumor type and location.

It would be erroneous to consider the latency period to be a period of absolute quiescence. Several studies were undertaken to evaluate sequential changes in the nervous system of rats from day 1 to 6 months following transplacental exposure to ENU (75,76). Increased cellularity of the trigeminal nerve was found as early as 20 days postpartum, and by 1 month more than half of the trigeminal nerves exhibited hypercellularity, termed *early neoplastic proliferation* (ENP) (Figs. 4 and 5). Transplantation of such lesions into syngeneic rats resulted in neurinoma development at the transplantation sites. ENP of spinal nerve roots was also detected at one month following ENU exposure whereas that of the brain took 4 months to become demonstrable. Correspondingly tumors in the PNS, particularly those of the trigeminal nerve, peak several months earlier than those of the CNS.

There is no clear definition of promotion following a single transplacental exposure to ENU. ENP can be observed several weeks after exposure, and both micro and macro tumors gradually develop from these clusters of proliferating cells. Burger et al. (40) first presented *in vivo* evidence for a multistep development of neural tumors. Grafting of forebrain tissue from transplacentally ENU-exposed fetuses into the cerebrum of syngeneic rats did not produce a single tumor from the initiated

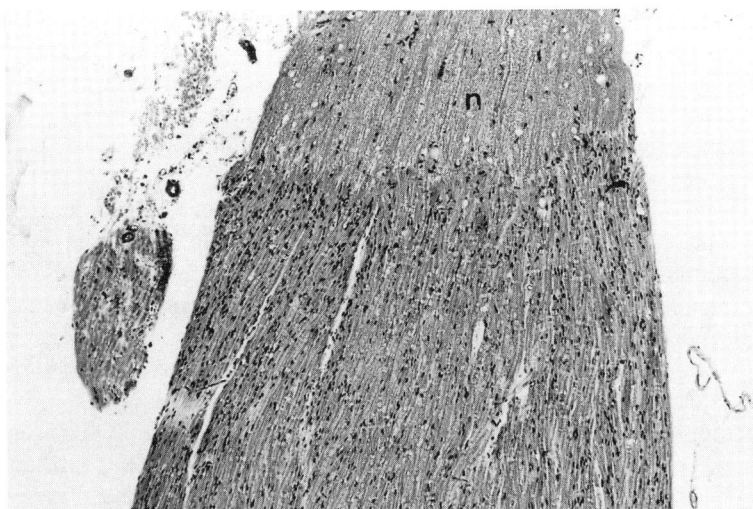

FIG. 4. ENP (early neoplastic proliferation) of trigeminal nerve in a rat at 3 weeks following transplacental exposure to ENU. Note difference in cellularity when compared to normal portion of nerve (n).

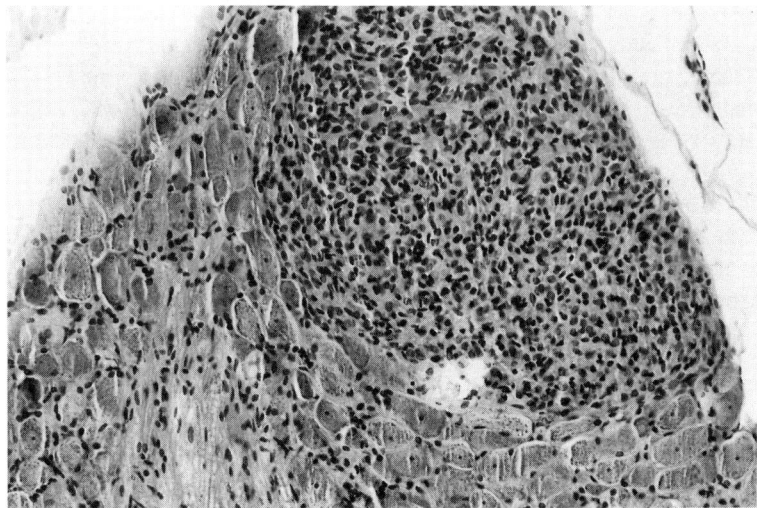

FIG. 5. Neurinoma; clearly defined microtumor of the trigeminal nerve separated from neurons of the ganglion Gasseri 90 days following transplacental exposure to ENU. [Reprinted with permission from Vinores and Koestner (180).]

glial cells within the graft. However, a subsequent exposure of the recipient rat to ENU resulted in a 100% incidence of oligodendrogliomas in the graft and only a 22% to 40% tumor incidence in the recipient brain outside the graft. The authors considered the promotional effect of the second ENU exposure responsible for tumor development within the graft and for the significantly higher incidence of tumors within the graft compared to the recipient's own brain.

It is essential to use multiple MNU exposures to produce brain tumors in adult rats. One could assume that every additional exposure will lead to new initiations and promotion of already initiated cells. As a consequence, multiple tumors at various stages of development are found in individual MNU-treated rats when they are sacrificed. What causes promotion remains a puzzle in the single transplacental ENU exposure model. The most obvious conclusion is that the high proliferation rate of cells in the fetus causes the clonal outgrowth of initiated cells.

Tumor development following transplacental ENU exposure is possible even when target cells are removed from fetal brains 1 h after exposure and implanted subcutaneously into syngeneic hosts. Under these conditions clinically detectable mixed glial tumors developed subcutaneously in 2 of 11 implanted rats following a latency period of 10 to 12 months (77).

Progression

During the stage of progression focal preneoplastic lesions develop into benign or malignant neoplasms. The triggering mechanisms for the uncontrolled proliferation of transformed cells during progression have not yet been fully defined. Additional mutational events may be the heart of this process. The original multihit concept developed by Knudson (78) which has been adapted to hepatocarcinogenesis by Scherer (79) and further refined by Pitot et al. (80,81), is one interpretation. Recent work points to the activation of protooncogenes and the inactivation of suppressor genes as underlying this process. The importance of these events to the progression phase of neurocarcinogenesis has been studied during the past decade but needs considerably more exploration.

Role of Protooncogenes and Suppressor Genes in Neurocarcinogenesis

Normal expression of N-*myc* is known to occur predominantly in immature human neural cells and disappears with differentiation (82). Amplification of N-*myc* has been detected in human neuroblastoma cells (83,84) as well as retinoblastoma cells (85). The amplification is frequently associated with DNA rearrangements (86) and may be related to the loss of a critical region on the short arm of chromosome 1 (87). N-*myc* amplification appears to be highly correlated with the advanced stage of disease, as the amplification is not found in the tumor tissue of patients with stage 1 or 2 of neuroblastoma but is present in 50% of patients with stage 3 or 4

(88). Seeger et al. (89) have demonstrated that the presence of N-*myc* amplification has prognostic significance and is associated with rapid tumor progression. Brodeur et al. (90) have further shown that the N-*myc* copy number is consistent within a given tumor, as well as tumor tissue obtained from different sites or from different tissues in each patient. High N-*myc* expression in rat neuroblastoma cells causes downregulation of class I histocompatibility antigens, which may contribute to tumor progression by decreasing antitumor immunoresponse (91). The rearrangement and amplification of the protooncogene c-*myc* have been found in double-minutes in cells from a patient with glioblastoma multiforme (92).

There is a growing body of evidence that an autocrine secretion of growth factors may operate in neoplastic transformation and tumor development (93). Tumors of the nervous system may express increased levels of the c-*erb*B/EGF receptor. Immunoprecipitation of functional EGF receptor kinase complexes revealed high levels of EGF receptor in human brain tumors of nonneuronal origin such as gliomas and meningiomas (94). Increased expression of EGF receptors in human gliomas was invariably associated with gene amplification and possible rearrangements (95,96). Polysomy of chromosome 7 was correlated with overexpression of c-*erb*B gene in a human glioblastoma cell line (97). In human gliomas, EGF receptor expression appears to be correlated with the WHO grade of malignancy (98). In two cases of human glioblastoma multiforme, cells carried amplified c-*erb*B genes bearing short deletion mutations within the ligand-binding domain of the EGF receptor (99). The products of these mutated genes were about 30 kDa smaller than the normal 170-kDa EGF receptor and showed a significant constitutive elevation of tyrosine kinase activity without its ligand, which may have contributed to the carcinogenic process.

Long-term culturing of neonatal rat brain cells, transplacentally treated with ENU results in phenotypic transformation, the timing of which correlates with expression of the c-*sis* protooncogene encoding the B-chain of PDGF (100). Since glial cells possess PDGF receptors, an autocrine mechanism could play an important role in ENU-induced neurooncogenesis in rats. Transcripts of the c-*sis* were also detected in human glioblastoma cell lines (101). Cultured human glioblastoma cells produce a PDGF-like mitogenic protein (102,103) and possess PDGF receptors (104). The expression of PDGF A chain, PDGF B chain/c-*sis*, and PDGF receptor mRNA has also been demonstrated in biopsies of human glioblastoma multiforme (105).

Investigation of a large panel of human glioblastoma cell lines (106) revealed that they expressed the PDGF receptor gene together with either the PDGF A chain gene, B chain gene, or both at high frequency. Most cell lines were found to express high levels of EGF/TGF-α receptor mRNA and TGF-α mRNA and displayed EGF/TGF-α receptor sites. Moreover, acidic FGF and the corresponding receptor were also expressed in human glioma cells (107,108). These findings suggest that there are multiple autocrine loops in human glioma cells (106).

The human genome contains a number of loci where mutations or deletions predispose to the development of tumors (109). They had been termed *recessive on-*

cogenes or *antioncogenes* (108) and perhaps better, suppressor genes. The RB1 gene on chromosome 13q is crucial for tumorigenesis of retinoblastoma and also for that of osteosarcoma, which commonly arises as a second tumor in children who survive retinoblastoma (110–112). The RB1 suppressor gene cannot only be deleted in tumor cells (113) but can also be inactivated by single point mutations (114). This gene encodes a mRNA of 4.6 kb (115) and produces a nuclear phosphoprotein with DNA binding activity (116). Introduction of a cloned wild-type RB1 gene into cultured retinoblastoma and osteosarcoma cells suppresses the neoplastic phenotype (117).

Both low- and high-malignancy-grade astrocytomas frequently display loss of distinct regions on chromosome 17p (118). This region may thus contain an antioncogene, the loss, deletion, or inactivation of which is associated with tumor initiation or early tumor progression in astrocytomas. Loss of constitutional heterozygosity for loci on chromosome 10 was observed in 28 of 29 tumors histologically classified as glioblastoma (malignancy grade IV), whereas similar losses were not observed in any of 22 gliomas of lower malignancy grade (119).

Partial monosomy of the short arm of chromosome 1 was the most consistent cytogenetic abnormality in human neuroblastomas (120,121). Meningiomas and acoustic neurinomas, both of which occur frequently in bilateral acoustic neurofibromatosis, are specifically associated with loss of genes of human chromosome 22 (122–126). In von Reckinghausen neurofibromatosis, none of the benign tumors, but almost all of the malignant neurofibrosarcomas, were associated with loss or deletions on chromosome 17 (127). The target of these deletions appears to be the p53 suppressor gene, which was found to be mutated in several neurofibrosarcomas (127).

Both protooncogene activation and tumor suppressor gene deletion play a significant role in cancer progression. They must be considered to be decisive factors in the sequential multistep process of cancer development. The recently acquired capability of gene transfer by replication-defective retroviral vectors permits selective examination of the effects of individual oncogenes or combinations of two or more oncogenes. Kleihues et al. (39) and Aguzzi et al. (128) infected fetal rat brain cells with oncogene-encoding retroviral vectors and transplanted these cells into the caudoputamen of syngeneic adult hosts. Rats carrying transplants transfected with polyoma middle T-antigen DNA sequence developed hemangiomas, while those transfected with the *src* gene developed astrocytic and mesenchymal tumors after latency periods of 2 to 6 months. Transplants of cells infected with v-*myc* oncogene encoded vectors remained free of neurogenic neoplasms with the exception of an embryonal tumor in one rat. Exposure to v-H-*ras*, in contrast, resulted in a low incidence of gliomas. The combined effect of v-*myc* and c-H-*ras* resulted in multiple undifferentiated neoplasms (some definitely of glial origin) which the investigators classified as primitive neuroectodermal tumors. With the application of these advanced molecular techniques, a more precise understanding of the role of oncogenes and suppressor genes will continue to emerge.

Role of Host Factors in the Progression Phase of Neurocarcinogenesis

Host factors have been recognized to play a significant role in all phases of carcinogenesis. They may influence susceptibility to cancer induction so that equal exposure will affect only a portion of the individuals at risk (77,129). The presence of activating and deactivating enzymes and the speed of their mobilization influences formation of the ultimate carcinogen and/or its speedy breakdown into harmless catabolites and thus facilitates or prevents cancer induction. The level of repair capability of carcinogen-damaged DNA is an important factor in preventing promutagenic lesions from causing mutations. Mutations are a crucial step in the process of initiation. It is certain, however, that not all initiated cells progress to cancer and that malignant neoplasms may spontaneously regress. The following discussion concentrates on two areas where host factors may play a potential role in the postinitiation stages of neurocarcinogenesis. They are immune mechanisms and growth and differentiation factors.

Immune Mechanisms

The principle of immune defense against cancer is based on Burnet's concept of immunological surveillance (130). An immune reaction of the allograft type was visualized as the primary and most important line of defense against neoplasia. It was suggested that most neoplasms are eliminated by this immunological surveillance at the early stages of development based on their content of tumor-specific antigens. Successful progression of transformed cells to grossly recognized tumors was considered possible by some undefined escape mechanisms or in immuno-oncologically compromised individuals such as fetuses, infants, the elderly, and persons subjected to immunosuppressive therapy (129).

The theory of immunological surveillance has been challenged seriously by Prehn (131), who presented evidence that the immunological surveillance of nascent tumors, as originally conceived, may not exist for most tumor types and that late-acting immunological defense was inefficient. The evidence for this challenge is limited and the immunological elimination of transformed cells cannot be discounted absolutely. With respect to experimental brain tumor production, our work indicates that immune mechanisms play an insignificant role in that process. Antilymphocyte serum treatment had no effect on the incidence of central and peripheral nervous system tumors, nor on the survival times of MNU-treated rats (Table 3). However, the experiment demonstrated that failure of immune defense in one organ may not be applicable to tumors of other organs or systems. Although the incidence of tumors of the nervous system were not affected, 25% of the antilymphocyte serum-treated rats in this experiment developed carcinomas of the bladder, while all untreated rats were free of bladder neoplasms. Tumors of the bladder were, to our knowledge, never reported in MNU experiments. These results suggest that immu-

TABLE 3. *Comparison of survival time and tumor incidence of the nervous system and bladder in rats treated with MNU alone and MNU + ALS[a]*

	Incidence (%)	
	MNU-treated	MNU–ALS-treated
CNS	14/37 (38)	10/37 (27)
PNS	34/37 (92)	31/37 (84)
Bladder	0/37 (0)	9/37 (24)
Mean survival time	262 ± 66 days	256 ± 71 days

Extracted from Denlinger et al. (138).
[a]MNU, methylnitrosourea; ALS, antilymphocytic serum; CNS, central nervous system; PNS, peripheral nervous system.

nological surveillance was a factor in bladder tumor development but not with neuroectodermal neoplasms. The conclusion that there is ineffective immune surveillance of neurogenic tumors is further supported by another experiment (132) in which neonatal rats were thymectomized (or sham-operated) and treated with 20 mg/kg ENU at 30 days of age, at which time immunologic competence is well developed. Thymectomy did not result in a higher incidence of tumors of the nervous system (compared to sham-operated rats) as would have been expected if immunological surveillance was an effective suppressor of neurogenic tumor development (Table 4).

The brain has long been considered as an immunologically privileged site, particularly because of its lack of direct lymphatic drainage. In a review article, Wikstrand and Bigner (133) present evidence that the immunologic privilege of the brain should be changed to "partial privilege." This change is justified according to these authors, because (a) graft rejection, although retarded, does occur intracerebrally; (b) intracerebral transplants induce a systemic immune response; and (c) effectors of systemic origin enter the brain parenchyma. The "immune privilege" of the brain compared to other organ sites is therefore best described in quantitative terms relative to differences in rates of antigenic recognition and the afferent limb of the immune response rather than in any absolute sense.

It should be mentioned that immunosuppression is often recognized in glioma patients, particularly involving cell-mediated immunologic function (134–137). A similar condition exists in MNU-treated rats. Skin graft survival time in rats treated

TABLE 4. *Effect of thymectomy on survival times of 30-day-old BD IX rats treated with 20 mg ENU/kg*

Group	Number of rats	Survival time (days)	Brain	Spinal cord	Peripheral nervous system
Thymectomized	42	642.5 ± 117.7	10	4	2
Sham-operated	38	592.1 ± 155.1	9	1	5
Control	9	835.2 ± 122.5	0	0	0

Selected data from Swenberg (132).

with tumor-inducing doses of MNU was increased significantly compared to controls (138). It is doubtful, however, that the MNU-induced immune suppression had any influence on the incidence of neurogenic tumors. As illustrated in Table 3, the antilymphocytic serum (ALS)-treated rats actually had a lower tumor incidence than the ALS-untreated rats, which speaks against immune protection. The ALS used in that study had a high potency and prolonged survival of skin grafts indefinitely (138).

The apparent lack of an effective immune surveillance as a significant host factor in neurocarcinogenesis may not preclude future use of immune mechanisms for diagnostic, monitoring, and therapeutic purposes. Although large batteries of glioma-associated monoclonal antibodies have been produced in various laboratories, progress is still hampered by the remarkable antigenic heterogeneity of human anaplastic gliomas and glioma-derived cell lines. Wikstrand et al. (134) expressed confidence that clear differences in lymphoid marker expression and the identification of widely and rarely expressed glioma-associated antigens, and the potential of immunological differentiation between glioblastoma multiforme and astrocytomas, will serve to reduce this complexity and may be of potential diagnostic or prognostic significance.

Therapy of brain tumors is not an objective of this chapter. Immunotherapy trials have been widely attempted, but to date, they have been, at best, inconclusive. Recent trials using intracompartmental and intralesional applications of radioisotopes attached to monoclonal antibodies have been very encouraging (D. Bigner, Duke University, personal communication). Considerable ongoing work in brain tumor biology and definition of tumor-specific antigens will provide a better basis for future immunotherapeutic purposes.

Growth and Differentiation Factors

Growth factors such as EGF, PDGF, and TGF thought to be involved in tumor development were discussed above. Maxwell et al. (108) recently reported overexpression of angiogenic growth factors (acidic FGF and TFG-α) and EGF/TGF-α receptors in 30 primary human astrocytomas. The authors propose that the overexpression of angiogenic growth factors may underlie the intense neovascularization characteristic of astrocytomas.

In this section we concentrate primarily on differentiation factors which, in contrast to the growth factors mentioned above, may inhibit progression and tumor development and act as reverse transformation agents. The most prominent and most thoroughly investigated differentiation factor is the nerve growth factor (NGF). NGF is essential for the maturation and maintenance of the autonomic nervous system. Development, but not maintenance, of the sensory portion of the nervous system also depends on NGF activity. Evidence has been presented during the past 5 years that NGF activity is not restricted to the autonomic and sensory nervous systems. It has been demonstrated that motor neurons in the brain stem and spinal cord express nerve growth factor receptors (NGFRs) during development (139). Although NGFRs cannot be identified in motor neurons of adult rats, these receptors reappear following injury to peripheral axons. Diverse activities have been proposed or demonstrated for NGF in the adult nervous system. NGF was shown to influence neurofilament gene expression in mature primary sensory neurons (140), stimulate function of cholinergic neurons (141,142), be involved in Schwann cell–neuronal interactions (143), and play a role in oxidant–antioxidant balance and neuronal injury (144,145). The promotion of differentiation and retardation of growth are the most important functions of NGF in the carcinogenic process. If an agent were capable of stimulating a cancer cell to terminally differentiate and consequently to lose its ability to divide continuously, the cell would eventually be eliminated. NGF has shown this capability in transformed cells of neuronal, glial, and Schwann cell origin in *in vitro* and *in vivo* studies.

In vitro *Studies.* PC12 pheochromocytoma cells respond to physiologic levels of NGF by developing a number of phenotypic properties of sympathetic neurons. They include neurite outgrowth, cessation of cell division, and the development of electrical excitability (146–148). Several human and murine neuroblastoma cell lines respond similarly to NGF by neurite outgrowth and development of electrical excitability (149).

The effect of NGF is not restricted to tumor cells of neuronal origin. Several cell lines and clones from human and rodent neoplasms of glial cell origin also respond to NGF (150–153). In these studies it has been reported that most differentiated glioma cell lines and clones were not visibly affected by NGF, while undifferentiated glioma cell lines and clones developed a more differentiated phenotype (150, 152). This effect on responsive cells was characterized by restoration of surface inhibition, decrease in nuclear cytoplasmic ratio, flattening of cellular surfaces with numerous protruding cellular processes, and retardation of growth (Fig. 6). Ultrastructural studies revealed that these cells were interconnected by junctional devices (bridges) and their cytoskeletal organization exhibited features similar to those observed during maturation of normal glia cells (154).

Five human neurogenic tumor cell lines responded similarly to NGF treatment (153). The human tumor cell lines were one mixed glioma, two glioblastoma multiforme, one medulloblastoma (all generous gifts from Darrell Bigner, Duke University), and a malignant melanoma obtained from the American Type Culture Collection. All four cell lines possessed NGF receptors; the melanoma had the most receptors and the glial tumors the least, while the medulloblastoma had a slightly higher receptor density than gliomas.

NGF treatment of these cell lines resulted in cellular compactness and process formation accompanied by a diminished or arrested growth. In both the rat and human neurogenic tumor cell lines the phenotypical change induced by NGF persisted following withdrawal of NGF (152,153). This persistence was best demonstrated in the human glioblastoma cell line U251 because of its longest survival in culture (153). The persistence of the NGF-induced morphological changes could be followed in this cell line for 53 days after removal of NGF from the culture medium (Fig. 7).

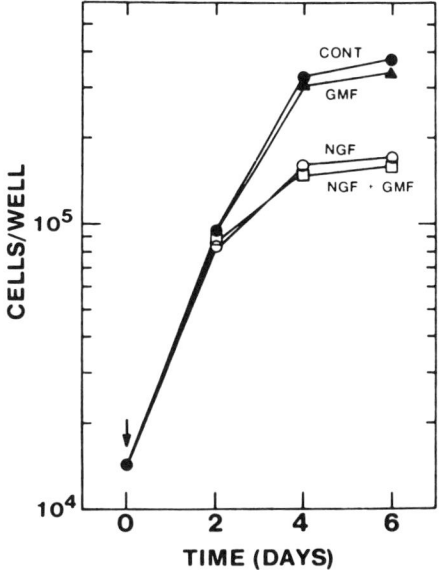

FIG. 6. Effects of NGF and GMF (glia maturation factor) on cell growth. T9 cells were first seeded in Dulbecco's modified Eagle's medium containing 10% fetal bovine serum. One day after seeding (day 0), the medium was changed to HL-1 (a chemically defined serum-free medium) with or without NGF, GMF, or both. Retardation of growth was attributable to NGF alone or to NGF in combination with GMF. [Reprinted with permission from Marushige et al. (152).]

Two procedures were used to determine if the morphological changes were the result of binding of NGF to specific surface receptors. In one procedure, 2.0 μg/mL cytochrome c, a protein similar to NGF in both size and charge (155), was added to the medium to determine if the changes attributed to NGF could be produced by the addition of a similar molecule. No changes were produced with cytochrome c. In the second procedure, cultured cells were preincubated with ME20.3, an antibody that binds specifically to the human NGFR (156). This procedure greatly diminished the development of NGF-induced morphological changes, indicating that the morphologic transformation induced by NGF was the result of NGF binding to specific receptors. Second messengers, particularly ionomycin, were able to simulate some morphological changes recognized with NGF treatment; however, their withdrawal resulted in quick reversion of these changes. The apparent differentiating effect of ionomycin indicates that calcium mobilization plays a role in the mechanism of NGF action (157).

The mechanism of action of NGF related to these changes is only partially understood. NGF action is initiated by the interaction with a specific receptor on the cell surface. Equilibrium binding analyses (158–160) have indicated that there are two receptor sites displaying high-affinity binding ($K_d = 10^{-11}$) and low-affinity binding ($K_d = 10^{-9}$) in neuroblastoma cells (161,162) as well as neuronal-like PC12 pheochromocytoma cells (163). The biological response to NGF is known to depend on interactions with the high-affinity receptor. The first NGF receptor molecular clones isolated (164,165) encode an intrinsic membrane protein of 75 to 80 kDa (p75^{NGFR}). When expressed in mammalian cells, p75^{NGFR} generates only low-affinity NGF binding (164,165). Generation of both high- and low-affinity receptor sites is, however, achieved by introduction of p75^{NGFR} cDNA into selected cell

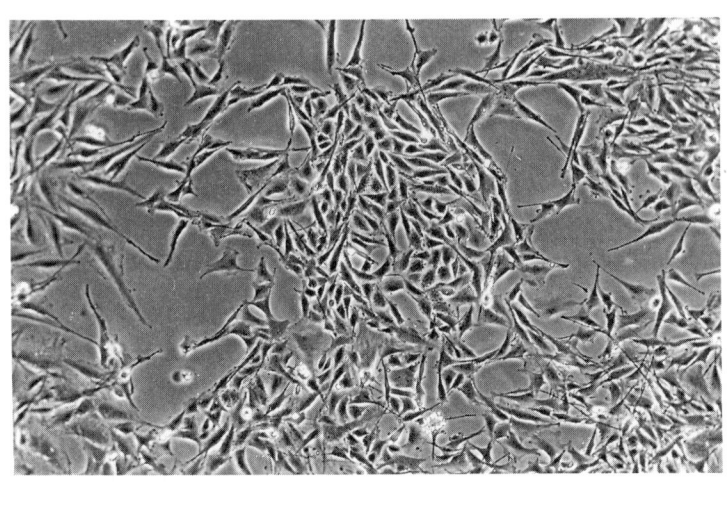

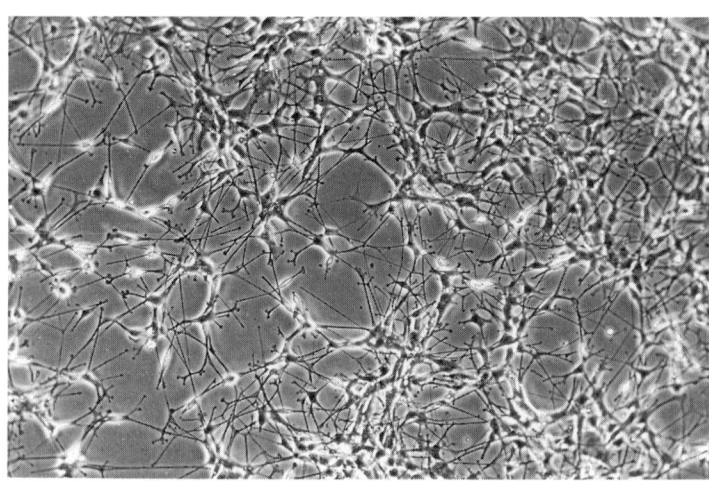

lines of neuronal origin such as an $p75^{NGFR}$-deficient variant of the PC12 pheochromocytoma cell line (166), a neuroblastoma cell line that does not express $p75^{NGFR}$ (167), and a medulloblastoma cell line (168). In addition to tumor cells of neuronal origin, $p75^{NGFR}$ has also been found in neurogenic tumor cells of nonneuronal origin, including melanoma and neurofibroma (156), schwannoma (169), and glioma (170) cells.

It has recently been shown that NGF induces tyrosine phosphorylation and tyrosine kinase activity of the *trk* protooncogene product of 130 to 140 kDa ($p140^{trk}$) in PC12 cells (171). Moreover, antibodies directed against NGF immunoprecipitate a 130- to 135-kDa protein with tyrosine kinase activity from NGF-treated PC12 cells (172). It has further been demonstrated that $p140^{trk}$ binds NGF, generating a NGF-receptor complex of approximately 160 kDa (173,174). Klein et al. (173) have reported that $p140^{trk}$ binds NGF with high affinity. Hempstead et al. (175) have, on the other hand, shown that high-affinity NGF binding requires both $p75^{NGFR}$ and $p140^{trk}$. These results suggest that activation of tyrosine kinase may be a critical early component of the cellular response to NGF. While equilibrium binding assays have indicated that C6 glioma cells possess high-affinity NGF receptors (170), cells of nonneuronal origin are generally known to express only low-affinity NGF receptors (176,177). The questions as to whether the *trk* protooncogene is expressed in neurogenic tumor cells of nonneuronal origin, and whether retardation of cell growth and morphological changes inducible by NGF in these cells utilize the same mechanism involved in the NGF response in neuronal cells remain to be investigated.

In vivo *Studies*. Two models were used to explore the reverse transformation effect of NGF upon neurogenic tumors *in vivo*: (a) NGF treatment of rats transplacentally inoculated with ENU, and (b) NGF treatment of tumors developing from transplantation of established tumor cell lines or clones.

NGF treatment of rats transplacentally inoculated with ENU. This model is useful because of the development of a predictable high number of neurogenic tumors in rats with a single transplacental inoculation of ENU. Tumor incidence and survival time depend on the age of fetal inoculation and dose. Earlier studies (178,179) using NGF and anti-NGF suggested that the level of NGF may modulate the carcinogenic response of the nervous system to ENU. These suggestions were substantiated by three consecutive experiments in our laboratory selecting intracranial and peripheral neurinomas (schwannomas) as the target tumor type for evaluation of the reverse transformation effect of ENU upon neurogenic tumors (180–182). The main advantages of selecting schwannomas were (a) their location outside the blood-brain

FIG. 7. Phase contrast of NGF-induced morphological changes in the U251 human glioblastoma multiforme cell line. **A:** Untreated control, day 11; **B:** NGF-treated, day 11: cells are more compact, developed a network of slender branching processes with the tendency to form intercellular connections; **C:** NGF-induced changes show persistence and further development by day 43. [Reprinted with permission from Yaeger et al. (153).]

barrier allowing systemic inoculation of NGF, and (b) their earlier appearance in comparison to gliomas. As discussed earlier, more than 50% of transplacentally ENU-exposed rats developed ENP (early neoplastic proliferation) in the trigeminal nerve by 3 weeks of age rising to 80% by 3 months, while ENP of glioma cells within the brain is demonstrable only 4 months after exposure.

Two experiments (180,181) targeted day 90 after treatment for the evaluation of NGF; the third (182) extended the target date to 1 year. In both 90-day experiments, pregnant rats received ENU i.v. (50 or 20 mg/kg) on day 21 of gestation. NGF was administered to one group of pregnant rats in each experiment preceding ENU exposure, while in other groups the offspring were treated with NGF following transplacental exposure to ENU (Table 5). In both experiments there was a significant reduction of neurinomas in the groups of rats treated with NGF following transplacental ENU exposure (Table 6). There was also a significantly reduced number of neurinomas in rats treated with NGF prior to ENU exposure. It was concluded that postnatal NGF treatment of rats exposed transplacentally to ENU resulted in reduction of the incidence of ENP and neurinomas at 90 days of age, presumably by differentiating initiated cells, which led eventually to their elimination. The significant reduction of neurinomas in rats treated with NGF prior to ENU exposure suggests a protective effect of NGF based on its capability to promote maturation of the target cell population.

The third experiment (182) was designed to determine the persistence of the effect of NGF upon neurinoma development over a 12-month period and to investigate whether the effect of NGF on the ENU-transformed cells was dependent on the presence of NGFR. Two groups of transplacentally ENU exposed rats were used in that study, one NGF treated and one left untreated (Table 7). The results revealed a significant reduction of neurinomas in the NGF-treated group at the termination of the experiment. When all neurinomas (trigeminal and peripheral) were counted the p value was <0.01, a reduction from 85% of untreated to 47% of NGF-treated rats (Table 8). An immunohistochemical evaluation for the presence of NGF receptor protein revealed that 24% of the neurinomas in the untreated group contained NGFR

TABLE 5. *Treatment schedule to determine effect of NGF on trigeminal nerve neoplasia induced by transplacental exposure to ENU*

Group	ENU	NGF
A1	50 mg/kg day 21 of gestation	Untreated control
A2	50 mg/kg day 21 of gestation	0.02 mg NGF (7S) on days 18–20 of gestation
A3	50 mg/kg day 21 of gestation	0.03 mg NGF (7S) on days 7–9 postpartum
B1	20 mg/kg day 20 of gestation	Untreated control
B2	20 mg/kg day 20 of gestation	0.2 mg total NGF (2.5 S) microinfusion starting day 14 of gestation[a]
B3	20 mg/kg day 20 of gestation	0.4 mg total NGF (2.5 S) microinfusion starting day 15 postpartum[a]

[a] The implanted osmotic microinfusion pump was designed to deliver 1.05 μL/h and the total dose within 1 week. Compilation of results from two studies designated as A (180) and B (181).

TABLE 6. *Effect of NGF treatment upon ENU-induced trigeminal neurinomas in Sprague–Dawley rats: 90-day studies*

Group	Treatment	Number of offspring	Offspring with trigeminal neurinomas		Clear significance[a]
			Number	%	
A1	ENU 50 mg/kg	10	9	90	
A2	ENU 50 mg/kg, NGF preceding ENU	13	9	69	Trend
A3	ENU 50 mg/kg, NGF to offspring	9	4	44	Trend
B1	ENU 20 mg/kg	19	11	58	
B2	ENU 20 mg/kg, NGF preceding ENU	19	5	26	$p \leq 0.025$
B3	ENU 20 mg/kg, NGF to offspring	18	5	28	$p \leq 0.05$

[a]Statistically significant differences from the control group B1. Compilation of results from two studies designated as A (180) and B (181).

protein, while none of the neurinomas of the NGF-treated group did. These results support the hypothesis that NGF has the capability to reduce the oncogenic consequences of ENU exposure by the process of growth retardation and differentiation of transformed cells; this effect depends on the presence of receptor binding sites (182).

NGF treatment of tumors developing from transplantation of established tumor cell lines and clones. The transplantation model has some advantages over the model of autochthonous tumor production. Experiments can be completed within a considerably shorter period of time; intracerebrally implanted tumor cells may kill the animals within 30 days; implanted cell lines or clones are well characterized and their rate of growth has been established. Furthermore, when subcutaneous transplantation is used, daily measurements of tumors can be accomplished and become a quantitative monitoring device for the effect of therapeutic measures. This model is readily adaptable to screening for prospective effects of therapeutic measures on human brain tumors.

NGF treatment of rats bearing intracerebrally implanted cells of an anaplastic glioma clone (F-98) led to a decreased tumor growth rate and increased survival

TABLE 7. *Treatment schedule for 1-year NGF-effect study on neurinomas induced transplacentally with a single i.v. administration of 50 mg/kg ENU into pregnant Sprague–Dawley rats*

Group	ENU	Number of offspring	NGF (2.5 S)
A	50 mg/kg transplacentally	34	0
B	50 mg/kg transplacentally	34	40 µg days 12–16 60 µg days 90–94 80 µg days 210–214[a]

Tabulated with permission from Raju et al. (182)
[a]40, 60, and 80 µg are total doses administered in five daily subcutaneous inoculations.

TABLE 8. Effect of NGF on neurinoma development in rats 1 year following transplacental exposure to 50 mg/kg ENU[a]

Group	Number of rats	Number of rats with trigeminal neurinomas	Number of rats with peripheral neurinomas	Total neurinomas
A (untreated)	34	18 (53%)[b]	11 (32%)	29 (85%)[c]
B (NGF treated)	34	11 (32%)[b]	5 (15%)	16 (47%)[c]

Reprinted with permission from Raju et al. (184).
[a]*Immunohistochemistry*: positive for NGFR: group A, 7 of 29 (24%); group B, 0 of 16 (0%).
[b]$p<0.05$.
[c]$p<0.01$.

time. Similar but less pronounced effects were observed when the cells were pretreated with NGF 24 h before implantation (150). Rats receiving intracerebral implants composed of a mixture of F-98 anaplastic glioma cells and NGF-producing C-6 cells survived longer than those receiving only F-98 cells, and 30% of the rats receiving the F-98/C-6 cell mixture were tumor-free at 90 days (151). For the reasons discussed above, several experiments were accomplished using subcutaneous implantation. In these experiments, rat tumor cell lines were implanted exclusively into syngeneic recipients and the tumors were allowed 10 days to become established before treatment was initiated. Two neurogenic tumor cell sources were used: an established anaplastic glioma cell line (T9) and an anaplastic neurinoma clone (clone 16). Treatment of both resulted in significant decreases in tumor growth rates (Fig. 8) (183). Unexpectedly, the tumor growth rate was not significantly different when a second series of NGF treatments was applied (Fig. 9). A plausible explanation for this phenomenon is that although NGF causes persistent growth suppression and differentiation of a NGF-responsive subpopulation of cells, a nonsensitive subpopulation of cells accounts for continuous growth of the tumor. The therapeutic potential of NGF may depend on the proportion of NGF-sensitive cells in a given tumor.

Implants of the human tumor cell lines into athymic mice displayed a much less dramatic decrease in growth rate in response to NGF than did the animal tumor implants, although their response *in vitro* was similar (183). No full explanation for this disparity is yet available; however, several prospective contributory factors have been identified. It has been established that addition of serum or α_2-macroglobulin, which is a component of serum to the culture medium, is capable of diminishing or preventing NGF-induced changes *in vitro* (183). Mouse serum is more potent than rat serum in accomplishing this. Furthermore, the delicate nature of the subcutaneous tissue in athymic mice usually results in serum transudation and/or slight hemorrhage following injection. Rats do not exhibit such a tendency. This aspect of the nude mouse model requires further investigation.

In conclusion, NGF must be considered as an effective reverse transformation agent for anaplastic tumor cells of neural crest origin possessing NGF receptors. It may act under natural conditions as a protective host factor in tumor development and prospectively may play a role in brain cancer therapy in the future.

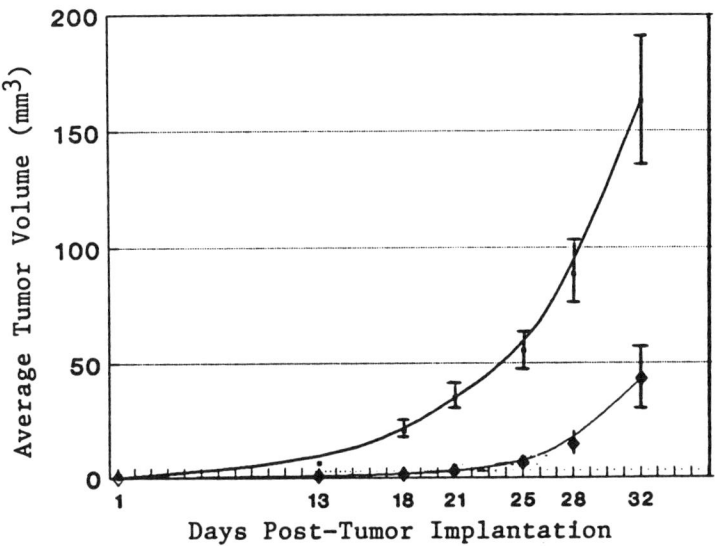

FIG. 8. Effect of NGF treatment on the growth rate of subcutaneous implants of anaplastic neurinoma cells from clone 16 in recipient rats. On days 10 to 15 postimplantation, 40 μg of NGF was administered directly at the implantation site. Note the significantly reduced growth rate of the NGF-treated compared to the saline-treated group. Each group contained seven experimental subjects. [Reprinted with permission from Yaeger et al. (183).]

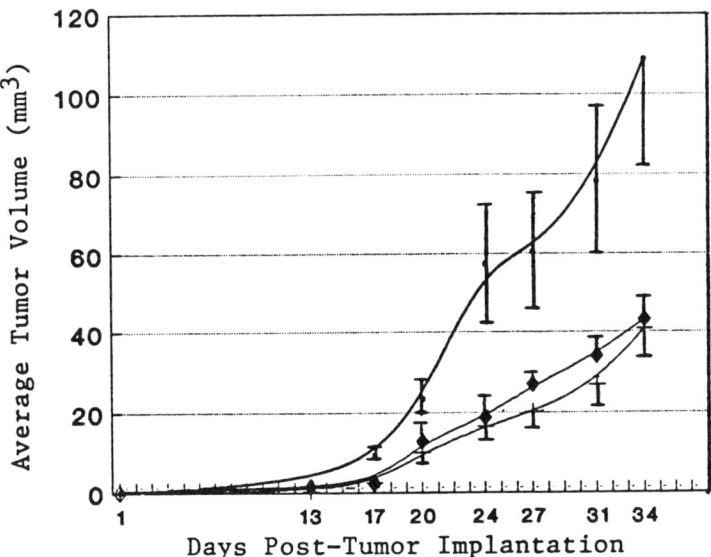

FIG. 9. Effect of repeated series of NGF treatments on the growth rate of subcutaneous implants of anaplastic neurinoma cells from clone 16. The top curve represents the growth rate of the control, the middle curve represents a single series of 40 μg of NGF administration on days 8 to 12, and the bottom curve represents two series of 40 μg of NGF administration on days 8 to 12 and 22 to 26. There is no significant difference between single and multiple series of NGF administration. [Reprinted with permission from Yaeger et al. (183).]

APPLICABILITY OF ANIMAL DATA TO THE PROBLEM OF HUMAN BRAIN TUMORS

Animal experimentation is used to investigate disease processes under controlled conditions with the purpose of defining the phenomena involved in agent–host interactions and their consequences, therefore providing the basis for a better understanding of comparable human diseases. The study of neoplasia, and specifically neoplasms of the nervous system, may benefit from the use of animals, particularly because of the difficulty of tracing human brain tumors to a principal causative agent. The major obstacles are the long latency periods and the multifactorial exposures. The exceptions are the genetically determined tumors of the nervous system, including the retinoblastoma and the inherited predisposition for neurogenic tumor development linked to neurofibromatosis, tuberous sclerosis, and Turcot's and Li-Fraumeni syndromes (184). There should be little doubt that some neurooncogenic compounds capable of producing brain tumors in animals may also produce such tumors in humans. As in animals, we should expect a broad range of susceptibility or resistance toward these agents. Tumor-prone animal strains exist and host factors may in addition protect individual animals from cancer development. Thus even with equal exposure, only a portion of the individuals at risk should be affected. In a survey, Mahaley et al. (185) found that 16% of patients with primary brain tumors have a family history of cancer. The many genetic possibilities responsible for this predisposition have not yet been fully investigated; however, the loss of tumor suppressor sequences such as the Rb1, the recessive locus responsible for the development of retinoblastoma and osteosarcoma, may serve as a good model for investigations of genetic predisposition for human cancer. In addition to genetic predisposition, there is now some evidence linking exposure to extrinsic agents to human brain tumor development. Radiotherapy of a craniopharyngioma apparently resulted in the development of a malignant astrocytoma (186). A cerebellar malignant glioma was attributed to previous radiation therapy of a glomus jugular tumor (187). In reviewing some chemicals known to cause brain tumors in animals, Wikstrand and Bigner (133) directed attention to vinyl chloride, which was incriminated as the possible cause of a four- to fivefold increase in the incidence of glioblastoma multiforme among workers heavily exposed to vinyl chloride (188). These authors also pointed out that the increased tumor incidence of the central nervous system, liver, lung, and lymphatic sites in individuals exposed to vinyl chloride closely paralleled those in experimental animal models. Investigations of potential linkages of brain tumors in workers exposed to known carcinogenic agents previously tested in animals, such as nitroso compounds, have not provided convincing evidence of a causal relationship. Although the link of human brain tumors to neurocarcinogenic chemicals has not yet been broadly established, it is very likely that such a relationship exists, as the vinyl chloride case indicates. Chemical carcinogens have been shown to cause tumors in extraneural organs. It may just be more difficult to document this in the brain because of the reduced access and the absence of enzymes capable of activating precarcinogens into ultimate carcinogens. Carcinogenic metabolites may gain access to the brain only in very small doses, and thus development of neoplasms may require repeated and perhaps multifactorial exposures. Small doses may, as in animals, greatly extend the latency period. With the advancement of molecular biology it may be possible in the near future to trace some chemical causes of brain tumors through their specific molecular interactions with nuclear macromolecules and the chemical lesions they produce.

The pathogenesis of brain tumor development has been established principally in animal models. Knowledge gained from these models is broadly applicable to human brain tumor development. Oncogenes, suppressor genes, and growth factors have been studied extensively in human brain tumors and have been reviewed in this chapter. Current experiments using sophisticated methods of molecular genetics, such as cell-specific tumor induction in neural grafts by retrovirus-mediated oncogene transfer (39), will further define the specific functions of individual oncogenes. The role of NGF as a protective host factor is probably similar in humans and animals, and the possible use of NGF as a therapeutic measure will be initially determined in animal studies. It is hoped that preventive measures and more effective therapeutic devices will be established as the causes of human brain tumors become better identified.

ACKNOWLEDGMENT

This work was supported in part by the National Cancer Institute Grant CA 32594.

REFERENCES

1. Rubinstein LJ. Tumors of the central nervous system. *Atlas of tumor pathology*. AFIP fascicle 6, Washington, DC: Armed Forces Institute of Pathology, 1972.
2. Peller S. *Cancer in childhood and youth*. Bristol, Gloucestershire, England: John Wright; 1960.
3. Kleihues P, Lantos PL, Magee PN, Chemical carcinogenesis in the nervous system. *Int Rev Exp Pathol* 1976;15:153–232.
4. Kleihues P, Rajewsky MF. Chemical neuro-oncogenesis: Role of structural DNA modifications, DNA repair and neural target cell population. *Prog Exp Tumor Res* 1984;27:1–16.
5. Koestner A. Characterization of N-nitrosourea-induced tumors of the nervous system; their prospective value for studies of neurocarcinogenesis and brain tumor therapy. *Toxicol Pathol* 1990;18:186–192.
6. Thompson SW, Hunt RD. Spontaneous tumors in the Sprague–Dawley rat. Incidence rates of some types of neoplasms as determined by serial section versus single section techniques. *Ann NY Acad Sci* 1963;108:832–845.
7. Koestner A. The brain tumour issue in long-term toxicity studies in rats. *Food Chem Toxicol* 1986;24:139–143.
8. Ward JM, Rice JM. Naturally occurring and chemically induced brain tumors of rats and mice in carcinogenesis bioassays. *Ann NY Acad Sci* 1982;381:304–319.
9. Sumi N, Stavrou D, Frohberg H, Jochman G. The incidence of spontaneous tumours of the central nervous system in Wistar rats. *Arch Toxicol* 1976;35:1–13.
10. Solleveld HA, Haseman JK, McConnell EM. Natural history of body weight gain, survival and neoplasia in the F344 rat. *J Natl Cancer Inst* 1984;72:929–940.
11. Druckrey H, Ivankovic S, Preussmann R. Selektive Erzeugung von Hirntumoren bei Ratten durch Methylnitrosoharnstoff. *Naturwissenschaften* 1964;50:44.

12. Druckrey H, Ivankovic S, Preussmann R. Teratogenic and carcinogenic effects in the offspring after a single injection of ethylnitrosourea to pregnant rats. *Nature* 1966;210:1378–1379.
13. Wechsler W, Koestner A. Developmental biology related to oncology. In: Raven RW ed. *Principles of surgical oncology*. New York: Plenum Press; 1977:93–108.
14. Denlinger RH, Koestner A, Wechsler W. Induction of neurogenic tumors in C3HeB/FeJ mice by nitrosourea derivatives: Observations by light microscopy, tissue culture, and electron microscopy. *Int J Cancer* 1974;13:559–571.
15. Wechsler W, Rice JM, Vesselinovitch SD. Transplacental and neonatal induction of neurogenic tumors in mice: comparison with related species and with human pediatric neoplasm. In: Rice JM, ed. *Perinatal carcinogenesis*. NCI monograph 51. Bethesda, MD: National Cancer Institute; 1979: 219–226.
16. Jurgelski W Jr, Hudson P, Tark HL. Tissue differentiation and susceptibility to embryonal tumor induction by ethylnitrosourea in the opossum. In: Rice JM, ed. *Perinatal carcinogenesis*. NCI monograph 51. Bethesda, MD: National Cancer Institute; 1979:123–158.
17. Zu Rhein GM, Varakis JN. Perinatal induction of medulloblastomas in Syrian golden hamsters by a polyoma virus (J.C.). In: Rice JM, ed. *Perinatal carcinogenesis*. NCI monograph 51. Bethesda, MD: National Cancer Institute; 1979:205–208.
18. Bigner DD, Odom GL, Mahaley MS, Day ED. Brain tumors induced in dogs by the Schmidt–Ruppin strain of Rouse sarcoma virus. Neuropathological and immunological observations. *J Neuropathol Exp Neurol* 1969;28:648–680.
19. Warzok R, Schneider J, Schreiber D, Jänisch W. Experimental brain tumors in dogs. *Experientia* 1970;26:303–304.
20. Denlinger RH, Koestner A, Swenberg JA. Neoplasms in pure-bred Boxer dogs following long-term administration of N-methyl-N-nitrosourea. *Cancer Res* 1978;38:1711–1717.
21. Jänisch W, Schreiber D. *Experimental tumors of the central nervous system*. English edition edited by Bigner DD, Swenberg JA. Kalamazoo, MI: Upjohn Co.; 1972.
22. Druckrey H, Landschütz CH, Ivankovic S. Transplacentare Erzeugung maligner Tumoren des Nervensystems. II. Äthylnitrosoharnstoff an 10 genetisch definierten Rattenstämmen. *Z Krebsforsch* 1970;73:371–386.
23. Warkany J, Mandybur TI, Kalter H. Oncogenic response of rats with x-ray-induced microcephaly to transplacental ethylnitrosourea. *J Natl Cancer Inst* 1976;56:59–64.
24. Camp RC, Koestner A, Vinores SA, Capen CC. The effect of nerve growth factor and antibodies to nerve growth factor on ethylnitrosourea-induced neoplastic proliferation in rat trigeminal nerve. *Vet Pathol* 1984;21:67–73.
25. Koestner A, Swenberg JA, Wechsler W. Experimental tumors of the nervous system induced by resorptive N-nitrosourea compounds. *Prog Exp Tumor Res* 1972;17:9–20.
26. Swenberg JA, Koestner A, Wechsler W, Bounden MN, Abe H. Differential oncogenic effects of methylnitrosourea. *J Natl Cancer Inst* 1975;54:89–96.
27. Swenberg JA, Wechsler W, Koestner A. Sequential development of transplacentally induced neuroectodermal tumors. *J Neuropathol Exp Neurol* 1972;31:202–203.
28. Denlinger RH, Koestner A, Swenberg JA. An experimental model for selective production of neoplasms of the peripheral nervous system. *Acta Neuropathol* 1973;23:219–228.
29. Koestner AW, Ruecker FA, Koestner A. Morphology and pathogenesis of tumors of the thymus and stomach in Sprague–Dawley rats following intragastric administration of methylnitrosourea. *Int J Cancer* 1977;20:418–428.
30. Stoica G, Koestner A. Diverse spectrum of tumors in male Sprague–Dawley rats following single high doses of N-ethyl-N-nitrosourea (ENU). *Am J Pathol* 1984;116:319–326.
31. Stoica G, Koestner A, Capen CC. Neoplasms induced with high single doses of N-ethyl-N-nitrosourea in 30-day-old Sprague–Dawley rats, with special emphasis on mammary neoplasia. *Anticancer Res* 1984;4:5–12.
32. Stoica G, Koestner A, Capen CC. Testicular (Sertoli's cell-like) tumors of the ovary induced by N-ethyl-N-nitrosourea (ENU) in rats. *Vet Pathol* 1985;22:483–491.
33. Kleihues P, Margison GP. Carcinogenicity of N-methyl-N-nitrosourea: possible role of repair excision of O^6-methylguanine from DNA. *J Natl Cancer Inst* 1974;53:1839–1841.
34. Goth R, Rajewsky MF. Persistence of O^6-ethylguanine in rat-brain DNA: correlation with nervous system–specific carcinogenesis by ethylnitrosourea. *Proc Natl Acad Sci USA* 1974;71:639–643.
35. Chang MJW, Koestner A, Hart RH. Interrelationships between cellular proliferation, DNA alkylation and age as determinants of ethylnitrosourea-induced neoplasia. *Cancer Lett* 1981;13:39–45.

36. Cohen SM, Ellwein LB. Cell proliferation in carcinogenesis. *Science* 1990;249:1007–1011.
37. Rajewsky MF. Chemical carcinogenesis in the developing nervous system. In: Zardi L, Santi L, eds. *Theories and models in cellular transformation.* New York: Academic Press; 1985:155–171.
38. Pilkington GJ, Lantos PL. The development of experimental brain tumours. A sequential light and electron microscope study of the subependymal plate. *Acta Neuropathol* 1979;45:177–185.
39. Kleihues P, Aguzzi A, Wiestler OD. Cellular and molecular aspects of neurocarcinogenesis. *Toxicol Pathol* 1990;18:193–203.
40. Burger PC, Shibata T, Aguzzi A, Kleihues P. Selective induction by N-nitrosourea of oligodendrogliomas in fetal forebrain transplants. *Cancer Res* 1988;48:2871–2875.
41. Rajewsky MF. Tumorigenesis by exogenous carcinogens: role of target-cell proliferation and state of differentiation (development). In: Likhachev A, Anisinov V, Montesano R, eds. *Age-related factors in carcinogenesis.* Lyon, France: International Agency for Research on Cancer; 1986:215–224.
42. Kleihues P, Wiestler O. Structural DNA modifications and DNA repair in organ-specific tumor induction. In: Cohen GM, ed. *Target organ toxicity.* Vol II. Boca Raton, FL: CRC Press; 1986: 159–180.
43. Potter VR. Phenotypic diversity in experimental hepatomas: the concept of partially blocked ontogeny. *Br J Cancer* 1978;38:1–23.
44. Trosko JE, Chang CC, Madhukar BV. Cell-to-cell communication: relationship of stem cells to the carcinogenic process. *Prog Clin Biol Res* 1990;331:259–276.
45. Rajewsky MF. Chemical carcinogenesis in the developing nervous system. In: Zardi L, Sariti L, eds. *Theories and models in cellular transformation.* New York: Academic Press; 1985:155–171.
46. Eadie JS, Conrad M, Toorchen D, Topal MD. Mechanism of mutagenesis by O^6-methylguanine. *Nature* 1984;308:201–203.
47. Loechler EL, Green CL, Essigman JM. *In vivo* mutagenesis by O^6-methylguanine built into a unique site in a viral genome. *Proc Natl Acad Sci USA* 1984;81:6271–6275.
48. Richardson KK, Richardson FC, Crosby RM, Swenberg JA, Skopek TR. DNA base changes and alkylation following *in vivo* exposure of *Escherichia coli* to N-methyl-N-nitrosourea or N-ethyl-N-nitrosourea. *Proc Natl Acad Sci USA* 1987;84:344–348.
49. Singer B, Spengler SJ, Fraenkel-Conrat H, Kusmierek JT. O^4-methyl, -ethyl, or -isopropyl substituents on thymidine in poly (dA-dT) all lead to transitions upon replication. *Proc Natl Acad Sci USA* 1986;83:28–32.
50. Preston BD, Singer B, Loeb LA. Mutagenic potential of O^4-methylthymine *in vivo* determined by an enzymatic approach to site specific mutagenesis. *Proc Natl Acad Sci USA* 1986;83:8501–8505.
51. Dosanjh MK, Essigman JM, Goodman MF, Singer B. Comparative efficiency of forming m^{4}T•G versus m^{4}T•A base pairs at unique site by use of *Escherichia coli* DNA polymerase I (Klenow fragment) and *Drosophila melanogaster* polymerase-α-primase complex. *Biochemistry* 1990;29: 4698–4703.
52. Olsson M, Lindahl T. Repair of alkylated DNA in *Escherichia coli.* Methyl group transfer from O^6-methylguanine to a protein cysteine residue. *J Biol Chem* 1980;255:10569–10571.
53. Pegg AE, Wiest L, Foote RS, Mitra S, Perry W. Purification and properties of O^6-methylguanine-DNA transmethylase from rat liver. *J Biol Chem* 1983;258:2327–2333.
54. Koike G, Maki H, Takeya H, Hayakawa H, Sekiguchi M. Purification, structure, and biochemical properties of human O^6-methylguanine-DNA methyltransferase. *J Biol Chem* 1990;265:14754–14762.
55. Sassanfar M, Dosanjh MK, Essigmann JM, Samson L. Relative efficiencies of the bacterial, yeast, and human DNA methyltransferase for the repair of O^6-methylguanine and O^4-methylthymine. Suggestive evidence for O^4-methylthymine repair by eukaryotic methyltransferases. *J Biol Chem* 1991;266:2767–2771.
56. Brennard J, Margison GP. Reduction of the toxicity and mutagencity of alkylating agents in mammalian cells harboring the *Escherichia coli* alkyltransferase gene. *Proc Natl Acad Sci USA* 1986; 83:6292–6296.
57. Ellison KS, Dogliotti E, Connors TD, Basu AK, Essigman JM. Site-specific mutagenesis by O^6-alkylguanines located in the chromosomes of mammalian cells: Influence of the mammalian O^6-alkyguanine-DNA alkyltransferase. *Proc Natl Acad Sci USA* 1989;76:8620–8624.
58. Thomale J, Huh N-M, Nehls P, Eberle G, Rajewsky MF. Repair of O^6-ethylguanine in DNA protects rat 208F cells from tumorigenic conversion by N-ethyl-N-nitrosourea. *Proc Natl Acad Sci USA* 1990;87:9883–9887.

59. Sukumar S, Notario V, Martin-Zanca D, Barbacid M. Induction of mammary carcinomas in rats by nitroso-methylurea involves malignant activation of H-*ras*-1 locus by single point mutations. *Nature* 1983;306:658–661.
60. Zarbl H, Sukumar S, Arthur AV, Martin-Zauca D, Barbacid M. Direct mutagenesis of Ha-*ras*-1 oncogenes by *N*-nitroso-*N*-methylurea during initation of mammary carcinogenesis in rats. *Nature* 1985;315:382–385.
61. Miyamoto S, Sukumar S, Guzman RC, Osborn RC, Nandi S. Transforming c-Ki-*ras* mutation is a preneoplastic event in mouse mammary carcinogenesis induced *in vitro* by *N*-methyl-*N*-nitrosourea. *Mol Cell Biol* 1990;10:1593–1599.
62. Kumar R, Sukumar S, Barbacid M. Activation of *ras* oncogenes preceding the onset of neoplasia. *Science* 1990;248:1101–1104.
63. Taparowsky E, Shimizu K, Coldfarb M, Wigler M. Structure and activation of the human N-*ras* gene. *Cell* 34;1983:581–586.
64. Padua RA, Barrass NC, Currie CA. Activation of N-*ras* in a human melanoma cell line. *Mol Cell Biol* 1985;5:582–585.
65. Schechter AL, Stern DF, Vaidyanathan L, et al. The *neu* oncogene: an *erb*-B-related gene encoding a 185,000-Mr tumour antigen. *Nature* 1984;312:513–516.
66. Bargmann CI, Hung M-C, Weinberg RA. The *neu* oncogene encodes an epidermal growth factor receptor-related protein. *Nature* 1986;319:226–230.
67. Yamamoto T, Ikawa S, Akiyama I, et al. Similarity of protein encoded by the human c-*erb*-B-2 gene to epidermal growth factor receptor. *Nature* 1986;319:230–234.
68. Bargmann CI, Hung M-C, Weinberg RA. Multiple independent activations of the *neu* oncogene by a point mutation altering transmembrane domain of p185. *Cell* 1986;45:649–657.
69. Weiner DB, Liu J, Cohen JA, Williams WV, Greene MI. A point mutation in the *neu* oncogene mimics ligand induction of receptor aggregation. *Nature* 1989;339:230–231.
70. Perantoni AO, Rice JM, Reed CD, Watatani M, Wenk ML. Activated *neu* oncogene sequences in primary tumors of the peripheral nervous system induced in rats by transplacental exposure to ethylnitrosourea. *Proc Natl Acad Sci USA* 1987;84:6317–6321.
71. Kokunai T, Korosue K, Tamaki N, Matsumoto S. Promoting effect of 12-*O*-tetradecanoylphorbol-13-acetate on neurogenic microtumors initiated by transplacental exposure to *N*-ethyl-*N*-nitrosourea. *Jpn J Cancer Res (Gann)* 1987;78:534–536.
72. Naito M, Naito Y, Ito A. Effect of phenobarbital on the development of tumors in mice treated neonatally with *N*-ethyl-*N*-nitrosourea. *Gann* 1982;73:111–114.
73. Walker VE, Swenberg JA. Phenobarbital lacks promoting activity for neurogenic tumors in F344 rats transplacentally exposed to ethylnitrosourea. *J Neuropathol Exp Neurol* 1989;48:263–269.
74. Herbst AL, Ulfelder H, Poskanzer DC. Adenocarcinoma of the vagina: association of maternal stilbestrol therapy with tumor appearance in young women. *N Engl J Med* 1971;284:878–881.
75. Swenberg JA, Koestner A, Wechsler W, Denlinger RH. Quantitative aspects of transplacental tumor induction with ethylnitrosourea in rats. *Cancer Res* 1972;32:2656–2660.
76. Swenberg JA, Clendenon N, Denlinger R, Gordon WA. Sequential development of ethylnitrosourea-induced neuriomas: morphology, biochemistry and transplantability. *J Natl Cancer Inst* 1975;55:147–152.
77. Koestner A, Swenberg JA, Denlinger RH. Host factors affecting perinatal carcinogenesis by resorptive alkylnitrosoureas in rats. In: Rice JM, ed. *Perinatal carcinogenesis*. NCI monograph 51. Bethesda, MD: National Cancer Institute; 1979:211–217.
78. Knudson AG. Mutation and cancer: Statistical study of retinoblastoma. *Proc Natl Acad Sci USA* 1971;68:820–823.
79. Scherer E. Neoplastic progression in experimental hepatocarcinogenesis. *Biochim Biophys Acta* 1984;738:219–236.
80. Pitot HC, Beer DG, Hendrich S. Gene expression during multistage hepatocarcinogenesis. *Scand J Gastroenterol* 1988;151:52–61.
81. Pitot HC, Campbell HA, Maronpot R, et al. Critical parameters in the quantitation of the stages of initiation, promotion, and progression in one model of hepatocarcinogenesis in the rat. *Toxicol Pathol* 1989;17:594–612.
82. Grady EF, Schwab M, Rosenau W. Expression of N-*myc*- and c-*src* during the development of fetal human brain. *Cancer Res* 1987;47:2931–2936.
83. Schwab M, Alitalo K, Klempnauer K-H, et al. Amplified DNA with limited homology to *myc* cellular oncogene is shared by human neuroblastoma cell lines and a neuroblastoma tumour. *Nature* 1983;305:245–248.

84. Montgomery KT, Biedler JL, Spengler BA, Melera PW. Specific DNA sequence amplification in human neuroblastoma cells. *Proc Natl Acad Sci USA* 1983;80:5724–5728.
85. Lee W-H, Murphree AL, Benedict WF. Expression and amplification of the N-*myc* gene in primary retinoblastoma. *Nature* 1984;309:458–460.
86. Shiloh Y, Korf B, Kohl NE, et al. Amplification and rearrangement of DNA sequences from the chromosomal region 2p24 in human neuroblastomas. *Cancer Res* 1986;46:5297–5301.
87. Fong C-T, Dracopoli NC, White PS, et al. Loss of heterozygosity for the short arm of chromosome 1 in human neuroblastoma: correlation with N-*myc* amplification. *Proc Natl Acad Sci USA* 1989; 86:3753–3757.
88. Brodeur GM, Seeger RC, Schwab M, Varmus HE, Bishop JM. Amplification of N-*myc* in untreated human neuroblastomas correlates with advanced disease stage. *Science* 1984;224:1121–1124.
89. Seeger RC, Brodeur GM, Sather H, et al. Association of multiple copies of the N-*myc* oncogene with rapid progression of neuroblastomas. *N Engl J Med* 1985;313:1111–1116.
90. Brodeur GM, Hayes FA, Green AA, et al. Consistent N-*myc* copy number in simultaneous or consecutive neuroblastoma samples from sixty individual patients. *Cancer Res* 1987;47:4248–4253.
91. Bernards R, Dessain SK, Weinberg RA. N-*myc* amplification causes down modulation of MHC class I antigen expression in neuroblastoma cells. *Cell* 1986;47:667–674.
92. Trent J, Meltzer P, Rosenblum M, et al. Evidence for rearrangement, amplification, and expression of c-*myc* in a human glioblastoma. *Proc Natl Acad Sci USA* 1986;83:470–473.
93. Sporn MB, Roberts AB. Autocrine growth factors and cancer. *Nature* 1985;313:745–747.
94. Libermann TA, Razon N, Bartal AD, Yarden Y, Schlessinger J, Soreq H. Expression of epidermal growth factor receptors in human brain tumors. *Cancer Res* 1984;44:753–760.
95. Liberman TA, Nusbaum HR, Razon N, et al. Amplification, enhanced expression and possible rearrangement of EGF receptor gene in primary human brain tumours of glial origin. *Nature* 1985; 313:144–147.
96. Wong AJ, Bigner SH, Bigner DD, Kinzler KW, Hamilton SR, Vogelstein B. Increased expression of the epidermal growth factor receptor gene in malignant gliomas is invariably associated with gene amplification. *Proc Natl Acad Sci USA* 1987;84:6899–6903.
97. Henn W, Blin N, Zang KD. Polysomy of chromosome 7 is correlated with overexpression of the *erb* B oncogene in human glioblastoma cell lines. *Hum Genet* 1986;74:104–106.
98. Reifenberger G, Prior R, Deckert M, Wechsler W. Epidermal growth factor receptor expression and growth fraction in human tumours of the nervous system. *Virchows Arch A Pathol Anat* 1989; 414:147–155.
99. Yamazaki H, Fukui Y, Ueyama Y, et al. Amplification of the structurally and functionally altered epidermal growth factor receptor gene (c-*erb* B) in human brain tumors. *Mol Cell Biol* 1988; 8:1816–1820.
100. Lens PF, Altena B, Nusse R. Expression of c-*sis* and platelet-derived growth factor in *in vitro*-transformed glioma cells from rat brain transplacentally treated with ethylnitrosourea. *Mol Cell Biol* 1986;6:3537–3540.
101. Eva A, Robbins KC, Andersen PR, et al. Cellular genes analogous to retroviral *onc* genes are transcribed in human tumour cells. *Nature* 1982;295:116–119.
102. Nistér M, Heldin CH, Wasteson A, Westermark B. A glioma-derived analog to platelet-derived growth factor: demonstration of receptor competing activity and immunological cross reactivity. *Proc Natl Acad Sci USA* 1984;81:926–930.
103. Pantazis P, Pelicci PG, Dalla-Favera R, Antoniades HN. Synthesis and secretion of proteins resembling platelet-derived growth factor by human glioblastoma and fibrosarcoma cells in culture. *Proc Natl Acad Sci USA* 1985;82:2404–2408.
104. Nistér M, Heldin CH, Westermark B. Clonal variation in the production of platelet-derived growth factor-like protein and expression of corresponding receptors in a human malignant glioma. *Cancer Res* 1986;46:332–340.
105. Hermansson M, Nistér M, Betscholtz C, Heldin CH, Westermark B, Funa K. Endothelial cell hyperplasia in human glioblastoma: coexpression of mRNA for platelet-derived growth factor (PDGF) B chain and PDGF receptor suggests autocrine growth stimulation. *Proc Natl Acad Sci USA* 1988;85:7748–7752.
106. Nistér M, Libermann TA, Betscholtz C, et al. Expression of messenger RNA for platelet derived growth factor and transforming growth factor-α and their receptors in human malignant glioma cell lines. *Cancer Res* 1988;48:3910–3918.

107. Libermann TA, Friesel R, Jaye M, et al. An angiogenic growth factor is expressed in human glioma cells. *EMBO J* 1987;1627–1632.
108. Maxwell M, Naber SP, Wolfe HJ, et al. Expression of angiogenic growth factor genes in primary human astrocytomas may contribute to their growth and progression. *Cancer Res* 1991;51:1345–1351.
109. Knudson AG. Hereditary cancer, oncogenes, and antioncogenes. *Cancer Res* 1985;45:1437–1443.
110. Benedict WF, Murphree AL, Banerjee AR, Spina CA, Sparkes MC, Sparkes RS. Patient with 13 chromosome deletion: evidence that retinoblastoma gene is a recessive cancer gene. *Science* 1983;219:973–975.
111. Hansen MF, Koufos A, Gallie BL, et al. Osteosarcoma and retinoblastoma: a shared chromosomal mechanism revealing recessive predisposition. *Proc Natl Acad Sci USA* 1985;82:6216–6220.
112. Friend SH, Bernards R, Rogelj S, et al. A human DNA segment with properties of the gene that predisposes to retinoblastoma and osteosarcoma. *Nature* 1986;323:643–646.
113. Friend SH, Horowitz JM, Gerber MR, Wang X-F, Bogenmann E, Li FP, Weinberg RA. Deletions of a DNA sequence in retinoblastomas and mesenchymal tumors: organization of the sequence and its encoded protein. *Proc Natl Acad Sci USA* 1987;84:9059–9063.
114. Horowitz JM, Yandell DW, Park S-H, et al. Point mutational inactivation of the retinoblastoma antioncogene. *Science* 1989;243:937–940.
115. Lee W-H, Bookstein R, Hong F, Young L-J, Shew J-Y, Lee EY-H. Human retinoblastoma susceptibility gene: cloning, identification, and sequence. *Science* 1987;235:1394–1399.
116. Lee W-H, Shew J-Y, Hong FD, et al. The retinoblastoma susceptibility gene encodes a nuclear phosphoprotein associated with DNA binding activity. *Nature* 1987;329:642–645.
117. Huang H-JS, Yee J-K, Shew J-Y, et al. Suppression of the neoplastic phenotype by replacement of the RB gene in human cancer cells. *Science* 1988;242:1563–1566.
118. El-Azouzi M, Chung RY, Farmer GE, et al. Loss of distinct regions on the short arm of chromosome 17 associated with tumorigenesis of human astrocytomas. *Proc Natl Acad Sci USA* 1989;86:7186–7190.
119. James CD, Carlbom E, Dumanski JP, et al. Clonal genomic alterations in glioma malignancy stages. *Cancer Res* 1988;48:5546–5551.
120. Brodeur GM, Green AA, Hayes FA, Williams KJ, Williams DL, Tsiatis AA. Cytogenetic features of human neuroblastomas and cell lines. *Cancer Res* 1981;41:4678–4686.
121. Gilbert F, Feder M, Balaban G, et al. Human neuroblastomas and abnormalities of chromosomes 1 and 17. *Cancer Res* 1984;44:5444–5449.
122. Dumanski JP, Carlbom E, Collins VP, Nordenskjöld M. Deletion mapping of a locus on human chromosome 22 involved in the oncogenesis of meningioma. *Proc Natl Acad Sci USA* 1987;84:9275–9279.
123. Seizinger BR, Martuza RL, Gusella JF. Loss of genes on chromosome 22 in tumorigenesis of human acoustic neuroma. *Nature* 1986;322:644–647.
124. Seizinger BR, de la Monte S, Atkins L, Gusella JF, Martuza RL. Molecular genetic approach to human meningioma: loss of genes on chromosome 22. *Proc Natl Acad Sci USA* 1987;84:5419–5423.
125. Rouleau GA, Wertelecki W, Haines JL, et al. Genetic linkage of bilateral acoustic neurofibromatosis to a DNA marker on chromosome 22. *Nature* 1987;329:246–248.
126. Seizinger BR, Rouleau G, Ozelius LJ, et al. Common pathogenic mechanism for three tumor types in bilateral accoustic neurofibromatosis. *Science* 1987;236:317–319.
127. Menon AG, Anderson KM, Riccardi VM, et al. Chromosome 17p deletions and p53 gene mutations associated with the formation of malignant neurofibrosarcomas in von Recklinghausen neurofibromatosis. *Proc Natl Acad Sci USA* 1990;87:5435–5439.
128. Aguzzi A, Kleihues P, Heckl K, Wiesler OD. Cell type-specific tumor induction in neural transplants by retrovirus-mediated oncogene transfer. *Oncogene* 1991;6:113–118.
129. Koestner A. Potential factors in carcinogenesis and tumor regression. *Biol Res Pregnancy Perinatol* 1983;4:17–21.
130. Burnet FM. *Immunological surveillance*. Oxford: Pergamon Press; 1970.
131. Prehn RT. Pitfalls in tumor immunology. In: *Proceedings of the 10th Canadian cancer research conference*. Toronto: University of Toronto Press; 1973:136–146.
132. Swenberg JA. Chemical induction of brain tumors. In: Thompson AA, Green JR, eds. *Neoplasms of the central nervous system*. New York: Raven Press; 1976:85–99.
133. Wikstrand CJ, Bigner DD. Immunobiological aspects of the brain and human gliomas. *Am J Pathol* 1980;98:517–568.

134. Wikstrand CJ, Grahmann FC, McComb RD, Bigner DD. Antigenic heterogenecity of human anaplastic gliomas and glioma-derived cell lines defined by monoclonal antibodies. *J Neuropathol Exp Neurol* 1985;44:229–241.
135. Brooks WH, Netsky MG, Normansell DE, Horwitz DA. Depressed cell-mediated immunity in patients with primary intracranial tumors: characterization of a humoral immunosuppressive factor. *J Exp Med* 1972;136:1631–1647.
136. Brooks WH, Caldwell HD, Mortara RH. Immune response in patients with gliomas. *Surg Neurol* 1974;2:419–423.
137. Brooks WH, Netsky MG, Levine JE. Immunity and tumors of the nervous system. *Surg Neurol* 1975;3:184–186.
138. Denlinger RH, Swenberg JA, Koestner A, Wechsler W. Differential effect of immunosuppression on the induction of nervous system and bladder tumors by N-methyl-nitrosourea. *J Natl Cancer Inst* 1973;50:87–93.
139. Word SJ, Pritchard J, Sofrouiew MV. Reexpression of nerve growth factor receptor after axonal injury recapitulates a developmental event in motor neurons: differential regulation when regeneration is allowed or prevented. *Eur J Neurosci* 1990;2:650–657.
140. Verge VMK, Tetzlaff W, Bisby MA, Richardson PM. Influence of nerve growth factor on neurofilament gene expression in mature primary sensory neurons. *J Neurosci* 1990;10:2018–2025.
141. Williams LR, Jodelis KS, Donald MR. Regional stimulation of cholinergic function by nerve growth factor in an animal model of Alzheimer's disease. In: Iqbal K, Wisniewski HM, Winblad B, eds. *Alzheimer's disease and related disorders*. New York: Alan R Liss; 1989:1179–1192.
142. Tuszynski MH, U HS, Amaral DG, Gage FH. Nerve growth factor infusion in the primate brain reduces lesion-induced cholinergic neuronal degeneration. *J Neurosci* 1990;10:3604–3614.
143. Urschel BA, Hulsebosch CE. Schwann cell-neuronal interactions in the rat involve nerve growth factor. *J Comp Neurol* 1990;296:114–122.
144. Jackson GR, Apffel L, Werrback-Perez K, Perez-Polo JR. Role of nerve growth factor in oxidant-antioxidant balance and neuronal injury. I. Stimulation of hydrogen peroxide resistance. *J Neurosci Res* 1990;25:360–368.
145. Jackson GR, Werrback-Perez K, Perez-Polo JR. Role of nerve growth factor in oxidant–antioxidant balance and neuronal injury. II. A conditioning lesion paradigm. *J Neurosci Res* 1990;25:369–374.
146. Greene LA, Tischler AS. Establishment of a noradrenergic clonal line of rat adrenal pheochromocytoma cells which respond to nerve growth factor. *Proc Natl Acad Sci USA* 1976;73:2424–2428.
147. Dichter MA, Tischler AS, Greene LA. Nerve growth factor induced increase in electrical excitability and acetylcholine sensitivity of a rat pheochromocytoma cell line. *Nature* 1977;268:501–504.
148. Reed JK, England D. The effect of nerve growth factor on the development of sodium channels in PC12 cells. *Biochem Cell Biol* 1986;69:1153–1159.
149. Perez-Polo JR, Reynolds CP, Tiffani-Castiglioni E, Ziegler M, Schulz I, Werrback-Perez K. NGF effects on human neuroblastoma lines: a model system. In: Haber B, Perez-Polo JR, Coulter JD, eds. *Proteins in the nervous system: structure and function*. New York: Alan R Liss; 1982:285–299.
150. Vinores SA, Koestner A. The effect of nerve growth factor on undifferentiated glioma cells. *Cancer Lett* 1980;10:309–318.
151. Vinores SA, Koestner A. Effect of nerve growth factor producing cells on anaplastic glioma and pheochromocytoma clones: involvement of other factors. *J Neurosci Res* 1981;6:389–401.
152. Marushige Y, Raju N, Marushige K, Koestner A. Modulation of growth and of morphological characteristics in glioma cells by nerve growth factor and glia maturation factor. *Cancer Res* 1987;47:4109–4115.
153. Yaeger MJ, Koestner A, Marushige K, Marushige Y. The reverse transforming effects of nerve growth factor on five human neurogenic tumor cell lines: *in vitro* results. *Acta Neuropathol* 1991;83:72–80.
154. Marushige Y, Marushige K, Okazaki DL, Koestner A. Cytoskeletal reorganization induced by nerve growth factor and glia maturation factor in anaplastic glioma cells. *Anticancer Res* 1989;9:1143–1148.
155. Korshing S, Thoenen H. Nerve growth factor in sympathetic ganglia and corresponding target organs of the rat: correlation with density of sympathetic innervation. *Proc Natl Acad Sci USA* 1983;80:3513–3516.

156. Ross AH, Grob P, Bothwell M, et al. Characterization of nerve growth factor receptor in neural crest tumors using monoclonal antibodies. *Proc Natl Acad Sci USA* 1984;81:6681–6685.
157. Marushige Y, Marushige K, Koestner A. Chemical control of growth and morphological characteristics of anaplastic glioma cells. *Anticancer Res* 1989;9:1729–1736.
158. Sutter A, Riopelle RJ, Harris-Warrick RM, Shooter EM. Nerve growth factor receptors. Characterization of two classes of binding sites on chick embryo sensory ganglia cells. *J Biol Chem* 1979; 254:5972–5982.
159. Landreth GE, Shooter EM. Nerve growth factor receptors on PC12 cells: ligand-induced conversion from low-to high-affinity states. *Proc Natl Acad Sci USA* 1980;77:4751–4755.
160. Schechter AL, Bothwell MA. Nerve growth factor receptors on PC12 cells: evidence for two receptor classes with differing cytoskeletal association. *Cell* 1981;24:867–874.
161. Sonnenfeld KH, Ishii DN. Nerve growth factor effects and receptors in cultured human neuroblastoma cell lines. *J Neurosci Res* 1982;8:375–391.
162. Sonnenfeld KH, Ishii DN. Fast and slow nerve growth factor binding sites in human neuroblastoma and rat pheochromocytoma cell lines: relationship of sites to each other and to neurite formation. *J Neurosci* 1985;5:1717–1728.
163. Green SH, Rydel RE, Connolly JL, Greene LA. PC12 cell mutants that possess low- but not high-affinity nerve growth factor receptors neither respond to nor internalize nerve growth factor. *J Cell Biol* 1986;102:830–843.
164. Chao MV, Bothwell MA, Ross AH, et al. Gene transfer and molecular cloning of the human NGF receptor. *Science* 1986;232:518–521.
165. Radeke MJ, Misko TP, Hsu C, Herzenberg LA, Shooter EM. Gene transfer and molecular cloning of the rat nerve growth factor receptor. *Nature* 1987;325:593–597.
166. Hempstead BL, Schleifer LS, Chao MV. Expression of functional nerve growth factor receptors after gene transfer. *Science* 1989;243:373–375.
167. Matsushima H, Bogenmann E. Nerve growth factor (NGF) induces neuronal differentiation in neuroblastoma cells transfected with the NGF receptor cDNA. *Mol Cell Biol* 1990;10:5015–5020.
168. Pleasure SJ, Reddy UR, Venkatakrishnan G, et al. Introduction of nerve growth factor (NGF) receptors into a medulloblastoma cell line results in expression of high- and low-affinity NGF receptors but not NGF-mediated differentiation. *Proc Natl Acad Sci USA* 1990;87:8496–8500.
169. DiStefano PS, Johnson EM Jr. Identification of a truncated form of the nerve growth factor receptor. *Proc Natl Acad Sci USA* 1988;85:270–274.
170. Kumar S, Huber J, Pena LA, Perez-Polo JR, Werrback-Perez K, de Vellis J. Characterization of functional nerve growth factor-receptors in a CNS glial cell line: monoclonal antibody 217C recognizes the nerve growth factor-receptor on C6 glioma cells. *J Neurosci Res* 1990;27:408–417.
171. Kaplan DR, Martin-Zanca D, Parada LF. Tyrosine phosphorylation and tyrosine kinase activity of the *trk* protooncogene product induced by NGF. *Nature* 1991;350:158–160.
172. Meakin SO, Shooter EM. Tyrosine kinase activity coupled to the high-affinity nerve growth factor-receptor complex. *Proc Natl Acad Sci USA* 1991;88:5862–5866.
173. Klein R, Jing S, Nanduri V, O'Rourke E, Barbacid M. The *trk* proto-oncogene encodes a receptor for nerve growth factor. *Cell* 1991;65:189–197.
174. Kaplan DR, Hempstead BL, Martin-Zanca D, Chao MV, Parada LF. The *trk* proto-oncogene product: a signal transducing receptor for nerve growth factor. *Science* 1991;252:554–558.
175. Hempstead BL, Martin-Zanca D, Kaplan DR, Parada LF, Chao DR. High-affinity NGF binding requires coexpression of the *trk* protooncogene and the low-affinity NGF receptor. *Nature* 1991; 350:678–683.
176. Hosang M, Shooter EM. Molecular characteristics of nerve growth factor receptor on PC12 cells. *J Biol Chem* 1985;260:655–662.
177. Yasuda T, Sobue G, Makuno K, Kreider B, Pleasure D. Cultured rat Schwann cells express low affinity receptors for nerve growth factor. *Brain Res* 1987;436:113–119.
178. Stahn R, Rose S, Sanborn S, Wert G, Herschmenn H. Effects of nerve growth factor administration on *N*-ethyl-*N*-nitrosourea carcinogenesis. *Brain Res* 1987;436:113–119.
179. Vinores SA, Perez-Polo JR. Growth and differentiation of fetal primary nervous tissue in the presence of ethylnitrosourea, nerve growth factor, and anti-nerve growth factor. *Tex J Sci* 1976; Spec Publ 1:101–111.
180. Vinores SA, Koestner A. Reduction of ethylnitrosourea-induced neoplastic proliferation in rat trigeminal nerve by nerve growth factor. *Cancer Res* 1982;42:1038–1040.
181. Camp RC, Koestner A, Vinores SA, Capen CC. The effect of nerve growth factor on ethylnitrosourea-induced neoplastic proliferation in rat trigeminal nerves. *Vet Pathol* 1984;21:67–73.

182. Raju NR, Koestner A, Marushige K, Lovell KL, Okazaki D. Effect of nerve growth factor on the transplacental induction of neurinomas by ethylnitrosourea in Sprague–Dawley rats. *Cancer Res* 1989;49:7120–7123.
183. Yaeger MJ, Koestner A, Marushige K, Marushige Y. The use of nerve growth factor as a reverse transforming agent for the treatment of neurogenic tumors: *in vivo* results. *Acta Neuropathol* 1992;83:624–629.
184. Black PMcL. Brain tumors. *N Engl J Med* 1991;324:1471–1476.
185. Mahaley MS Jr, Mettlin C, Narajan N, et al. National survey of pattern of care for brain-tumor patients. *J Neurosurg* 1989;71:826–836.
186. Sogg RL, Donaldson SS, Yorke CH. Malignant astrocytoma following radiotherapy of a craniopharyngioma: case report. *J Neurosurg* 1978;48:622–627; cited by Wikstrand and Bigner (133).
187. Preissig SH, Bohmfalk GL, Reichel GW, Smith MT. Radiation-induced malignant glioma in the cerebellum. *Cancer* 1979;43:2243–2247; cited by Wikstrand and Bigner (133).
188. Waxweiler RJ, Stringer W, Wagoner JK, Jones J. Neoplastic risk among workers exposed to vinyl chloride. *Ann NY Acad Sci* 1976;271:40–48; cited by Wikstrand and Bigner (133).
189. Koestner A. *N*-Nitrosourea-induced neurogenic tumors in the rat. Animal model of human disease. *Comp Pathol Bull* 1978;10:2–3.
190. Koestner A, Swenberg JA, Wechsler W. Transplacental production with ethylnitrosourea of neoplasms of the nervous system in Sprague–Dawley rats. *Am J Pathol* 1971;63:37–50.

Carcinogenesis, edited by
M.P. Waalkes and J.M. Ward.
Raven Press, Ltd., New York © 1994.

11

Male Reproductive System

Maarten C. Bosland

Institute of Environmental Medicine, New York University Medical Center, Tuxedo, New York 10987

This chapter addresses the male reproductive system as a target of carcinogenesis. The male reproductive organs include the testis with its efferent duct system, including the epididymis, the accessory sex glands, the preputial gland, and the penis. Although of these reproductive tissues the preputial gland is the most frequent site of tumor formation in carcinogenesis bioassays (1,2), the discussion on target-organ carcinogenesis in this chapter focuses primarily on the testis and the prostate, because more information is available about these sites than about the other tissues. The preputial gland, the testicular efferent duct system, and the male accessory sex glands other than the prostate are discussed only briefly. The penis is not included, because it has never been reported as a target of chemical carcinogenesis, and in humans penile cancer probably has a predominantly viral etiology (3), which is outside the scope of this chapter.

The male reproductive tract is not a common site of tumor development in carcinogenesis bioassays in rodents (1,2), and reproductive system tumors are uncommon in male farm and companion animals and in laboratory rodents, with the exception of Leydig cell and ventral prostatic neoplasms in some rat strains (4–12). However, in most Western countries, carcinoma of the prostate is the most commonly diagnosed cancer in men (not counting nonmelanoma skin cancer) (13). Testicular tumors are the leading cancer in men between 20 and 34 years of age (13–16), accounting for about 20% of neoplasms, but for all age groups combined testis cancer comprises less than 1% of cases (13). Tumors of other male reproductive organs are very infrequent in humans.

The main purpose of this chapter is to give an overview, albeit not all-inclusive, of factors that determine susceptibility to carcinogenesis in male reproductive tract tissues. Although chemical and physical agents that are carcinogenic for the male reproductive tract will be discussed, it is not the purpose of this chapter to provide a complete review of these.

TESTES

The testis is a complex tissue, and testicular tumors can be derived from a variety of cell types. These neoplasms are usually classified as either germ cell tumors, accounting for 90% to 95% of testicular tumors, or the more uncommon sex cord–stromal tumors and testicular adnexal tumors (Table 1). Testicular lymphoma, which is the predominant testicular tumor in men over 60 years of age, is not discussed here. Although testicular tumors are the most common neoplasms in men between 20 and 39 years of age (14–16), their etiology is basically not understood.

Epidemiology of Testicular Cancer

The epidemiology of testicular cancer has been reviewed by Muir and Nectoux (17), Schottenfeld et al. (16), and Henderson et al. (18) in 1979–1983, but there are no recent reviews. Therefore, those aspects relevant to the topic of this chapter are discussed here in some detail.

TABLE 1. *Classification of human testicular tumors, including their approximate frequency*

Type	Occurrence (%), all ages	Age-specific occurrence
Germ cell tumors	95	85% of testicular tumors in infants and children
		60% of testicular tumors in men ages 20–39
Seminoma	40	4% of testicular tumors in infants and children
		≥50% of testicular tumors in men ages 20–39
Embryonal carcinoma	24	
Teratocarcinoma	25 ⎫	31% of testicular tumors in infants and children
Teratoma	5 ⎭	
Choriocarcinoma	1	
Yolk sac tumor	<1	50% of testicular tumors in infants and children
Non-germ cell tumors	5	15% of testicular tumors in infants and children
Sex cord-stromal tumors	3	
Leydig cell tumor	2	
Sertoli cell tumor (androblastoma)		
Granulosa cell tumor		
Other sex cord-stromal tumors		
Adnexal tumors	<2	
Rete testis carcinoma		
Mesothelioma		
Other adnexal tumors		

Adapted from Morse and Withmore (15).

Incidence Patterns

There is a considerable variation in the frequency of occurrence of testicular cancer between countries and among populations. High incidence rates are found in white populations in the United States, Canada, and northwest Europe, and in white and Maori populations in New Zealand and Australia, whereas rates are low in most African, Asian, and South American populations and in U.S. blacks. Data from migrant studies suggest at least some role of environmental factors in the etiology of testicular cancer, although not as strongly as for prostate cancer, for example (see later). A role of environmental factors in the causation of testicular cancer is supported by the sometimes-marked increasing time trends in incidence in many of the high-risk populations; the increase in incidence of testicular cancer in 20- to 40-year-old U.S. men increased a dramatic 275% to 300% from 1935–1939 to 1975–1979 (19).

Risk Factors

Few risk factors for cancer of the testis have been found consistently; these are discussed in this section. Contradictory or inconsistent findings have been reported for a number of other risk factors. These include urban-rural differences in occurrence, familial aggregation of risk, or genetic predisposition for developing testicular cancer, mumps-orchitis, testicular trauma, inguinal hernia, and religion (16,17, 19–29). Vasectomy does not seem to affect testicular cancer risk (30,31). There is a poorly understood higher risk for non-seminoma testis cancer in single than in married men over the age of 25 years (14).

Cryptorchidism

Cryptorchidism is the most consistently found risk factor for testicular cancer. Relative risks between 2.5 and 9.0 have been reported (16,20–26,28,32). Thus the attributable risk estimated for cryptorchidism approaches but does not exceed 10% (16). Although not found in all studies (21), the excess risk in unilateral cryptorchidism is confined predominantly to the ipsilateral testis, indicating a direct effect of the condition of not being descended on the propensity of a testicle to develop cancer (16,24,26,27). This hypothesis is supported by reports of a positive correlation between risk and duration of the cryptorchidic condition before correction (orchiopexy) (26,28), as well as by the lower frequency of both cryptorchidism and testis cancer in African-American men than in U.S. Caucasians (16,17,27,33,68). Two studies (24,25) indicated that particularly risk for developing seminoma was associated with cryptorchidism, but other studies have not confirmed this (16,28). Cryptorchidism may also be a risk factor for the development of Leydig cell tumors, but this has not been well studied because this type of testicular tumor is very rare in men (34). Prenatal exposure to estrogens, specifically diethylstilbestrol (DES), has been shown to be a risk factor for cryptorchidism (35–37), although not in all studies (38). This elevated risk for testicular cancer in cryptorchid men is widely believed to be involved in the association between cryptorchidism and testicular cancer risk (16,20–23,25,28,39). However, although cryptorchidism is the most consistently found and strongest risk factor for testicular cancer in men, it accounts for less than 10% of cases. Unfortunately, the frequency of testicular cancer in cohorts of men with and without a history of cryptorchidism has not been determined in prospective or retrospective studies.

Hormone Exposure

Prenatal Hormone Exposure. The hypothesis that prenatal exposure to estrogens, including DES as well as maternal estrogens, is related to the development of testicular cancer has been examined in several epidemiologic studies (16,20–23,25,28). Moss et al. (25) combined the data from their own study with those of previous studies by Depue et al. (21) and Schottenfeld et al. (16). They concluded that there is weak evidence that prenatal exposure to hormones is related to risk for cancer of the testis ($p=0.0220$, one-sided χ^2 test), and little evidence for a similar relation between prenatal DES exposure and risk ($p>0.1$).

Combination of the case-control data presented by Moss et al. (25) with those of the only newer study examining this question (20) and two other earlier studies (23,40) strengthens the evidence that prenatal exposure to any type of hormone is related to increased testis cancer risk (Table 2). However, there is little consistency between these studies, inasmuch as only the four earliest studies (16,21,23,40) show the association, whereas it is completely absent in the two more recent studies (20,25). Combination of all data (Table 2) weakens the evidence for DES exposure ($p>>0.1$). On the other hand, there are case reports (see ref. 40) of men who were exposed to DES *in utero* and later developed testicular cancer (42) or seminoma (43). Furthermore, studies of this type probably have considerable recall bias, which in all likelihood leads to underestimation of prenatal hormone use, particularly for specific drugs such as DES (20,25). Therefore, the results of these studies taken together do not discount the hypothesis that prenatal DES exposure is a risk factor for developing testicular cancer, and they provide moderately strong evidence that hormone exposure in general is a weak risk factor for cancer of the testis.

Only a small fraction of cases (i.e., less than 5%) is potentially attributable to prenatal exposure to exogenous hormones. The role of maternal (endogenous) hormones, particularly estrogen, in the development of testicular cancer in male offspring has not been examined specifically. Very interesting in this regard are reports indicating that Leydig cell hyperplasia occurs in males that have been exposed to DES prenatally (41; see also ref. 40). There is, however, no evidence that *in utero* DES exposure leads to Leydig cell tumors.

Postnatal Hormone Exposure. There are a few case reports of a variety of testicular tumors (seminoma, teratoma, embryonal carcinoma, and Leydig cell neoplasia)

TABLE 2. *Hormone exposure during pregnancy in mothers of testicular cancer cases and controls*

Exposure as reported by the mothers	Henderson et al. (23)		Schottenfeld et al. (16)		Loughlin et al. (40)		Depue et al. (21)		Moss et al. (25)		Morris Brown et al. (20)		Combined data	
	n	%	n	%	n	%	n	%	n	%	n	%	n	%
All hormones														
Cases	6/78	7.6	11/190	3.6	2/28	7.1	9/97[a]	9.3	8/222	3.6	4/202	2.0	40/817[b]	4.9
Controls	1/78	1.3	3/141	2.1	0/28	0	2/105	1.9	9/224	4.0	5/206	2.4	24/945	2.5
			4/163	2.5										
Diethylstilbestrol only														
Cases					1/28	3.6	2/97	2.1	4/222	1.8	2/202	1.0	9/549	1.7
Controls					0/28	0	1/105	1.0	2/224	0.9	2/206	1.0	5/563	0.9

[a] Significantly higher than in controls when tested by χ^2 test ($p = 0.0433$, one-sided, $\chi^2 = 3.9883$).
[b] Significantly higher than in controls when tested by χ^2 test ($p = 0.0084$, one-sided, $\chi^2 = 6.9502$).

arising in men that had been treated with estrogenic compounds for either prostate cancer (DES) or infertility (clomiphene) (45–48). Although these reports suggest that postnatal exposure to estrogens may induce testicular neoplasms, there is no evidence for this from epidemiological studies. Furthermore, the estrogen treatments were of relatively short duration, 9 to 21 months for clomiphene and 11 to 28 months for DES. Therefore, it is likely that, if anything, the estrogen exposures enhanced the development of already present (pre)neoplastic testicular lesions rather than induced them *de novo* (48).

Low Birth Weight and Premature Birth

Low birth weight (≤ 5 or 6 lb) and/or premature delivery have been found to be strongly associated with testis cancer risk in three studies, with significantly elevated relative risks or odds ratios of between 3.2 and 21.0 (20–22). An association between testis cancer risk and low birth weight (<2.7 kg) was not observed in one study (25). The former studies suggest that low birth weight and testicular cancer share common, as yet unknown, risk factors (20). A Japanese study on maternal factors and testis cancer found significantly fewer live births for mothers of testicular cancer cases than for control mothers (49).

Occupation

Elevated risk for testis cancer has been reported for farmers, farm workers, and/or farming as an occupation in several studies (50–55). However, in only one of these studies (53) was the excess risk statistically significant, and there are several other studies that did not find an elevated risk (56–60). Wiklund et al. (55) reported a nonsignificant elevation of testicular cancer risk among licenced pesticide applicators, and Hayes et al. (57) found a similar association between risk and self-reported pesticide exposure for non-seminoma testis tumors, but no association with risk for seminoma and all types of testis tumors.

Significantly elevated testis cancer risk was found for professional/managerial job categories in three U.S. studies (27,57,60), but not in three British studies (32,51,59). Army personnel have been found to have a significant excess testis cancer risk in several studies (51,56,61,62) but not in all (59). A relation between occupational exposure to dimethylformamide and other chemicals has been suggested but not substantiated (61,63,64). Hayes et al. (57) found an association between testis cancer risk and self-reported exposure to microwaves and radio waves among military personnel. However, they did not observe a correlation between testis cancer risk and level of exposure as assessed from job titles. Significant excess risk for testicular cancer has been reported for U.S. Army Vietnam veterans (65) and, interestingly, military dogs that were used in Vietnam (66). The authors of both studies suggested a relation with exposure to Agent Orange (65,66). Elevated risks for testicular cancer have been reported for production workers (non-seminoma, particularly teratocarcinoma) (57) and for workers in the mining and natural gas/crude petroleum extraction industries (53). These associations, however, have not been confirmed by other studies (51,53,56–58,60).

In summary, the available data seem to suggest that occupational exposure to a wide variety of potentially carcinogenic substances is possibly related to the development of testicular cancer. However, there is considerable inconsistency among these data, and no specific chemical or physical exposures have been found to be related to elevated risk for testicular cancer.

Race

One of the most striking racial differences in the occurrence of cancer of the testis is the four times lower incidence among black men than in white males in the United States (14,16,17,19,27,33,67). Testicular cancer incidence rates among black men living in Africa and the Caribbean are also low (17,33). In contrast, testis cancer rates are low among Japanese and Chinese men living in Asia, whereas rates among Japanese and, particularly, Chinese migrants to the United States are distinctly higher (17,33). Interesting also are the very high testicular cancer rates in New Zealand among both white immigrants as well as the indigenous people, the Maoris (17,33). These data suggest that environmental as well as genetically determined racial factors may be involved in testicular tumorigenesis.

The low testis cancer risk among African-American men correlates well with the lower frequency of cryptorchidism in this group (68). However, the association observed between risk for testicular cancer and low birth weight is not in line with the low testicular cancer rates in U.S. blacks and the high rates in Caucasians (20–22), because low birth weights are twice as frequent among blacks than among whites in the United States (69).

Socioeconomic Status

Invariably, a positive correlation has been found between a high socioeconomic status and risk for testicular cancer (16,27,58). This finding is compatible with the elevated risks found for professional–managerial job categories in some studies (27,57,59).

Conclusions

The only risk factors for testicular cancer found consistently in epidemiological studies are cryptorchidism and, examined in fewer studies, a high socioeconomic status. Less consistent are the associations observed between testis cancer risk and low birth weight, premature birth, and prenatal exposure to hormones, particularly estrogens. The evidence for postnatal estrogen exposure and occupational exposures as risk factors for testicular cancer is inconclusive. The association between testis cancer risk and cryptorchidism accounts for only approximately 10% of cases and may be related to prenatal estrogen exposure. The reasons for the observed correlations between testicular cancer risk, on the one hand, and high socioeconomic status and, possibly, low birth weight and premature birth, on the other hand, are not understood.

Induction of Testis Tumors in Experimental Animals

The induction of testicular tumors in rodents has been reviewed by Boorman et al. (70,71), Kirkman and Kempson (10), Mostofi and Bresler (11), and Mostofi et al. (12). A number of chemicals have been shown to induce testicular tumors in rodent carcinogen bioassays (see, e.g., refs. 1,2). The tumors induced in these bioassays were in all but a very few cases Leydig cell neoplasms. The mechanisms by which tumors of interstitial cell origin are produced is not known for most of these chemicals. Only for estrogens and cadmium is there information in this regard, which is detailed in later paragraphs. Interestingly, Leydig cell tumors are also the most common spontaneous testicular neoplasms in rodents, while other types of testis tumors are exceedingly rare in untreated aging rodents (7,10–12,70,71). The exception to this apparent rule is the occurrence of teratomas/embryonal carcinomas in strain 129 mice (1% incidence) and its 129/Sv-Sl (5–10% incidence) and 129/terSv sublines (32% incidence) (11,72–76).

Induction of Non-Leydig Cell Tumors

Chemical induction of testicular tumors of non-Leydig cell origin has only been observed after treatment of rats with a nitrosamine (77), after prenatal treatment with estrogens in mice (78–80), and after cadmium administration to adult rats (81). In addition, induction of such tumors has been reported resulting from a variety of treatments (10,12), including intratesticular administration of zinc chloride in hamsters (82) or some irritants in mice (11).

Pour (77) observed a 29% to 32% incidence of testicular tumors following a single *in utero* treatment of Wistar-derived rats with 20 mg/kg maternal body weight of N-nitrosobis(2-oxopropyl)amine (BOP) on days 14, 18, or 20 of gestation. Three treatments with 10 mg/kg BOP on days 14, 18, and 20 resulted in a 53% incidence. The first tumors were observed when the animals were 82 weeks old. The incidence of testicular tumors in control rats was 8%, all of which were Leydig cell tumors. The histology of the BOP-induced tumors was not well described. Many of these tumors (no exact incidences were given) were Leydig cell tumors with "epithelial cell components in the form of mixed stromal-glandular elements," and these "glandular elements were most probably ductal differentiation of Sertoli cells." BOP administered at a dose of 10 mg/kg twice weekly for the first 5.5 weeks of life resulted in the development of gonadal stromal tumors (not otherwise specified) in 13 of 19 F344 rats (68%) (83). BOP given to adult Wistar-derived rats produced Leydig cell tumors in 5 of 15 animals (33%) provided that the dose was sufficiently low to avoid reduced survival; there were no such tumors in 15 control rats (84). The mechanism for the effective induction of testicular tumors by transplacental BOP administration is not known.

Adenocarcinomas of the rete testis have been found in 11 of 233 (5%) mice after prenatal treatment with 100 μg/kg maternal body weight DES on days 9 to 16 of gestation (78). Hyperplastic lesions of the rete testis occurred in 56% of these animals. Hyperplasia of Sertoli cells occurred in 6 of 18 mice that had received the same *in utero* treatment; one of these 6 mice also had a "Sertoli cell carcinoma *in situ*" (85,86).

Prenatal exposure to the potent estrogen ethinyl estradiol at doses of 20 or 200 μg/kg maternal body weight increased the incidence of teratomas/embryonal carcinomas in 129/Sv-Sl mice from 4 of 107 (3.7%) in controls to 11 of 109 (10.1%) and 8 of 115 (7.0%), respectively; these increases were not statistically significant, and there was no relationship between estrogen dose and tumor incidence (80). Such tumors can also be induced by transplantation of fetal genital ridges to adult mouse testes (87; reviewed in ref. 12). A 100% incidence of tumors that probably originate from Sertoli cells has been reported to result from transplantation of neonatal testis into the spleen of adult rats (88).

Waalkes and co-workers (70,81,89,90) reported that a single subcutaneous or intramuscular injection with 10 to 40 μmol/kg cadmium chloride in a total of 264 adult Wistar rats (some of which also received 0.1 to 1.0 mmol zinc/kg) resulted in the induction of one seminoma, one rete testis adenocarcinoma, and one mixed Sertoli-Leydig cell tumor. Additionally, one seminoma was found in 1 of 30 rats that had received four injections with 5 μmol/kg cadmium chloride at 2- to 3-day intervals (70,81,89). The overall incidence of non-Leydig cell tumors in these studies was four in a total of 473 cadmium-exposed rats (0.8%). Two additional rats had hyperplastic lesions of the rete testis (81). There were no such tumors or hyperplasias in a total of 128 control rats.

Induction of Leydig Cell Tumors

Prenatal Estrogen Treatment

Prenatal exposure of CD-1 mice to DES (100 μg/kg maternal body weight on days 9 to 16 of gestation) has been shown to result in an almost 100% frequency of cryptorchidism and impairment of spermatogenesis, as well as a lower incidence of testicular fibrosis and inflammatory lesions (79,85,86,91). Leydig cell tumors were found following prenatal DES treatment from 10 months of age onward in 7 of 277

CD-1 mice (2.5%) in one study (79) and in 4 of 18 CD-1 mice (22%) in another (85). As indicated earlier, the latter study also reports some Sertoli cell lesions.

In utero exposure of strain 129/Sv-Sl mice to ethinyl estradiol (20 or 200 μg/kg maternal body weight) resulted in a much lower incidence of cryptorchidism than in the cited studies with DES in CD-1 mice [i.e., 10 of 109 mice (9.2%) and 23 of 115 mice (20%) as compared to 4 of 107 controls (3.7%)]; the relationship between estrogen dose and incidence of cryptorchidism was highly significant (p value for trend $= 0.0001$) (80). However, no Leydig cell neoplasms were found in this study, although there was a slightly, but not significantly, increased incidence of teratomas/embryonal carcinomas in the estrogen-exposed mice of this strain, as indicated earlier (73,80).

Cryptorchidism following prenatal estrogen treatment in rats has been found in some studies (92) but not in others (85). Leydig cell hyperplasia or tumors have not been described in these studies of prenatal estrogen treatment in rats (85,92).

Adult Estrogen Treatment

Subcutaneous implantation of DES-containing cholesterol pellets induces Leydig cell tumors with high efficiency in some mouse strains, such as BALB/c mice, but not in other strains, such as C3H mice (93). DES treatment did not induce Leydig cell tumors in testes that were neonatally transplanted from C3H to BALB/c mice, but it did induce such tumors in testes neonatally transplanted from BALB/c to C3H mice, which indicates that the susceptibility to estrogen induction of Leydig cell tumors in mice is determined by factors localized within the testis (93). Similar to DES, subcutaneously implanted estradiol-17β induces Leydig cell tumors in mice, whereas following estradiol-17β implantation in the spleen, no such tumors are induced (94). Moreover, if testicular grafts are placed in close proximity of an estradiol-17β pellet in the mouse spleen, Leydig cell tumors are formed in the grafts, whereas if the grafts are placed in the spleen at a distance from the pellets, no tumors develop (94). These data clearly indicate that a direct effect of the estrogen is responsible for the induction of Leydig cell tumors in mice, and not, for example, an estrogen metabolite or estrogen-controlled pituitary factor.

Both Syrian golden hamsters and European hamsters also develop Leydig cell tumors following estrogen treatment (95). In contrast to mice and hamsters, treatment of rats with estradiol-17β does not induce Leydig cell tumors, and it prevents the development of spontaneous Leydig cell tumors in the typically high-incidence F344 strain (96,97). The latter effect of estradiol-17β is probably related to elevation of circulating prolactin concentrations, since grafting of pituitary tissue under the kidney capsule, which markedly elevates prolactin, also inhibited spontaneous Leydig cell tumor formation, as shown by Bartke et al. (96). These authors suggest that hyperprolactinemia suppresses Leydig cell tumor development by lowering circulating LH levels.

Pituitary Factors and Cryptorchidism and Rodent Leydig Cell Tumor Formation

The presence of a functioning pituitary is necessary for estrogen induction of Leydig cell tumors in the mouse, since hypophysectomy is preventive, but it is not clear what pituitary factor(s) is (are) involved (93). Hypergonadotrophic stimulation of the testes as such does not seem to lead to formation of Leydig cell tumors in mice, and there is no clear correlation between induction of Leydig cell tumors and pituitary tumors (probably producing prolactin) in estrogen-treated mice (93). In hamsters, on the other hand, there seems to be a partial correlation between the presence of pituitary tumors and Leydig cell tumors (95). Surgically produced cryptorchidism in mice leads to development of small Leydig cell tumors with a long latency, and surgical cryptorchidism enhances the induction of these neoplasms in mice treated with estrogen (93).

In rats, on the other hand, elevation of circulating LH by, for example, transplantation of the testes to the spleen or parabiosis of intact with castrated rats, is known to enhance the spontaneous formation of Leydig cell tumors (98,99). Furthermore, reduction of circulating LH by treatment with LH-RH agonists inhibits the formation of these tumors in the high-incidence F344 rat strain (100). Coincidently, DES treatment, which inhibits Leydig cell tumor formation in F344 rats, also lowers circulating LH (96). However, circulating estradiol levels increase, and serum and particularly pituitary levels of LH decrease, with aging in the F344 rat, in parallel with the development of Leydig cell hyperplasias and tumors (101). Huseby (97) demonstrated that parabiosis of F344 rats with castrated male partners does not influence Leydig cell tumorigenesis, whereas surgically created cryptorchidism in F344 rats, even when parabiosed to castrated partners, almost completely abolishes the formation of Leydig cell hyperplasia and tumors. This suggests that local testicular factors present under cryptorchid conditions can override the enhancement of the spontaneous formation of Leydig cell tumors by elevated levels of LH in rats.

In conclusion, while the mechanisms of Leydig cell tumorigenesis in rats and mice seem to be quite dissimilar, pituitary factors appear to play a decisive role in the formation of Leydig cell tumors in both species.

Cadmium-Induced Leydig Cell Tumors in Rodents

Cadmium is a firmly established tumorigenic agent for the rodent testis, producing predominantly Leydig cell tumors, as recently reviewed by Waalkes and Oberdörster (102). Gunn and co-workers (103,104) and Roe et al. (105) first demonstrated that a single subcutaneous injection of cadmium chloride induces a high incidence of Leydig cell tumors in rats and mice when given in doses of ≥ 2 to 2.5 mg/kg (approximately 11 to 14 μmol cadmium/kg); these doses are also minimally required for acute testicular toxicity of cadmium (see later). This has been confirmed by several other investigators (e.g., refs. 89,90,106) in rats; mice remain a less well-studied species. A single oral cadmium administration to rats produced Leydig cell hyperplasia within 6 months, indicative of Leydig cell tumor formation at later time points which were not studied, but only when given in a very high dose (over the LD_{50}) (106). The testicular tumorigenicity of cadmium does not appear to differ considerably among rat strains with a low spontaneous incidence of these neoplasms; cadmium does not seem to enhance Leydig cell tumor formation in rats of the high-incidence F344 strain (107). Strain differences have not been studied in mice, but the acute effects of cadmium (see later) seem to depend on the strain used, but this has not been well studied (104,136). Most cadmium-induced Leydig cell tumors are benign, but high doses can induce malignant Leydig cell neoplasms, as manifested by local invasion and distant metastases (102,106). Repeated subcutaneous injection and repeated oral administration of low cadmium doses have failed to induce Leydig cell tumors (89,106). The induction of testicular tumors by cadmium can be effectively inhibited by pretreatment with a low dose of cadmium or with dimethylnitrosamine, and by treatment with high doses of zinc (zinc/cadmium total dose ratio of 100:1) around the time of cadmium injection (90,103,104; for a review, see ref. 102).

Other Chemicals That Induce Leydig Cell Tumors

A number of other chemicals have been reported to induce Leydig cell tumors in carcinogen bioassays in rats or mice (1,2,108), including metronidazole in rats (109), reserpine in rats (110), o,p'-dichlorodiphenyldichloroethane in rats (111), and cyclophosphamide and skin painting with methylcholanthrene in mice (see ref. 11).

Conclusions

Induction of a significant incidence of testicular tumors of non-Leydig cell origin has been reported for prenatal treatment of rats with N-nitrosobis(2-oxopropyl)amine (mixed stromal tumors). Low to very low incidences of non-Leydig cell tumors resulted from (a) prenatal exposure to estrogens (rete testis carcinoma, and Sertoli cell hyperplasia in DES-treated mice, and teratoma/embryonal carcinoma in ethinyl estradiol-treated mice of a strain that spontaneously develops such neoplasms), and (b) single parenteral administration of cadmium in rats (seminoma, rete testis carcinoma, mixed stromal tumor).

Leydig cell tumors can effectively be induced by pre- and postnatal estrogen treatment in mice, depending on the strain used, and in (adult) hamsters, but not in rats. Prenatal estrogen administration also causes cryptorchidism in mice and probably also in rats, a condition which in and of itself produces Leydig cell tumors in mice but probably not in rats. In rat strains with a high spontaneous incidence of Leydig cell tumors (postnatal), estrogen treatment and surgical cryptorchidism in fact inhibit the formation of these neoplasms. Elevation of circulating LH seems to enhance Leydig cell tumor formation in rats, whereas reduction of LH may inhibit it. In mice, LH *per se* does not seem to induce Leydig cell tumors, and the presence of an intact pituitary is essential for tumor induction by estrogens.

Cadmium induces a high incidence of Leydig cell tumors when given at doses that cause acute testicular toxicity, irrespective of the route of administration and rodent species. Treatment with cadmium below these doses, even when administered repeatedly, does not induce Leydig cell tumors.

Target-Organ-Specific Mechanisms of Testicular Tumorigenesis

The possible target-organ-specific mechanisms of testicular tumorigenesis are discussed in the following sections for the major risk factors in humans and major causative agents/conditions of testicular cancer identified in animal studies: cryptorchidism, hormones, and cadmium exposure.

Cryptorchidism

Cryptorchidism is the most consistent risk factor for testicular cancer in humans. Prenatal estrogen exposure has been proposed as a causative factor in the pathogenesis of both cryptorchidism and testis cancer (17). Some investigators have hypothesized that prenatal estrogen exposure induces testicular cancer by first causing cryptorchidism (16,20–23,25,28,39). Indeed, a higher-than-expected frequency of cryptorchid testes has been found in men exposed *in utero* to DES (35,37). In addition, in comparison with controls ($n = 24$), serum of mothers of males born with cryptorchid testes ($n = 24$) was found to contain significantly greater percentages of free ($p = 0.010$) and non-SHBG-bound estradiol-17β ($p = 0.014$), as well as, on average, 16% more free ($p = 0.066$) and 16% more albumin-bound estradiol-17β ($p = 0.038$) during the first trimester of pregnancy (39). These findings appear to contrast with the slightly higher amounts of circulating total ($p = 0.09$) and free estradiol-17β ($p = 0.10$) found in 20 black women pregnant with a male fetus during the first trimester than in 20 Caucasian controls (112); African-Americans have a considerably lower risk for both cryptorchidism and testicular cancer than do U.S. whites, as indicated earlier.

Prenatal estrogen exposure effectively induces cryptorchidism in animal studies with rodents. Particularly in mice, a high incidence of retained testes results from prenatal estrogen treatment (79). In most mouse studies with prenatal estrogen exposure only tumors of Leydig cell and Sertoli cell origin have been found, and their incidence was low (79,85,86). However, in humans, germ cell tumors are by far the most common testicular tumor types, and stromal tumors are very uncommon. The only animal study in which prenatal estrogen exposure caused germ cell tumors, albeit at low incidence, was conducted with a mouse strain that spontaneously develops teratomas/embryonal carcinomas (80). There was, however, no significant correlation between the occurrence of cryptorchidism and the presence of these tumors in this study.

Overall, neither in epidemiological studies, nor in animal experiments, is there consistency in the correlation between prenatal estrogen exposure and the joint occurrence of cryptorchidism and testicular tumors. This raises the possibility that cryptorchidism and testicular tumorigenesis induced by prenatal estrogen exposure are independent processes. It is also possible that cryptorchidism is responsible for only a fraction of testicular tumors, in which case it is unknown whether prenatal estrogen-induced cryptorchidism is the underlying cause of the development of this fraction of testicular tumors. Sato et al. (113) found that the estrogen receptor content of the scrotal testis is approximately 25% of that of surgically produced cryptorchid testes in BALB/c mice. This finding suggests that estrogen induction of tumors in cryptorchid mouse testes may involve estrogen-receptor mediation.

Testicular descent in mammals has been proposed to be a biphasic process (114,115), consisting of a transabdominal migration phase, probably involving the gubernaculum and under control of Müllerian inhibiting substance (MIS) (114, 115), followed by a transinguinal migration stage that is predominantly under androgen control (114). Although the precise mechanism of induction of cryptorchidism by prenatal estrogen exposure is unknown, it appears that the transabdominal phase is affected selectively (114,116). Suppression of androgen production by prenatal estrogen has been demonstrated (116), and inhibition of the secretion of MIS by the developing testis has been proposed (35). However, direct inhibition of the action of MIS on the Müllerian duct seems the most likely mechanism of prenatal estrogen induction of cryptorchidism (114). The *in vitro* regression of Müllerian duct structures induced by MIS is inhibited by prenatal DES treatment in mice (117), and DES and other estrogens completely protect Müllerian duct structures in male chicken embryos from regression, probably via direct inhibition of the action of MIS (for a summary, see ref. 114). In addition, estrogens cause atrophy of the gubernaculum (115,118), and in the testicular feminization mouse model, prenatal DES administration inhibits transabdominal testicular descent to the same extent as in controls, ruling out that androgens are involved (114).

The mechanism whereby cryptorchidism *per se* may lead to testicular tumor development in humans and rodents is not known. In most epidemiologic studies, the excess risk for testis cancer was confined to the cryptorchid testicle (16,24,26,28). Therefore, local factors are probably responsible for the increased risk for cancer development in the undescended testis. The cryptorchid testis is exposed to a higher temperature than a scrotal testis, and this elevated temperature has been suggested to be involved in testicular tumorigenesis. However, there is no consistent epidemiologic evidence for raised testicular temperatures as a risk factor for testis cancer (29,119). Cryptorchidism causes and enhances Leydig cell tumorigenesis in mice, but it inhibits this process in rats. Unfortunately, with one exception, all research on the mechanisms of the influence of cryptorchidism on Leydig cell structure and function and on testicular tumorigenesis in rodents has used rats (e.g., ref. 120), and therefore provides no useful data in relation to enhancement of testicular tumorigenesis in humans.

Hormones

There is, as pointed out earlier, limited evidence that prenatal hormone exposure is related to testicular cancer development in men, including Leydig cell hyperplasia, and only some case reports suggesting that postnatal estrogen exposure may lead to testis tumors. Furthermore, in comparison with pregnant U.S. Caucasian women, pregnant African-American women have been shown to have slightly, but not significantly, higher circulating levels of estrogens (see earlier), whereas U.S. black men have a considerably lower risk for testicular cancer than that of Caucasian men (112). Thus it is at present not at all clear whether prenatal estrogen exposure leads to testicular cancer development in men.

In laboratory mice, however, prenatal estrogen treatment results, depending on the strain used, in hyperplasia and tumors of Leydig cell and/or Sertoli cell origin, and/or teratomas/embryonal carcinomas and rete testis hyperplasia and carcinomas, albeit in low incidence. As indicated earlier, estrogen administration to adult rodents induces exclusively Leydig cell tumors in mice (and hamsters), whereas in rats Leydig cell tumor development is actually suppressed. Furthermore, elevation of circulating LH enhances spontaneous Leydig cell tumor development in rats, but seems to have no effect on estrogen-induced Leydig cell tumor formation in mice. Thus the hormonal factors involved in Leydig cell tumor development in rats appear to be almost the opposite of those in mice, and they are not very relevant in the context of human testicular carcinogenesis.

As summarized earlier, ingenious studies by Huseby (94) have demonstrated that direct effects of estrogen on the testis are responsible for induction of Leydig cell tumors in mice. In other studies, Huseby and Samuels (121) showed that stimulation of DNA synthesis in mouse Leydig cells by estrogen administration was independent of the presence of the pituitary. Huseby and associates (113,122) have further demonstrated that testicular nuclear estrogen receptor content is markedly up-regulated by acute and chronic estrogen treatment in a mouse strain that is sensitive to estrogen induction of Leydig cell tumors (BALB/c), whereas this does not occur in a resistant strain (C3H). Subsequent experiments (123) with a variety of (putative) estrogenic compounds revealed that Leydig cell hyperplasia could only be induced with chronic treatment of those substances that acutely stimulated Leydig cell DNA synthesis and increased nuclear estrogen-receptor content and reduced cytosolic estrogen-receptor content in the testis. These results strongly suggest that the induction of Leydig cell tumors by estrogen in sensitive mice involves estrogen-receptor-mediated, nongenotoxic mechanisms. However, they do not rule out that genotoxic mechanisms are also involved, similar to estrogen induction of kidney tumors in the male hamster, which involves both estrogen genotoxicity and estrogen-receptor mediation (124–126).

Cadmium

The mechanisms of cadmium carcinogenicity have recently been reviewed by Waalkes and Oberdörster (102) and Snow (127). Cadmium is genotoxic in several manners, including DNA damage, inhibition of DNA repair, and alteration of DNA replication fidelity and gene expression (see refs. 127,128). However, the testicular tumorigenicity of cadmium may be entirely based on nongenotoxic mechanisms as discussed in the following paragraphs.

Cadmium is a well-established testicular toxicant that selectively causes widespread hemorrhagic necrosis due to degenerative effects on testicular blood vessels (89,105,129–131). Simple total or partial ligation of afferent and efferent testicular vasculature has the same acute effects as cadmium, and it also causes a high incidence of Leydig cell tumors (132). Cadmium will only induce Leydig cell tumors when given in doses that exceed the dose minimally required for testicular toxicity (5 to 10 μmol cadmium/kg), and testicular tumorigenicity of cadmium is dose-dependent above this dose (89). It is therefore possible that the testicular tumorigenicity of cadmium is entirely attributable to its toxic effects on the testicular vasculature. Pretreatment with zinc prevents cadmium-induced tumors, but not tumors induced by ligation of testicular vasculature, suggesting dissimilar mechanisms of testicular tumorigenicity of cadmium and vascular ligation (132). However, zinc treatment also inhibits the atrophying effect of cadmium on the rat testes in a dose-dependent manner (90,103,104), and so does treatment with a low dose of cadmium in mice (133). Zinc (and perhaps low-dose cadmium pretreatment) may therefore prevent cadmium-induced Leydig cell tumor formation by interfering with the toxic effects of cadmium on testicular vasculature (90,103,104).

The selective sensitivity of the rodent testis for cadmium toxicity and tumorigenicity is probably related to a deficiency of metallothionein in that tissue (134–136). Although there are proteins in the rodent testis that bind cadmium and other metals (134,135), they are distinct from metallothionein and they are not inducible, unlike metallothionein (136). These observations also indicate that the mechanisms whereby high-dose zinc and low-dose cadmium pretreatments inhibit testicular tumorigenicity by cadmium do not involve induction of metallothionein (90,102). Recently, Wahba et al. (137) observed that low-dose cadmium *in vivo* pretreatment increased glutathione levels in isolated Leydig cells and prevented glutathione depletion following *in vitro* cadmium exposure. Thus the recruitment of non-heavy-metal-specific intracellular defense mechanisms may be responsible for the remarkable preventive effects of zinc and cadmium pretreatment.

The mechanism of the vascular toxicity of cadmium in the rodent testis is unknown. The degenerative effects of cadmium on the testis may be due in part to a high sensitivity of Leydig cells, and particularly, Sertoli cells, for cadmium cytotoxicity as indicated by *in vitro* studies with isolated cell types (138–141). The cadmium-induced vascular changes in the testis could be secondary to these cytotoxic effects of cadmium. However, cadmium induces vascular changes within minutes following its administration, suggesting a direct effect on the testicular blood vessels (130,131). This "direct" effect may be mediated by catecholaminergic mechanisms, because reserpine pretreatment and prior adrenalectomy inhibit the acute toxic effects of cadmium on the rat testis (142). Isolated Leydig cells from zinc- or low-dose cadmium-pretreated rats are refractory to cadmium cytotoxicity

(139–141). Therefore, the preventive effects of zinc on the testicular toxicity and tumorigenicity of cadmium may be due to intracellular interactions between these two metals, such as competition for macromolecular binding (127), or induction of non-heavy-metal-specific intracellular defense mechanisms, as mentioned earlier.

Following the severe testis damage that results from exposure to cadmium doses that induce Leydig cell tumors, testicular testosterone production drastically diminishes (143) due to reduced progesterone utilization for testosterone biosynthesis and increased catabolism of progesterone (100,144). As a result, pituitary LH secretion is markedly elevated, which has been proposed to be the central factor in the induction by cadmium of Leydig cell tumors in rodents (98). However, in mice, LH does not affect Leydig cell tumor formation, whereas in rats LH induces these neoplasms or enhances their formation, but cadmium induces Leydig cell tumors and causes testicular toxicity in both species (see earlier). Furthermore, the testes of treated rats do not produce testosterone in response to LH (103). On the other hand, cadmium-induced Leydig cell hyperplasia seems to be prevented by testosterone treatment, which probably reduces LH secretion (102). Thus although testicular toxicity appears to be an absolute requirement for cadmium to cause Leydig cell tumors, the role of LH remains unclear.

In conclusion, the precise mechanism whereby cadmium causes the formation of Leydig cell tumors in rats and mice is not known at present.

Conclusions

The etiology of human testicular tumors is poorly defined, as indicated earlier. With the possible exception of prenatal estrogen exposure, no specific chemical exposures have been associated with testicular cancer risk in men. Prenatal as well as postnatal estrogen treatments induce testicular tumors in some mouse strains but not in other mouse strains or in rats. Prenatal estrogen exposure also causes cryptorchid testes in mice and possibly rats. Cryptorchidism is a consistent risk factor for testicular cancer in men, and estrogen- or surgically induced cryptorchidism is associated with Leydig cell tumorigenesis in mice. In rats, however, surgically induced cryptorchidism inhibits Leydig cell tumor formation. Cadmium administration induces Leydig cell tumors in both rodent species, but cadmium exposure is not known to be associated with testicular tumor formation in men. Overall, it appears that the mouse may be the most appropriate species as an animal model for testicular tumorigenesis in humans.

From the preceding discussion it appears that any of the following treatments or conditions may cause testicular tumor formation: (a) severe acute testicular toxicity in mice and rats; (b) chronic exposure to estrogenic compounds of adult mice and hamsters; (c) prenatal exposure to estrogenic compounds of mice and possibly humans; and (d) any treatment or condition that induces cryptorchidism in mice and humans. The mechanisms whereby these treatments or conditions may cause testicular tumorigenesis are largely poorly understood.

PROSTATE

Epidemiology of Prostate Cancer

Prostate cancer incidence and mortality rates have increased in the United States over the past two decades (145,146). It is currently the most frequently diagnosed cancer and the second most frequent cause of death due to cancer in U.S. males (13). The epidemiology of prostatic cancer has recently been reviewed in depth elsewhere (147–151). Environmental and hormonal factors, particularly androgens, are almost certainly involved in human prostatic carcinogenesis, as demonstrated in these reviews.

The following conditions were among those ruled out by Bosland (147) as possible risk factors for prostate cancer: smoking, alcohol use, prior prostatitis or benign prostatic hyperplasia, transmissible factors such as viruses, cadmium exposure, and most exposures in the rubber industry. The data concerning dietary intake of vitamin A and/or β-carotene were found to be contradictory. However, since this review was composed, new studies have been published concerning, among other aspects, dietary factors, vasectomy, smoking, cadmium exposure, farming, radiation exposures, and hormonal factors in relation with human prostate cancer risk. These are summarized in the following sections, with emphasis on those factors that are of interest in the context of this chapter; it is not the purpose of this section to provide a detailed update of the previous review by Bosland (147), since more recent reviews by Meikle and Smith (148), Muir et al. (149), Nomura and Kolonel (150), and van der Gulden et al. (151) are available.

Diet and Nutrition

The association between dietary patterns and prostate cancer risk has been studied in a variety of populations using a range of epidemiological approaches. These studies, which have been extensively summarized in previous reviews (147,152), in general found a high intake of dietary fat and, to a lesser extent, protein and energy to be associated with increased risk for prostate cancer, whereas the influence on prostate cancer risk of vitamin A and its precursors was not clear. Associations with prostate cancer risk observed for individual nutrients or foods are not very strong. However, the change in risk with migration from low-risk areas such as Japan to high-risk countries such as the United States is considerable. These changes in risk are thought to be due to differences in environment including lifestyle, particularly dietary habits (see ref. 147). It is therefore conceivable that the combined effects of dietary factors on prostate carcinogenesis are more important than the separate effects of the individual factors. Studies specifically addressing this possibility have not been conducted. The apparent relation between dietary habits and prostate cancer risk is further supported by the observation that the current Westernization of lifestyle in Japan is associated with an increasing incidence of prostate cancer (153) and by the correlation between rates of prostate cancer and other diet-associated cancers such as colon cancer (154; see also ref. 147).

Recent studies concerning prostate cancer risk and intake of dietary fat and vitamin A and its precursors are discussed briefly in subsequent sections. Not previously summarized case-control studies concerning associations between intake of nutrients other than fat and vitamin A and its precursors (155–157) or the consumption of foods (158–164) provide some, but inconsistent, support for the notion that intake of fatty foods is a risk factor and that the consumption of dietary fiber, carrots, certain (leafy) vegetables, pulses, tomatoes, and fish may be protective. Similar findings were reported from one recent cohort study (165), whereas another cohort study did not find any significant associations with risk for major food groups (166). A "dose"-related positive association with prostate cancer risk was found for amount of milk intake and for milk fat level by Mettlin et al. (159) and by LaVecchia et al. (158), whereas other recent studies found no influence of milk or dairy intake (160,163,165–167). This confirms an earlier conclusion (147) that the data on the effect of milk consumption are inconsistent. Two case-control studies found significant elevation of risk with increasing (estimated) intake of zinc (156,157). West et al. (157) also found increases in risk with increases in estimated dietary intake of cadmium and selenium; selenium showed a positive gradient in risk elevation. The observation that selenium is a possible risk factor contrasts with earlier summarized findings suggesting a protective effect (see ref. 147). A protective effect on prostate cancer development has been proposed for vitamin D (168). This was based on the inverse correlation between the geographic distribution of exposure to ultraviolet radiation and prostate cancer mortality in the United States (169), and on the presence of receptors for $1\alpha,25$-dihydroxyvitamin D_3 on LNCaP human prostate cancer cells and biological responsivity of these cells to this active vitamin D metabolite (170).

Dietary Fat

Earlier conclusions (147) that fat is the dietary risk factor most strongly associated with prostate cancer risk are supported by recent international correlation studies (171,172), and by case-control and cohort studies recently summarized by LaVecchia (173), Mettlin et al. (159), Nomura and Kolonel (150), and Prentice and Sheppard (172). A recent prospective study (163) and a case-control study (155) did not find a positive association between risk and fat intake, but this lack of association may be related to the populations studied, Hawaiian Japanese and Canadians in Alberta, respectively. Thus there is considerable consistency across studies for indications that fat intake is a risk factor for prostate cancer, but the strength of the associations found is not very strong, with relative risks in the range 1.5 to 2.0. Where gradients of risk in relation with fat intake have been studied, they were often reasonably monotonous and, if tested for trend, significant in some studies (156,157,174), but not in others (159,163,165). The positive association between risk and dietary fat intake appears to be limited predominantly to men who develop prostate cancer at an older age (≥ 67 to 70 years) (156,157,159,174), and to saturated or animal fat intake (156,157,159,165,174), although positive associations with risk have occasionally been observed for mono- and polyunsaturated fat and cholesterol (156,157). One of the very few studies that has attempted to estimate dietary fat intake patterns from determination of adipose tissue fatty acid composition indicated a higher intake of saturated fat and a lower intake of monounsaturated fat intake in U.S. blacks than in whites (175).

Using data from three case-control studies conducted in Hawaii, Hankin et al. (176) calculated an attributable risk of 13% for the highest saturated fat intake quartile, setting the attributable risk at 0% for the lowest quartile. The attributable risk for the highest saturated fat intake quartile was 23.9% for Caucasian Hawaiians and 8.8% for Japanese Hawaiians. Considering that fat consumption in Hawaii is slightly lower than in U.S. mainland Caucasians and African-Americans, these data suggest that as much as 25% of prostate cancer in the United States may be attributable to a high saturated fat intake. There is one animal model study that found an enhancing effect of adding 20% corn oil by weight to a natural ingredient diet (not equicaloric) on induction of prostate carcinomas in rats by testosterone (177,178). More recent studies, several of which used equicaloric, semipurified diets, did not find any effect of either amount or type of dietary fat on prostate cancer induction in rats by testosterone or a combination of chemical carcinogens and testosterone (179–182; Bosland, unpublished observations). Interestingly, linoleic acid complexed with bovine serum albumin has been shown to stimulate the *in vitro* growth of the human prostate carcinoma cell line PC-3, but not the DU-145 line, whereas omega-3 fatty acids inhibited the growth of both cell lines (183). A biological mechanism that could explain an enhancing effect of (saturated) fat on prostate carcinogenesis is not known. Several hypotheses in this regard, including hormonal mediation, have been discussed elsewhere (147,184), but the biological plausibility of fat as a risk factor of prostate cancer remains uncertain.

Vitamin A and β-Carotene

As stated earlier, epidemiologic data on the association between prostate cancer risk and dietary intake of vitamin A and/or carotenes are conflicting, as is apparent from recent reviews on this issue (147,150,159,185,186). In 4 of 16 (25%) case-control and cohort studies that studied the possible relation between prostate cancer risk and intake of carotenes and/or vitamin A, or foods rich in carotenes and/or vitamin A, negative associations were found, which were significant in three studies (159,160,162) and not in one (187). Seven (44%) of these studies reported a *positive* association that was significant in three studies (156,174,188,189), and not in four (157,163,190,191). In two studies (12%) there was no association (192[1],193). In three studies (19%) both positive and negative associations were found (166, 194[2]), or both negative and no associations occurred (165), depending on the age of the cases. The prostate is the only human cancer site for which positive associations between risk and vitamin A intake have been found in several studies. Among the studies in which a positive association between risk and dietary vitamin A intake was found, there are three case-control studies (156,157,174,189) and one prospective study (194) in which the association was only present for men that were 68 to 70 years and older at the time of diagnosis, but not for younger men. In a recent reanalysis of one of the case-control studies (156,189), the positive association appeared due entirely to the consumption of papaya, which is a major source of carotenes in Hawaii, the location of this study (195). However, it seems highly unlikely that papaya intake explains the positive associations found in studies conducted elsewhere. Therefore, one or more unmeasured factors, the intake of which correlates with that of papaya, may be responsible for this association. In a recent cohort study, a positive association between risk and β-carotene intake was only found for men that were younger than 75 years at the time of diagnosis (166).

In retrospective case-control and cohort studies of cancer risk and serum levels of vitamin A and β-carotene, either no association (196–200) or an inverse relation with prostate cancer risk was found (185,201,202), but never a positive correlation. A synthetic retinoid, N-(4-hydroxyphenyl)retinamide, when tested for its chemopreventive potential, inhibited prostate cancer induction in rats by methylnitrosourea and testosterone (203) and growth of the MLL Dunning R-3327 rat prostate adenocarcinoma subline *in vitro* and *in vivo* and human PC-3 cells (204). On the other hand, the growth of the androgen-independent DU-145 human prostate cancer cell line was stimulated by retinyl acetate added to the diet at a dose of 61,400 IU/kg diet (205). These studies require further confirmation and extension, particularly in view of the limited description of the results of the tumor induction study (203), the small number of prostate cancer cell lines tested thus far, and the lack of data concerning the effects of natural retinoids; for example, it is presently not known whether the synthetic retinoid acts via the same molecular and cellular mechanisms as natural retinoids would. Parenthetically, enhancing effects of retinoids have been reported before in experimental studies. For example, tumor promotion by retinoids, rather than inhibition, has been found in some animal models of liver and skin tumorigenesis (206,207) at dietary retinoid concentrations that were not toxic but were effectively chemopreventive in other systems, such as models of bladder and mammary cancer (208,209).

In conclusion, there is a complete lack of consistency among epidemiologic studies of prostate cancer risk and dietary vitamin A and β-carotene intake. Thus these data raise the possibility that retinoids and/or carotenes may enhance rather

---

[1] This is the most recent report of this study; earlier reports were published by Paganini-Hill et al. in 1985 (*Natl Cancer Inst Monogr* 69:133–135) and 1987 (*J Natl Cancer Inst* 79:443–448).

[2] An earlier report indicated only a protective effect of green-yellow vegetable intake (*Natl Cancer Inst Monogr* 1979;53:149–155).

than inhibit prostatic carcinogenesis under certain circumstances or in certain populations, although there is some evidence from animal and *in vitro* studies suggesting a protective effect of retinoids. There is no known mechanism by which retinoids and/or carotenoids may inhibit or enhance prostate carcinogenesis, but inhibition is biologically more plausible than enhancement, as discussed previously (147). It will be essential in future epidemiologic studies to consider separately such factors as race, genetic (familial) predisposition, and, particularly, age, since it is possible that they may, in part, determine whether retinoids and carotenes cause inhibition or enhancement of prostate carcinogenesis. The observation that papaya intake explains the positive association between risk and carotene intake found in studies conducted in Hawaii (195) raises the possibility that unmeasured other factors, correlating with papaya intake, may be involved.

Physical Activity and Anthropometric Correlates of Risk

A number of studies in the last few years have implicated the level of physical activity as a possible risk factor for prostate cancer (210–213). There are large differences in type of study, populations studied, methodology used, and index of physical activity determined between these and older studies (214–216). The results of these studies are summarized in Table 3, and they demonstrate that a possible relation between the level of physical activity and prostate cancer risk is unclear at

TABLE 3. *Summary of studies on the relation between the level of physical activity and prostate cancer risk*

Ref.	Type of study	Measure of physical activity	Association[a]
Albanes et al. (210)	Cohort (NHANES I follow-up)	Recreational activity level Nonrecreational activity level	Negative None
Brownson et al. (211)	Retrospective case control	Estimated frequency of occupational physical activity	Negative
LeMarchand et al. (212)	Case control	No. years with sedentary/light work No. years with moderate/heavy work	Negative None
Paffenbarger et al. (214)	Cohorts of:		
	Longshoremen	Estimated energy expenditure	None
	College alumni	≥ 5 h/wk of sports activity during college years	Positive
	College alumni	Physical activity index during college years	Negative[b]
Polednak (215)	Cohort of college alumni	Major athletes vs. nonathletes	Positive
Severson et al. (213)	Cohort (Hawaiian Japanese)	Physical activity index Physical activity level at home or at work	None None
Yu et al. (216)	Case control	Level of exercise activity U.S. whites U.S. blacks	 Negative None

[a] Only statistically significant positive or inverse relationships are indicated.
[b] The level of significance for this association was borderline ($0.1 > p > 0.05$).

present. In addition, unmeasured exposures related to activity on the job may be confounding factors (217).

Interestingly, sports exercise may decrease as well as increase circulating androgen concentrations or have no effect, depending on such factors as the time of blood sampling in relation to the exercise, the level of exercise, and the training protocol followed (218,219). Thus the type and extent of physical activity may influence circulating androgen concentrations and thereby, perhaps, prostate cancer risk.

Obesity was found to be a possible risk factor for prostate cancer in a previous summary of the literature (147). This association was observed in two cohort studies and one case-control study, but not in four other case-control studies (see ref. 147). A relation between prostate cancer risk and body mass index [Quetelet index: weight (kg)/height (cm)^2] was absent in all but two more recent studies in a variety of populations: four cohort studies (165,220–222) and six case-control studies (156,157,162,164,212,223). Only Yu et al. (216) found significantly elevated odds ratios for high body mass index in U.S. Caucasians, but not African-Americans, while a "dose"-response gradient was absent. Thompson et al. (167) found that prostate cancer cases had a nonsignificantly higher body mass index than that of controls ($p = 0.06$). Garfinkel (224) confirmed earlier findings (225) from a cohort study indicating that prostate cancer mortality is higher in overweight men than in men of normal weight, but they did not present statistical analysis of the data. Fincham et al. (155), on the other hand, found a significant negative relation between risk and weight ($p = 0.05$ for trend) in a Canadian Caucasian population. In conclusion, there is presently no evidence that obesity is a prostate cancer risk factor.

Severson et al. (221) observed a significant increase in prostate cancer risk with increasing upper arm circumference and (calculated) upper arm muscle area ($p = 0.026$ for trend) but not fat area; the increase in risk with increasing upper arm muscle area was not linear but reached a plateau similar to the relation between risk and upper arm circumference. This finding is at variance with findings of Denmark-Wahnefried et al. (223) that suggest a relation between prostate cancer risk and amount of upper body fat: a significant ($p = 0.0332$) positive relation between risk and the ratio of waist-to-thigh circumference. The latter group also found a significant ($p = 0.0146$) positive relation between risk and sitting-to-standing height ratio. A positive association between prostate cancer risk and muscle mass, but not fat mass, could be suggestive of exposure to endogenous or exogenous androgenic hormones or other anabolic factors (221,226). Indeed, there is evidence that body mass index correlates inversely with plasma testosterone levels and positively with estradiol-17β levels, as discussed elsewhere (147,227).

Smoking

Smoking has never been found to be associated with prostate cancer risk (see refs. 147,228). Some recent studies, however, have found a relationship between smoking and risk for prostate cancer (166,228,229). Honda et al. (229) found a relative risk of 1.9 [95% confidence interval (CI): 1.2 to 3.0] for ever versus never smoking cigarettes in a study with 216 case-control pairs. The relative risk increased with increasing duration of smoking cigarettes from nonsignificant to 1.9 (CI: 1.1 to 3.1) for 20 to 39 years of smoking and to 2.6 (CI: 1.4 to 4.9) for smoking for 40 years or longer; this trend was significant ($p=0.001$). Hsing et al. (166) studied a relatively rural cohort of men belonging to an insurance society, (17,633) 68.5% of which responded to a questionnaire about smoking habits. After a follow-up of 10 years, 149 cases of fatal prostate cancer occurred in this cohort. Significant elevated relative risks of between 1.7 and 2.9 were found for ever using tobacco, and ever smoking cigarettes, with or without smoking pipe or cigars. Men who ever used smokeless tobacco, with or without smoking, also had significantly elevated relative risks of between 2.1 and 4.5, and the relative risk increased with increasing frequency of use from nonsignificant to significant, but no statistical elevation of this trend was given. Snuff dipping and tobacco chewing were associated with the highest relative risks. Another study by Hsing et al. (228) concerned a 26-year follow-up of a cohort of 293,916 U.S. veterans, 85% (almost 250,000) of which responded to inquiries about smoking habits. Among the respondents, 4,607 prostate cancer deaths occurred. The relative risk for prostate cancer was slightly, but significantly, elevated among former cigarette smokers (1.13, CI: 1.03 to 1.24), and current smokers of any form of tobacco (1.18, CI: 1.09 to 1.28). The number of years during which cigarettes were smoked was significantly related to increased relative risk ($p<0.005$ for trend). Use of smokeless tobacco was not associated with risk in this study.

The studies by Hsing et al. (166,228) have been criticized on methodological and interpretational grounds (230,277). Furthermore, in addition to older studies that demonstrated an absence of a relation between smoking and prostate cancer risk (see refs. 147,228), no such association was found in a number of recent studies: seven case-control studies (155,157,158,162,164,216,231,232) and two cohort studies (163,233).

In summary, although there are some recent studies that indicate a possible association between smoking, and perhaps also smokeless tobacco use, and prostate cancer risk, the vast majority of studies found no such relationship, and those studies that did only found slightly elevated relative risks. However, the risk of prostate cancer as a second primary cancer is 2 and 1.5 times higher in men with lung cancer or another smoking-related cancer (pancreas, urinary bladder, upper aerodigestive tract), respectively (154), perhaps suggesting a commonality in etiology between prostate cancer and smoking-related cancers. In addition, smoking appears to have no effect on circulating levels of testosterone and other hormones that may be involved in prostate carcinogenesis (227,234).

Familial Aggregation of Risk

Prostate cancer occurs more frequently in men with a family history of prostate cancer, as summarized elsewhere (147,150). Confirming this rather consistent finding, the great majority of recent studies found excess risks of between 2- and 11-fold (155–157,229,235–237). In a case-control study of 691 prostate cancer patients, Steinberg et al. (236) observed that risk tended to increase with increasing number of affected blood relatives from twofold for men with one affected first-degree relative, to fivefold and 11-fold for those with two and three affected first-degree relatives, respectively. A further analysis of this study (238) indicated that the familial clustering of prostate cancer risk in this population was best explained by autosomal dominant inheritance of a single risk-conferring allele. In conclusion, familial aggregation of prostate cancer risk is a consistent finding across studies, and the risk for prostate cancer may increase with an increasing number of affected blood relatives. However, inherited risk for prostate cancer could only explain a small proportion of prostate cancer cases (i.e., less than 10%) (238). Although a variety of genetic alterations have been identified with varying frequency in human prostate carcinomas (summarized in refs. 239,240), none of these have thus far been linked to the inheritability of prostate cancer.

Vasectomy

Vasectomy has been identified as a possible risk factor for prostate cancer in several recent case-control studies (229,241–245) and two cohort studies (246, 247). Relative risks in the range 1.4 to 5.3 were found in the case-control studies, including several with over 200 cases, and some with over 600 cases and/or multiple control groups. Three of the studies with over 200 cases systematically investigated risk in relation to time interval between vasectomy and prostate cancer diagnosis; two of these found a significant positive trend for this interval (229,242), whereas one did not (241).

A retrospective cohort study of 13,034 vasectomized husbands of U.S. nurses with 59 cases of prostate cancer and 12,306 nonvasectomized men with 37 cases found relative risks of 1.11 (95% CI: 0.46 to 2.70), 1.26 (0.75 to 2.10), and 1.89 (1.14 to 3.14) for men vasectomized 1 to 9 years (8 cases), 10 to 19 years (24 cases), or ≥20 years earlier (27 cases), respectively (31,246). This trend of increasing risk with increasing interval since vasectomy was significant ($p = 0.03$). If cases with stage A and/or stage B prostate cancer were excluded, similar relative risks were observed. A prospective study was conducted by the same group (247) on a cohort of 47,855 health professionals, 10,055 of which had undergone vasectomy. When stage A1 cases were excluded, 225 nonvasectomized and 54 vasectomized cases were found. Relative risks of 1.23 (95% CI: 0.60 to 2.53), 1.37 (0.83 to 2.27), and 1.85 (1.26 to 2.72) were observed for men vasectomized 1 to 11 years (8 cases), 12 to 21 years (17 cases), or ≥22 years earlier (29 cases), respectively.

Risk for prostate cancer following vasectomy was not elevated in two case-control studies (220,248) and two retrospective cohort studies (249–251). The first cohort study (249) concerned 13,246 British vasectomized men with a mean follow-up of 6.6 years, and 22,196 men that did not have this procedure with a follow-up of 7.5 years. Relative risk was 0.44 (95% CI: 0.1 to 4.0), but the number of cases found (6) was very small. The most recent report of the second cohort study (251) included 135 cases in a total cohort of 5,119 vasectomized men and 15,996 nonvasectomized men followed for 6.8 years. Relative risk for prostate cancer was 1.0.

In summary, the majority of epidemiologic studies concerning vasectomy and prostate cancer have found an excess risk. There are many potential sources of bias for such studies (242,252,253). However, elevated risks were observed in several studies that carefully addressed this problem (229,241), particularly the reports by Mettlin et al. (242) and Giovanucci et al. (246,247). However, the observed associations are weak at best, and they are not found consistently (six out of eight case-control studies, and two out of four cohort studies) (253). Further studies, particularly cohort studies, will be required to further establish whether vasectomy is a true risk factor for prostate cancer (252,253).

The biological plausibility of an association between prostate cancer and vasectomy is not clear since there are no known biologic mechanisms by which vasectomy could lead to prostate cancer (253). Three potential mechanisms have been proposed: elevation of circulating androgens, immunologic mechanisms involving antisperm antibodies, and reduction of seminal fluid production (229,241,242,246, 253). Antibodies against sperm develop in approximately half of all vasectomized men (254,255), but there is to date no clear evidence suggesting that their presence plays a role in prostate cancer development (256). Vasectomy leads to a permanent reduction of seminal fluid production and prostatic secretion (257; see also ref. 246), and the resulting stagnation of secretion in the prostate has been postulated to contribute to prostatic carcinogenesis (258). However, reduction of prostatic secretion could equally well be a protective mechanism (253).

Several studies that investigated the effect of vasectomy on pituitary–gonadal function did not find any effect (258–263). For example, de la Torre et al. (259) conducted a thorough statistical analysis but did not find any systematic effects of vasectomy on peripheral levels of LH, FSH, or a large number of steroid hormones. In some other studies, however, slight, but statistically significant changes were found in circulating levels of some hormones (255,264–266). Three groups reported slightly elevated circulating testosterone levels (229,265,267), but in only one study was the increase statistically significant (265). The latter study had a larger sample size than any of the other earlier quoted studies, as well as a longer follow-up period (17% elevation, $p<0.001$, $n=229$ for 6 months; 25% elevation, $p<0.001$, $n=212$ for 1 year; 43% elevation, $p<0.001$, $n=152$ for 2 years; 14% elevation, $p>0.05$, $n=59$ for 3 years). Only the study by Honda et al. (229) concerned a longer interval between vasectomy and blood sampling (17.7 ± 8.3 years; mean $\pm$ SD of 30 vasectomized men and 30 controls). Serum testosterone levels were 6.7% increased in the vasectomized group ($p=0.056$, one-sided; repeated measures analysis of covariance). The binding capacity of testosterone binding globulin was not influenced, but the ratio of testosterone to testosterone binding globulin binding capacity was significantly increased by 13.6% after vasectomy ($p=0.029$). These data from the only study that attempted to estimate unbound testosterone suggest that elevation of free circulating testosterone following vasectomy might be a critical factor associated with prostate cancer risk. A possible mechanism whereby vasectomy could influence the hypothalamic–pituitary–gonadal axis is not known.

Prostatitis and Benign Prostatic Hypertrophy

Two recent case-control studies found significantly elevated relative risks for a history of prostatitis or prostatitis plus benign prostatic hypertrophy (BPH) [i.e., 2.2 (95% confidence interval: 1.2 to 4.3) and 1.57 (95% CI: 1.14 to 2.15; $p = 0.004$), respectively] (165,229). These results are in agreement with observations from some earlier, not convincing, case-control studies (see ref. 147), but not with a case-control study by Ross et al. (220). The evidence for an association between prostate cancer risk and the prior occurrence of BPH was previously deemed inconclusive and biologically unlikely (147). The observation of a relative risk of 3.6 (95% CI: 2.0 to 7.1) for BPH in a recent case-control study (229) provides more support for a possible association. Other studies reported a nonsignificant higher frequency of BPH in prostate cancer cases than controls (156) and a significantly increased relative risk for BPH plus prostatitis in cases (165). Additional support for such an association is derived from recent data indicating that prostate carcinoma develops not only in the peripheral zone of the prostate, but also from the transition zone, which is the predominant site of origin of BPH (268).

Venereal Disease

A history of venereal disease was previously found to be a consistent risk factor across studies, except in Japan (147). Three case-control studies in the United States have confirmed the association between venereal disease and prostate cancer risk (162,229,269). Mandel and Schuman (269) found odds ratios of between 1.90 (95% CI: 1.30 to 2.47) and 2.71 (95% CI: 1.14 to 6.46) for a history of venereal disease, whereas Honda et al. (229) reported a nonsignificant elevation of relative risk (1.5; 95% CI: 0.8 to 2.7). Ross et al. (162) found that risk was significantly elevated in both black and white men with a history of venereal disease: In the black population (179 case-neighborhood control pairs of available incident cases of prostate cancer diagnosed from January 1977 to August 1980 in Los Angeles County black residents between the ages of 60 and 75) 49% of cases and 37% of controls had a history of venereal disease; the matched relative risk was 1.7 ($p = 0.03$). Eleven percent of cases and 5% of controls in the white population (142 case-control pairs of all available incident cases of prostate cancer diagnosed from January 1977 to August 1980 in a Los Angeles area, all white, retirement community) reported a history of venereal disease; the matched relative risk was 2.3 ($p = 0.07$). Thus the prevalence of a venereal disease history was considerably higher in the African-American group than in the Caucasians, but there were major socioeconomic differences between these two populations. The lack of association between venereal disease and prostate cancer risk in Japan has been confirmed in two recent case-control studies (232,270). There was also no such association in Dutch men (270). Nevertheless, most studies, and all studies in U.S. populations, found a history of venereal disease to be positively associated with prostate cancer risk.

Marital Status and Sexual Factors

A previous summary of the literature (147) revealed that in comparison with married men, single men had in general a lower risk, and widowed or divorced men a higher risk, except in African-American men, where single men had the highest risk. Newell et al. (271), using U.S. SEER data on 48,106 men with prostate cancer, reported that married Caucasian and Hispanic men had a higher prostate cancer risk than that of separated and divorced men and to a lesser extent, widowed men, regardless of age. They confirmed, however, the earlier data that African-American single men have the highest risk. Yu et al. (216) found a significantly lower risk in single than in married U.S. black men, but their results were based on very few cases. Other recent studies found no clear relation between prostate cancer risk and marital status in Japanese and Dutch men (270), and a significantly higher risk in single than in married Caucasian men in Canada (155). In conclusion, with the exception of the high risk in single African-American men, there appears no consistent, clear association between marital status and prostate cancer risk.

A variety of recent studies have addressed the possible role of sexual factors in prostate cancer etiology (155,162,229,269,270). The results of these studies in general support earlier conclusions (147) that prostate cancer risk appears related with (1) an early age of onset of sexual activity; (2) high sexual drive, particularly at a young age; and (3) a low frequency of intercourse, especially in old age, or a high frequency of intercourse up to 50 years of age and a low frequency thereafter. Mandel and Schuman (269) found significantly lower risk for prostate cancer (odds ratios were 0.54 and 0.68 for hospital and neighborhood controls, respectively) for a high estimated total lifetime frequency of intercourse (>3000 for all ages combined), but multiple logistic regression analysis did not substantiate this finding (odds ratio = 0.92; 95% CI: 0.82 to 2.06). They also found elevated risk for a history of homosexual partners (odds ratio = 2.33; 95% CI: 0.90 to 6.07), and for the number of homosexual partners (odds ratio = 3.71; 95% CI: 1.35 to 10.18; multiple logistic regression analysis). In addition, they found a significantly less frequent history of problems with erection in prostate cancer patients than in controls (odds ratios 0.53 and 0.76 for hospital and neighborhood controls, respectively). Yoshida et al. (270) found a significantly elevated relative risks (3.17 to 6.16) for a perceived low quality of sex life or sexual excitement in Japanese, but not Dutch men. In contrast to the results of Mandel and Schuman (269), Ross et al. (162) compared African-American and U.S. Caucasian men and found that in the former population, but not the latter, frequency of intercourse was higher in cases than in controls, which was significant only for men diagnosed at 60 years of age and older. None of a number of other factors related to sexual activity was associated with prostate cancer risk in the recent studies quoted.

Interestingly, Tsitouras et al. (272) observed a significant positive association between the level of sexual activity (intercourse and masturbation) and circulating total testosterone in men between the ages of 60 and 79, in the absence of a decrease in testosterone levels with aging. These data suggest a possible hormonal mechanism underlying the earlier quoted associations between prostate cancer risk and frequency of intercourse observed in case-control studies.

Hormones

A causal relation between androgens and prostate carcinoma development in human and animal models is biologically plausible (see ref. 147). There are, indeed, a few case reports of prostate cancer in men in which androgenic steroids were used as anabolic agents or for medical purposes (273–276). On the other hand, prostate cancer appears to occur in castrated dogs and may even be more prevalent in those animals than in intact dogs (278). Endocrine studies comparing human prostate cancer patients with control subjects are not very appropriate for exploring this relationship for two reasons: The presence of a prostate carcinoma may interfere with the subject's endocrine status; and it is probable that the hormonal status of patients does not reflect very well their exposure to (endogenous) androgens earlier in life, which may be more relevant as risk determinant. These studies will therefore not be discussed here. A number of studies compared healthy males in populations that are at high risk for prostate cancer with populations at lower risk. These studies are summarized in the following.

Ross et al. (279) compared 50 healthy young African-American men (very high-risk group) and 50 young Caucasian males (at half the risk of the black men) in the Los Angeles area. They found that total circulating testosterone was 19% higher and free testosterone 21% higher in the black group than in the whites ($p=0.02$; two-sided t-test). Serum estrone concentrations were also higher (16%) in the blacks than in the white group ($p=0.05$). There were no significant differences between the groups in circulating estradiol-17β (estradiol) and sex hormone–binding globulin (SHBG) levels. Ross et al. (279) contend that the observed 19% to 21% difference in circulating testosterone is sufficiently large to explain the twofold difference in prostate cancer risk between U.S. white and black men. In a recent repeat analysis of the same serum samples (280), the difference in circulating testosterone was 11%, which was statistically significant ($p=0.018$); SHBG was also again somewhat higher (9%); estrogens were not measured. These findings suggest an association between prostate cancer risk and high concentrations of circulating androgens and, perhaps, estrogens.

Circulating hormone levels in 20 pregnant African-American and 20 white women in their first trimester were compared by Henderson et al. (112). Serum testosterone levels were 47% higher in black than in white women ($p=0.0009$; two-sided paired t-test), and estradiol levels were 37% higher ($p=0.09$). There were no differences in circulating SHBG and human chorionic gonadotrophin, or in relevant pregnancy characteristics, including the sex ratio of the offspring. Adjustment for the sex of the offspring did not influence the hormonal differences between black and white women. These findings indicate that U.S. black males are exposed to higher androgen concentrations than are white men, even before birth.

In their more recent study, Ross et al. (280) also compared U.S. black and white men with 54 Japanese men of the same age (mean age: 19 to 23 years). The Japanese men had serum testosterone levels that were not lower than, but intermediate between, those of U.S. whites and blacks, whereas their SHBG levels were significantly lower. This suggests a higher percentage of free testosterone in the Japanese (low risk) than in the U.S. men (high risk). In comparison with the Japanese, the U.S. groups had significantly higher ($p<0.05$; two-sided t-test) serum concentrations of the conjugated testosterone metabolites androsterone glucuronide (41% to 50% higher) and $3\alpha,17\beta$-androstanediol glucuronide (25% to 31% higher). This suggests that in comparison with the high-risk U.S. groups, the low-risk Japanese population has a lower testosterone metabolism, probably a lower activity of the enzyme 5α-reductase that converts testosterone to 5α-dihydrotestosterone (DHT).

A similar observation was made by Lookingbill et al. (281) comparing 53 normal healthy U.S. Caucasians and 57 Chinese males in Hong Kong between the ages (mean age) of 24 and 26 years. In comparison with the Chinese men, the Caucasians had considerably higher ($p<0.001$) serum levels of androsterone glucuronide (67% higher) and $3\alpha,17\beta$-androstanediol glucuronide (76% higher). There was no significant difference in circulating testosterone, free testosterone, or DHT, but Caucasian men had higher ($p<0.001$) serum levels of the androgen precursors dehydroepiandrosterone sulfate (46%) and androstenedione (32%). These data were interpreted to indicate a higher 5α-reductase activity in the high-risk Caucasians than in the low-risk Chinese men, and additionally, an increased production of androgen precursors in the Caucasians.

In contrast to the observations of Ross et al. (279,280) and those of Lookingbill et al. (281), de Jong and co-workers (282) found higher (17%; $p<0.05$) circulating total testosterone levels in 123 high-risk Caucasian men (Dutch) than in a low-risk Asian population (91 Japanese men). The subjects in these studies were considerably older than those studied by the two other groups, namely 50 to 79 years (mean age: 63 to 70 years). DHT levels were not different, but the ratio of DHT to testosterone was 10% lower ($p<0.05$) in the Dutch than in the Japanese men, perhaps reflecting lower 5α-reductase activity, at least peripherally, in the Dutch than the Japanese; no data were collected on androgen metabolites. Serum levels of estradiol were significantly higher (15%) in the Dutch than the Japanese men. SHBG levels were comparable, while the ratio of testosterone to SHBG concentrations was 34% higher in Dutch than Japanese men ($p<0.001$), suggesting higher amounts of free testosterone (which was not measured separately) in the high-risk Dutch.

Nomura and colleagues (283) compared 98 prostate cancer cases with matched controls from a cohort of 6,860 Hawaiian Japanese men followed for an average of 14 years. There were no differences between cases and controls in serum levels of testosterone, DHT, estrone, estradiol, and SHBG measured once at the start of the cohort study (free testosterone levels were not determined). The serum hormone concentrations were divided into tertiles, and relative risks were calculated. An elevation in relative risk was observed only for an increasing ratio of testosterone to DHT, which was borderline significant ($p=0.06$ for trend; conditional logistic regression analysis). When the interval between blood collection and the diagnosis of prostate cancer was taken into account, the elevation in risk for this ratio appeared to be confined to an interval of 5.5 years or less. This was probably due to a significant ($p = 0.03$) decrease in risk with increasing serum DHT concentration that occurred only during that interval. These data may suggest an inverse relation between (peripheral) 5α-reductase activity and prostate cancer risk.

Barrett-Connor et al. (222) followed a cohort of 1,008 white upper-middle-class men between the ages of 40 and 79 for a period of 14 years, during which 57 prostate cancer cases occurred, 26 deaths, and 31 incident cases. There was no relation between risk for prostate cancer and baseline serum concentrations of testosterone, estrone, and SHBG. However, relative risk increased linearly with increasing serum level of androstenedione, a testosterone precursor, from 1.00 in the lowest tertile to 1.38 in the highest tertile, after adjustment for age and body mass index ($p<0.05$ for trend). Relative risk also increased linearly with increasing serum level of estradiol, but this was not statistically significant ($p = 0.11$ for trend).

Older studies by Hill and co-workers, which were previously summarized and discussed (147), compared the endocrine status of healthy U.S. black and white men, 12 to 15 or 40 to 55 years of age, and endocrine patterns in 40- to 55-year-old U.S. black and white men with those of age-matched South African black men. The endocrine differences between the very high-risk U.S. black and high-risk U.S. white men were not consistent in the two age groups, and they were not similar to the differences observed between the high-risk U.S. populations and the low-risk South African black men. These inconsistencies raise the possibility that the factors and endocrine mechanisms that determine the difference in risk between African black men and African-Americans are dissimilar to those that determine the risk difference between white and black Americans (147).

Taken together, the results of the above-summarized studies do not provide unequivocal evidence for any particular association between circulating levels of hormones and prostate cancer risk. In interpreting these observations, one should bear several points in mind: Young Japanese and Chinese from Hong Kong, who are likely to be at least partially Westernized in their lifestyle (153), cannot simply be compared with older Asian men; young men that are hormonally studied today may have a prostate cancer risk that is different than the currently recorded risk in older men of the same population (e.g., prostate cancer rates are rising in Japan) (153); the causes of the white–black difference in prostate cancer risk in the United States may be different from those that determine prostate cancer risk differences between Asian or African populations and Western countries; and most important, circulating hormone levels provide very little information about concentrations at the molecular targets of these hormones in the prostate gland.

Nevertheless, four hypotheses seem to emerge supported by data from some of the studies summarized above. Prostate cancer risk may be positively associated with (a) bioavailable testosterone serum levels as indicated by studies comparing healthy low- and high-risk men (279,280,282); (b) serum levels of androgen precursors as indicated by a cohort study and a study comparing healthy Chinese and U.S.

Caucasian men (222,281); (c) peripheral and/or prostatic activity of 5α-reductase (280,281); and (4) serum levels of estrogens as indicated by studies comparing healthy low- and high-risk men (279,282; Hill et al., see ref. 147). However, there are some contradictory data for each of these three hypotheses (222,279,281–283; Hill et al., see ref. 147). The risk-increasing effects of elevated circulating levels of androgens and estrogens may act early in life (279–281) or even before birth (112), rather than in the 10 to 30 years preceding the diagnosis of prostate cancer.

Two of the four hypotheses implicate higher bioavailable circulating androgen levels in high-risk men in comparison with low-risk populations. However, this may not be universally true in all high-risk populations. Meikle and co-workers (284,285) found that circulating levels of testosterone and DHT were significantly lower in blood relatives of prostate cancer patients, brothers (age 47 to 75) and sons (age 22 to 43), who have a three- to fourfold excess risk, than in unrelated control subjects of the same age ranges. Zumoff et al. (286) observed that circulating concentrations of testosterone, but not DHT, in prostate cancer patients were markedly lower in those younger than 65 years than in those 65 years and older; control subjects had testosterone levels that were similar to those of prostate cancer patients of 65 years and older. These data indicate the possibility that the role of androgens in prostatic carcinogenesis is different depending on age, and different in men who are at high risk because of familial predisposition and those at high risk for ethnic or other (environmental) reasons.

Occupation

An in-depth review of some of the current literature on occupational factors and prostate cancer risk was recently presented by van der Gulden and co-workers (151). Their findings confirm one of the conclusions of an earlier literature review on this subject (147): Although several studies have observed increased risk for a variety of occupations (some recent studies: 151,155,212,231,232,270,288,289), this is consistently found for only a few occupational categories, among them farmers and farm workers. Other conclusions of the earlier literature review (147) were that (a) armed services personnel are consistently at increased risk, (b) the evidence for an association between cadmium exposure and prostate cancer risk is at best very weak, and (c) an association between exposures in the rubber industry and prostate cancer risk is limited to one or a few plants. There are no new studies concerning armed services personnel. The one new study concerning rubber industry workers found, if anything, a lower-than-expected risk for prostate cancer in these workers (290). On the other hand, there are two studies that found higher-than-expected rates of prostate cancer among workers exposed to acrylonitrile in textile fiber production plants (291,292). Rates were highest in workers exposed to the highest levels and with the longest period between onset of exposure and cancer diagnosis. These studies were, however, based on only a few cases (4–6), but exposure to dimethylformamide, a possible confounder in these workers, does not appear to be associated with prostate cancer risk (293). Recent studies about risk in farmers or farm workers and in cadmium-exposed populations is summarized in the following sections. In addition, recent data concerning the earlier observed (see ref. 147) relation between ionizing radiation exposure and prostate cancer risk are discussed. A possible elevated prostate cancer risk in mechanics, repairmen, and machine operators, a very diverse group of occupations with a large range of potential exposures to carcinogenic agents, is discussed by van der Gulden et al. (151).

Farming

Farmers and farm workers were found to have a slightly increased risk for prostate cancer in many, but not all studies (see refs. 147,151,294,295). Van der Gulden et al. (151) listed 14 incidence studies and 17 mortality studies relevant to this subject. Prostate cancer risk was significantly higher than expected in three of the incidence studies (21%) and six of the mortality studies (35%). The measure of prostate cancer risk (PIR, SIR, odds ratio, SMR, or PMR) was equal or higher than 1.10 in 9 of the incidence studies (64%) and 10 of the mortality studies (58%). Several of these studies were included in a meta-analysis on 22 mortality and incidence studies conducted by Blair et al. (294). A significantly elevated meta-relative risk of 1.08 was calculated, with a 95% confidence interval of 1.06 to 1.11 for a range of relative risks from 0.9 to 2.7. From recent epidemiologic studies in farmers, Burmeister (296) and Fincham et al. (297) reported additional data indicating increased prostate cancer risk, whereas Stark et al. (298), Ronco et al. (299), and Gunnarsdottir and Rafnsson (300) found no significantly elevated risk. From these studies and those summarized by Blair et al. (294) and van der Gulden et al. (151), it appears that there is weak to inconclusive evidence for a positive association between farming and prostate cancer risk.

Revelant to this subject are recent conclusions that there is no association between prostate cancer risk and occupational exposure to insecticides or pesticides (301) or to herbicides (302). Van der Gulden et al. (151), Morrison et al. (302), and Pearce and Reif (295) list a number of studies showing excess risk for prostate cancer in populations exposed to pesticides, herbicides, and/or fertilizers, as well as several studies in which no such association was found; this is consistent with the aforementioned weak-to-inconclusive association between farming and prostate cancer risk.

Cadmium Exposure

The literature on cadmium exposure and prostate cancer risk has recently been summarized by Waalkes and Oberdörster (102) and by Boffetta (303), who confirm earlier conclusions that there is very little if any evidence that cadmium exposure is associated with elevation of prostate cancer risk (147,304). In none of the few more recent studies (212,305,306) were elevated risks for prostate cancer observed in (potentially) cadmium-exposed groups. On the other hand, a high incidence of prostate cancer has recently been found to correlate with high cadmium levels in groundwater available for drinking purposes (307). This is in contrast with an earlier found absence of a correlation between prostate cancer risk and cadmium levels in drinking water (see ref. 147), but in line with a positive correlation observed for cadmium levels in food products (157; see also ref. 147).

Radiation

A number of previously summarized (147) reports suggest that exposure to ionizing radiation increases risk for prostate cancer in workers in the nuclear industry, and that prostate cancer risk in survivors of the 1945 atomic bomb explosions in Japan may also be elevated. An additional study of nuclear industry workers confirms this, but the elevation in risk was not significant (308). However, the most recent update on cancer risk among 76,000 survivors of the 1945 atomic bomb explosions in Japan, including revised estimates of radiation dose received, indicates that prostate cancer risk is not elevated in this population (309,310). Interestingly, a strong international correlation between prostate cancer incidence and indoor radon levels in 14 countries ($r = 0.72$, $p < 0.01$) has recently been reported (311). Some of these recent studies provide some additional support for the earlier found (147) association between prostate cancer risk and exposure to ionizing radiation, but the current evidence for this is equivocal.

Socioeconomic Status

Recent studies in a variety of countries about the relation between socioeconomic status (SES; measured as level of education, income, or occupation/socioeconomic class) and prostate cancer risk largely confirm an earlier conclusion (147) that some studies find an increasing risk with higher SES (216,248,289), whereas in others a decreasing risk with higher SES (155,165) or no association with SES was observed (164,213,231,269,270). The black–white difference in prostate cancer risk in the United States does not appear to be related to differences in SES as measured by percent of the population living below the poverty level (312). However, overall mortality, which is also higher in African-American men than in U.S. Caucasians, is similar in both groups after controlling for SES (313).

Conclusions

There are few risk factors for prostate cancer that have consistently been found in epidemiologic studies. These are summarized in Table 4. They are similar to those previously identified (147), with the following exceptions: There is to date no credible evidence that exposures to ionizing radiation or specific chemicals are risk

TABLE 4. Summary of risk factors for prostate cancer derived from epidemiologic studies

Risk factor	Association Strength (risk increase)	Consistency	Mechanism (plausibility)
Western lifestyle	5- to 10-fold (American vs. Asiatic lifestyles)	Very high	Environmental (dietary) causes suspected
Prostate cancer in blood relatives	3- to 4-fold (vs. no family history)	High	Possibly single dominant autosomal risk-conferring allele responsible
High bioavailable plasma or prostatic androgen levels	2-fold (U.S. blacks vs. whites) to 10-fold (Asian vs. American men)	Not conclusive[a]	High biological plausibility
African-American descent[b]	2-fold (vs. U.S. Caucasians)	Very high	Unknown
Western dietary habits, particularly high fat intake	1.25- to 2-fold (high vs. low fat intake in the U.S.)	High	Unknown
History of venereal disease	1.5- to 2-fold (vs. no history of venereal disease)	High	Unknown
Employment in the armed services	2- to 3-fold (vs. no armed forces employment)	High but limited to few studies	Unknown
Vasectomy	No or 1.2- to 1.9-fold (vs. no vasectomy)	Weak	Unknown
Farm work (farmer or farm worker)	No or 1.1- to 2-fold (vs. no involvement in farming)	Weak to inconclusive	Unknown (no clear relation with exposure to agricultural chemicals)
Prostatitis	No or 1.5- to 2-fold (vs. no history of prostatitis)	Weak to inconclusive	Unknown

[a]Animal studies strongly corroborate this association.
[b]African-American men have the highest risk in the world for prostate cancer.

factors for prostate cancer (151). Obesity is also not a risk factor, but there are some indications that muscle mass is positively correlated with risk, perhaps reflecting exposure to endogenous androgens or anabolic steroids (221).

The single most important combination of risk factors is to be black and residing in the United States. Whereas genetic factors are highly unlikely to be involved, environmental exposures (in the broadest sense of the term) are most probably responsible for this as discussed in depth previously (147). African-Americans are, as most U.S. populations, genetically a very heterogeneous "ethnic" group, because of interracial reproductive patterns. Yet, as a group, their risk is twice that of white Americans. The lack of an association between risk and SES, on the other hand, argues against a role of environmental factors. However, current SES, particular income or occupation, does not well reflect SES in the past, which may be more relevant. Moreover, most studies on SES and cancer occurrence have used census tract or similar data, and they have, therefore, little power in detecting individual differences. To date there are no definite reasons known for the black–white disparity in prostate cancer rates in the United States, but a relation with similar racial disparities in exposure to potential carcinogens and high-risk dietary habits has been proposed (147).

The strongest single risk factor is a Western lifestyle, including Western dietary habits. It is conceivable that this risk factor exerts its risk-enhancing effects mediated by a hormonal mechanism involving androgens (147). Elevation of bioavailable and bioactive androgens in the circulation or the target tissue may be an important risk factor, and this would be biologically very plausible. The results of several animal model studies support this contention. However, more research is needed to confirm and further define this association and to establish its underlying biological mechanisms.

Familial aggregation of prostate cancer risk is very consistently observed and confers a considerable (three- to fourfold or more) increase in risk. However, it explains fewer than 10% of all cases. Other possible risk factors listed in Table 4 are, if anything, weak and/or not very consistently observed, and they lack biological plausibility.

In conclusion, with the exception of exposure to a Western lifestyle, venereal disease, and perhaps, to androgenic hormones, there are no known specific chemical or other exposures that are associated with prostate cancer risk. This lack of risk-enhancing exposures is remarkable in view of the high frequency of this malignancy in Western countries. The following hypotheses can be suggested: (a) The factor(s) responsible for a high risk of clinically evident prostate cancer is (are) very ubiquitously present in Western countries, but not at all in, for example, Asian countries; (b) there are a large number of different prostate cancer–causing factors, probably present in different combinations throughout the world, that require an appropriately conducive setting (i.e., a Western lifestyle environment), to produce clinical prostate cancer; and (c) a combination of these two hypotheses, in which the ubiquitously present risk factor in (a) is the Western lifestyle environment in (b).

The last hypothesis is fully consistent with the observation that early prostate cancer that is not clinically evident (so-called "latent" cancer) occurs at similar rates throughout the world, whereas there are large geographic differences in the frequency of clinically evident prostate cancer (see refs. 147,314). This implies that exposure to a Western lifestyle causes or enhances progression from latent to clinically evident cancer by an unknown, perhaps hormonal mechanism that permits required additional genetic alterations to occur in the target cells (314). The existence of a large number of different prostate cancer–causing factors could explain why no specific exposures have been found to be related to prostate cancer risk. This could also contribute to the very high frequency of latent prostate cancer in aging men throughout the world (see ref. 147). Alternatively, the aging process itself (e.g., accumulating oxidative DNA damage) may specifically affect the human prostate. However, the earlier mentioned divergent data on diet and prostate cancer risk in men of different ages, and on hormonal patterns in men with and without a family history of prostate cancer, suggest that the prostate cancer–causing factors and prostate cancer risk-enhancing settings may differ for men who develop clinically evident prostate cancer at a younger or at an older age, and for men who develop prostate cancer because of genetic predisposition and men with prostate cancer who are not genetically predisposed (see ref. 147).

Induction of Prostate Tumors in Experimental Animals

Unlike the human or canine prostate, the rodent prostate consists of distinct paired lobes: the ventral, dorsal, lateral, and anterior lobes; the dorsal and lateral lobes are frequently referred to as the *dorsolateral prostate*; and the anterior lobe is more commonly termed the *coagulating gland*. In the human and canine prostate, these lobes have merged into one gland, in which different zones have been defined (268). A homolog of the rodent ventral lobe is not present in the human gland (315). The various lobes of the rat prostate differ in their propensity to develop prostate carcinomas, either spontaneously or induced by carcinogens or hormones (316). However, the exact lobe location of prostate tumors has often not been reported accurately in the literature. Spontaneously occurring prostate tumors are rare in most species (4,5,315), with the exception of the dog and, particularly, humans. It is not clear why prostate cancer is so common in men, whereas it very rare in almost all other species.

There are two rat strains in which prostate carcinomas are more or less common. In inbred rats from the ACI/Seg subline of the ACI strain the incidence of (non-metastasizing) carcinomas of the ventral prostate is 35% to 50% at 30 months of age, while almost every rat has carcinoma precursor lesions, atypical hyperplasia, in their prostate at that time (317,318). At 36 months of age approximately 20% of ACI/Seg rats have grossly manifest prostate carcinomas. The exact mechanism of prostate carcinoma development in the ACI/Seg rat is not known, but some genetically determined factor(s) appear(s) to be involved since the parent ACI strain does not develop prostate cancer (319). Metastasizing adenocarcinomas, allegedly developing in or from the area of the dorsolateral prostate, have been reported in the Lobund Wistar rat; a 10% incidence in germ-free rats of this strain and approximately 25% in non–germ free rats (320,321).

Induction of Prostate Tumors by Carcinogenic Agents

Prostatic neoplasms have not been found to be induced in carcinogenicity bioassays (1,2,108). The only reports of induction of such tumors are from experimental studies on prostatic carcinogenesis and the effects of perinatal and adult treatment with hormones.

Organic Chemical Carcinogens

Direct application of chemical carcinogens to prostate tissue in experimental animals can produce sarcomas or squamous cell carcinomas (see refs. 4,322). Induction of prostate tumors by chemical carcinogens administered systemically or via the oral or inhalation routes is very rare; in fact, there are only two carcinogens that, without any additional concomitant or subsequent treatment, induce prostate tumors, both upon systemic administration, N-nitrosobis(oxopropyl)amine (BOP) and 3,2'-dimethyl-4-aminobiphenyl (DMAB). Pollard and co-workers (323,324) reported induction of prostate carcinomas in 2/20 (10%) and 4/20 (20%) of Lobund Wistar rats given a single i.v. injection of N-methyl-N-nitrosourea (MNU), but this was not confirmed by Hoover et al. (325) in a group of 45 rats of the same strain.

Weekly gavage administration of 10 mg/kg BOP to MRC rats resulted in a 33% incidence of squamous cell carcinomas in the ventral prostate with an average latency of 50 weeks (326). In this study there was a high incidence of atypical glandular hyperplasia that seemed to progress to a squamous differentiation. Administration for no longer than 20 weeks did not produce prostate tumors, and subcutaneous administration was less effective than intragastric treatment (326,327).

Katayama et al. (328) first reported induction of epithelial proliferative lesions of the F344 rat prostate by 20 or 50 mg/kg DMAB for 37 or 20 weeks. This was subsequently confirmed by Shirai and co-workers (329). The induced lesions, referred to as carcinomas *in situ*, were noninvasive atypical epithelial proliferations confined to one or a few adjacent alveoli, and they occurred exclusively in the ventral prostate (328,329). The highest reported incidence was 32% (328). One invasive adenocarcinoma apparently originating from the dorsolateral lobe was found in one of 293 DMAB-exposed rats (0.34%) by Katayama et al. (328). It is not clear whether this tumor was induced or, in fact, occurred spontaneously.

The age at which DMAB is administered did not influence its prostatic carcinogenicity since similar *in situ* carcinoma responses were obtained in rats aged 5, 35, or 65 weeks (330). However, there are important strain differences in the carcinogenic potential of DMAB for the rat prostate, the F344 and ACI/N strains being very susceptible, and the LEW, Sprague–Dawley, and Wistar strains developing few or no *in situ* prostate carcinomas (331). No such strain differences were, however, found in the formation of DMAB-DNA adducts (331). Administration of the N-hydroxy metabolite of DMAB to F344 rats at a weekly dose of 5 mg/kg for 20 weeks produced a 42% incidence of *in situ* carcinoma and atypical hyperplasia in 84% of the animals in one experiment; Wistar rats did not develop *in situ* carcinomas (332). In a subsequent experiment the same treatment did not produce *in situ* carcinomas, and only 46% hyperplasia; a dose of 20 mg/kg, however, produced *in situ* carcinomas in 67% of animals and hyperplasia in 100% (333). Notwithstanding this inconsistency (perhaps due to instability of the carcinogen), these data indicate that N-hydroxy-DMAB is more carcinogenic for the rat prostate than DMAB itself, DMAB at a dose of 25 mg/kg resulting in incidences of 25% for *in situ* carcinomas and 50% for atypical hyperplasia (333).

Cadmium

Very little evidence of carcinogenicity of cadmium for the rodent prostate was found in a previous review of the literature (147). More recently, Waalkes and co-workers (89,90) have documented that a single injection of cadmium chloride in rats produces *in situ* carcinomas in the ventral prostate when cadmium-induced testicular toxicity is avoided, either by lowering the cadmium dose to under 5 mg/kg, by administering cadmium intramuscularly rather than subcutaneously, or by antagonizing cadmium by simultaneous administration of a sufficient amount of zinc. The incidence of these noninvasive, intraalveolar lesions was at best between 30% and 40%. Oral cadmium exposure also resulted in such *in situ* lesions, but relatively few of these lesions (in less than 10% of the animals) qualified as adenoma (334), and no invasive carcinomas have been found in any of these studies (89,90,334). No proliferative lesions were found in other parts of the rat prostate than the ventral lobe. These data indicate that only when testicular function, most likely testosterone production, is intact, cadmium induces proliferative lesions in the rat ventral prostate. Interestingly, cadmium has been shown to be capable of producing *in vitro* transformation of rat ventral prostate epithelial cells (335). These transformed cells develop into squamous cell carcinomas, but not adenocarcinomas, when injected in syngeneic rats (336).

Ionizing Radiation

Local exposure to x-rays of the pelvic area has been shown to produce prostate carcinomas in rodents. Eight 1,000-rad exposures at different intervals induced a 3.7% incidence of prostate carcinomas in ICR/JCL mice; at least some of these tumors occurred in the ventral prostate (337). Five exposures to 1,000 rad of Sprague–Dawley rats only produced prostate carcinomas, in a 33% incidence, when the animals were castrated and received androgen replacement prior to irradiation (338). Intact and only castrated rats did not develop prostate carcinomas following irradiation, indicating that testosterone treatment may be required for tumor development. Whole-body x-irradiation at a single dose of 1,000 rad of NEDH rats parabiosed to not-irradiated male partners produced prostate carcinomas in 2.2% of animals (339). The incidence of prostate carcinomas in nonirradiated partners and parabiosed controls was 0.2% to 0.3%. These studies indicate that x-irradiation can produce prostate cancer in rodents, providing support for the epidemiologic indications for an association between exposure to ionizing radiation and prostate cancer risk.

Induction of Prostate Tumors by Stimulation of Cell Proliferation and Exposure to Chemical Carcinogens

Stimulation of cell proliferation in the prostate at the time of carcinogen administration has been shown to be an effective way to increase the sensitivity of the target tissue for tumor induction. Several chemical carcinogens that do not induce prostate carcinomas when administered alone have been shown to produce these tumors in a low incidence (5% to 25%) following stimulation of prostatic cell proliferation. This has been demonstrated for a single-dose administration of the indirect-acting carcinogens DMAB and 9,12-dimethylbenz[a]anthracene, and the direct-acting MNU (340–342). Furthermore, treatments that stimulate prostatic cell proliferation have been shown to enhance the carcinogenic potential of DMAB markedly (343,344). However, other studies found only a very small or no enhancing effect of stimulation of prostatic cell proliferation on prostate carcinoma induction by MNU (182,345,346) and BOP (327). The site of carcinoma formation within the prostate was the ventral lobe for the DMAB studies of Shirai et al. (343) and Ito et al. (344), and the dorsolateral prostate and coagulating gland for the experiments with MNU, DMAB, and 9,12-dimethylbenz[a]anthracene conducted by Bosland et al. (340–342).

Induction of Prostate Tumors by Hormones

Testosterone

Chronic administration of testosterone has been shown to induce a low-to-moderate (5% to 56%) incidence of prostate carcinomas in several rat strains, the Wistar WU, Wistar MRC, Lobund Wistar, and NBL strain (177,178,239,325,327,347,348), but not in the F344 strain (349). In all studies the carcinomas seemed to develop from the dorsolateral prostate and/or coagulating gland, but not the ventral prostate (177,178,239,325,327,347,348), and these tumors were adenocarcinomas in all studies, but one in which some squamous cell carcinomas were also observed (327). The prostate carcinoma incidence in most of these studies was low (i.e., between 5% and 20%) (239,325,327,347). Only in the studies by Pollard and co-workers with the Lobund Wistar strain were higher carcinoma incidences sometimes found, but the reported incidences varied considerably from 0% (178) to 16% (324), to 35% to 40% (177,350) to 56% to 60% (323,348). The only other study with the Lobund Wistar strain found a 7% incidence (325). The dose of testosterone fluctuated considerably over time in many of these studies, from 5 to 10 times control values down to control values (325), but even when circulating testosterone was steadily elevated by only two- to threefold, prostate carcinomas were induced (351). In conclusion, testosterone is a weak complete carcinogen for the rat prostate (352).

Estrogens and Testosterone

Noble, in pioneering studies summarized in 1982 (347), first established that testosterone is carcinogenic for the rat prostate, and that sequential treatment with testosterone and estradiol-17β was even more effective, resulting in a 50% prostate carcinoma incidence in the NBL rat strain that he developed. In a modification of Noble's protocol, Drago (353) demonstrated that combined long-term treatment with testosterone and estradiol-17β produced prostate carcinomas, which was confirmed by Leav et al. (354). It was shown subsequently that this combined treatment of NBL rats leads to a 100% incidence of adenocarcinomas that appeared to develop from the periurethral ducts of the dorsolateral and anterior prostate and were of microscopic size and therefore easily missed if the periurethral portion of the prostate is not examined histologically (239,355). The development of these tumors is preceded by the appearance of epithelial dysplasia in the ducts and acini of the dorsolateral prostate in 100% of treated animals (354,356). When estradiol-17β was replaced by diethylstilbestrol (DES), combined treatment with testosterone resulted in widespread dysplasia in the ventral prostate and less or no dysplasia in the dorsolateral prostate (356).

Long-term treatment of NBL rats with DES plus testosterone produces a low carcinoma incidence in the dorsolateral prostate and some early-stage carcinomas (carcinoma *in situ*) in the ventral lobe (M. Bosland et al., unpublished observations). When these treatments were given to rats from another strain, Sprague–Dawley, dysplasia occurred equally frequently as in the NBL rats, but carcinoma incidence was considerably lower (354; M. Bosland et al., unpublished observations). In conclusion, combined long-term treatment with testosterone and estradiol-17β is strongly carcinogenic for the dorsolateral prostate in the NBL rat, and weaker in other strains. The sensitivity for the carcinogenic effects of testosterone and estradiol-17β exposure seems to be confined to the periurethral, proximal ducts of the dorsolateral and anterior prostate.

Perinatal Estrogen Exposure

Carcinogenic effects of perinatal exposure to DES in male experimental animals have been described in mice, rats, and hamsters. McLachlan and Newbold (86,91) studied the effects in male offspring of CD-1 mice that had been treated with DES on days 9 to 16 of gestation at a daily dose of 100 μg/kg. At the age of 9 to 10 months, 6 of 24 (25%) of the animals had nodular enlargements of the coagulating gland, ampullary glands, and colliculus seminalis. In one animal (4%) a hyperplastic and squamous metaplastic lesion was found in the area of the coagulating gland and colliculus seminalis that showed a high degree of cellular atypia, resembling early neoplasia (91). When eight prenatally DES-exposed male mice were allowed to live for 20 to 26 months, one animal had an adenocarcinoma of the coagulating gland, three animals had hyperplasia of coagulating gland, two had hyperplasia of the ventral prostate, one had a carcinoma of the seminal vesicle, and two had squamous metaplasia of the seminal vesicle (85,86). No such lesions were found in control animals.

The long-term effects of neonatal exposure of Han:NMRI mice to DES or estradiol-17β was studied by Pylkkänen and co-workers (357,358). DES at a dose of

2 μg/pup/day and estradiol-17β at doses of 20 to 200 μg/pup/day, for the first 3 days of life, resulted after 12 to 18 months in a high incidence (90% to 100%) of moderate to severe epithelial dysplasia of a region that included the periurethral glands and the periurethral proximal parts of the dorsolateral prostate, coagulating glands, and seminal vesicles. Additional treatment with DHT and estradiol-17β from 9 to 12 months of age increased severity for the dysplasia examined at 12 months.

Arai et al. (85,359,360) studied the effects in Wistar rats of neonatal exposure to DES. The rats were treated with DES from birth for 30 days at a dose of 1 μg/rat/day for the first 10 days, 2 μg/rat/day for the next 10 days, and 4 μg/rat/day for days 21 to 30. One group was neonatally castrated and the second group was left intact. Two of 11 (18%) castrated, DES-exposed rats developed squamous cell carcinomas in the area of the dorsolateral prostate, coagulating gland, and ejaculatory ducts, and all 11 animals had papillary hyperplastic and squamous metaplastic lesions of the coagulating gland and ejaculatory duct area. Squamous metaplasia was also found in some of eight noncastrated, DES-exposed rats, but hyperplastic or neoplastic lesions were not observed. Vorherr et al. (92) exposed a very small number of rats pre- and/or neonatally to DES, and found nonneoplastic lesions, but no tumors, in the genital tract of male offspring that survived for 9 to 23 months. There are some data indicating that prenatal DES exposure also results in male genital tract abnormalities and tumors in hamsters (109).

In conclusion, perinatal estrogen exposure is carcinogenic for the male accessory sex glands in rodents. The sensitivity for the carcinogenic effects of perinatal estrogen exposure seems to be highest in the periurethral, proximal ducts of the dorsolateral and anterior prostate and seminal vesicle, and the intraprostatic urethral epithelium. Interestingly, Driscoll and Taylor (44) reported hypertrophy and squamous metaplasia of the prostatic utricle and prostatic ducts in 55% to 71% of 31 infants exposed to DES *in utero* that had died perinatally from unrelated causes. Squamous metaplastic changes were also found in human fetal prostatic tissue transplanted into DES-treated nude mice (361). The changes were confined to the prostatic utricle and urethra in tissue grown to a gestational age equivalent of 16.5 weeks or less, but included the prostatic ducts in tissue grown to a gestational age equivalent of 17 weeks or more.

Induction of Prostate Tumors by Chemical Carcinogens and Hormones

Prostatic carcinogenesis is markedly enhanced by long-term administration of testosterone to rats initially treated with chemical carcinogens that target the prostate because of their tissue-specific metabolism (DMAB, BOP) and/or concurrent hormonal stimulation of prostatic cell proliferation, or because of the specific sensitivity of the rat strain (Lobund–Wistar rat) to a particular carcinogen (MNU) (239,316,323–325,327,349,350,362). If all requirements are not met adequately, this enhancement may not occur (316,327). For example, when a single injection of

BOP or MNU was given to F344 rats without concurrent stimulation of prostatic cell proliferation, testosterone treatment did not enhance prostatic carcinogenesis (182). Chronic testosterone administration was given following a single administration of MNU or BOP during stimulation of prostatic cell proliferation in Wistar WU or Wistar MRC rats, or during and after 10 repeated biweekly injections of DMAB in F344 rats; this treatment produced carcinomas of the dorsolateral and/or anterior prostate, but not the ventral prostate, in 66% to 83% of the animals (239,316,327, 349,362). However, when the same treatments were given to Lobund–Wistar rats, rather variable incidences of between 50% and 97% were reported by Pollard and co-workers (323,324,350,362) and only a 24% incidence was found by Hoover et al. (325). Thus, as was the case with prostate carcinoma induction by testosterone, induction using combined treatment with MNU and testosterone produces highly variable prostate cancer yields in the Lobund–Wistar rat strain (316).

It is remarkable that the enhancing effect of testosterone on prostate carcinogenesis is confined to the dorsolateral and anterior prostate, and does not occur for the ventral prostate. In fact, long-term testosterone administration shifts the site of DMAB- and BOP-induced carcinoma occurrence from exclusively the ventral lobe to predominantly the dorsolateral and anterior lobes (327,349,363). The dose-response relationship between testosterone dose and prostate carcinoma yield is extremely steep; only very little (less than 1.5-fold) elevation of circulating testosterone levels is sufficient for a near-maximal increase in tumor response, and a two- to threefold elevation is sufficient for a maximal response (239). Testosterone is thus a very powerful tumor promoter for the rat prostate at near-physiological plasma concentrations.

Target-Organ-Specific Mechanisms of Prostate Carcinogenesis

Metabolism of Chemical Carcinogens

Metabolism of specific chemical carcinogens selectively in the prostate may determine the sensitivity of this target tissue for these agents in rats and humans, as reviewed previously (147). The prostate is rich in certain drug-metabolizing enzymes, some of which are highly inducible. For example, the rat ventral prostate has a level of mRNA expression of the P450PCN gene that is similar to that in the liver (364). Although the activity of aryl hydrocarbon hydroxylase in the rat ventral prostate is 1,000-fold lower than in the liver, it can be induced 1,000-fold by β-naphthoflavone in the prostate but only eightfold in the liver (365). Furthermore, there is a specific high-affinity receptor for phorbol esters in the rat ventral prostate (366). Also, two TCDD-binding proteins have been found in the rat ventral prostate, one of which has similarities with the TCDD receptor, and the other with the androgen-dependent prostatic binding/secretory protein (367). Thus there are multiple mechanisms whereby carcinogenic agents and tumor promoters can affect the rat and, perhaps, human prostate.

Of the two carcinogens that specifically target the prostate in the rat, BOP and DMAB, only the metabolism and genotoxicity of the latter agent has been studied. DMAB is activated by initial N-hydroxylation in the liver or prostate followed by acetyl CoA-linked O-acetylation. O-acetylation occurs only in the ventral, but not the dorsolateral prostate in the rat, which may explain why DMAB selectively targets the ventral lobe (368). DMAB–DNA adduct formation was studied by Shirai and co-workers (331,363,369) using polyclonal antibodies. The ventral prostate was a major site of adduct formation, and the adducts persisted longer at that site than in any of the other tissues examined, including dorsal and lateral prostate, seminal vesicle, liver, and colon. However, when several rat strains that differed in susceptibility to the induction of carcinoma *in situ* of the ventral prostate were compared, there was only little correlation with both O-acetylation (368) and DMAB–DNA adduct formation in the ventral prostate (331). Thus, although there appears to be preferential O-acetylation of DMAB and DMAB–DNA adduct formation in the ventral prostate, the only prostate lobe target of DMAB, differences in these two processes do not explain differences among rat strains in sensitivity for prostate carcinoma induction by this compound. This suggests that there are additional, as yet unknown, determinants of the carcinogenicity of DMAB for the rat prostate.

Protective Mechanisms

Metallothionein is a high-affinity metal-binding protein that is considered to play a major role in determining tissue sensitivity to the toxic and carcinogenic effects of cadmium. The rat prostate has been shown to lack metallothionein but has some other cadmium-binding proteins that are distinct from metallothionein in their amino acid composition (370). The ventral prostate contains one isoform, and the dorsolateral prostate five other separate forms of cadmium-binding proteins (370). Total cadmium-binding protein levels in both prostate lobes were not inducible by cadmium treatment, unlike in the liver, where a 25-fold increase was found 24 h after a single 20 μmol/kg cadmium injection (370). Total cadmium-binding protein levels in the ventral prostate were approximately 30% of those in the dorsolateral prostate (370). This severe lack of cadmium binding in the ventral prostate and its noninducibility in comparison with the dorsolateral prostate and other tissues may explain why this prostate lobe is a selective target for the carcinogenic action of cadmium.

DNA repair is another potential protective mechanism that may determine the susceptibility of the prostate for chemical carcinogens. As mentioned earlier, differences in persistence of DMAB–DNA adducts in rats correlated with differences in prostate lobe susceptibility, but not rat strain susceptibility, to carcinoma induction by DMAB. No such rat prostate lobe differences were found in unscheduled DNA synthesis following MNU injection, which is indicative of both DNA damage and repair (342).

Cell Proliferation

Increased prostatic cell proliferation at the time of exposure to carcinogens may enhance the sensitivity of the tissue to the carcinogenic effects of these agents (340–344). As indicated earlier, not all studies observed this effect (182,327,345,346). One possible cause of these contrasting results is differences between rat strains in their sensitivity to enhancement of prostatic carcinogenesis by stimulation of prostatic cell proliferation. Bosland et al. (340,341) obtained their results using Wistar WU rats, while Takai et al. (345) and Shirai et al. (182) used F344 rats, and Pour and Stepan (327) used Wistar MRC rats. Bosland et al. (342) compared Wistar, F344, and Sprague–Dawley rats, and found MNU following stimulation of prostatic cell proliferation induced a 3% to 10% incidence of prostate carcinomas in the Wistar and Sprague–Dawley rats, but not in the F344 rats.

The method of stimulation of prostatic cell proliferation also differed among these studies; some used sequential treatment with an antiandrogen (3 weeks) and testosterone (3 days) (340,341,345), while others employed sequential dietary administration of ethinyl estradiol (2 to 3 weeks) and either methyl testosterone or basal diet (for 5 days) (182,343,344,346), or treatment with testosterone only (for 2 to 5 days) (327). However, regardless of the method used, the levels of stimulation of prostatic cell proliferation obtained were of the same order of magnitude (327, 349,351,371). This stimulation of cell proliferation may be cocarcinogenic for prostate cancer induction by many chemical carcinogens.

A third possible source of variation between these studies is the carcinogen used. It is possible that enhancement of prostatic cell proliferation differentially influences the effectiveness of direct- and indirect-acting carcinogens, particularly those that are metabolized in the prostate itself, such as DMAB and perhaps BOP.

The hormonally manipulated increases in cell proliferation found in the various prostate lobes (327,342,371; Bosland et al., unpublished observations) did not correlate well with the earlier mentioned remarkable selectivity of the sites of carcinoma formation within the prostate and with rat strain susceptibility (342). Only when chronic testosterone administration was given during and after repeated injections of DMAB in F344 rats was cell proliferation in the dorsolateral prostate, the target tissue, markedly higher than in the ventral prostate, but only for the first 2 weeks of treatment (349).

In summary, there may be multiple, as yet only partially known factors that determine lobe and strain selectivity of prostate carcinoma induction by chemical carcinogens in rats, only one of which is the rate of cell proliferation at the time of carcinogen exposure. Stimulation of cell proliferation during carcinogen exposure increases the likelihood that promutagenic DNA damage, such as carcinogen–DNA adducts, gets "fixed" as permanent mutations. For example, a high percentage of rat prostate carcinomas induced by MNU plus chronic testosterone treatment contain activating G-to-A mutations in codon 12 of the K-*ras* gene (372). This suggests that base mispairing due to formation of O^6-methylguanine is the first step in the process of multistage prostatic carcinogenesis by MNU.

Hormonal Mechanisms

Carcinogenic and Tumor-Promoting Effects of Androgens

The mechanism of the carcinogenic and tumor-promoting effects of androgens on rat prostatic carcinogenesis is presently not known. It is most conceivable that the normal androgen-receptor-mediated mechanisms are involved. For example, it has been hypothesized (372) that prostate cells carrying critical genetic alterations may be selectively sensitive to the cell proliferative actions, rather than to the cell differentiating actions, of androgen. These cells would then have a selective growth advantage over normal cells, which do not respond to chronic testosterone treatment with sustained proliferation (349). The activation by a G-to-A transition in codon 12 of K-*ras* genes in a high percentage of rat prostate carcinomas induced by MNU plus chronic testosterone treatment may be one such critical genetic alteration (372). The shape of the very steep relationship between testosterone dose and prostate carcinoma response also suggests the involvement of an androgen-receptor-mediated mechanism (239).

As indicated earlier, chronic testosterone administration following carcinogen treatment is required for a high carcinoma response of the rat prostate. This strongly suggests that the developing carcinomas are androgen-dependent or, at least, androgen-sensitive. This is supported by findings indicating that castration early after carcinogen exposure prevents prostate carcinoma induction (342, 362). Paradoxically, the currently available information indicates that, once developed, most of the resulting carcinomas are androgen-insensitive for unknown reasons (347,362, 373). The causes of the specificity of the prostate carcinogenesis-enhancing effect of testosterone for the dorsolateral lobe are also not known. It is unlikely that the short-lived elevated cell proliferative response observed selectively in that lobe by Shirai et al. (349) is responsible for this.

Intact testicular androgen production is required for cadmium to produce proliferative lesions in the rat ventral prostate (89,90,334). This suggests that androgen may act as a tumor promoter in this system as well, but this hypothesis has not been tested specifically. Another effect of testosterone relevant in this respect is that it considerably increases cadmium disposition and retention in the rat ventral prostate (374).

The role of androgens and other hormones in the spontaneous formation of carcinomas of the ventral prostate of ACI/Seg rats (317) and the dorsolateral prostate of Lobund–Wistar rats (320,375) is not clear. Circulating levels of testosterone and prolactin and the ratio of testosterone to total serum estrogen are somewhat higher throughout life in ACI/Seg rats than in COP rats that do not develop ventral prostatic carcinomas, but testosterone treatment did not affect carcinoma formation in the ACI/Seg rats (317). Food restriction inhibits prostatic carcinoma formation in Lobund–Wistar rats (320,321), but it decreases circulating testosterone levels and increases serum prolactin levels (375).

Prostate Carcinoma Induction by Estrogens With or Without Androgens

Testosterone Plus Estrogen Exposure. In dorsolateral prostatic tissue with epithelial dysplasia from NBL rats treated with testosterone and estradiol-17β for 16 weeks, two estrogenic species have been shown to accumulate, estradiol-17β and 5α-androstane-3β,17β-diol (354,356); this did not occur in the ventral lobe, which does not develop dysplasia. In rats treated with testosterone and DES for 16 weeks, dysplasia developed more distinctly in the ventral than in the dorsolateral prostate, as indicated earlier. This coincided with a preferential accumulation of estradiol-17β and 5α-androstane-3β,17β-diol in the ventral prostate (356). These observations suggest that the increased levels of estrogenic species in prostatic target tissue may be causally related to the development of hormone-induced dysplasia and perhaps carcinomas (356).

Dorsolateral prostatic tissue with epithelial dysplasia from rats treated with testosterone and estradiol-17β for 16 weeks also had elevated levels of nuclear, but not cytosolic, type II (intermediate-affinity) estrogen binding sites, but not type I (high-affinity) binding sites (354,376). The type II estrogen receptor is a cell proliferation marker believed to be a key factor in normal and aberrant growth regulation in female estrogen target tissues (354,376). These observations may indicate that protracted stimulation of cell proliferation is involved in the formation of hormone-induced rat prostate dysplasia. Indeed, mitotic indices in testosterone plus estrogen-treated NBL rat dorsolateral prostate were seven- to ninefold increased over control values; this increased mitotic activity was confined largely to the dysplastic lesions (376,377).

Estrogens have been shown to be capable of producing DNA damage in estrogen-carcinogenicity target tissues (125,126,378), independent of their interaction with the estrogen receptor (124,126). A direct DES-DNA adduct (379) and indirect (endogenous) DNA adducts of undetermined structure detectable by ^{32}P-postlabeling have been found in the kidney of male hamsters treated with DES (125). Recently, 16-week treatment with testosterone plus estradiol-17β has been found to enhance the formation of a chromatographically unique endogenous adduct selectively in the periurethral region of the rat dorsolateral prostate, which is the site of the carcinogenic effect of this treatment (355). The enhancement of the adduct formation selectively at the site of tumor formation and preceding it suggests that the adduct is causally involved in the carcinogenic effect of treatment with testosterone plus estradiol-17β. However, it is at present not certain whether these hormones act via a genotoxic mechanism and/or via other mechanisms, including receptor mediation. Thus the exact mechanisms whereby exposure to testosterone and estrogens leads to prostate cancer in rats remain unknown.

Perinatal Estrogen Exposure. Perinatal estrogen exposure of mice resulted in a high incidence of epithelial dysplasia of the periurethral proximal parts of the dorsolateral and anterior prostate, and seminal vesicles (357,358), and carcinomas in these areas (91). Mice that were neonatally estrogenized responded to secondary estrogen treatment (at 2 months of age) with the development of considerable squamous metaplasia in the same periurethral tissues, whereas controls responded with little or no squamous changes (357). These same areas selectively have immunohistochemically detectable estrogen receptors indicative of selective estrogen sensitivity (357). However, the activity of estradiol-17β hydroxysteroid oxidoreductase, a marker of estrogen sensitivity, and epithelial tritiated thymidine incorporation in response to secondary treatments with estradiol-17β, DHT, or estradiol-17β plus DHT, were not changed in neonatally estrogenized mice (357,358). On the other hand, tritiated thymidine incorporation was markedly increased in response to secondary treatment with DHT, but not estradiol-17β or estradiol-17β plus DHT, selectively in stromal cells of the anterior and ventral prostate, indicating a lasting effect of neonatal estrogen exposure on the stromal component of the mouse prostate (357). In all, the exact role of target tissue estrogen sensitivity in the carcinogenic effects of perinatal estrogen exposure in mice remains unclear.

Perinatal estrogen treatment also may act via inducing permanent alterations in the secretion of pituitary hormones and testicular androgen, and in the accessory sex gland androgen and prolactin receptors, resulting in impaired growth of these glands (380–383). LH and FSH plasma levels were elevated in neonatally estrogenized mice (383), while circulating testosterone levels were decreased (380,381) or unaltered (383). Nuclear androgen receptor levels in these mice were decreased in dorsal and ventral prostate but unchanged in the lateral lobe (380). However, there was an increase in the numbers of stromal cells with immunohistochemically detectable androgen receptors in all three lobes (380). The significance of these findings for the carcinogenic effects of perinatal estrogen exposure is not clear. No abnormalities in circulating estrogen and androgen levels were found in boys who had been exposed to DES *in utero* (384).

Other mechanisms, including disturbed morphogenesis of the target tissues (91), and genotoxic effects of estrogens are possibly involved in the carcinogenic effects for the prostate of perinatal estrogen treatment of mice. Interesting in this respect is that in comparison with control animals, a twofold elevation in the expression of the c-*myc* protoonocogene was found in all accessory sex gland tissues of 9-month-old neonatally estrogenized mice, but not in other tissues (358). It was not clear, however, whether the increased protooncogene expression observed was cause or effect.

PREPUTIAL GLAND

The preputial gland is a not infrequent site of tumor induction in rodent carcinogenicity bioassays (1). A variety of chemicals have been shown to induce such neoplasms, which are most often adenomas and adenocarcinomas, and less frequently squamous cell carcinomas (385). Among the chemicals that induced such tumors in carcinogen bioassays in mice and/or rats are 2,4-diaminoanisole sulfate, 1,5-naphthalenediamine, 5-nitroacenaphthene, 5-nitro-*o*-anisidine, glycidol, chlorendic acid, dimethylvinyl chloride, nitrofurazone, and tris(aziridinyl)phosphine sulfate (1,2). Preputial gland tumors have also been found in a variety of tumor induction experiments with a variety of chemical carcinogens in mice (see ref. 8). In rats, such tumors have been observed following treatment with DMAB (329, 343), 7,12-dimethylbenz[a]anthracene (386), azoxymethane (387), and 2-acetylaminofluorene and heterocyclic amines (see ref. 9).

OTHER ACCESSORY SEX GLANDS

Seminal Vesicle

Spontaneous seminal vesicle tumors in rodents are extremely rare (6). With the exception of reserpine, which induced some seminal vesicle tumors in mice, no such neoplasms have been observed in carcinogen bioassays (1,2,108). Several of the treatments that induce carcinomas of the dorsolateral and anterior prostate, but not those that produce ventral prostatic tumors, have been shown to result in adenocarcinomas of the seminal vesicle as well (6,325,341,342,349,363). Treatment with 2-acetylaminofluorene of intact male rats parabiosed with castrated male or female partners leading to elevated levels of androgens also produced seminal vesicle adenocarcinomas (388). Although the same potential mechanisms and enhancing effects of testosterone and cell proliferation described earlier for the prostate may also be involved in the induction of adenocarcinomas of the seminal vesicle, there are some differences. Unlike prostate carcinomas, once developed, seminal vesicle carcinomas seem to be androgen-dependent (342).

There is a high frequency of atypical hyperplasia of the seminal vesicle in rats exposed to chemical carcinogens, but this lesion is not necessarily a precursor of carcinoma (6). High incidences of this lesion can be found in both the presence and absence of carcinomas (182,341,346,363). Levels of DMAB-DNA adducts do not correlate with the seminal vesicle carcinoma response to DMAB treatment (363). Differences between the seminal vesicle and the dorsolateral/anterior prostate in the level of cell proliferation at the time of carcinogen administration also do not correlate with the carcinoma response in the seminal vesicle in comparison with the dorsolateral/anterior prostate (182; Bosland et al., unpublished observations).

Perinatal estrogen exposure may also be carcinogenic for the seminal vesicle. In eight prenatally DES-exposed male CD-1 mice that were allowed to live for 20 to 26 months, one had a carcinoma of the seminal vesicle, and two had squamous metaplasia of the seminal vesicle (85,86).

Bulbourethral Gland

There are no reports of induction of bulbourethral gland tumors in rats or mice. These tumors occur spontaneously with some frequency in Syrian golden hamsters and have been induced by a variety of carcinogens (389; see ref. 10).

ACKNOWLEDGMENTS

This work was supported in part by NIH Grants CA43151, CA48084, CA58088, and CA13343. The very dedicated assistance of Judy Battista and Tracy Kimmel in preparing this manuscript is gratefully acknowledged.

REFERENCES

1. Huff J, Cirvello J, Haseman J, et al. Chemicals associated with site-specific neoplasia in 1934 long-term carcinogenesis experiments in laboratory rodents. *Environ Health Perspect* 1991;93:247–270.
2. Swirsky Gold L, Slone TH, Manley NB, et al. Target organs in chronic bioassays of 533 chemical carcinogens. *Environ Health Perspect* 1991;93:233–246.
3. McCance DJ. Human papillomavirus types 16 and 18 in carcinomas of the penis in Brazil. *Int J Cancer* 1986;37:59.
4. Bosland MC. Adenocarcinoma, prostate, rat. In: Jones TC, Mohr U, Hunt RD, eds. *Genital system*. Berlin: Springer-Verlag; 1987:252–260.
5. Bosland MC. Adenoma, prostate, rat. In: Jones TC, Mohr U, Hunt RD, eds. *Genital system*. Berlin: Springer-Verlag; 1987:261–266.
6. Bosland MC. Adenocarcinoma, seminal vesicle/coagulating gland, rat. In: Jones TC, Mohr U, Hunt RD, eds. *Genital system*. Berlin: Springer-Verlag; 1987:272–275.
7. Mitsumori K, Elwell MR. Proliferative lesions in the male reproductive system of F344 rats and B6C3F1 mice: incidence and classification. *Environ Health Perspect* 1988;77:11–21.
8. Franks LM. Tumours of the accessory male sex glands. In: Turusov VS, ed. *Pathology of tumours in laboratory animals*. Vol II. *Tumours of the mouse*. IARC scientific publication 23. Lyon, France: International Agency for Research on Cancer; 1979:351–357.
9. Ito N, Shirai T. Tumours of the accessory male sex organs. In: Turusov V, Mohr U, eds. *Pathology of tumours in laboratory animals*. Vol I. *Tumors of the rat*. IARC scientific publication 99. Lyon, France: International Agency for Research on Cancer; 1990:421–431.
10. Kirkman H, Kempson RL. Tumours of the testis and accessory male sex gland. In: Turusov V, ed. *Pathology of tumours in laboratory animals*. Vol 3. *Tumours of the hamster*. IARC scientific publication 34. Lyon, France: International Agency for Research on Cancer; 1982;175–190.
11. Mostofi FK, Bresler VM. Tumours of the testis. In: Turusov VS, ed. *Pathology of tumours in laboratory animals*. Vol II. *Tumours of the mouse*. IARC scientific publication 23. Lyon, France: International Agency for Research on Cancer; 1979:327–338.
12. Mostofi FK, Sesterhenn IA, Bresler VM. Tumors of the Testis. In: Turusov VS, Mohr U, eds. *Pathology of tumours in laboratory animals*. Vol 1. *Tumours of the rat*. IARC scientific publication 99. Lyon, France: International Agency for Research on Cancer; 1990:399–407.
13. ACS. *Cancer facts and figures*. Atlanta, GA: American Cancer Society; 1992.
14. Newell GR, Spitz MR, Sider JG, et al. Incidence of testicular cancer in the United States related to marital status, histology and ethnicity. *J Natl Cancer Inst* 1987;78:881–885.
15. Morse MJ, Whitmore WF. Neoplasms of the testis. In: Walsh PC, Gittes RF, Perlmutter AD, et al., eds. *Campbell's urology*. Vol 2. Philadelphia: WB Saunders; 1986:1535–1583.
16. Schottenfeld D, Warshauer ME, Sherlock S, et al. The epidemiology of testicular cancer in young adults. *Am J Epidemiol* 1980;112:232–246.
17. Muir CS, Nectoux J. Epidemiology of cancer of the testis and penis. *Natl Cancer Inst Monogr* 1979;53:157–164.
18. Henderson BE, Ross RK, Pike MC, et al. Epidemiology of testis cancer. In: Skinner DG, ed. *Urological cancer*. New York: Grune & Stratton; 1983:237–250.
19. Morris Brown L, Pottern LM, Hoover RN, et al. Testicular cancer in the United States: trends in incidence and mortality. *Int J Epidemiol* 1986;15(2):164–170.
20. Morris Brown L, Pottern LM, Hoover RN. Prenatal and perinatal risk factors for testicular cancer. *Cancer Res* 1986;46:4812–4816.
21. Depue RH, Pike MC, Henderson BE. Estrogen exposure during gestation and risk of testicular cancer. *J Natl Cancer Inst* 1983;71:1151–1155.

22. Gershman ST, Stolley PD. A case-control study of testicular cancer using Connecticut tumour registry data. *Int J Epidemiol* 1988;17:738–742.
23. Henderson BE, Benton B, Jing J, et al. Risk factors for cancer of the testis in young men. *Int J Cancer* 1979;23:598–602.
24. Morrison AS. Cryptorchidism, hernia and cancer of the testis. *J Natl Cancer Inst* 1976;56:731–733.
25. Moss AR, Osmond D, Bacchetti P, et al. Hormonal risk factors in testicular cancer. *Am J Epidemiol* 1986;124:39–52.
26. Pottern LM, Morris Brown L, Hoover RN, et al. Testicular cancer risk among young men: role of cryptorchidism and inguinal hernia. *J Natl Cancer Inst* 1985;74:377–381.
27. Ross RK, McCurtis JW, Henderson BE, et al. Descriptive epidemiology of testicular and prostatic cancer in Los Angeles. *Br J Cancer* 1979;39:284–292.
28. Strader CH, Weiss NS, Daling JR, et al. Cryptorchidism, orchiopexy, and the risk of testicular cancer. *Am J Epidemiol* 1988;127:1013–1018.
29. Swerdlow AJ, Huttly SRA, Smith PG. Is the incidence of testis cancer related to trauma or temperature? *Br J Urol* 1988;61:518–521.
30. Strader CH, Weiss NS, Daling JR. Vasectomy and the incidence of testicular cancer. *Am J Epidemiol* 1988;128:56–63.
31. Giovannucci E, Tosteson TD, Speizer FE, et al. A long-term study of mortality in men who have undergone vasectomy. *N Engl J Med* 1992;326:1392–1398.
32. Mills PK, Newell GR, Johnson DE. Testicular cancer associated with employment in agriculture and oil and natural gas extraction. *Lancet* 1984;1:207–210.
33. Kolonel LN, Ross RK, Thomas DB, et al. Epidemiology of testicular cancer in the Pacific Basin. *Natl Cancer Inst Monogr* 1982;62:157–160.
34. Kim I, Young RH, Scully RE. Leydig cell tumors of the testis. *Am J Surg Pathol* 1985;9:177–192.
35. Cosgrove MD, Benton B, Henderson BE. Male genitourinary abnormalities and maternal diethylstilbestrol. *J Urol* 1977;117:220–222.
36. Gill WB, Schumacher GFB, Bibbo M. Structural and functional abnormalities in the sex organs of male offspring of mothers treated with diethylstilbestrol (DES). *J Reprod Med* 1976;16:147–153.
37. Whitehead ED, Leiter E. Genital abnormalities and abnormal semen analyses in male patients exposed to diethylstilbestrol *in utero*. *J Urol* 1980;125:47–50.
38. Beard CM, Melton LJ, O'Fallon VM, et al. Cryptorchidism and maternal estrogen exposure. *Am J Epidemiol* 1984;120:706–716.
39. Bernstein L, Pike MC, Depue RH, et al. Maternal hormone levels in early gestation of cryptorchid males: a case-control study. *Br J Cancer* 1988;58:379–381.
40. Loughlin JE, Robboy SJ, Morrison AS. Risk factors for cancer of the testis. *N Engl J Med* 1980;303:112.
41. Gill WB. Effects on human males of *in utero* exposure to exogenous sex hormones. In: Mori T, Nagasawa H, eds. *Toxicity of hormones in perinatal life*. Boca Raton, FL: CRC Press; 1988:161–184.
42. Gill WB, Schumacher GFB, Bibbo M, Straus FH, et al. Association of diethylstilbestrol exposure *in utero* with cryptorchidism, testicular hypoplasia, and semen abnormalities. *J Urol* 1979;122:36–39.
43. Conley CR, Sant GR, Ucci AA. Seminoma and epididymal cysts in a young man with known diethylstilbestrol exposure *in utero*. *JAMA* 1983;249:1325–1326.
44. Driscoll SG, Taylor SH. Effects of prenatal maternal estrogen on the male urogenital system. *Obstet Gynecol* 1980;56:537–542.
45. Deshmukh AS, Hartung WH. Leydig cell tumor in patient on estrogen therapy. *Urology* 1983;21:538–539.
46. Hem E, Attramadal A, Tveter KJ. Synchronous bilateral primary germ cell tumors in patient receiving estrogen therapy. *Urology* 1988;31:70–71.
47. Nilsson A, Nilsson S. Testicular germ cell tumors after clomiphene therapy for subfertility. *J Urol* 1985;134:560–562.
48. Neoptolemos JP, Locke TJ, Fossard DP. Testicular tumor associated with hormonal treatment for oligospermia. *Lancet* 1981;2:754.
49. Mori M, Davis TW, Miyake H, et al. Maternal factors in testicular cancer: a case-control study in Japan. *Jpn J Clin Oncol* 1990;20:72–77.

50. Decoufle P, Stanislawizyk K, Houten L, et al. *A retrospective survey of cancer in relation to occupation.* DHEW (NIOSH) publication. Cincinnati, OH: National Institute for Occupational Safety and Health; 1977;77–178.
51. Logan WPD. *Cancer mortality by occupational and social class, 1951–1971.* IARC scientific publication 36. Lyon, France: International Agency for Research on Cancer; 1982. *Studies on medical and population subjects no 44.* London: HMSO; 1982.
52. McDowall M, Balarajan R. Testicular cancer and employment in agriculture. *Lancet* 1984;1:510–511.
53. Mills PK, Newell GR. Testicular cancer risk in agriculture occupations. *J Occup Med* 1984;26:798–799.
54. Wiklund K, Holm LE. Trends in cancer risks among Swedish agricultural workers. *J Natl Cancer Inst* 1986;77:657–664.
55. Wiklund K, Dich J, Holm LE. Testicular cancer among agricultural workers and licensed pesticide applicators in Sweden. *Scand J Work Environ Health* 1986;12:630–631.
56. Dubrow R, Wegman DH. Setting priorities for occupational cancer research and control: synthesis of the results of occupational disease surveillance studies. *J Natl Cancer Inst* 1983;71:1123–1142.
57. Hayes RB, Morris Brown L, Pottern LM, et al. Occupation and risk for testicular cancer: a case-control study. *Int J Epidemiol* 1990;19:825–831.
58. Sewell CM, Castle SP, Hull HF. Testicular cancer and employment in agriculture and oil and natural gas extraction. *Lancet* 1986;1:553.
59. Swerdlow AJ, Douglas AJ, Huttly SRA, et al. Cancer of the testis, socioeconomic status and occupation. *Br J Ind Med* 1991;48:670–674.
60. Williams RR, Stegens NL, Goldsmith JR. Associations of cancer site and type with occupation and industry from the third National Cancer Survey Interview. *J Natl Cancer Inst* 1977;59:1147–1185.
61. Ducatman A. Dimethylformamide, metal dyes and testicular cancer. *Lancet* 1989;332:1253–1254.
62. Olson JH, Jensen OM. Occupation and risk of cancer in Denmark. *Scand J Work Environ Health* 1987;13:1–91.
63. Calvert GM, Fajen JM, Hills BW, et al. Testicular cancer, dimethylformamide, and leather tanneries. *Lancet* 1990;336:1253–1254.
64. Gollins WJF. Dimethylformamide and testicular cancer. *Lancet* 1991;337:306–307.
65. Tarone RE, Hayes HM, Hoover RN, et al. Service in Vietnam and risk of testicular cancer. *J Natl Cancer Inst* 1991;83:1497–1499.
66. Hayes HM, Tarone RE, Casey WH, et al. Excess of seminomas observed in Vietnam services U.S. military working dogs. *J Natl Cancer Inst* 1991;82:1042–1046.
67. Van Den Eeden SK, Weiss NS. Is testicular cancer incidence in blacks increasing? *Am J Public Health* 1989;79:1553–1554.
68. Heinonen OP, Slone D, Shapiro S. Malformation of the genitourinary system. In: Kaufman DW, ed. *Birth defects and drugs in pregnancy.* Littleton, MA: Publishing Sciences Group; 1977:176–199.
69. Physicians Task Force on Hunger in America. *Hunger in America.* Boston: Harvard School of Public Health; 1985.
70. Boorman GA, Abbot DP, Elwell MR, et al. Sertoli's cell tumor, testis, rat. In: Jones TC, Mohr U, Hunt RD, eds. *Genital system.* Berlin: Springer-Verlag; 1987:195–199.
71. Boorman GA, Rehm S, Waalkes MP, et al. Seminoma, testis, rat. In: Jones TC, Mohr U, Hunt RD, eds. *Genital system.* Berlin: Springer-Verlag; 1987:192–195.
72. Stevens LC. Embryology of testicular teratomas in strain 129 mice. *J Natl Cancer Inst* 1959;23:1249–1295.
73. Stevens LC. A new inbred subline of mice (129/terSv) with a high incidence of spontaneous congenital testicular teratomas. *J Natl Cancer Inst* 1973;50:234–242.
74. Stevens LC, Hummel KP. A description of spontaneous congenital testicular teratomas in strain 129 mice. *J Natl Cancer Inst* 1957;18:719–747.
75. Stevens LC, Little CC. Spontaneous testicular teratomas in an inbred strain of mice. *Proc Natl Acad Sci USA* 1954;40:1080–1087.
76. Stevens LC, Mackensen JA. Genetic and environmental influences on teratocarcinogenesis in mice. *J Natl Cancer Inst* 1961;27:443–453.
77. Pour PM. Transplacental induction of gonadal tumors in rats by a nitrosamine. *Cancer Res* 1986;46:4135–4138.
78. Newbold RR, Bullock BC, McLachlan JA. Lesions of the rete testis in mice exposed prenatally to diethylstilbestrol. *Cancer Res* 1985;45:5145–5150.

79. Newbold RR, Bullock BC, McLachlan JA. Testicular tumors in mice exposed *in utero* to diethylstilbestrol. *J Urol* 1987;138:1446–1450.
80. Walker AH, Bernstein L, Warren DW, et al. The effect of an *in utero* ethinyl oestradiol exposure on the risk of cryptorchid testis and testicular teratoma in mice. *Br J Cancer* 1990;62:599–602.
81. Rehm S, Waalkes MP. Mixed Sertoli–Leydig cell tumor and rete testis adenocarcinoma in rats treated with $CdCl_2$. *Vet Pathol* 1988;25:163–166.
82. Guthrie J, Guthrie O. Embryonal carcinomas in Syrian hamsters after intratesticular inoculation of zinc chloride during seasonal testicular growth. *Cancer Res* 1974;34:2612–2613.
83. Rao MS, Subbarao V, Scarpelli DG. Carcinogenic effect of *N*-nitrosobis(2-oxopropyl)amine in newborn rats. *Carcinogenesis* 1985;6:1395–1397.
84. Pour P, Salmasi S, Runge R, et al. Carcinogenicity of *N*-nitrosobis(2-hydroxypropyl)amine and *N*-nitrosobis(2-oxopropyl)amine in MRC rats. *J Natl Cancer Inst* 1979;63:181–190.
85. Arai Y, Mori T, Suzuki Y, et al. Long-term effects of perinatal exposure to sex steroids and diethylstilbestrol on the reproductive system of male mammals. *Int Rev Cytol* 1983;84:234–268.
86. McLachlan JA. Rodent models for perinatal exposure to diethylstilbestrol and their relation to human disease in the male. In: Herbst AL, Bern HA, eds. *Developmental effects of diethylstilbestrol (DES) in pregnancy*. Stuttgart: Thieme Verlag; 1981:141–157.
87. Stevens LC. Testicular teratomas in fetal mice. *J Natl Cancer Inst* 1962;28:247–267.
88. Kojima A, Yamashita K, Tsutsui K, et al. Development of "granulosa" cell tumors from intrasplenic testicular transplants in castrated ACI rats. *Jpn J Cancer Res* 1984;75:159–165.
89. Waalkes MP, Rehm S, Riggs CW, et al. Cadmium carcinogenesis in male Wistar [CRL:(WI)BR] rats: dose-response analysis of tumor induction in the prostate and testes and at the injection site. *Cancer Res* 1988;48:4656–4663.
90. Waalkes MP, Rehm S, Riggs C, et al. Cadmium carcinogenesis in male Wistar [CRL:(WI)BR] rats: dose-response analysis of effects of zinc on tumor induction in the prostate, in the testes and at the injection site. *Cancer Res* 1989;49:4282–4288.
91. McLachlan JA, Newbold RR. Reproductive tract lesions in male mice exposed prenatally to diethylstilbestrol. *Science* 1975;190:991–992.
92. Vorherr H, Messer RH, Vorherr UF, et al. Teratogenesis and carcinogenesis in rat offspring after transplacental and transmammary exposure to diethylstilbestrol. *Biochem Pharmacol* 1979;28:1865–1877.
93. Huseby RA. Estrogen-induced Leydig cell tumor in the mouse: a model system for the study of carcinogenesis and hormone dependency. *J Toxicol Environ Health* 1976;1:177–192.
94. Huseby RA. Demonstrations of a direct carcinogenic effect of estradiol on Leydig cells of the mouse. *Cancer Res* 1980;40:1006–1013.
95. Reznik-Schuller H. Carcinogenic effects of diethylstilbestrol in male Syrian golden hamsters and European hamsters. *J Natl Cancer Inst* 1979;62:1083–1088.
96. Bartke A, Sweeney CA, Johnson L, et al. Hyperprolactinemia inhibits development of Leydig cell tumors in aging Fisher rats. *Exp Aging Res* 1985;11:123–128.
97. Huseby RA. Effects of cryptorchidy, parabiosis, and estrogen administration upon Leydig cell tumorigenesis in Fisher rats. *Cancer Res* 1981;41:3172–3178.
98. Brown CE, Warren S, Chute RN, et al. Hormonally induced tumors of the reproductive system of parabiosed male rats. *Cancer Res* 1979;39:3971–3976.
99. Jones A. Experimental production of interstitial cell tumors. *Br J Cancer* 1955;9:640–645.
100. Chatani F, Nonoyama T, Katsuichi S, et al. Stimulatory effect of luteinizing hormone on the development and maintenance of 5α-reduced steroid-producing testicular interstitial cell tumors in Fisher 344 rats. *Anticancer Res* 1990;10:337–342.
101. Turek FW, Desjardins C, Development of Leydig cell tumors and onset of changes in the reproductive and endocrine systems of aging F344 rats. *J Natl Cancer Inst* 1979;63:969–975.
102. Waalkes MP, Oberdörster G. Biological effects of heavy metals. In: Foulkes ED, ed. *Metal carcinogenesis*. Boca Raton, FL: CRC Press; 1990:129–158.
103. Gunn SA, Gould TC, Anderson WA. Cadmium-induced interstitial cell tumors in rats and mice and their prevention by zinc. *J Natl Cancer Inst* 1963;31:745–759.
104. Gunn SA, Gould TC, Anderson WAD. Effect of zinc on cancerogenesis by cadmium. *Proc Soc Exp Biol Med* 1964;115:653–657.
105. Roe FJ, Dukes CE, Cameron KM, et al. Cadmium neoplasia: testicular atrophy and Leydig cell hyperplasia and neoplasia in rats and mice following the subcutaneous injection of cadmium salts. *Br J Cancer* 1964;18:674–681.

106. Bomhard E, Vogel O, Löser E. Chronic effects on single and multiple oral and subcutaneous cadmium administrations on the testes of Wistar rats. *Cancer Lett* 1987;36:307-315.
107. Waalkes MP, Rehm S, Sass B. Chronic carcinogenic and toxic effects of a single subcutaneous dose of cadmium in the male Fisher rat. *Environ Res* 1991;55:40-50.
108. Marselos M, Vainio H. Carcinogenic properties of pharmaceutical agents evaluated in the IARC Monographs programme. *Carcinogenesis* 1991;12:1751-1766.
109. Rustia M, Shubik P. Experimental induction of hepatomas, mammary tumors, and other tumors with metronidazole in noninbred Sas:MRC(WI)BR rats. *J Natl Cancer Inst* 1979;63:863-868.
110. Owen PE, Glaister JR. Inhalation toxicity and carcinogenicity of 1,3-butadiene in Sprague-Dawley rats. *Environ Health Perspect* 1990;86:19-25.
111. La Cassagne A. Revue critique des tumeurs expérimentales des cellules de Leydig, plus particulièrement chez le rat. *Bull Cancer* 1971;58:235-276.
112. Henderson BE, Bernstein L, Ross RK, et al. The early *in utero* oestrogen and testosterone environment of blacks and whites: potential effects on male offspring. *Br J Cancer* 1988;57:216-218.
113. Sato B, Spomer W, Huseby RA. The testicular estrogen receptor system in two strains of mice differing in susceptibility to estrogen-induced Leydig cell tumors. *Endocrinology* 1979;104:822-831.
114. Hutson JM, Donahoe PK. The hormonal control of testicular descent. *Endocr Rev* 1986;7:270-283.
115. Wensing CJG, Colenbrander B. Normal and abnormal testicular descent. *Oxford Rev Reprod Biol* 1986;8:136-164.
116. Hadziselimovic F, Herzog B, Kruslin E. Estrogen-induced cryptorchidism in animals. *Clin Androl* 1989;3:166-174.
117. Newbold RR, Carter DB, McLachlan JA. Müllerian duct maintenance in heterotypic organ culture after *in vivo* exposure to diethylstilbestrol. *Endocrinology* 1984;115:1863-1868.
118. Wensing CJG, Colenbrander B, Bosma AA. Testicular feminization syndrome and gubernacular development in the pig. *Proc Kon Ned Akad Wet* 1975;C78:402-405.
119. Morris Brown L, Pottern LM, Hoover RN. Testicular cancer in young men: the search for causes of epidemic increase in the United States. *J Epidemiol Community Health* 1987;41:349-354.
120. Kerr JB, Risbridger GP, Murray PJ, et al. Effect of unilateral cryptorchidism on the intertubular tissue of the adult rat testis: evidence for intracellular changes within the Leydig cells. *Int J Androl* 1988;11:209-223.
121. Huseby RA, Samuels LT. Lack of influence of hypophysectomy on estrogen-induced DNA synthesis in Leydig cells of BALB/c mice. *J Natl Cancer Inst* 1977;58:1047-1049.
122. Terakawa N, Huseby RA, Fang SM, et al. Quantitative changes in estrogen receptor produced by chronic DES treatment of two mouse strains differing in susceptibility to Leydig cell tumor induction. *J Steroid Biochem* 1982;16:643-652.
123. Juriansz RL, Huseby RA, Wilcox RB. Interactions of putative estrogens with the intracellular receptor complex in mouse Leydig cells: relationship to preneoplastic hyperplasia. *Cancer Res* 1988;48:14-18.
124. Liehr JG. 2-Fluoroestradiol: separation of estrogenicity from carcinogenicity. *Mol Pharmacol* 1983;23:278-281.
125. Liehr JG, Avitts TA, Randerath E. Estrogen-induced endogenous DNA adduction: possible mechanism of hormonal cancer. *Proc Natl Acad Sci USA* 1986;83:5301-5305.
126. Liehr JG, Sirbasku DA, Jurka E, et al. Inhibition of estrogen-induced renal carcinogenesis in male Syrian hamsters by tamoxifen without decrease in DNA adduct levels. *Cancer Res* 1988;48:779-783.
127. Snow ET. Metal carcinogenesis: mechanistic implications. *Pharmacol Ther* 1992;53:31-65.
128. Rossman TG, Roy NK, Lin WC. Is cadmium genotoxic? In: Nordberg GF, Alessio L, Herber RSM, eds. *Cadmium in the human environment: toxicity and carcinogenicity*. Lyon, France: International Agency for Research on Cancer; 1992:367-375.
129. Gunn SA, Gould TC, Anderson WAD. The selective injurious response of testicular and epididymal blood vessels to cadmium and its prevention by zinc. *Am J Pathol* 1963;42:685-702.
130. Clegg EJ, Carr I. Changes in the blood vessels of the rat testis and epididymis produced by cadmium chloride. *J Pathol Bacteriol* 1967;94:317-322.
131. Waites GM, Setchell BP. Changes in blood flow and vascular permeability of the testis, epididymis and accessory reproductive organs of the rat after administration of cadmium chloride. *J Endocrinol* 1966;34:329-342.

132. Gunn SA, Gould TC, Anderson WAD. Comparative study of interstitial cell tumors of rat testis induced by cadmium injection and vascular ligation. *J Natl Cancer Inst* 1965;35:329–334.
133. Yoshikawa H. Preventive effect of pretreatment with low dose of metals in the acute toxicity of metals in mice. *Ind Health* 1970;8:184–191.
134. Deagen JT, Whanger PD. Properties of cadmium-binding proteins in rat testes: characteristics unlike metallothionein. *Biochem J* 1985;231:279–283.
135. Waalkes MP, Perantoni A. Isolation of a novel metal-binding protein from rat testes: characterization and distinction from metallothionein. *J Biol Chem* 1986;261:13097–13103.
136. Waalkes MP, Perantoni A, Bhave MR, et al. Strain dependence in mice of resistance and susceptibility to the testicular effects of cadmium: assessment of the role of testicular cadmium-binding proteins. *Toxicol Appl Pharmacol* 1988;93:47–61.
137. Wahba ZZ, Hernandez L, Issaq HJ, et al. Involvement of sulfhydryl metabolism in tolerance to cadmium in testicular cells. *Toxicol Appl Pharmacol* 1990;104:157–166.
138. Clough SR, Welsh MJ, Payne AH, et al. Primary rat Sertoli and interstitial cells exhibit a differential response to cadmium. *Cell Biol Toxicol* 1990;6:63–79.
139. Espevik T, Lamvik MK, Sunde A, et al. Effects of cadmium on survival and morphology of cultured rat Sertoli cells. *J Reprod Fertil* 1982;65:489–495.
140. Wahba ZZ, Waalkes MP. Effect of *in vivo* low-dose cadmium pretreatment on the *in vitro* interactions of cadmium with isolated interstitial cells of the rat testes. *Fundam Appl Toxicol* 1990;15:641–650.
141. Koizumi T, Waalkes MP. Interactions of cadmium with rat testicular interstitial cell nuclei: alterations induced by zinc pretreatment and cadmium binding proteins. *Toxicol in Vitro* 1989;3:215–220.
142. Chatterjee RP. Reserpine, adrenalectomy and the reversal of the early action of cadmium on scrotal and cryptorchid testes in the rat. *J Reprod Fertil* 1973;33:523–526.
143. Favino A, Baillie AH, Griffiths K. Androgen synthesis by the testes and adrenal glands of rats poisoned with cadmium chloride. *J Endocrinol* 1966;35:185–192.
144. Lucis OJ, Lucis R, Aterman K. Tumorigenesis by cadmium. *Oncology* 1972;26:53–67.
145. Carter B, Coffey D. Prostate: an increasing medical problem. *Prostate* 1990;16:39–48.
146. Anonymous. Trends in prostate cancer: United States, 1980–1988. *Morbid Mortal Weekly Rep* 1992;41:401–404.
147. Bosland MC. The etiopathogenesis of prostatic cancer with special reference to environmental factors. *Adv Cancer Res* 1988;51:1–106.
148. Meikle AW, Smith JA Jr. Epidemiology of prostate cancer. *Urol Clin North Am* 1990;17:709–718.
149. Muir CS, Nectoux J, Staszewski J. The epidemiology of prostatic cancer. *Acta Oncol* 1991;30:133–139.
150. Nomura AMY, Kolonel LN. Prostate cancer: a current perspective. *Am J Epidemiol* 1991;13:200–227.
151. van der Gulden JWJ, Kolk JJ, Verbeek ALM. Prostate cancer and work environment. *J Occup Med* 1992;34:402–409.
152. Bosland MC. Diet and cancer of the prostate: epidemiologic and experimental evidence. In: Reddy BS, Cohen LA, eds. *Diet, nutrition, and cancer: a critical evaluation*. Vol 1. *Macronutrients and cancer*. Boca Raton, FL: CRC Press; 1986;125–149.
153. Wynder EL, Fujita Y, Harris RE, et al. Comparative epidemiology of cancer between the United States and Japan. *Cancer* 1991;67:746–763.
154. Schatzkin A, Baranovsky A, Kessler LG. Evidence from associations of multiple primary cancers in the SEER program. *Cancer* 1988;62:1451–1457.
155. Fincham SM, Hill GB, Hanson J, et al. Epidemiology of prostatic cancer: a case-control study. *Prostate* 1990;17:189–206.
156. Kolonel LN, Yoshizawa CN, Hankin JH. Diet and prostatic cancer: a case-control study in Hawaii. *Am J Epidemiol* 1988;127:999–1012.
157. West DW, Slattery ML, Robison LM, et al. Adult dietary intake and prostate cancer risk in Utah: a case-control study with special emphasis on aggressive tumors. *Cancer Causes Control* 1991;2:85–94.
158. LaVecchia C, Negri E, Avanzo BD, et al. Dairy products and risk of prostatic cancer. *Oncology* 1991;48:406–410.
159. Mettlin C, Selenskas S, Natarajan N, et al. Beta-carotene and animal fats and their relationship to prostate cancer risk. *Cancer* 1989;64:605–612.

160. Ohno Y, Yoshida O, Oishi K, et al. Dietary β-carotene and cancer of the prostate: a case-control study in Kyoto, Japan. *Cancer Res* 1988;48:1331–1336.
161. Oishi K, Okada K, Yoshida O, et al. A case-control study of prostatic cancer with reference to dietary habits. *Prostate* 1988;12:179–190.
162. Ross RK, Shimizu H, Paganini-Hill A, et al. Case-control studies of prostate cancer in blacks and whites in southern California. *J Natl Cancer Inst* 1987;78:869–874.
163. Severson RK, Nomura AMY, Grove JS, et al. A prospective study of demographics, diet, and prostate cancer among men of Japanese ancestry in Hawaii. *Cancer Res* 1989;49:1857–1860.
164. Walker ARP, Walker BF, Tsotetsi NG, et al. Case-control study of prostate cancer in black patients in Soweto, South Africa. *Br J Cancer* 1992;65:438–441.
165. Mills PK, Beeson WL, Phillips RL. Cohort study of diet, lifestyle and prostate cancer in Adventist men. *Cancer* 1989;64:598–604.
166. Hsing AW, McLaughlin JK, Schuman LM, et al. Diet, tobacco use, and fatal prostate cancer: results from the Lutheran Brotherhood cohort study. *Cancer Res* 1990;50:6836–6840.
167. Thompson MM, Garland C, Barrett E, et al. Heart disease risk factors, diabetes, and prostatic cancer in an adult community. *Am J Epidemiol* 1989;129:511–517.
168. Schwartz GG, Hulka BA. Is vitamin D deficiency a risk factor for prostate cancer? *Anticancer Res* 1990;10:1307–1311.
169. Hanchette CL, Schwartz GC. Geographic patterns of prostate cancer mortality. *Cancer* 1992; 70:2861–2869.
170. Miller GJ, Stapleton GE, Ferrara JA, et al. The human prostatic carcinoma cell line LNCaP expresses biologically active, specific receptors for 1α,25-dihydroxyvitamin D receptors in normal human tissues. *Cancer Res* 1992;52:515–520.
171. Hursting SD, Thornquist M, Henderson MM. Types of dietary fat and the incidence of cancer at five sites. *Prev Med* 1990;19:242–253.
172. Prentice RL, Sheppard L. Dietary fat and cancer: consistency of the epidemiologic data, and disease prevention that may follow from a practical reduction in fat consumption. *Cancer Causes Control* 1990;1:81–97.
173. LaVecchia C. Cancers associated with high-fat diets. *Natl Cancer Inst Monogr* 1992;12:79–85.
174. Graham S, Haugey B, Marshall J, et al. Diet in the epidemiology of carcinoma of the prostate gland. *J Natl Cancer Inst* 1983;70:687–692.
175. Bhattacharya AK, Malcom GT, Guzman MA. Differences in adipose tissue fatty acid composition between black and white men in New Orleans. *Am J Clin Nutr* 1987;46:41–46.
176. Hankin JH, Zhao LP, Wilkens LR, et al. Attributable risk of breast, prostate and lung cancer in Hawaii due to saturated fat. *Cancer Causes Control* 1992;3:17–23.
177. Pollard M, Luckert PH. Promotional effects of testosterone and dietary fat on prostate carcinogenesis in genetically susceptible rats. *Prostate* 1985;6:1–5.
178. Pollard M, Luckert P. Promotional effects of testosterone and high fat diet on the development of autochthonous prostate cancer in rats. *Cancer Lett* 1986;32:223–227.
179. Carroll KK, Noble RL. Dietary fat in relation to hormonal induction of mammary and prostatic carcinoma in Nb rats. *Carcinogenesis* 1987;8:851–853.
180. Kroes R, Beems RB, Bosland MC, et al. Nutritional factors and cancer: some aspects and possible mechanisms. *Fed Proc* 1986;45:136–141.
181. Pour PM, Groot K, Kazakoff F, et al. Effects of high-fat diet on the patterns of prostatic cancer induced in rats by N-nitrosobis(2-oxopropyl)amine and testosterone. *Cancer Res* 1991;51:4757–4761.
182. Shirai T, Yamamoto A, Iwasaki S, et al. Induction of invasive carcinomas of the seminal vesicles and coagulating glands of F344 rats by administration of N-methyl-nitrosourea or N-nitrosobis(2-oxopropyl)amine and followed by testosterone propionate with or without high-fat diet. *Carcinogenesis* 1991;12:2169–2173.
183. Rose DP, Connolly JM. Effects of fatty acids and eicosanoid synthesis inhibitors on the growth of two human prostate cancer cell lines. *Prostate* 1991;18:243–254.
184. National Research Council, Committee on Diet and Health. *Diet and health: implications for reducing chronic disease risk.* Washington, DC: National Academy Press, National Academy of Sciences; 1989.
185. Hsing AW, Comstock GW, Abbey H, et al. Serologic precursors of cancer. Retinol, carotenoids, and tocopherol and risk of prostate cancer. *J Natl Cancer Inst* 1990;82:941–946.
186. Steinmetz KA, Potter JD. Vegetables, fruits, and cancer. I. Epidemiology. *Cancer Causes Control* 1991;2:325–357.

187. Schuman LM, Mandel JS, Radke A, et al. Some selected features of the epidemiology of prostatic cancer: Minneapolis–St. Paul, Minnesota case-control study, 1976–1979. In: Magnus K, ed. *Trends in cancer incidence: causes and practical implications.* Washington, DC: Hemisphere; 1982:345–354.
188. Heshmat MY, Kaul L, Kovi J, et al. Nutrition and prostate cancer: a case-control study. *Prostate* 1985;6:7–17.
189. Kolonel LN, Hankin JH, Yoshizawa CN. Vitamin A and prostate cancer in elderly men: enhancement of risk. *Cancer Res* 1987;47:2982–2985.
190. Middleton B, Byers T, Marshall J, et al. Dietary vitamin A and cancer: a multisite case-control study. *Nutr Cancer* 1986;8:107–116.
191. Talamini R, La Vecchia C, Decarli A, et al. Nutrition, social factors and prostate cancer in a northern Italian population. *Br J Cancer* 1986;53:817–821.
192. Shibata A, Paganini-Hill A, Ross RK, et al. Intake of vegetables, fruits, beta-carotene, vitamin C and vitamin supplements and cancer incidence among the elderly: a prospective study. *Br J Cancer* 1992;66:673–679.
193. Snowdon DA, Phillips RL, Choi W. Diet, obesity, and risk of fatal prostate cancer. *Am J Epidemiol* 1984;120:244–250.
194. Hirayama T. A large scale cohort study on cancer risks by diet—with special reference to the risk reducing effects of green-yellow vegetable consumption. In: Hiyasashi Y, Nagao M, Sugimura T, et al, eds. *Diet, nutrition, and cancer.* Tokyo: Japan Scientific Societies Press; 1986:41–53.
195. Le Marchand L, Hankin JH, Kolonel LN, et al. Vegetable and fruit consumption in relation to prostate cancer risk in Hawaii: a reevaluation of the effect of dietary beta-carotene. *Am J Epidemiol* 1991;133:215–219.
196. Biesalski HK, Hafner G, Gross M, et al. Vitamin A in Serum gesunder Probander und klinischer Kollektive. *Infusionstherapie* 1985;12:109–114.
197. Coates RJ, Weiss NS, Daling JR, et al. Serum levels of selenium and retinol and subsequent risk of cancer. *Am J Epidemiol* 1988;128:515–523.
198. Peleg I, Heyden S, Knowles M, et al. Serum retinol and risk of subsequent cancer: extension of the Evans County, Georgia, study. *J Natl Cancer Inst* 1984;73:1455–1458.
199. Whelan P, Walker BE, Kelleher J. Zinc, vitamin A and prostatic cancer. *Br J Urol* 1983;55:525–528.
200. Willet WC, Polk BF, Underwood BA, et al. Relation of serum vitamins A and E and carotenes to the risk of cancer. *N Engl J Med* 1984;310:430–434.
201. Hayes RB, Bogdanovicz JF, Schroeder FH, et al. Serum retinol and prostate cancer. *Cancer* 1988;62:2021–2026.
202. Reichman ME, Hayes RB, Ziegler RG. Serum vitamin A and subsequent development of prostate cancer in the first National Health and Nutrition Examination Survey epidemiologic follow-up study. *Cancer Res* 1990;50:2311–2315.
203. Pollard M, Luckert PH, Sporn MB. Prevention of primary prostate cancer in Lobund–Wistar rats by *N*-(4-hydroxyphenyl)retinamide. *Cancer Res* 1991;51:3610–3611.
204. Pienta KJ, Nguyen NM, Lehr J. Treatment of prostate cancer in the rat with the synthetic retinoid fenretinide. *Cancer Res* 1993;53:224–226.
205. Rose DP, Cohen LA. Effects of dietary menhaden oil and retinyl acetate on the growth of DU 145 human prostatic adenocarcinoma cells transplanted into athymic nude mice. *Carcinogenesis* 1988; 9:603–605.
206. McCormick DL, Bagg BJ, Hultin TA. Comparative activity of dietary or typical exposure to three retinoids in the promotion of skin tumor induction in mice. *Cancer Res* 1987;47:5989–5993.
207. McCormick DL, Hollister JL, Bagg BJ. Enhancement of murine hepatocarcinogenesis by all-*trans*-retinoic acid and two synthetic retinamides. *Carcinogenesis* 1990;11:1605–1609.
208. McCormick DL, Mehta RG, Thompson CA, et al. Enhanced inhibition of mammary carcinogenesis by combined treatment with *N*-(4-hydroxyphenyl)retinamide and ovariectomy. *Cancer Res* 1982;42:508–512.
209. Moon RC, McCormick DL, Becci PJ, et al. Influence of 15 retinoic acid amides on urinary bladder carcinogenesis in the mouse. *Carcinogenesis* 1982;3:1469–1472.
210. Albanes D, Blair A, Taylor PH. Physical activity and risk of cancer in the NHANES I population. *Am J Public Health* 1989;79:744–750.
211. Brownson RC, Chang JC, Davis J, et al. Physical activity on the job and cancer in Missouri. *Am J Public Health* 1991;81:630–642.

212. LeMarchand L, Kolonel LN, Yoshizawa CN. Lifetime occupational physical activity and prostate cancer risk. *Am J Epidemiol* 1991;133:103–111.
213. Severson RK, Nomura AMY, Grove JS, et al. A prospective analysis of physical activity and cancer. *Am J Epidemiol* 1989;130:522–529.
214. Paffenbarger RS, Hyde RT, Wing AL. Physical activity and incidence of cancer in diverse populations: a preliminary report. *Am J Clin Nutr* 1987;45:312–317.
215. Polednak AP. College athletics, body size and cancer mortality. *Cancer* 1976;38:382–387.
216. Yu H, Harris RE, Wynder EL. Case-control study of prostate cancer and socioeconomic factors. *Prostate* 1988;13:317–325.
217. Coughlin SS. Re: Lifetime occupational physical activity and prostate cancer. *Am J Epidemiol* 1991;134:672–673.
218. Adlercreutz H, Harkonen M, Kuoppasalmi K, et al. Effect of training on plasma anabolic and catabolic steroid hormones and their response during physical exercise. *Int J Sports Med* 1986;7:27–28.
219. Keizer H, Janssen GME, Menheere P. Changes in basal plasma testosterone, cortisol and dehydroepiandrosterone sulfate in previously untrained males and females preparing for a marathon. *Int J Sports Med* 1989;10:S139–S145.
220. Ross RK, Paganini-Hill A, Henderson BE. The etiology of prostate cancer: what does the epidemiology suggest? *Prostate* 1983;4:333–344.
221. Severson RK, Grove JS, Nomura AMY, et al. Body mass and prostatic cancer: a prospective study. *Br Med J* 1988;287:713–715.
222. Barrett-Connor E, Garland C, McPhilips JB, et al. A prospective, population-based study of androstenedione, estrogens, and prostatic cancer. *Cancer* 1990;50:169–173.
223. Denmark-Wahnefried W, Paulson DF, Robertson CN, et al. Body dimension differences in men with or without prostate cancer. *J Natl Cancer Inst* 1992;84:1363–1364.
224. Garfinkel L. Overweight and mortality. *Cancer* 1986;58:1826–1829.
225. Lew EA, Garfinkel L. Variations in mortality by weight among 750,000 men and women. *J Chron Dis* 1979;32:563–567.
226. Landry GL, Primos WA. Anabolic steroid abuses. *Adv Pediatr* 1990;37:185–205.
227. Meikle AW, Bishop DT, Stringham JD, et al. Relationship between body mass index, cigarette smoking, and plasma sex steroids in normal male twins. *Genet Epidemiol* 1989;6:399–412.
228. Hsing AW, McLaughlin JK, Hrubec Z, et al. Tobacco use and prostate cancer: 26-year follow-up of US veterans. *Am Epidemiol* 1991;133:437–441.
229. Honda GD, Bernstein L, Ross RK, et al. Vasectomy, cigarette smoking, and age at first sexual intercourse as risk factors for prostate cancer in middle-aged men. *Br J Cancer* 1988;57:326–331.
230. Muscat JE, Taioli E, Hsing AW et al. Re: diet, tobacco use and fatal prostate cancer: results from the Lutheran Brotherhood cohort study. *Cancer Res* 1991;51:3067.
231. Abd Elghany N, Schumacher MC, Slattery ML. Occupation, cadmium exposure, and prostate cancer. *Epidemiology* 1990;1:107–115.
232. Oishi K, Okada K, Yoshida O, et al. Case-control study of prostatic cancer in Kyoto, Japan: demographic and some lifestyle risk factors. *Prostate* 1989;14:117–122.
233. Mills PK, Beeson WL. Re: Tobacco use and prostate cancer: 26-year follow-up of US veterans. *Am J Epidemiol* 1992;135:326–327.
234. Handelsman DJ, Conway AJ, Boylan LM, et al. Testicular function in potential sperm donors: normal ranges and the effects of smoking and varicocele. *Int J Androl* 1984;7:369–382.
235. Ghardirian P, Cadotte M, Lacroiz A, et al. Family aggregation of cancer of the prostate in Quebec: the tip of the iceberg. *Prostate* 1991;19:43–52.
236. Steinberg GD, Carter BS, Beaty TH, et al. Family history and the risk of prostate cancer. *Prostate* 1990;17:337–347.
237. Spitz MR, Currier RD, Fueger JJ, et al. Familial patterns of prostate cancer: a case-control analysis. *J Urol* 1991;146:1305–1307.
238. Carter BS, Beaty TH, Steinberg GD, et al. Mendelian inheritance of familial prostate cancer. *Proc Natl Acad Sci USA* 1992;89:3367–3371.
239. Bosland MC, Dreef-Van Der Meulen H, Sukumar S, et al. Multistage prostate carcinogenesis: the role of hormones. In: Harris CC, Hirohasi S, Ito N, et al, eds. *Multistage carcinogenesis*. Boca Raton, FL: CRC Press; 1992:109–123.
240. Sandberg AA. Chromosomal abnormalities and related events in prostate cancer. *Hum Pathol* 1992;23:368–380.

241. Rosenberg L, Palmer JR, Zauber AG, et al. Vasectomy and the risk of prostate cancer. *Am J Epidemiol* 1990;132:1051–1055.
242. Mettlin C, Natarajan N, Huben R. Vasectomy and prostate cancer risk. *Am J Epidemiol* 1990; 132:1056–1061.
243. Peterson DE, Remington PL, Anderson HA. Re: "Vasectomy and the risk of prostate cancer." *Am J Epidemiol* 1992;135:324–325.
244. Perlman JA, Spirtas R, Kelaghan J. Re: vasectomy and the risk of prostate cancer. *Am J Epidemiol* 1991;134:107–108.
245. Spitz MR, Fueger JJ, Babaian JR. Re: vasectomy and the risk of prostate cancer. *Am J Epidemiol* 1991;134:108–109.
246. Giovannucci E, Tosteson D, Speizer FE, et al. A retrospective cohort study of vasectomy and prostate cancer in US men. *JAMA* 1993;269:878–882.
247. Giovannucci E, Ascherio A, Rimm EB, et al. A prospective cohort study of vasectomy and prostate cancer in US men. *JAMA* 1993;269:873–877.
248. Newell GR, Fueger JJ, Spitz MR, et al. A case-control study of prostate cancer. *Am J Epidemiol* 1989;130:395–398.
249. Nienhuis H, Goldacre M, Segroatt V, et al. Incidence of disease after vasectomy: a record linkage retrospective cohort study. *Br Med J* 1992;304:743–746.
250. Sidney S. Vasectomy and the risk of prostatic cancer and benign prostatic hypertrophy. *J Urol* 1987;138:795–797.
251. Sidney S, Quesenberry CP, Sadler MC, et al. Vasectomy and the risk of prostate cancer in a cohort of multiphasic health-checkup examinees: second report. *Cancer Causes Control* 1991;2:113–116.
252. Guess HA. Invited commentary: vasectomy and prostate cancer. *Am J Epidemiol* 1990;132:1062–1065.
253. Howards SS, Peterson HB. Vasectomy and prostate cancer. Chance, bias, or a causal relationship. *JAMA* 1993;269:913–914.
254. Anderson DJ, Alexander NJ, Fuigham DL, et al. Immunity to tumor associated antigens in vasectomized men. *J Natl Cancer Inst* 1982;69:551–555.
255. Alexander NJ, Free MJ, Paulsen CA, et al. A comparison of blood chemistry, reproductive hormones, and the development of antisperm antibodies after vasectomy in men. *J Androl* 1980;1:40–50.
256. Ablin R, Kulikauskas V, Gonder MJ. Antibodies to sperm in benign and malignant diseases of the prostate in man: incidence, disease-associated specificity, and implications. *Am J Reprod Immunol Microbiol* 1988;16:42–45.
257. Jakobsen H, Rui H, Thomassen Y, et al. Polyamines and other accessory sex gland secretions in human seminal plasma 8 years after vasectomy. *J Reprod Fertil* 1989;87:39–45.
258. Isaacs JT. Prostatic structure and function in relation to the etiology of prostatic cancer. *Prostate* 1983;4:351–366.
259. de la Torre B, Hedman M, Jensen F, et al. Lack of effect of vasectomy on peripheral gonadotrophin and steroid levels. *Int J Androl* 1983;6:125–134.
260. Johnsonbaugh RE, O'Connell K, Engel SB, et al. Plasma testosterone, luteinizing hormone, and follicle-stimulating hormone after vasectomy. *Fertil Steril* 1975;26:329–330.
261. Rosemberg E, Marks SC, Howard PJ, et al. Serum levels of follicle stimulating and luteinizing hormones before and after vasectomy in men. *J Urol* 1974;111:626–629.
262. Varma MM, Varma RR, Johanson AJ, et al. Long-term effects of vasectomy on pituitary-gonadal function in man. *J Clin Endocrinol Metab* 1975;40:868–871.
263. Wieland RG, Hallberg MC, Zorn EM, et al. Pituitary–gonadal function before and after vasectomy. *Fertil Steril* 1972;23:779–781.
264. Kobrinsky NL, Winter JSD, Reyes FI, et al. Endocrine effects of vasectomy in man. *Fertil Steril* 1976;27:152–156.
265. Smith KD, Tcholakian RK, Chowdhury M. Endocrine studies in vasectomized men. In: Lepow IH, Crozier R, eds. *Vasectomy: immunologic and patho-physiologic effects in animals and men.* New York: Academic Press; 1979:183–197.
266. Whitby M, Gordon RD, Seeney N, et al. Vasectomy: a long-term study of its effects on testicular endocrine function in man. *Andrologia* 1976;8:55–59.
267. Skegg DCG, Mathews JD, Guillebaud J, et al. Hormonal assessment before and after vasectomy. *Br Med J* 1976;1:621–622.

268. McNeal JE, Redwine EA, Freiha FS, et al. Zonal distribution of prostatic adenocarcinoma. Correlation with histologic pattern and direction of spread. *Am J Surg Pathol* 1988;12:897–906.
269. Mandel JS, Schuman LM. Sexual factors and prostatic cancer: results from a case-control study. *J Gerontol* 1987;42:259–264.
270. Yoshida O, Oishi K, Ohno Y, et al. A comparative study in prostatic cancer in the Netherlands and Japan. In: Sasaki R, Aoki K, eds. *Proceedings Monbusho 1989 international symposium. Comparative study of etiology and prevention of cancer.* Nagoya, Japan: Nagoya Press; 1990:73–84.
271. Newell GR, Pollack ES, Spitz MR, et al. Incidence of prostate cancer and marital status. *J Natl Cancer Inst* 1987;79:259–262.
272. Tsitouras PD, Martin CE, Harman SM. Relationship of serum testosterone to sexual activity in healthy elderly men. *J Gerontol* 1982;37:288–293.
273. Guinan PD, Sadoughi W, Alsheik H, et al. Impotence therapy and cancer of the prostate. *Am J Surg* 1976;131:599–600.
274. Jackson JA, Waxman J, Spiekerman AM. Prostatic complications of testosterone replacement therapy. *Arch Intern Med* 1989;149:2365–2366.
275. Roberts JT, Essenhigh DM. Adenocarcinoma of prostate in 40-year-old body-builder. *Lancet* 1986;2:742.
276. Sandeman TF. The possible dangers of androgens used for male climacteric. *Med J Aust* 1975;2:571.
277. Mantel N. Re: Tobacco use and prostate cancer: 26 year follow-up of US veterans. *Am J Epidemiol* 1992;135:326–327.
278. Bell FW, Klausner JS, Hayden DW, et al. Clinical and pathologic features of prostatic adenocarcinoma in sexually intact and castrated dogs: 31 cases (1970–1987). *J Am Vet Med Assoc* 1991;11:1623–1630.
279. Ross R, Bernstein L, Judd H, et al. Serum testosterone levels in healthy young black and white men. *J Natl Cancer Inst* 1986;76:45–48.
280. Ross RK, Bernstein L, Lobo RA, et al. 5 Alpha-reductase and risk of prostate cancer among Japanese and US white and black males. *Lancet* 1992;339:887–889.
281. Lookingbill DP, Demers LM, Wand C, et al. Clinical and biochemical parameters of androgen action in normal healthy Caucasian versus Chinese subjects. *J Clin Endocrinol Metab* 1991;72:1242–1248.
282. de Jong FH, Oishi K, Hayes RB, et al. Peripheral hormone levels in controls and patients with prostatic cancer or benign prostatic hyperplasia: results from the Dutch–Japanese case-control study. *Cancer Res* 1991;51:3445–3450.
283. Nomura A, Heilbrun LK, Stemmermann GN, et al. Prediagnostic serum hormones and the risk of prostate cancer. *Cancer Res* 1988;48:3515–3517.
284. Meikle AW, Stanish WM, Taylor N, et al. Familial effects on plasma sex-steroid content in man: testosterone, estradiol and sex-hormone-binding globulin. *Metabolism* 1982;31:6–9.
285. Meikle AW, Smith JA, West DW. Familial factors affecting prostatic cancer risk and plasma sex steroid levels. *Prostate* 1985;6:121–128.
286. Zumoff B, Levin J, Strain GW, et al. Abnormal levels of plasma hormones in men with prostate cancer: evidence toward a "two-disease" theory. *Prostate* 1982;3:579–588.
287. Brownson RC, Chang JC, Davis JR, et al. Occupational risk of prostate cancer: a cancer registry-based study. *J Occup Med* 1988;30:523–526.
288. Checkoway H, DiFerdinanco G, Hulka BS, et al. Medical life-style and occupational risk factors for prostate cancer. *Prostate* 1987;10:79–88.
289. Pearce NE, Sheppard RA, Fraser J. Case-control study of occupation and cancer of the prostate in New Zealand. *J Epidemiol Community Health* 1987;41:130–132.
290. Sorahan T, Parkes HG, Veys CA, et al. Mortality in the British rubber industry. *Br J Ind Med* 1989;46:1–10.
291. O'Berg MT, Chen JL, Burke CA, et al. Epidemiologic study of workers exposed to acrylonitrile: an update. *J Occup Med* 1985;27:835–840.
292. Chen JL, Walrath J, O'Berg MT, et al. Cancer incidence and mortality among workers exposed to acrylonitrile. *Am J Ind Med* 1987;11:157–163.
293. Walrath J, Fayerweather WE, Gilby PG, et al. A case-control study of cancer among Du Pont employees with potential for exposure to dimethylformamide. *J Occup Med* 1989;31:432–438.
294. Blair A, Zahm SH, Pearce NE, et al. Clues to cancer etiology from studies of farmers. *Scand J Work Environ Health* 1992;18:209–215.

295. Pearce N, Reif JS. Epidemiologic studies of cancer in agricultural workers. *Am J Ind Med* 1990; 18:133–148.
296. Burmeister LF. Cancer in Iowa farmers: recent results. *Am J Ind Med* 1990;18:295–301.
297. Fincham SM, Hanson J, Berkel J. Patterns and risks of farmers in Alberta. *Cancer* 1992;69:1276–1285.
298. Stark AD, Chang H, Fitzgerald EF, et al. A retrospective cohort study of cancer incidence among New York State Farm Bureau members. *Arch Environ Health* 1990;45:155–162.
299. Ronco G, Costa G, Lynge E. Cancer risk among Danish and Italian farmers. *Br J Ind Med* 1992; 49:220–225.
300. Gunnarsdottir H, Rafnsson V. Cancer incidence among Icelandic farmers. *Scand J Soc Med* 1991; 19:170–173.
301. IARC. *IARC monographs on the evaluation of carcinogenic risks to humans.* Vol 53. *Occupational exposures in insecticide application, and some pesticides.* Lyon, France: International Agency for Research on Cancer; 1991.
302. Morrison HI, Wilkins K, Semenciw R, et al. Herbicides and cancer. *J Natl Cancer Inst* 1992; 84:1866–1874.
303. Boffetta P. Methodological aspects of the epidemiological association between cadmium and cancer in humans. In: Nordberg GF, Herber RFM, Alessio L, eds. *Cadmium in the human environment: toxicity and carcinogenicity.* Lyon, France: International Agency for Research on Cancer; 1992:425–435.
304. IARC. *IARC monographs on the evaluation of carcinogenic risks to humans.* Suppl 7. *Overall evaluations of carcinogenicity: an updating of IARC monographs vols 1–42.* Lyon, France: International Agency for Research on Cancer; 1987:139–142.
305. Kazantzis G, Lam TH, Sullivan KR. Mortality of cadmium-exposed workers, a five-year update. *Scand J Work Environ Health* 1988;14:220–223.
306. Kazantzis G, Blanks RG, Sullivan KR. Is cadmium a human carcinogen? In: Nordberg GE, Herber RFM, Alessio L, eds. *Cadmium in the human environment: toxicity and carcinogenicity.* Lyon, France: International Agency for Research on Cancer; 1992:435–446.
307. Garcia Sanchez A, Anotona JF, Urrutia M. Geochemical prospection of cadmium in a high incidence area of prostate cancer, Sierra de Gata, Salamanca, Spain. *Sci Total Environ* 1992;116:243–251.
308. Checkoway H, Mathew RM, Shy CM, et al. Radiation, work experience, and cause specific mortality among workers at an energy research laboratory. *Br J Ind Med* 1985;42:525–533.
309. Shimizu Y, Kata H, Schull WJ. Studies of the mortality of A-bomb survivors. *Radiat Res* 1990; 121:120–141.
310. Shimizu Y, Kato H, Schull WJ. Risk of cancer among atomic bomb survivors. *J Radiat Res* 1991; 2:54–63.
311. Eatough JP, Henshaw DL. Radon and prostate cancer. *Lancet* 1990;335:1292.
312. McWhorter WP, Schatzkin AG. Horm JW, et al. Contribution of socioeconomic status to black/white differences in cancer incidence. *Cancer* 1989;63:982–987.
313. Keil JE, Sutherland SE, Knapp RG. Does equal socioeconomic status in black and white men mean equal risk of mortality? *Am J Public Health* 1992;82:1133–1136.
314. Carter HB, Piantodosi S, Issacs JT. Clinical evidence for and implications of multistep development of prostate cancer. *J Urol* 1990;143:742–746.
315. Price D. Comparative aspects of development and structure in the prostate. In: Vollmer EP, Kauffman G, eds. *The biology of the prostate and related tissues.* National Cancer Institute monograph 12. Washington, DC: NIH;1962:1–28.
316. Bosland MC. Animal models for the study of prostate carcinogenesis. *J Cell Biochem* 1992;(Suppl) 16H:89–98.
317. Isaacs JT. The aging ACI/Seg versus Copenhagen male rat as a model system for the study of prostatic carcinogenesis. *Cancer Res* 1984;44:5785–5796.
318. Ward JM, Reznik G, Stinson SF. Histogenesis and morphology of naturally occurring prostatic carcinoma in the ACI/SegHapBR rat. *Lab Invest* 1980;43:517–522.
319. Maekawa A, Odashima S. Spontaneous tumors in ACI/N rats. *J Natl Cancer Inst* 1975;55:1437–1445.
320. Snyder DL, Pollard M, Wostmann BS, et al. Life span, morphology, and pathology of diet-restricted germ-free and conventional Lobund Wistar rats. *J Gerontol* 1990;45:B52–B58.
321. Pollard M, Luckert PH, Snyder D. Prevention of prostate cancer and liver tumors in L-W rats by moderate dietary restriction. *Cancer* 1989;64:686–690.

322. Rivenson A, Silverman J. The prostatic carcinoma in laboratory animals: a bibliographic survey from 1900 to 1977. *Invest Urol* 1979;16:468–472.
323. Pollard M, Luckert PH. Autochthonous prostate adenocarcinomas in Lobund–Wistar rats: a model system. *Prostate* 1987;11:219–227.
324. Pollard M, Luckert PH, Snyder D. The promotional effect of testosterone on induction of prostate-cancer in MNU sensitized L-W rats. *Cancer Lett* 1989;45:209–212.
325. Hoover DM, Best KL, McKenney BK. Experimental induction of neoplasia in the accessory sex organs of male Lobund–Wistar rats. *Cancer Res* 1990;50:142–146.
326. Pour PM. Prostatic cancer induced in MRC rats by N-nitrosobis(2-oxopropyl)amine and N-nitrosobis(2-hydroxypropyl)amine. *Carcinogenesis* 1983;4:49–55.
327. Pour PM, Stepan K. Induction of prostatic carcinomas and lower urinary tract neoplasms by combined treatment of intact and castrated rats with testosterone propionate and N-nitrosobis(2-oxopropyl)amine. *Cancer Res* 1987;47:5699–5706.
328. Katayama S, Fiala E, Reddy BS, et al. Prostate adenocarcinoma in rats: induction by 3,2'-dimethyl-4-aminobiphenyl. *J Natl Cancer Inst* 1982;68:867–873.
329. Shirai T, Sakata T, Fukushima S, et al. Rat prostate as one of the target organs for 3,2'-dimethyl-4-aminobiphenyl-induced carcinogenesis: effects of dietary ethinyl estradiol and methyltestosterone. *Jpn J Cancer Res* 1985;76:803–805.
330. Shirai T, Nakamura A, Fukushima S. Effects of age on multiple organ carcinogenesis induced by 3,2'-dimethyl-4-aminobiphenyl in rats, with particular reference to the prostate. *Jpn J Cancer Res* 1989;80:312–316.
331. Shirai T, Nakamura A, Fukushima S. Different carcinogenic responses in a variety of organs, including the prostate, of five different rat strains given 3,2'-dimethyl-4-aminobiphenyl. *Carcinogenesis* 1990;5:793–797.
332. Shirai T, Nakamura A, Fukushima S. Selective induction of prostate carcinomas in F344 rats treated with intraperitoneal injections of N-hydroxy-3,2'-dimethyl-4-aminobiphenyl. *Jpn J Cancer Res* 1990;81:320–323.
333. Shirai T, Iwasaki S, Naito H, et al. Dose dependence of N-hydroxy-3,2'-dimethyl-4-aminobiophenyl-induced rat prostate carcinogenesis. *Jpn J Cancer Res* 1992;83:695–698.
334. Waalkes MP, Rehm S. Carcinogenicity of oral cadmium in the male Wistar (WF/Ncr) rat; effect of chronic dietary zinc deficiency. *Fundam Appl Toxicol* 1992;19:512–520.
335. Terracio L, Nachtigal M. Transformation of prostatic epithelial cells and fibroblasts with cadmium chloride *in vitro*. *Arch Toxicol* 1986;58:141–151.
336. Terracio L, Nachtigal M. Oncogenicity of rat prostate cells transformed *in vitro* with cadmium chloride. *Arch Toxicol* 1988;61:450–456.
337. Hirose F, Takizawa S, Watanabe H, et al. Development of adenocarcinoma of the prostate in ICR mice locally irradiated with x-rays. *Jpn J Cancer Res* 1976;67:407–411.
338. Takizawa S, Hirose F. Role of testosterone in the development of radiation-induced prostate carcinoma in rats. *Jpn J Cancer Res* 1978;69:723–736.
339. Brown CE, Warren S. Carcinoma of the prostate in irradiated parabiotic rats. *Cancer Res* 1978;38:159–162.
340. Bosland MC, Prinsen MK, Kroes R. Adenocarcinomas of the prostate induced by N-nitroso-N-methylurea in rats pretreated with cyproterone acetate and testosterone. *Cancer Lett* 1983;18:69–78.
341. Bosland MC, Prinsen MK. Induction of dorsolateral prostate adenocarcinomas and other accessory sex gland lesions in male Wistar rats by a single administration of N-methyl-N-nitrosourea, 7,12-dimethylbenz(a)anthracene, and 3,2'-dimethyl-4-aminobiphenyl after sequential treatment with cyproterone acetate and testosterone propionate. *Cancer Res* 1990;50:691–699.
342. Bosland MC, Prinsen MK, Rivenson A, et al. Induction of proliferative lesions of ventral prostate, seminal vesicle, and other accessory sex glands in rats by N-methyl-N-nitrosourea: effect of castration, pretreatment with cyproterone acetate and testosterone propionate, and rat strain. *Prostate* 1992;20:339–353.
343. Shirai T, Fukushima S, Ikawa E, et al. Induction of prostate carcinoma *in situ* at high incidence in F344 rats by combination of 3,2'-dimethyl-4-aminobiphenyl and ethinyl estradiol. *Cancer Res* 1986;46:6423–6426.
344. Ito N, Shirai T, Tagawa Y, et al. Variation in tumor yield in the prostate and other target organs of the rat in response to varied dosage and duration of administration of 3,2'-dimethyl-4-aminobiphenyl. *Cancer Res* 1988;48:4629–4632.

345. Takai K, Kakizoe T, Tobisu K, et al. Sequential changes in the prostate of rats treated with chlormadinone acetate, testosterone and N-nitroso-N-methylurea. *J Urol* 1988;139:1363–1366.
346. Shirai T, Ikawa E, Tagawa Y, et al. Lesions of the prostate glands and seminal vesicles induced by N-methylnitrosourea in F344 rats pretreated with ethinyl estradiol. *Cancer Lett* 1987;35:7–15.
347. Noble RL. Prostate carcinoma of the Nb rat in relation to hormones. *Int Rev Exp Pathol* 1982; 23:113–159.
348. Pollard M, Luckert PH, Schmidt MA. Induction of prostate adenocarcinomas in Lobund Wistar rats by testosterone. *Prostate* 1982;3:563–568.
349. Shirai T, Tamano S, Kato T, et al. Induction of invasive carcinomas in the accessory sex organs other than the ventral prostate of rats given 3,2'-dimethyl-4-aminobiphenyl and testosterone propionate. *Cancer Res* 1991;51:1264–1269.
350. Pollard M, Luckert PH. Production of autochthonous prostate cancer in Lobund–Wistar rats by treatments with N-nitroso-N-methylurea and testosterone. *J Natl Cancer Inst* 1986;77:583–587.
351. Bosland MC, Scherrenberg PM, Ford H, et al. Promotion by testosterone of N-methyl-N-nitrosourea-induced prostatic carcinogenesis in rats. *Proc Am Assoc Cancer Res* 1989;30:272.
352. Bosland MC. Carcinogenic risk assessment of steroid hormone exposure in relation to prostate cancer. In: Li JJ, Nandi S, Li AA, eds. *Hormonal carcinogenesis*. Berlin: Springer-Verlag; 1992: 225–233.
353. Drago JR. The induction of Nb rat prostatic carcinomas. *Anticancer Res* 1984;4:255–256.
354. Leav I, Ho MS, Ofner P, et al. Biochemical alterations in sex hormone induced hyperplasia and dysplasia of the dorsolateral prostates of Noble rats. *J Natl Cancer Inst* 1988;80:1045–1053.
355. Bosland MC, Han X, Liehr JG. Enhancement of endogenous DNA adduct formation and induction of adenocarcinomas at the same site in the rat dorsolateral prostate by treatment with estradiol-17β and testosterone. *Proc Am Assoc Cancer Res* 1993;34:241.
356. Ofner P, Bosland MC, Vena RL. Differential effects of diethylstilbestrol and estradiol-17β in combination with testosterone on rat prostate lobes. *Toxicol Appl Pharmacol* 1992;112:300–309.
357. Pylkkänen L, Santti R, Newbold R, et al. Regional differences in the prostate of the neonatally estrogenized mouse. *Prostate* 1991;18:117–129.
358. Pylkkänen L, Santti R, Mäentausta O, et al. Distribution of estradiol-17β hydroxysteroid oxidoreductase in the urogenital tract of control and neonatally estrogenized male mice: immunohistochemical, enzymehistochemical, and biochemical study. *Prostate* 1992;20:59–72.
359. Arai Y, Chen CY, Nishizuka Y. Cancer development in male reproductive tract in rats given diethylstilbestrol at neonatal age. *Gann* 1978;69:861–862.
360. Arai Y, Suzuki Y, Nishizuka Y. Hyperplastic and metaplastic lesions in the reproductive tract of male rats induced by neonatal treatment with diethylstilbestrol. *Virchows Arch A Pathol Anat Histol* 1977;376:21–28.
361. Sugimura Y, Cunha GR, Yonemura GU, et al. Temporal and spatial factors in diethylstilbestrol-induced squamous metaplasia of the developing human prostate. *Hum Pathol* 1988;19:133–139.
362. Pollard M, Luckert PH, Snyder D. Prevention and treatment of experimental prostate cancer in Lobund–Wistar rats. 1. Effects of estradiol, dihydrotestosterone, and castration. *Prostate* 1989; 15:95–103.
363. Shirai T, Imaida K, Iwasaki S, et al. Sequential observation of rat prostate lesion development induced by 3,2'-dimethyl-4-aminobiphenyl and testosterone. *Jpn J Cancer Res* 1993;84:20–25.
364. Simmons DL, Kasper C. Quantitation of mRNAs specific for the mixed-function oxidase system in rat liver and extrahepatic tissues during development. *Arch Biochem Biophys* 1989;271:10–20.
365. Söderkvist P, Töftgård R, Gustafsson JA. Induction of cytochrome P-450 related metabolic activities in the rat ventral prostate. *Toxicol Lett* 1982;10:61–69.
366. Carmena MJ, Garcia-Paramio MP, Prieto JC. Receptors for tumor-promoting phorbol esters in rat ventral prostate. *Cancer Lett* 1993;68:143–147.
367. Söderkvist P, Poellinger L, Gustafsson JA. Carcinogen-binding proteins in the rat ventral prostate: Specific and nonspecific high-affinity binding sites for benzo(a)pyrene, 3-methylcholanthrene, and 2,3,7,8-tetrachlorodibenzo-p-dioxin. *Cancer Res* 1986;46:651–657.
368. Yamada H, Shirai T, Ito N, et al. Species- and strain-specific O-acetylation of N-hydroxy-3,2'-dimethyl-4-aminobiphenyl by liver and prostate cytosol. In: King CM, Schuetzle D, eds. *Carcinogenic and mutagenic responses to aromatic amines and nitroarenes*. New York: Elsevier; 1988: 223–227.

369. Shirai T, Nakamura A, Fukushima S, et al. Immunohistochemical demonstration of carcinogen-DNA adducts in target and non-target tissues of rats given a prostate carcinogen, 3,2'-dimethyl-4-aminobiphenyl. *Carcinogenesis* 1990;11:653–657.
370. Waalkes MP, Perantoni A. Apparent deficiency of metallothionein in the Wistar rat prostate. *Toxicol Appl Pharmacol* 1989;101:83–94.
371. Shirai T, Ikawa E, Imaida K. Proliferative response of rat accessory sex organs to dietary sex hormones after castration or initial dietary administration of estrogen. *J Urol* 1987;138:216–219.
372. Sukumar S, Armstrong B, Bruyntjes JP, et al. Frequent activation of the Ki-*ras* oncogene at codon 12 in *N*-methyl-*N*-nitrosourea-induced rat prostate adenocarcinomas and neurogenic sarcomas. *Mol Carcinog* 1991;4:362–368.
373. Condon MS, Horton L, Dennison J, Bosland MC. Rat prostatic adenocarcinomas induced by *N*-methyl-*N*-nitrosourea and chronic testosterone treatment are androgen-indepedent. *Proc Am Assoc Cancer Res* 1993;34:248.
374. Waalkes MP, Rehm S, Perantoni AO, et al. Cadmium exposure in rats and tumours of the prostate. In: Nordbert GF, Herber RFM, Alessio L, eds. *Cadmium in the human environment: toxicity and carcinogenicity*. Lyon, France: International Agency for Research on Cancer; 1992;391–400.
375. Snyder DL, Wostmann BS, Pollard M. Serum hormones in diet-restricted gnotobiotic and conventional Lobund-Wistar rats. *J Gerontol* 1988;43:168–173.
376. Ho SM, Yu M, Leav I, et al. The conjoint actions of androgens and estrogens in the induction of proliferative lesions in the rat prostate. In: Li JJ, Nandi S, Li SA, eds. *Hormonal carcinogenesis*. Berlin: Springer-Verlag; 1992:18–25.
377. Leav I, Merk FB, Kwan PWL, et al. Androgen-supported estrogen-enhanced epithelial proliferation in the prostate of intact Noble rats. *Prostate* 1989;15:23–40.
378. Banerjee SK, Banerjee S, Li SA, et al. Cytogenetic changes in renal neoplasms and during estrogen-induced renal tumorigenesis in hamsters. In: Li JJ, Nandi S, Li AA, eds. *Hormonal carcinogenesis*. Berlin: Springer-Verlag, 1992;247–253.
379. Gladek A, Liehr JG. Mechanism of genotoxicity of diethylstilbestrol *in vivo*. *J Biol Chem* 1989;264:16847–16852.
380. Prins GS. Neonatal estrogen exposure induces lobe-specific alterations in adult rat prostate androgen receptor expression. *Endocrinology* 1992;2401–2412.
381. Jean C, Andre JM, Berger JM, et al. Estimation of testosterone and androstenedione in the plasma and testes of cryptorchid off spring of mice treated with oestradiol during pregnancy. *J Reprod Fertil* 1975;44:235–247.
382. Edery M, Turner T, Dauder S. Influence of neonatal diethylstilbestrol treatment on prolactin receptor levels in the mouse male reproductive system. *Proc Soc Exp Biol Med* 1990;194;289–292.
383. Dalterio S, Bartke A, Steger R. Neonatal exposure to DES in BALB/c male mice: effects on pituitary–gonadal function. *Pharmacol Biochem Behav* 1985;22:1019–1024.
384. Ross RK, Gabeff P, Hill-Paganini A, et al. Effect of *in utero* exposure to diethylstilbestrol on age at onset of puberty and on postpubertal hormone levels in boys. *Can Med Assoc J* 1983;128:1197–1198.
385. Reznik G, Ward JM. Morphology of neoplastic lesions in the clitoral and prepucial gland of the F334 rat. *J Cancer Res Clin Oncol* 1981;101:249–263.
386. Yoshida H. Preputial tumours induced by intragastric intubation of 7,12-dimethylbenz(*a*)anthracene in gonadectomized female and male rats. *J Cancer Res Clin Oncol* 1983;105:299–302.
387. Ward JM. Dose response to a single injection of azoxymethane in rats. *Vet Pathol* 1975;12:165–177.
388. Bielschowsky F, Hall WH. Carcinogenesis in parabiotic rats. Tumours of liver and seminal vesicle induced by acetylaminofluorene in normal males joined to castrated males or females. *Br J Cancer* 1951;5:106–114.
389. Pour PM, Salmasi SZ, Runge RG. Selective induction of pancreatic ductular tumors by single doses of *N*-nitrosobis(2-oxopropyl)amine in Syrian golden hamsters. *Cancer Lett* 1978;4:317–323.

Carcinogenesis, edited by
M.P. Waalkes and J.M. Ward.
Raven Press, Ltd., New York © 1994.

12

Carcinogenesis of the Hematopoietic System

J. H. Harleman, *H. J. Schuurman, and †C. Frieke Kuper

*Department of Experimental Pathology, ASTA Medica AG,
Halle Westphalen, Germany 33790;
*Pharma Preclinical Research, Sandoz AG, CH-4002, Basel, Switzerland
†TNO-Toxicology and Nutrition Institute, 3700 AJ, Zeist, The Netherlands*

Tumors of the hematopoietic system occur spontaneously in most animal species, including humans. In an experimental animal setting they are known to be induced by a variety of agents in many different treatment schedules and are one of the earliest model systems in carcinogenesis research. Many experimental studies use the mouse as a model system. Tumors of the hematopoietic system are known to be induced by viruses, radiation, and chemicals. In addition, the pathogenesis of these tumors is influenced by a host of other factors, such as nutrition and immune status. In this chapter we discuss the classification of hematopoietic tumors, then focus our attention on the various agents, followed by a section on the pathogenesis of these tumors.

CLASSIFICATION OF HEMATOPOIETIC TUMORS

Classification of Hematopoietic Tumors in Humans

The classification of hematopoietic tumors is complicated. Various classification schemes have been proposed. In the literature on human tumors some of the classification schemes use surface marker immunophenotyping, such as T- and B-cells or the presence of lysosomal enzyme, to facilitate differentiation between the various lineages.

Leukemias

The classification of the leukemias is dominated by hematological criteria, as the diagnosis, evaluation of the progression, and effect of treatment of these tumors is generally made in the peripheral blood smear. Leukemia and myeloproliferative diseases are malignant neoplasms derived from hematopoietic stem cells characterized by a diffuse replacement of the bone marrow by tumor cells. Even though the morphological features of leukemias may be different on the cellular level, they share a similar progression and pathological/clinical presentation. The leukemic cell may infiltrate any tissue of the body, but the main changes are seen in the bone marrow, spleen, lymph nodes, and liver. The tumor cells replace and suppress the bone marrow cells, resulting in anemia, thrombocytopenia, and an enhanced susceptibility to infection due to an actual or functional lymphopenia. Generally, the spleen and to a lesser degree, the liver are markedly enlarged. Lymph node enlargement is more prominent in lymphocytic leukemia than in other forms of leukemia (1).

A simple, and commonly applied classification of human leukemias is based on conventional cytomorphology performed on blood or bone marrow smears. A rough differentiation of the more frequently occurring leukemias is in myelocytic and myeloblastic cell types, and lymphocytic and lymphoblastic cell types. The blastic cell types represent fast-growing cells: blastic leukemias are therefore mostly of acute clinical characteristics, associated with a rapid clinical course with a high mortality. On the other hand, chronic leukemias tend to have a slower progression. Associated with these growth features, acute lymphoblastic and myeloblastic leukemias show a good response to initial therapy but have a tendency to relapse. Chronic lymphocytic and myelocytic leukemias are less susceptible to therapy.

In addition to conventional cell morphology, other modalities have been introduced to classify hematologic neoplasms. Immunologic phenotyping is commonly applied. In this approach markers on the (malignant) cell are determined using monoclonal antibodies. Most of these reagents have been grouped according to their reactivity pattern in *clusters of differentiation* (CD) (2–5). There are three main groups of cell surface/cytoplasmic molecules on leucocytes excluded from the CD nomenclature: HLA antigens, Ig molecules, and T-cell receptors (TCR). Antibodies to antigens located only inside the cell are also not included; examples relevant for the present chapter are the Ki-67 antibody reacting to a nuclear antigen present in cells during the G1, S, G2, and M phases of the cell cycle, and antibodies to terminal deoxynucleotidyl transferase, an enzyme present in the nucleus of immature lymphocytes. Another approach in evaluation of hematopoietic cells is given by recent developments in molecular biology: for example, the assessment of T-cell receptor gene rearrangement in T-cell malignancies, immunoglobulin gene assessment in B-cell malignancies, and the Philadelphia Chromosome in myeloid malignancies. Also, the assessment of *onc* genes (e.g., c-*myc* and *bcl*-2 loci in non-Hodgkin's lymphomas in humans) is a recent development. These methods are not yet that common compared to immunologic phenotyping.

Based on expression of markers assessed with (monoclonal) antibodies, leukemic cells can be categorized with respect to cell lineage and stage of maturation or proliferation (6–8). In the differentiation between a malignant and reactive character of the cells under study immunologic phenotyping can also be helpful, as for instance in the assessment of a single immunoglobulin light-chain expression in B-lymphoid neoplasms. The phenotype of acute lymphoblastic leukemias is mainly that of immature (blastlike) cells in physiologic cell differentiation. On the other hand, the phenotype of lymphocytic leukemias is mainly that of more mature well-differentiated cells.

Lymphomas

The classification of the solid tumors of the hematopoietic system concerns mostly the lymphomas and histiocytic tumors. Lymphomas are separated in two groups: Hodgkin's disease and non-Hodgkin's lymphoma. *Hodgkin's disease* arises characteristically in a single node or chain of nodes and spreads to the anatomically contiguous nodes. It is morphologically characterized by the presence of a distinct neoplastic cell type, the Reed–Sternberg cell. The Reed–Sternberg cell is a large cell (15 to 40 μm), which has typically a binucleated or bilobed nucleus. This cell type is found in association with a variable mixed lymphoid and/or inflammatory cell infiltrate.

The classification of the *non-Hodgkin's lymphomas* is probably the most complicated and controversial in the classification of hematopoietic tumors. Several classification schemes have been proposed. Older schemes, such as the Rappaport scheme, relied only on morphological criteria (9,10). Newer classification schemes, such as the Lukes–Collins classification, also use immunological markers. In these classifications, immunological phenotyping has shown its value (11–17). The Kiel classification is widely applied in Europe and was developed by Lennert and colleagues (18). It is based on the resemblance of the tumor cells on lymphoid cells in the normal situation. These classification schemes resemble each other in some aspects but deviate from each other in emphasis. To enable a comparison between the various classification schemes and to link histology to clinical prognosis, a new and, in the United States, widely accepted classification was recently proposed, termed the Working Group classification (19). This scheme divides the tumors into low-, intermediate-, and high-grade malignant lymphomas, in which low-grade tumors have an indolent clinical course, nondestructive pattern of growth, and respond poorly to chemotherapy. On the other hand, high-grade tumors are characterized by an agressive destructive growth pattern, presence of atypia, and susceptibility to chemotherapy. Table 1 describes some of these classification schemes.

In addition to acute monocytic leukemia, the tumors of the mononuclear phagocytic system are malignant histiocytosis and histiocytic sarcoma. *Malignant histiocytosis* is a malignancy that involves the entire reticuloendothelial system. The cells frequently retain the phagocytic properties as well as surface markers of histiocytes. It is characterized by a diffuse proliferation of histiocytic cells. Some classifications include relatively rare conditions such as histiocytosis-x, which occurs in Letterer Siwe syndrome and Hand–Schueller–Christian disease as well as in eosinophilic granuloma (12). *Histiocytic sarcomas* are localized tumors that may or may not progress to disseminated disease. They have immunological and cytochemical markers of macrophages. Phagocytic activity and Langerhans cells/foreign body cells may be present (1).

TABLE 1. Comparison of classification schemes for human non-Hodgkin's lymphoma[a]

Working formulation	Rappaport classification		Luke–Collins classification	
Low-grade	Nodular		Undefined cell type	—
A. Small lymphocytic	Lymphocytic, poorly differentiated	B	T-cell type, small lymphocytic	A
—Consistent with CLL	Mixed, lymphocytic and histiocytic	C	T-cell type, Sézary mycosis fungoides (cerebriform)	—
—Plasmacytoid	Histiocytic	D		
B. Follicular predominantly small cleaved cell	Diffuse		T-cell type, convoluted lymphocytic	I
—Diffuse areas	Lymphocytic, well differentiated	A	T-cell type, immunoblastic sarcoma (T-cell)	H
—Sclerosis	Lymphocytic, well differentiated with plasmacytoid features	A	B-cell type, small lymphocytic	A
C. Follicular mixed, small cleaved and large cell	Lymphocytic, poorly differentiated	E	B-cell type, plasmacytoid lymphocytic	A
—Diffuse areas	Lymphoblastic, convoluted	I	Follicular center cells, small cleaved	B, E
—Sclerosis	Lymphoblastic, nonconvoluted	I	Follicular center cells, large cleaved	D, G
	Mixed, lymphocytic and histiocytic	F	Follicular center cells, small non-cleaved	J
Intermediate grade	Histiocytic	G, H		
D. Follicular predominantly large cell	Burkitt's tumor	J	Follicular center cells, large non-cleaved	D, G
—Diffuse areas	Undifferentiated, non-Burkitt's	J	Subtypes of follicular center cell lymphomas	
—Sclerosis			1. Follicular	
E. Diffuse small cleaved cell	Kiel classification		2. Follicular and diffuse	
—Sclerosis			3. Diffuse	
F. Diffuse mixed, small and large cell	Low-grade malignancy		4. Sclerotic with follicles	
—Sclerosis	Lymphocytic	A	5. Sclerotic without follicles	
—Epithelioid cell component	Immunocytoma			
G. Diffuse large cell	Lymphoplasmacytoid	A		
—Cleaved	Polymorphic	F		

—Noncleaved		
—Sclerosis		
High-grade		
H. Diffuse large cell, immunoblastic		
—Plasmacytoid	Centrocytic	E, F, G
—Clear cell	Centrocytic–centroblastic, follicular	B, C, D
—Polymorphous	Centrocytic–centroblastic, diffuse	F, G
—Epithelioid cell component	Plasmacytoma	Miscellaneous
I. Lymphoblastic	High–grade malignancy	
—Convoluted	Centroblastic	G
—Nonconvoluted	Lymphoblastic	J
J. Small noncleaved cell	Immunoblastic	H
—Burkitt's	Immunoblastic sarcoma (B-cell)	H
—Follicular areas	Histiocytic	—
Miscellaneous	Malignant lymphoma, unclassified	—
—Composite		
—Mycosis fungoides		
—Histiocytic		
—Extramedullary plasmacytoma		

[a]For each classification the letter in the Working Formulation is given.

Thymomas

Thymomas are neoplasms of the thymic epithelial cells, regardless of the abundance or paucity of the lymphoid component. True thymomas in humans are rare; most thymomas are benign. Thymomas are often associated with various system disorders, such as myasthenia gravis (15% to 44%), cytopenias (21%), carcinomas (17%), hypogammaglobulinemia (6%), polymyositis (5%), and SLE (2%) (20–22).

Classification of Hematopoietic Tumors in Rodents

Human classification schemes are generally not used in research and diagnosis of hematopoietic tumors in rodent carcinogenicity studies. This in part reflects a different emphasis in animal studies as treatment and progression are generally not as important as in human studies. Second, the immunohistochemical or immunological markers are often not an option in regulatory studies, particularly with formalin-base fixatives, which alter tissue antigens. Nevertheless, several schemes for the classification of rodent hematopoietic tumors have been published recently, some of which use immunologic markers as well as morphological criteria (23–26). Immunophenotyping showed that, especially in mice, the lymphomas closely resembled their human counterparts (23,27). The mouse lymphomas are therefore good models for the study of lymphoma development.

Although the objectives of the diagnosis of hematopoietic tumors are different in regulatory-type rodent carcinogenicity studies, it is nevertheless quite important to make an accurate diagnosis. Induction of lymphoid tumors often gives rise to a specific type of tumor (e.g., lymphoblastic lymphoma). In such cases, a more specific diagnosis would lead to a higher detection level. This is especially true in strains that have a high background incidence of lymphoid tumors.

The classification of hematopoietic tumors by Wogan et al. (25) in mice and modified by Harleman and Jahn (24) for rats is generally suited for routine carcinogenicity studies. If further, more detailed examination is needed, it may be expanded and subdivided further using specific immunological markers. Table 2 gives a comparison of the various classification schemes used in rodents. In rodent classifications, generally no distinction is made between lymphomas and lymphocytic leukemia, contrary to human classifications. In the combined rodent classification scheme for hematopoietic tumors, the malignant lymphomas are placed into six subdivisions. Additional modifiers may be used depending on the distribution of the tumor, such as thymic, mesenteric, and leukemic.

The *lymphocytic malignant lymphoma* is composed of relatively uniform small to medium-sized well-differentiated lymphocytes. The nuclear chromatin is generally densely organized, and only a narrow rim of cytoplasm is present. The cells differ little, if at all, from the normal circulating lymphocytes. The tumor sometimes also contains slightly larger cells with a somewhat irregular nuclei corresponding to small follicular center cells (Fig. 1).

TABLE 2. Comparison of classification schemes for lymphoid tumors[a]

Mice/rats[b]	Rats[c]	Mice[d]
Lymphatic	Small lymphocytic (T), Medium-sized lymphocytic (T)	Small lymphocyte (T/B)
Pleomorphic	Follicular center cell (B)	Follicular center cell (B)
Lymphoblastic	Lymphoblastic (T/B)	Immunoblastic (T/B)
	Immunoblastic (B)	Lymphoblast (T/B)
Plasmacytic	Plasmacytoma (B)	Plasma cell
Large granular cell	Large granular lymphocyte leukemia	

[a] T, T-cell origin; B, B-cell origin.
[b] From Harleman and Jahn (24) and Wogan et al. (25).
[c] From Ward et al. (26).
[d] From Pattengale and Taylor (23).

The *pleomorphic malignant lymphoma* consists of a heterogeneous population of medium to large cells, which express a variable degree of pleomorphia ranging from fairly uniform cells to considerably pleomorphic cells and nuclei. The degree of pleomorphism may also be present between different locations of the same tumor. The tumor contains cells resembling the large cells seen in germinal centers. Large cells with cleaved or centroblastic and generally angular or indented nuclei may be present as well as small cells with rounded nuclei and basophilic cytoplasm. The nuclear chromatin is frequently marginated and the cells may have prominent nucleoli. Occasionally, multinucleated cells occur that may resemble Reed–Steinberg cells (Fig. 2). This is the most common tumor type in many mouse strains.

The *lymphoblastic malignant lymphoma* consists of a homogeneous population of medium-sized to large lymphoblastic cells with a high nuclei/cytoplastic ratio. The nuclei are round to ovoid and not indented or twisted and have prominent nucleoli. The nuclei are surrounded by a small rim of basophilic cytoplasm with few if any granules. The tumor generally has a high mitotic index (Fig. 3).

Plasmacytic malignant lymphomas are relatively rare tumors that consist of a uniform population of predominantly plasma cells and/or cells with an obvious plasmacytoid differentiation. The mitotic activity is variable but generally low. The nuclei are round and occasionally show a cartwheel appearance. The cytoplasm is abundant, basophilic, and pyroninophilic, and a small pyroninophilic halo may be present (Fig. 4).

Large granular lymphocyte malignant lymphoma is a subtype of malignant lymphoma that occurs in rats but has not been described in mice. One could say that it is by definition characterized by a leukemic growth pattern. Early lesions are found in the spleen (28,29). It is very common in Fischer 344 rats, but has also been reported in Wistar and Sprague-Dawley strains. It is characterized by medium-sized cells that may show a slight degree of pleomorphism. The nuclei are round or reniform. They have clumped nuclear chromatin and nucleoli. The basophilic cytoplasm has in a variable number of cells relatively small numbers of reddish granules that can be seen in peripheral blood smears stained with Giemsa but not in routine H&E-

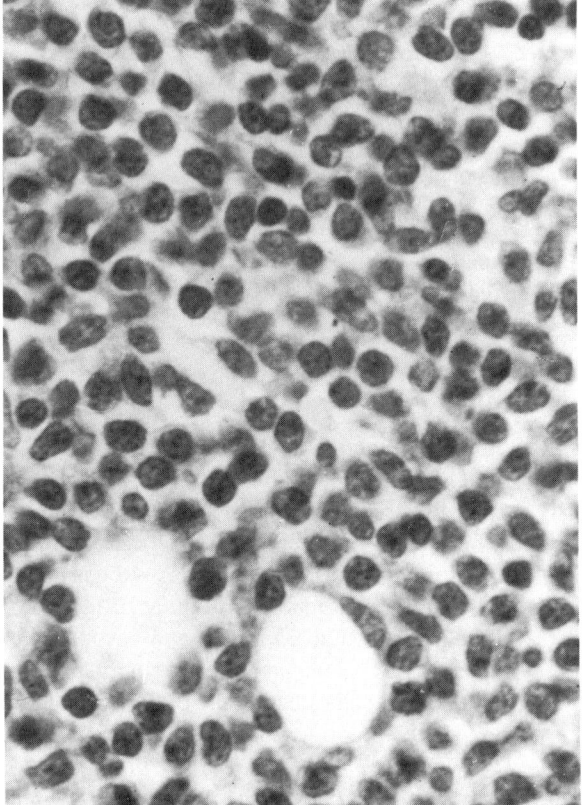

FIG. 1. Lymphocytic malignant lymphoma in Wistar rat.

stained sections. These cells react positively with OX-8 mouse monoclonal antibodies (26) (Fig. 5).

Malignant lymphoma NOS (not otherwise specified) is a subtype that is used in regulatory studies as a localized or generalized tumor of cells of the lymphocytic type, but further classification is precluded by the presence of autolysis, poor fixation, and so on. The leukemias are subdivided as described below, depending on their lineage.

Erythroid leukemia is a tumor derived from the erythroid lineage in the hematopoietic tissues. It has not been reported to occur spontaneously in rats, but can be induced. Like its human counterpart, it is characterized by a primarily erythroblastic cell population. The spleen tends to be the organ most often affected.

Granulocytic leukemia is derived from the myeloid lineage of the hematopoietic tissue. The tumor is generally characterized by increased numbers of granulocytes in the peripheral blood smear. The cells may show varying degrees of differentiation, ranging from myeloblasts, promyelocytes, and myelocytes, to mature granu-

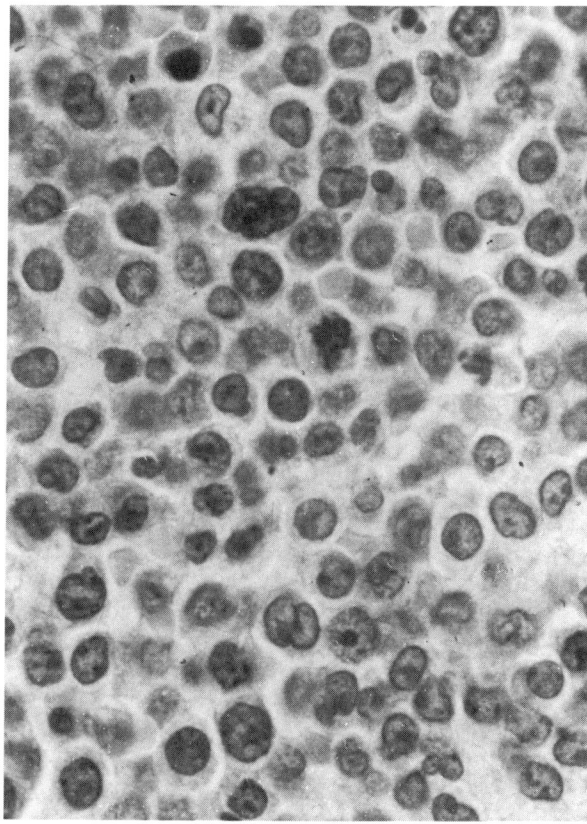

FIG. 2. Pleomorphic malignant lymphoma in Wistar rat.

locytes. The modifier *neutrophilic, basophilic,* or *eosinophilic* is used, based on tinctorial characteristics of the granules. Neutrophilic granulocytic leukemia is the most common form (Fig. 6). The granulocytic leukemia must be differentiated from the more commonly occurring reactive myeloid/extramedullary hyperplasia found in aging rodents as a reaction upon, for example, abscesses, pneumonia, acute pyelonephritis, neoplasms, or repeated blood loss. The latter has generally, in contrast to true granulocytic leukemia, foci of erythroid precursor cells and relatively large numbers of megakaryocytes. The liver is only mildly enlarged and the extramedullary hematopoietic tissue is noninvasive. Only in extreme cases are the adrenal, ovary, perirenal fat, and pituitary involved (30).

Mast cell tumor is a rare tumor in both rats and mice. In rats, two cases have been reported by Tuch and Puschner (31). Macroscopically, the rat tumors were found as small nodular masses in the mesentery. In mice the tumor consists of soft nodules that may be widely distributed in the lymphatic or other organs. Microscopically, they consist of a population of well-differentiated, uniform, large, round to polygo-

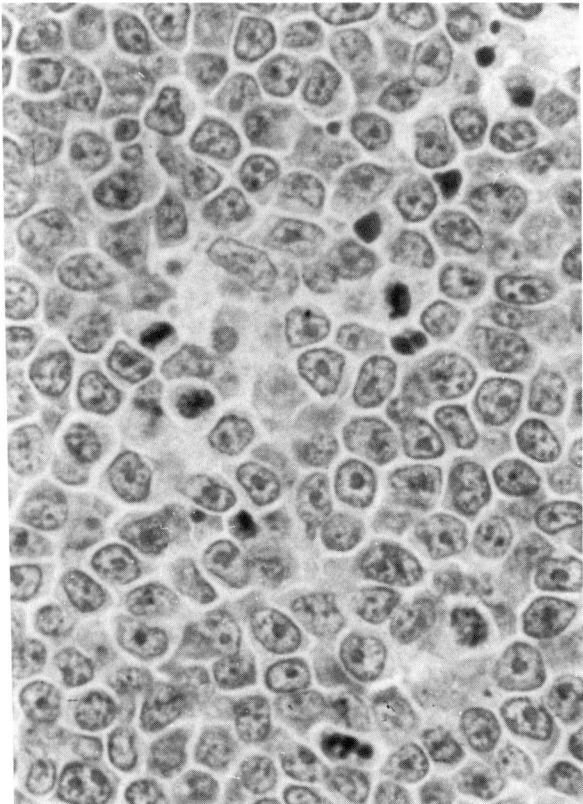

FIG. 3. Lymphoblastic malignant lymphoma in Wistar rat.

nal cells with round nuclei. The cells have generally abundant granular cytoplasm which shows the typical metachromatic staining of positive granules with the appropriate stains, such as toluidine blue (Fig. 7). This tumor is a bit more common and may also be leukemic in certain mouse strains (32).

Histiocytic sarcomas are tumors composed of cells of the mononuclear phagocytic system. Both are fairly common in rats and mice. In mice they are frequently found as nodules in the female genital tract (uterus, vagina) and the liver. In rats two types appear to exist. One type presents itself as a subcutaneous/subperitoneal nodule with mostly a hematogeneous metastasis, and another type is found in the liver which shows mostly metastasis via the lymphatics. The tumor growth in the liver tends to be diffuse in both species. The tumor is comprised of highly pleomorphic cells, ranging from fusiform cells with low amounts of cytoplasm to large cells with abundant eosinophilic cytoplasm. The latter cells frequently tend to fuse to foreign body type giant cells which are typically found around foci of necroses (Fig. 8). Tumor cells may show signs of phagocytic activity (e.g., erythrophagocytosis) (33–

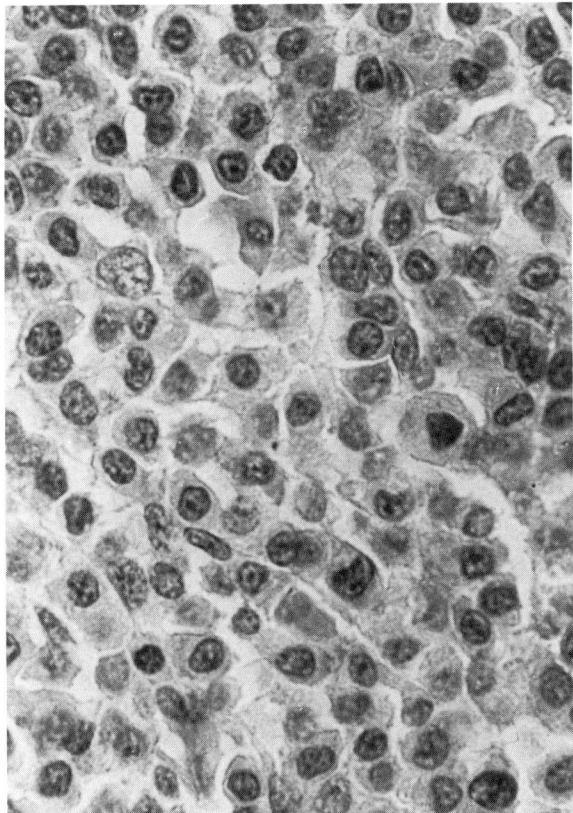

FIG. 4. Plasmacytic malignant lymphoma in Wistar rat.

35). This tumor must be differentiated from the malignant fibrous histiocytoma, which has also been described in both rats and mice (30,36). The latter tends to have a more fibrous character, with a storiform pattern of growth. The tumor may have areas with a mixture of fibroblasts and histiocytelike cells which may also have multinucleated cells, but lacks the typical foreign body cell appearance and necrosis with palisading characteristic of histiocytic sarcoma.

Thymomas

Thymomas are by definition tumors of the thymic epithelial cells. They may have variable amounts of lymphocytes. They are generally rare tumors in rats and mice, with exception of certain Wistar strains (24,30,37,38). The benign thymomas are generally well encapsulated but may show slight local invasiveness. Various levels of differentiation may be present, ranging from tumors with an almost normal thy-

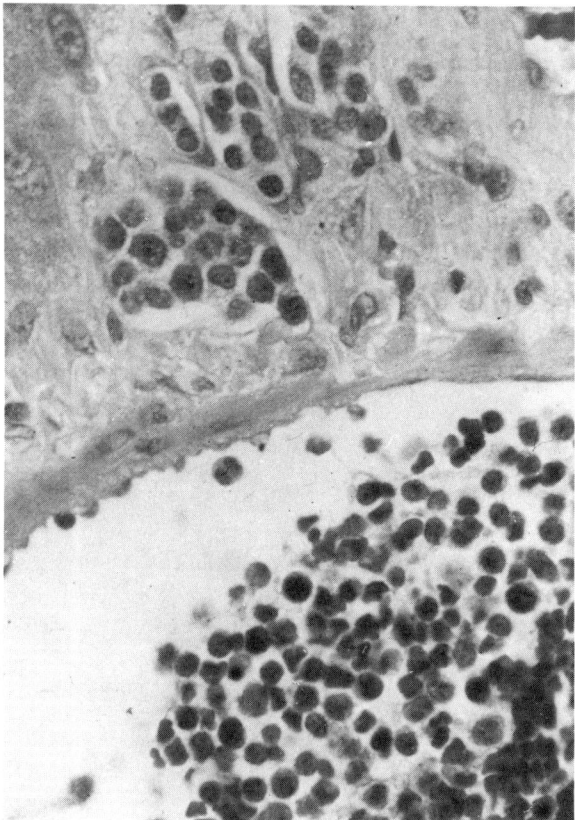

FIG. 5. Malignant lymphoma with large granular lymphocyte in F344 rat.

mic structure to tumors without medullary differentiation, composed of a mixture of epithelial cells and lymphocytes (39). This is the most common presentation of this tumor (Fig. 9). Occasionally, the tumor appears to consist almost exclusively (>80%) of thymic epithelial cells. In this case the modifier *epithelial* is used. Generally, the epithelial cells retain their normal structure, although fusiform spindle cell types have been observed in predominantly epithelial thymomas (38). The malignant thymomas are most frequently of the epithelial type and have a markedly invasive growth pattern, squamous metaplasia, and may develop metastasis (40). Thymomas are reported to be induced by urethan treatment in Buffalo rats (41).

The thymomas should not be confused with the hyperplasia of epithelial tubules and cords also commonly seen in certain aging rat strains, such as the Wistar. This lesion may also be intermixed with the thymomas. It is characterized by nests of epithelial tubules and cords. The tubules may be partially cystic and filled with a markedly eosinophilic colloid material. The cystic structures are lined by cuboidal or columnar epithelial cells, which occasionally are ciliated and contain some secre-

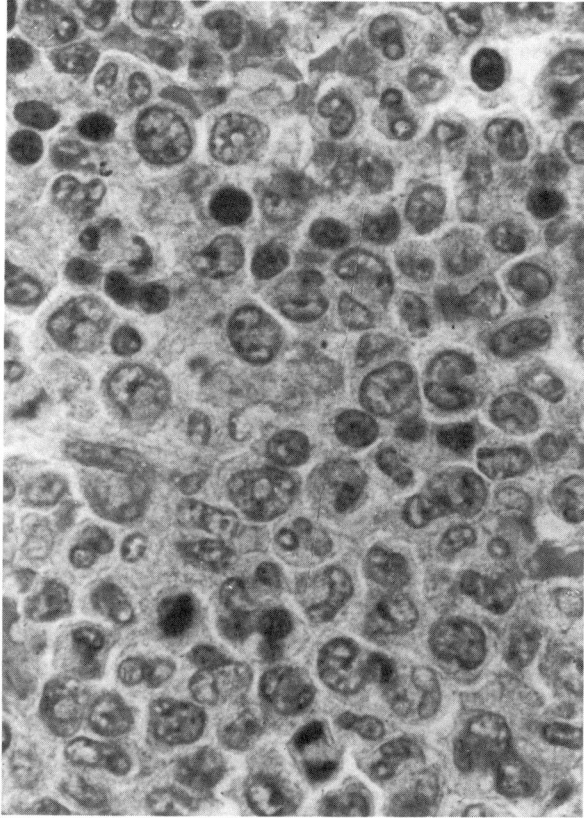

FIG. 6. Granulocytic leukemia in Wistar rat.

tory goblet cells (Fig. 10). They are postulated to be derived of bronchial epithelial remnants (42).

CHEMICAL-INDUCED HEMATOPOIETIC TUMORS

Tumors of the hematopoietic tissue are readily induced by a variety of chemical agents in rodents and in humans (43,44). Tumors of the hematopoietic system have been observed in early studies on chemical carcinogenesis in mice along with neoplasms of other organs. One of the first experimental models, which specifically and preferentially induced lymphoid tumors, were the studies of Pietra et al. (45). They recognized that the carcinogen administration to newborn or very young mice rapidly produced lymphosarcomas mostly of thymic origin. Pending the model system, predominantly lymphomas and/or preferentially myeloid leukemias could be induced. A whole range of carcinogens were found to have an affinity for the hema-

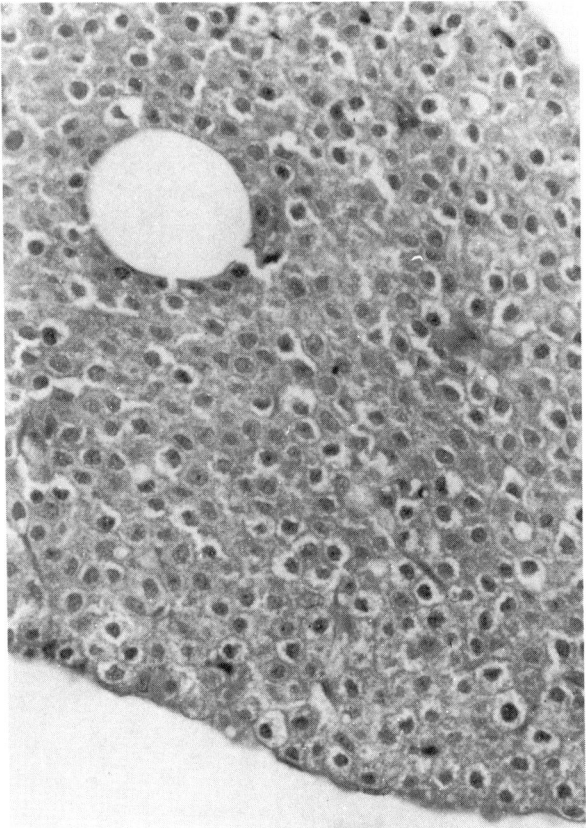

FIG. 7. Mast cell tumor in Wistar rat.

topoietic system. Potent carcinogens for the lymphoid system are N-nitrosomethylurea (NMU) and the 5-nitrofurans. One peculiar exception are the nitrosamines (46). The reason why certain carcinogens do have an affinity for the lymphoid system while others do not may be at least partially related to the metabolic potential of these agents.

Hematopoietic tumors are also induced in rats. In rats and mice, the route of administration and age are important factors in these models, as they determine whether a low or high incidence of these tumors are induced. The model conditions also influence whether lymphomas or myeloid leukemias are preferentially induced. Compounds, which show efficiency in inducing hematopoietic tumors, are 7,12-dimethylbenz[a]anthracene, methylcholanthracene, and benz[a]pyrene. Table 3 lists some compounds that induce hematopoietic neoplasms in rodents. Even though this list is by no means comprehensive, it does show the variety of chemical entities as well as the different types of tumors induced. In the National Toxicology Pro-

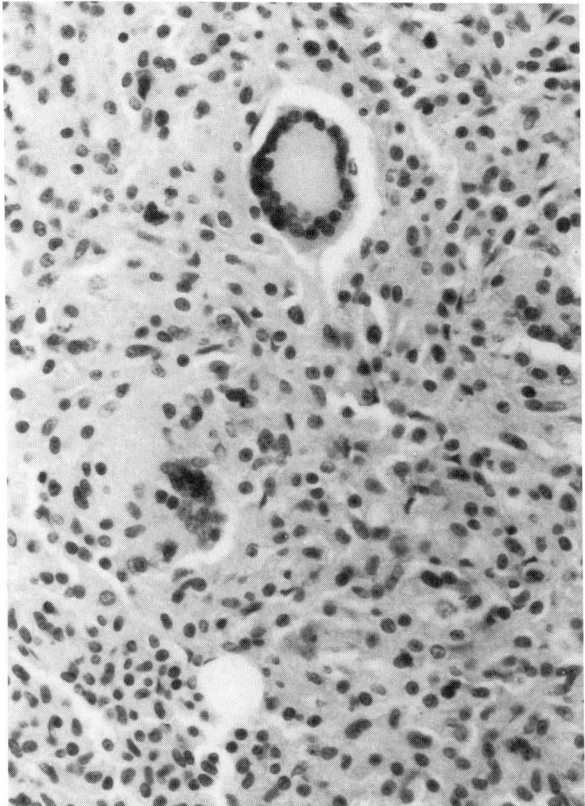

FIG. 8. Histiocytic sarcoma in Wistar rat.

gram (NTP), 35 of 354 (10%), chemicals evaluated positive as carcinogenic in rats had the hematopoietic system as a target organ. In mice, 39 of 229 chemicals tested showed this result (44).

The induction of hematopoietic tumors is also known in humans. This is a phenomenon seen especially as a late side effect after antitumor treatment (47,48). Acute nonlymphocytic leukemia is, among other tumors, a common consequence of antitumor treatment. One compound, to which this risk has been linked, is cyclophosphamide (49,50). Another agent, melphalan, has also been shown to induce lymphoid tumors, even with a higher potency than cyclophosphamide (51). Another well-known human hematopoietic carcinogen is benzene. Epidemiological studies found that chronic exposure to high concentrations of benzene resulted in a higher incidence of leukemia in some exponents, next to a more generalized bone marrow disorder (52,53). Although benzene as an hematopoietic carcinogen in humans is beyond doubt, the induction of leukemia in experimental animals has not been convincing, even though the bone marrow is a target organ of toxicity (54).

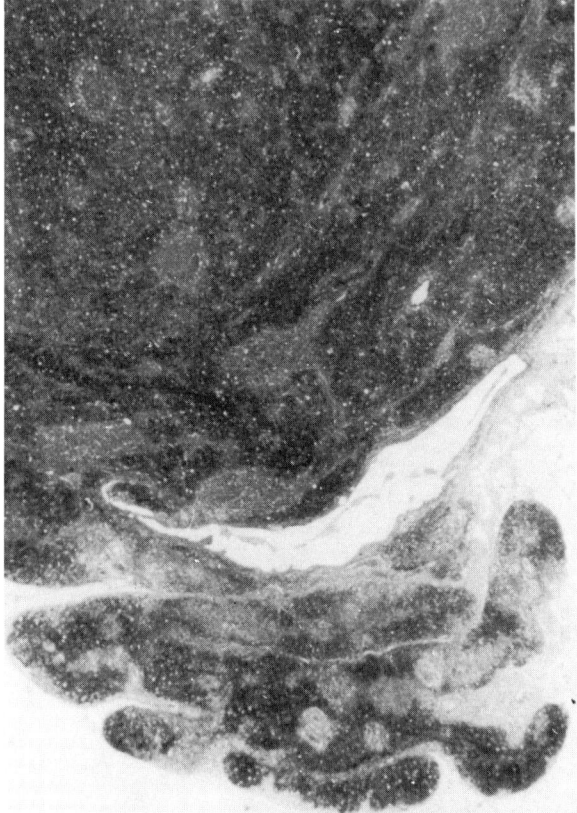

FIG. 9. Benign thymoma in Wistar rat.

Two other drugs associated with hematopoietic cancers in humans are phenytoin and chloramphenicol. Chronic phenytoin use is associated with a marginal increase in the incidence of non-Hodgkin's lymphomas (55,56). In mouse carcinogenicity studies, phenytoin also showed an increased incidence of lymphoreticular neoplasms. The animal studies for chloramphenicol are not adequate (54).

RADIATION-INDUCED HEMATOPOIETIC TUMORS

Radiation is a well-known cause of hematopoietic cancer in both animals and humans. Electromagnetic (x-rays, gamma rays) and particulate (α- and β-particles, protons, neutrons) radiation are all carcinogenic (1). All types of ionizing radiation induce hematopoietic tumors in mice after whole-body radiation. A wide range of susceptibility exists between the various strains of mice. Like chemicals, radiation most commonly induces thymic lymphomas and granulocytic leukemia. In radiation

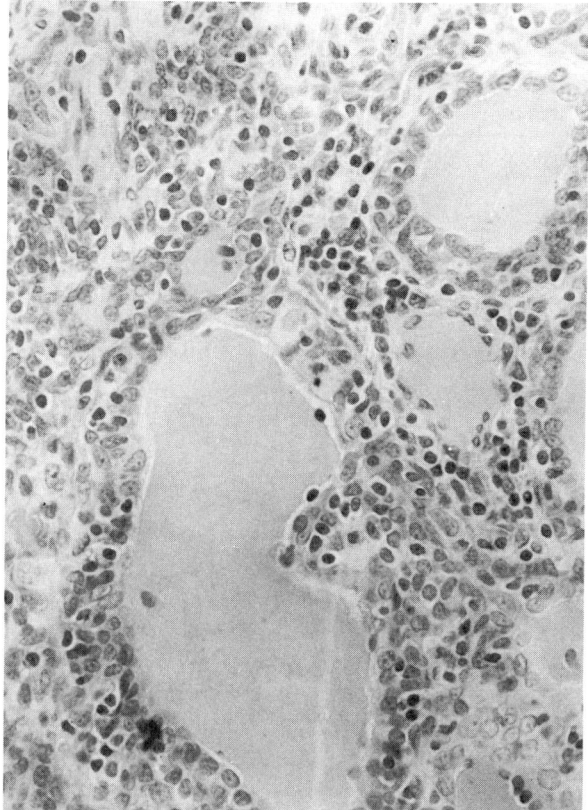

FIG. 10. Hyperplasia epithelial tubules and cords in Wistar rat.

model systems, the age and doses also determine whether lymphomas or myeloid leukemias are induced preferentially (57,58). Lymphomas are more readily induced in young mice of less than 1 month of age, while myeloid leukemias are more frequent after radiation treatment at a later age, greater than approximately 2 months (59,60). Cell-free preparation of radiation-induced lymphomas and myeloid leukemias are able to reproduce the disease in the susceptible models, indicating a role for viral involvement (61). The susceptibility for radiation induced tumors in most cases is linked to the presence of endogenous retroviral background of the mouse strains. The studies of induction of hematopoietic tumors in rats were not as successful as in mice (62).

The induction of hematopoietic tumors in humans was most tragically demonstrated in the studies that followed the survivors of the atomic bombs in Japan. They showed a marked increase in the incidence of hematopoietic tumors. Acute and chronic myelocytic leukemias, especially were frequently seen after an average latent period of 7 years. Decades later, the leukemia risk in this population is still

TABLE 3. Chemicals found to be associated with a higher incidence of hematopoietic tumors in a large-scale bioassay program[a]

	Mice		Rats	
Chemical	Male	Female	Male	Female
Acetaminophen (4-hydroxyacetanilide)	−	−	−	±
Allyl isovalerate	−	+ +	+ +	−
2-Aminoanthraquinone	+ +	+ +	+ +	IS
2-Amino-5-nitrothiazole	−	−	+ +	−
11-Aminoundcanoic acid	±	−	+ +	−
Ampicillin trihydrate	−	−	±	−
5-Azacytidine	IS	+ +	IS	IS
Benzene	+	+	+	+
Bisphenol A	−	−	±	−
1,3-Butadiene	+	+		
Butyl benzyl phthalate	−	−	IS	+ +
Chloraminated water	−	−	−	±
Chlorinated paraffins: C12, 60% chlorine	+	+	+	+
Chlorinated paraffins: C12, 43% chlorine	+	±	−	±
Chlorinated water	−	−	−	±
CI Acid Red 114			+	+
CI Basic Red 9 monohydrachloride	+	+	+	+
CI Direct Blue 15			+	+
CI Disperse Yellow 3	−	+ +	+ +	−
CI Vat Yellow 4	+ +	−	−	−
Diallyl phthalate	±	±	−	±
2,4-Diaminotoluene	−	+ +	+ +	+ +
2,7-Dichlorodibenzo-p-dioxin	±	−	−	−
Dichlorvos	±	+	±	±
3,3′-Dimethoxybenzidine-4,4′-diisocyanate	−	−	+ +	+ +
3,3′-Dimethylbenzidine dihydrochloride			+	+
Dimethyl methylphosphonate	IS	−	±	−
Dimethyl morpholinophosphoramidate	−	−	±	±
Estradiol mustard	+ +	+ +	−	−
Ethylene oxide	+	+		
Furan	+	+	+	+
Glycidol	+	+	+	+
Hydroquinone	−	±	±	±
ICRF-159	−	+ +	−	+ +
Iodinated glycerol	−	±	±	−
IPD (3,3′-iminobis-1-propanol dimethanesulfonate)	±	±	±	±
Isophorone	±	−	±	−
Isophosphamide	−	+ +	−	+ +
Lasiocarpine			+ +	+ +
2-Mercaptobenzothiazole	−	±	±	±
4,4′-Methylenedianiline dihydrochloride	+ +	+ +	+ +	+ +
Mirex			+	+
Phenesterin	+ +	+ +	−	+ +
Procarbazine hydrochloride	+ +	+ +	+ +	+ +
Propyl gallate	±	−	±	−
Tetrachloroethylene	+	+	+	±
2,4,6-Trichlorophenol	+ +	+ +	+ +	−
Tris(aziridinyl)phosphine sulfide	+ +	+ +	+ +	+ +
Tris(2-chloroethyl) phosphate	±	±	+	+

From Huff et al. (43).
[a] IS, inadequate study; + +, positive; +, clear evidence; ±, equivocal/some evidence; −, negative.

higher than average (63). Even therapeutic irradiation has proven to be carcinogenic. The previous practice of radiation of the spine affected with ankylosing spondylitis yielded a 10- to 12-fold higher risk for the development of leukemias 10 to 12 years later (64,65).

VIRAL-INDUCED HEMATOPOIETIC TUMORS

Several viruses are associated with the causation of tumors of the hematopoietic system in both humans and animals. Much of our knowledge of oncogenic viruses is derived from studies of murine lymphomas and leukemias. Inbred strains of mice have marked differences in the incidence of leukemias and lymphomas. The AKR strain, for example, shows a high incidence, while the C3H strain has a relatively low incidence. Viral-induced hematopoietic tumors in mice were one of the first model systems in this area of research. It is now known that several retroviruses are integrated in the mouse DNA as DNA proviruses. These proviruses are transmitted vertically from parents to offspring. Provirus expression leading to lymphoma or leukemia depends on various factors, one of which is the susceptibility of the hosts to viral infection (66).

The viruses known to induce hematopoietic tumors in mice turned out to be mostly retroviruses. Most of them belong morphologically to the C-type viruses. The particular type of tumor induced may, however, be influenced by factors such as strain, age, and route of inoculation. The virus isolated by Gross (67) causes the development of mostly thymic lymphomas after inoculation of newborn mice. The same virus inoculated in newborn thymectomized C3H mice leads to the development of granulocytic leukemia. The virus isolated by Friend and Rauscher induces erythroblastic leukemia. Other viruses, such as the Graffi virus, may also induce different types of lymphatic tumors, depending on the strain, age, and experimental manipulation. Thymectomy in this model system also increases the incidence of granulocytic leukemia. This virus is also able to induce histiocytic sarcomas. Thymic grafting in thymectomized mice after inoculation restored the susceptibility to lymphatic tumor induction. Not only thymic lymphomas are induced. Other viruses, such as the Abelson virus, caused lymphoma of the bone marrow (46).

The isolation of viruses and the induction of tumors by cell-free filtrates was less successful in rats compared to mice in spontaneous or induced hematopoietic tumors. On the other hand, the inoculation of mouse-derived viruses in rats was often successful and led almost always to thymic lymphoma development. The yield of granulocytic tumors was low and partially dependent on the presence of a thymus (62).

In humans, viruses are also known to be associated with the development of hematopoietic tumors. For two virus groups this relationship is firmly established. One, the Epstein–Barr virus (EBV), is a herpes virus, the other is the retrovirus, human T-cell leukemia virus I and II (HTLV-I and HTLV-II). The EBV viral infection is associated primarily with a B-cell lymphoma, which is the most common childhood tumor in Central Africa and New Guinea, but also with T-lymphoma

(68). In the vast majority of cases the DNA of the tumor contains EBV-viral genome sequences. However, the EBV virus is not limited to those geographic areas. EBV is present worldwide. The virus has a trophism for B-cells. Infection is frequently asymptomatic, but EBV is known to cause infectious mononucleosis. It is therefore likely that EBV is a major factor in the development of Burkitt's lymphoma, but that other factors, such as concomitant malaria infection, are also important in the probably multistep process (1) or immunosuppression (see the following section, on immunity and hematopoietic tumors). Another herpes virus associated with cutaneous T-lymphocyte proliferation is the human B-lymphotropic virus or human herpes virus-6 (69).

The HTLV-I virus is a human retrovirus. It is associated with a T-cell lymphoma/leukemia which is found in certain areas of Japan and the West Indies. Like the AIDS virus, it has a strong trophism for CD4 lymphocytes, but it also infects other T-cells. In addition, the HTLV-II virus can also infect B-cells. The HTLV-II virus is more associated with intravenous drug abuse. It has been linked to a small number of cases in the United States and Europe of hairy-cell leukemia, chronic T4-cell lymphoma, and chronic T-cell lymphocytic leukemia (70).

IMMUNITY AND HEMATOPOIETIC TUMORS

The function of the immune system in the pathogenesis of hematopoietic tumors seems paradoxical. Both inhibition and stimulation of the immune system can lead to a higher incidence of hematopoietic tumors, most notably lymphomas. Experimental studies in rodents and clinical studies in humans showed that suppression of the immune system with immunosuppressant drugs such as cyclosporine leads to a higher incidence of lymphomas as well as other tumors (47,71,72). Also, the induction of lymphomas by antitumor drugs has been postulated to be due partially to their immunosuppressive effects. The tumor-enhancing effects of inhibition of the immune system (T-cells) is also seen with AIDS. One of the tumors that is found in high frequency in chronic AIDS patients are lymphomas (73,74). Also, in congenital immunodeficiencies, such as the Wiskott–Aldrich syndrome, there is a high risk of developing malignant lymphomas (75).

Many non-Hodgkin's lymphomas that occur in patients with a suppressed immune system have an EBV etiology, including tumors occurring after bone marrow or organ (heart, kidney, etc.) transplantations, after infection with human immunodeficiency virus (AIDS lymphoma), or in patients with congenital immunodeficiency. In the group of Burkitt-type lymphomas about 60% have an EBV etiology. This is virtually 100% in posttransplantation lymphomas. Also, in Hodgkin's lymphomas an EBV etiology has been claimed based on expression of EBV components in Sternberg–Reed cells.

An extreme example of EBV-associated malignancy is the X-linked lymphoproliferative syndrome, where the defective host response to EBV is associated with an EBV-induced lymphoid malignancy (17,68). On the other hand, it is known that prolonged stimulation of the immune system may also lead to an increased risk of developing lymphoid tumors. This is true in rodents as well as in humans. In rodents this is demonstrated by the induction of malignant B-cell lymphomas by a graft-versus-host reaction in mice (76). Chronic infection of mycoplasm in rats is associated with a higher incidence of lymphomas, especially in the peribronchial lymphocytic tissues (62). Also in humans, the immunological stimulation provided by a concominant infection with malaria is thought to be a major factor in the development of Burkitt's lymphoma (1).

NUTRITION AND OTHER FACTORS IN HEMATOPOIETIC TUMORS

The incidence of hematopoietic tumors is influenced by a variety of factors in rodent carcinogenicity studies. The prevalence of lymphoma often varies between studies in control mice of the same strain housed under similar conditions (77–79). One major factor may be diet. Tucker (79) showed that diet restriction in mice led to a reduction in tumors of the hematopoietic system. This effect can also be shown in experimental models with induction of hematopoietic tumors by whole-body radiation. Fifty percent of the control group, fed an ad libitum diet, developed leukemia, while only 3% of the mice on a restricted diet developed this condition (80). Other factors, also shown to be of influence, are magnesium deficiency and cage size and shelving (81,82).

There appears to exist a negative correlation between nodular liver lesions and the occurrence of malignant lymphoma in both rats and mice. Animals without malignant lymphoma appear to have a higher incidence of hepatocellular tumors, which is not due entirely to lymphoma-induced early deaths (82).

MECHANISMS OF INDUCTION OF HEMATOPOIETIC TUMORS

The models of hematopoietic tumors in mice have been fundamental in the understanding of the development of tumors. Our understanding of the process of carcinogenesis has made tremendous progress with the development of molecular biological methods, but is still limited (83). This limited insight is amply demonstrated in the sometimes emotional discussions on the validity of carcinogenicity tests in rodents (84–86). In these discussions on carcinogenesis, the main issues are the role of mutagenesis and mitogenesis. Other key characteristics of carcinogenesis are the multistep process, role of oncogenic viruses, oncogenes, and karyotypes.

The role of mutagenesis and mitogenesis is emphasized by the fact that mitosis is the moment in the cell cycle that is inherently prone to mutations and initiating lesions (1,87). It is not only the sequence in the cell cycle, which is most sensitive to external influences such as chemicals and radiation, but it is also the critical period in the normal cell cycle and source of endogenous carcinogenesis (88). This explains why radiation and many chemical carcinogens are potent carcinogens for the hematopoietic system. This organ system is one of the most proliferative in the body. Lymphomas may be induced more frequently in young animals than in old animals based on the higher mitotic rate due to development of the lymphoid organs at early life. Mitogenesis is also likely to be a factor in the stimulation of the immune system as a contributory factor in the development of lymphoid tumors as postulated in Burkitt's lymphoma. Mitogenesis is therefore an important factor in the process of carcinogenesis as it increased the period of potential sensitivity to internal and external mutagens and may function as an important factor in tumor promotion.

Our current concepts of carcinogenesis describe this as a multistep process. The process is divided into initiation, promotion, and progression. These processes are also found in the carcinogenesis of the hematopoietic system. After the initiating effect, as seen in radiation, carcinogen treatment, or viral infection, there is a lag phase after which the tumors occur. During this phase, tumor promotion takes place (89,90).

The mutagenic processes in the initiation phase leading to tumor formation do not happen haphazardly but are linked to certain genes called the *oncogenes*. These were first detected in studies that led to their name, with the idea that their activation is a carcinogenic signal with leukemia and other retroviruses. Later it was found that many normal cells also contain DNA fragments, which are very similar to these viral oncogenes (91). These *protooncogenes* may become oncogenic by viral infection or mutagenic processes caused by, for example, radiation and chemical carcinogens. These mutations activate the protooncogene sequences into cellular oncogenes. The latter genes act dominantly to convert normal cells to transformed or malignant cells. These (proto)oncogenes also have a more general role in the differentiation and proliferation of the cell (92). Most oncogene products are growth factors necessary for normal growth and homeostasis. The oncogenes can be divided into several groups, such as protein kinases (*src, yes, abl*), GTP-binding proteins (*ras*), growth factors or their receptors (*sis, int, erb*-B), nuclear proteins (*myc, fos*), and others for which the role is still unknown (e.g., *met, raf*). Their association in hematopoietic and other tumors has been amply demonstrated (93–98). The oncogene *myc*, for example, has been associated with human Burkitt's lymphoma and mouse B-cell lymphomas (99). On the other hand, c-*myc* is necessary for the normal physiologic differentiation and proliferation in normal germinal centers of the peripheral lymphoid tissues. Some *onc* genes are rearranged in specific types of non-Hodgkin's lymphoma (e.g., *bcl*-2 in follicular lymphoma).

Next to these oncogenes other gene sequences were detected that inhibited the expression of the oncogenes; these gene sequences are termed *oncosuppressor genes* or *anti-oncogenes* (100–102). Interactions between oncogenes have been shown in studies with transgenic mice. These interactions are also important in the induction of hematopoietic tumors with either viruses or carcinogens (103,104).

Many tumors share a common karyotypic change, such as the Ph-chromosome in CML and the translocation seen in Burkitt's lymphoma. These karyotypic changes are caused by mutations and are often associated with the activation of particular oncogenes. Other changes include chromosomal deletions or cytogenetic manifestations of gene amplification (1).

REFERENCES

1. Cotran RS, Kumar V, Robbins SL. *Robbins pathologic basis of disease*. Philadelphia: WB Saunders; 1989.
2. Bernard A, Boumsell L, Dausset J, Milstein C, Schlossman SF, eds. *Leucocyte typing: human leucocyte differentiation antigens detected by monoclonal antibodies*. Berlin, Springer-Verlag; 1984.
3. Knapp W, Dörken B, Gilks WR, Rieber EP, Schmidt RE, Stein H, von dem Borne ADGKr, eds. *Leucocyte typing IV: white cell differentiation antigens*. Oxford: Oxford University Press; 1989.
4. McMichael AJ, et al, eds. *Leucocyte typing III*. Oxford: Oxford University Press; 1987.
5. Reinherz EL, Haynes BF, Nadler LM, Bernstein ID, eds. *Leucocyte typing II*. Vol 1. *Human T lymphocytes*. Vol 2. *Human B lymphocytes*. Vol 3. *Human myeloid and hematopoietic cells*. Berlin, Springer-Verlag; 1986.
6. Deegan MJ. Membrane antigen analysis in the diagnosis of lymphoid leukemias and lymphomas. Differential diagnosis, prognosis as related to immunophenotype, and recommendations for testing. *Arch Pathol Lab Med* 1989;113:606–618.
7. Foon KA, Todd RF III. Immunologic classification of leukemia and lymphoma. *Blood* 1986;68:1–31.
8. Greaves MF, Chan LC, Furley AJW, Watt SM, Molgaard HV. Lineage promiscuity in hemopoietic differentiation and leukemia. *Blood* 1986;67:1–11.
9. Rappaport H. Tumours of the hematopoietic system. In: *Atlas of tumour pathology*. Section 3, fascicle 8. Washington DC: US Armed Forces Institute of Pathology; 1966.
10. Berard CW, Dorfman RF. Histopathology of malignant lymphomas. In: Rosenberg SA, ed. *Clinics in hematology*. Vol 3, no 1. London: WB Saunders; 1974;39.
11. Lukes RJ, Collins RD. New approaches to the classification of lymphomata. *Br J Cancer* 1975;31 [Suppl 2]:1–28.
12. Jaffe ES. Lymph nodes, reactive and neoplastic conditions. In: Zucker-Franklin D, Greaves MF, Grossi CE, Marmont AM, eds. *Atlas of blood cells*. Vol 2. *Function and pathology*. Stuttgart: Gustav Fischer Verlag; 1988:549–598.
13. Picker LJ, Weiss LM, Medeiros LJ, Wood GS, Warnke RA. Immunophenotypic criteria for the diagnosis of non-Hodgkin's lymphoma. *Am J Pathol* 1987;128:181–201.
14. Stein H, Lennert K, Feller AC, Mason DY. Immunohistological analysis of human lymphoma. Correlation of histological and immunological categories. *Adv Cancer Res* 1984;42:67–147.
15. Sun T, Susin M. A practical approach to immunophenotyping of lymphomas. Comparison of immunohistologic and immunocytologic techniques. *Ann Clin Lab Sci* 1987;17:14–26.
16. Tubbs RR, Fishleder A, Weiss RA, Savage RA, Sebek BA, Weick JK. Immunohistologic cellular phenotypes of lymphoproliferative disorders. Comprehensive evaluation of 564 cases including 257 non-Hodgkin's lymphomas classified by the International Working Formulation. *Am J Pathol* 1983;113:207–221.
17. Schuurman H-J, Henzen-Logmans S, Kluin PhM. Non-Hodgkin's lymphomas. In: Sell S, ed. *Clinical cancer markers: diagnosis, prognosis and monitoring*. Totowa, NJ: Humana Press; 1994 [in press].
18. Lennert K, Mohri N. In: Lennert K, ed. *Histopathology and diagnosis of non-Hodgkin's lymphomas: malignant lymphomas other than Hodgkin's disease*. Berlin, Springer-Verlag; 1978:111–469.
19. Rosenberg SA, Berard CW, Brown BW, et al. National Cancer Institute sponsored study of classification of non-Hodgkin's lymphomas: summary and description of a Working Formulation for clinical usage. *Cancer* 1982;49:2112–2136.
20. Delellis RA. Thymus. In: Cotran RS, Kumar V, Robbins SL, eds. *Robbins pathologic basis of disease*. Philadelphia: WB Saunders; 1989:1268–1271.
21. Ashley DJB. Tumours of the thymus. In: Ashley DJB, ed. *Evans' histological appearances of tumours*. Edinburgh: Churchill Livingstone; 1990:239–248.
22. Müller-Hermelink HK, Kirchner T. The diagnosis of thymic epithelial tumors. In: Sarrazin R, Vrousos C, Vincent F, eds. *Thymic tumors*. Basel: S Karger; 1989:37–44.
23. Pattengale PK, Taylor CR. Experimental models of lymphoproliferative disease: the mouse as a model for human non-Hodgkin's lymphomas and related leukemias. *Am J Pathol* 1983;113:237–265.
24. Harleman JH, Jahn W. A morphologic classification of hematopoietic tumors, rats. In: Jones TC, Ward JM, Mohr U, Hunt RD, eds. *Hemopoietic system*. Berlin: Springer-Verlag; 1990:149–154.

25. Wogan GN, Clayson DB, Rapp F. Tumours of the mouse hematopoietic system: their diagnosis and interpretation in safety evaluation tests. Report of a study group. *CRC Crit Rev Toxicol* 1984; 13:161–181.
26. Ward JM, Rehm S, Reynolds CW. Tumours of the haematopoietic system. In: Turusov VS, ed. *Pathology of tumours in laboratory animals.* vol 1. *Tumours of the rat.* Lyon; France: International Agency for Research on Cancer; 1990:625–658.
27. Pattengale PK, Frith CH. Contribution of recent research to the classification of spontaneous lymphoid cell neoplasms in mice. *CRC Crit Rev Toxicol* 1986;16:185–212.
28. Stromberg PC, Vogtsberger M. Pathology of the mononuclear cell leukemia of Fischer rats. I. Morphological studies. *Vet Pathol* 1983;20:698–708.
29. Losco PE, Ward JM. The early stage of large granular lymphocytic leukemia in the F344 rat. *Vet Pathol* 1984;21:286–291.
30. Faccini JM, Abbott DP, Paulus GJJ. *Mouse histopathology: a glossary for use in toxicology and carcinogenicity studies.* Amsterdam: Elsevier; 1990.
31. Tuch K, Puschner H. Personal communication. 1991.
32. Lewis DJ, Offer JM. Malignant mastocytoma in mice. *J Comp Pathol* 1984;94:615–620.
33. Barsoum NJ, Hanna W, Gough AW, Smith GS, Sturgess JM, de la Inglesia FA. Histiocytic sarcoma in Wistar rats. *Arch Pathol Lab Med* 1984;108:802–807.
34. Wright JA, Goonetilleke UR, Waghe M, Horne M, Stewart MG. An immunohistochemical study of spontaneous histiocytic tumour in the rat. *J Comp Pathol* 1991;104:223–232.
35. Squire RA, Brinkous KM, Peiper SC, Grominger HI, Mann RB, Strandberg JD. Histiocytic sarcoma with a granuloma-like component occurring in a large colony of Sprague–Dawley rats. *Am J Pathol* 1981;105:21–30.
36. Greaves MF. Fibrous histiocytoma, malignant, subcutis, rat. Integument and mammary glands. In: Jones TC, Mohr U, Hunt RD, eds. *Monographs on pathology of laboratory animals.* New York: Springer-Verlag; 1989:66–112.
37. Kuper CF, Beems RB. Thymoma, epithelial, rat. Hematopoietic system. In: Jones TC, Ward JM, Mohr U, Hunt RD, eds. *Monographs on pathology of laboratory animals.* New York: Springer-Verlag; 1990:280–286.
38. Naylor DC, Krinke GJ, Ruefenacht HJ. Primary tumors of the thymus in the rat. *J Comp Pathol* 1988;99:187–203.
39. Kuper CF, Beems RB, Hollanders VMH. Spontaneous pathology of the thymus in aging Wistar (Cpb:Wu) rats. *Vet Pathol* 1986;23:270–277.
40. Abbott DP, Cherry CP. Malignant mixed thymic tumor with metastasis in a rat. *Vet Pathol* 1982; 19:721–723.
41. Matsuyama M, Suzuki H, Yamada S, Ito M, Nagayo T. Ultrastucture of spontaneous and urethane-induced thymomas in buffalo rats. *Cancer Res* 1975;35:2771–2779.
42. Cherry CP, Eisenstein R, Glucksmann A. Epithelial cords and tubules of the rat thymus. Effect of age, sex, castration, thyroid and other hormones and their incidence and secretory activity. *Br J Exp Pathol* 1966;48:90–106.
43. Huff J, Cirvello J, Haseman J, Bucher J. Chemicals associated with site specific neoplasia in 1394 long-term carcinogenesis experiments in laboratory rodents. *Environ Health Perspect* 1991;93: 247–270.
44. Gold LS, Slone TH, Manley NB, Bernstein L. Target organs in chronic bioassays of 533 chemical carcinogens. *Environ Health Perspect* 1991;93:233–246.
45. Pietra G, Spencer K, Shubrik P. Response of newly born mice to a carcinogen. *Nature* 1959; 183: 1689.
46. Della-Porta G, Chieco-Bianchi L, Penelli N. Tumours of the haematopoietic system. In: Turusov VS, ed. *Pathology of tumours in laboratory animals.* Vol 2. *Tumours of the mouse.* Lyon; France: International Agency for Research on Cancer, 1979;527–576.
47. Penn I. The occurrence of malignant tumors in immunosuppressed states. *Prog Allergy* 1986;37: 259–300.
48. Travis B, Curtis RE, Boice JD, Hankey BF, Fraumeni JF. Second cancers following non-Hodgkin's lymphoma. *Cancer* 1991;62:2002–2009.
49. Green MH, Young RC, Merrill JM, DeVita VT. Evidence of a treatment dose response in acute non-lymphocytic leukemia which occurs after therapy of non-Hodgkin's lymphoma. *Cancer Res* 1983;40:1891–1896.
50. Pedersen S, Bjergaard J, Ersboll J, Sorensen HM, et al. Risk of acute nonlymphocytic leukemia and preleukemia in patients treated with cyclophosphamide for non-Hodgkin's lymphoma. *Ann Intern Med* 1985;103:195–200.

51. Green MH, Harris EL, Gershenson DM, Malkasian GD, Melton LJ, Dembo AJ, Bennett JM, Moloney WS, Boice JD. Melphalan may be a more potent leukemogen than cyclophosphamide. *Ann Intern Med* 1986; 105:360–367.
52. Snyder R, Kocsis JJ. Current concept of chronic benzene toxicity. *CRC Crit Rev Toxicol* 1975; 3:265–288.
53. Vigliani EC, Forni A. Benzene and leukemia. *Environ Res* 1976;11:122–127.
54. Ayers PH, Taylor WD. Solvents. In: Hayes AW, ed. *Principles and methods of toxicology*. New York: Raven Press; 1989:111–135.
55. Vardiman JW, Variakojis D. The hematopoietic system. In: Riddell RH, ed. *Pathology of drug induced and toxic disease*. New York: Churchill Livingstone; 1982:87–118.
56. Shu XO, Luet MS, Goor N, et al. Chloramphenicol use and childhood leukemia in Shanghai. *Lancet* 1987;2:934–937.
57. Kaplan HS. Influence of age and susceptibility of mice to the development of lymphoid tumor after irradiation. *J Natl Cancer Inst* 1948;9:55–56.
58. Covelli V, Di Majo V, Coppola M, Rebessi S. The dose response relationship for myeloid leukemia and malignant lymphoma in BC3F1 mice. *Radiat Res* 1989;119:553–561.
59. Major IR. Induction of myeloid leukemia by whole body single exposure of CBA male mice to x-rays. *Br J Cancer* 1979;40:903–913.
60. Wolman SR, McMorrow LE, Cohen MW. Animal model of human disease: myelogeneous leukemia in the RF-mouse. *Am J Pathol* 1982;107:280–284.
61. Kaplan HS. On the natural history of murine leukemias. Presidential address. *Cancer Res* 1967; 27:1325–1340.
62. Swaen GJV, van Heerde P. Tumours of the hematopoietic system. In: Turusov VS, ed. *Pathology of tumours in laboratory animals*. Vol 1. *Tumours of the rat*. Lyon, France: International Agency for Research on Cancer; 1973:185–201.
63. Kohn HI, Fry RJM. Radiation carcinogenesis. *N Engl J Med* 1984;310:504.
64. Walter JB, Israel MS. The effects of ionizing radiation. In: Walter JB, Israel MS, eds. *General Pathology*. Edinburgh: Churchill Livingstone; 1974:408–417.
65. Mole RH, Major IR. Myeloid leukemia frequency after protracted exposure to ionizing radiation: experimental confirmation of the flat dose response found in ankylosing spondylitis after a single treatment course with x-rays. *Leuk Res* 1983;7:295–300.
66. Wyke JA. Oncogenic viruses. *J Pathol* 1981;135:39–45.
67. Gross L. Development of myeloid (chloro-) leukemia in thyrectomized C3H mice following inocculation of lymphatic leukemia virus. *Proc Soc Exp Biol* 1960;103:509–514.
68. Su I-J, Hsieh H-C, Lin K-H, Uen W-C, Kao C-L, Chen C-J, Cheng A-L, Kadin M, Chen J-Y. Aggressive peripheral T-cell lymphomas containing Epstein–Barr viral DNA: a clinicopathologic and molecular analysis. *Blood* 1991;77:799–808.
69. Biberfeld P, Kramarsky B, Saluhuddin SZ, Gallo RC. Ultrastructural characterization of a new human B lymphotropic DNA virus (human herpesvirus 6) isolated from patients with lymphoproliferative disease. *J Natl Cancer Inst* 1987;79:933–941.
70. Nerurkar LS, Gallo RC. Human retroviruses: Cancer and AIDS. *Int J Cancer* 1989;Suppl 4: 2–5.
71. Shinozuka H, Hattori A, Gill TJ, Kunz HW. Experimental models of malignancy after cyclosporin therapy. *Transplant Proc* 1988;22:893–899.
72. Kripke ML. Immunoregulation of carcinogenesis: past, present, and future. *J Natl Cancer Inst* 1988;80:722–727.
73. Reichert CM, O'Leary TJ, Levens DL, Simrell CR, Macher AM. Autopsy pathology in the acquired immune deficiency syndrome. *Am J Pathol* 1983;112:357–382.
74. Jaffe ES, Clark J, Steis R, et al. Lymph node pathology of HTLV and HTLV-associated neoplasms. *Cancer Res* 1985;45:4662–4664.
75. Cotelingan JD, Witebsky FG, Blaese RM, Jaffe ES. Malignant lymphoma in patients with the Wiskott–Alrich syndrome. *Cancer Invest* 1985;3:515.
76. Pals ST, Zijlstra M, Radaszkiewicz Th, et al. Immunologic induction of malignant lymphoma: graft-vs-host reaction induced B-cell lymphoma contain integrations of predominantly ecotropic murine leukemia proviruses. *J Immunol* 1986;136:331–339.
77. Clayson DB. Modulation of the incidence of murine leukemia and lymphoma. *CRC Crit Rev Toxicol* 1984;13:183–195.
78. Faccini JM, Irisarri E, Monro AM. A carcinogenicity study in mice of a beta-adrenergic antagonist primidolol: increased total tumour incidence without tissue specificity. *Toxicology* 1981;21:279–290.

79. Tucker M. Effect of diet on spontaneous disease in the inbred mouse strain C57B1/10J. *Toxicol Lett* 1975;25:131–135.
80. Gross L. Inhibition of the development of tumors or leukemia in mice and rats after reduction of food intake. *Cancer* 1988;62:1463–1465.
81. Greenman DL, Kodell RL, Sheldon WG. Association between cage shelf level and spontaneous and induced neoplasms in mice. *J Natl Cancer Inst* 1984;73:107–113.
82. Greaves MF. *Histopathology of preclinical toxicity studies.* Amsterdam: Elsevier; 1990.
83. Cline MJ. Biology of disease. Molecular diagnosis of human cancer. *Lab Invest* 1989;61:368–380.
84. Ames BN. Carcinogenesis mechanism: the debate continues. *Science* 1991;252:902.
85. Cohen SM, Ellwein LB. Carcinogenesis mechanism: the debate continues. *Science* 1991;252:902–903.
86. Perera F, Rall D, Weinstein IB. Carcinogenesis mechanism: the debate continues. *Science* 1991;252:903–904.
87. Weisburger JH, Williams GM. Chemical carcinogens. In: Doull J, Klaassen CD, Amdur MO, eds. *Casarett and Doull's toxicology: the basic science of poisons.* New York: Macmillan; 1980:84–138.
88. Loeb L. Endogenous carcinogenesis; molecular oncology into the twenty-first century: presidential address. *Cancer Res* 1989;49:5489–5496.
89. Boniver J, Humblet, C, Rongy AM, et al. Cellular aspects of the pathogenesis of radiation-induced thymic lymphomas in C57B1-mice (review). *In Vivo* 1990;4:41–44.
90. Weinberg RA. Oncogenes, antioncogenes and the molecular bases of multistep carcinogenesis. *Cancer Res* 1989;49:3713–3721.
91. Kaczmarek L. Protooncogene expression during the cell cycle. *Lab Invest* 1986;54:365–376.
92. Robert-Lézènes J, Meneceur P, Ray D, Moreau-Gachelin F. Protooncogene expression in normal, preleukemic, and leukemic murine erythroid cells and its relationship to differentiation and proliferation. *Cancer Res* 1988;48:3972–3976.
93. Mitani S, Sugawara I, Shiku H, Mori S. Expression of c-*myc* oncogene product and *ras*-family products in various human malignant lymphomas defined by immunohistochemical techniques. *Cancer* 1988;62:2085–2093.
94. Preisler HD, Kinniburgh AJ, Wei-Dong G, Khan S. Expression of the protooncogenes c-*myc*, c-*fos*, and c-*fms* in acute myelocytic leukemia at diagnosis and in remission. *Cancer Res* 1987;47:874–880.
95. Muschel RJ, McKenna WG. Oncogenes and tumor progression. *Anticancer Res* 1989;9:1395–2406.
96. Bos JL. Ras oncogenes in human cancer: a review. *Cancer Res* 1989;49:4682–4689.
97. Vousden KH, Marshall CJ. Three different activated ras genes in mouse tumours; evidence for oncogene activation during progression of a mouse lymphoma. *EMBO J* 1984;3:913–997.
98. Janowski M, Cox R, Strauss PG. The molecular biology of radiation-induced carcinogenesis, thymic lymphoma, myeloid leukemia and osteosarcoma. *Int J Radiat Biol* 1990;57:677–691.
99. Goldfarb MP. The role of cellular oncogenes in cancer of non-viral etiology. In: Grunberger D, Goff SP, eds. *International encyclopedia of pharmacology and therapeutics.* Vol 126. *Mechanisms of cellular transformation by carcinogenic agents.* Oxford: Pergamon Press; 1988.
100. Schäfer R. Suppression of the neoplastic phenotype and *"anti*-oncogenes." *Blut* 1987;54:257–265.
101. Anderson MCM, Spandidos DA. Onco-suppressor genes and their involvement in cancer. *Anticancer Res* 1988;8:873–880.
102. Den Otter W, Koten JW, van der Vegt BJH, et al. Oncogenesis by mutation in *anti*-oncogenes: a view. *Anticancer Res* 1990;10:475–488.
103. Berns A, Breuer M, Verbeek S, Van Lohuizen M. Transgenic mice as a means to study synergism between oncogenes. *Int J Cancer* 1989; Suppl 4:22–25.
104. van Lohuizen M, Verbeek S, Krimpenfort P, et al. Predisposition to lymphomagenesis in pim-1 transgenic mice: Cooperation with c-*myc* and n-*myc* in murine leukemia virus-induced tumors. *Cell* 1989;56:673–682.

13
Pathology Procedures in Laboratory Animal Carcinogenesis Studies

Deborah E. Devor, *John R. Henneman, **Yasushi Kurata,
†Sabine Rehm, Christopher M. Weghorst, and ††Jerrold M. Ward

*Laboratory of Comparative Carcinogenesis, National Cancer Institute,
Frederick Cancer Research and Development Center, Frederick, Maryland 21702;
*Carcinogenesis Studies Section, Biological Carcinogenesis and
Development Program, Program Resources Inc./DynCorp, National Cancer Institute,
Frederick Cancer Research and Development Center, Frederick, Maryland 21702;
**First Department of Pathology, Nagoya City University Medical School,
Nagoya, 467, Japan; †Division of Pharmaceuticals, Toxicology U.S.,
SmithKline Beecham Pharmaceuticals, King of Prussia, Pennsylvania 19406;
††Veterinary and Tumor Pathology Section, Office of Laboratory Animal Science,
National Cancer Institute, Frederick Cancer Research and Development Center,
Frederick, Maryland 21702*

au'topsy (G. *autopsia*, seeing with one's own eyes). 1. Postmortem examination; necropsy; necroscopy; thanatopsy; an examination of the internal organs of a dead body for the purpose of determining the cause of death or of studying the pathologic changes present. *Stedman's Medical Dictionary* (1)

The development of animal models of significant human illnesses provides the unique opportunity to initiate and follow a disease process from inception to any specified endpoint. The human clinical picture is all too often that of advanced or endstage disease or the loss of subjects to follow-up because of cure or patient indifference. Carcinogenesis and toxicology studies with laboratory animals yield data not only at autopsy but throughout the experimental duration in such parameters as latency to clinical illness, diagnostic markers, early tissue changes, potential reversibility of lesions, and ultimately, opportunities for treatment and cure.

The quality and completeness of a pathology evaluation in any oncologic or toxicologic study is dependent on a number of factors. Most of the factors that come readily to mind are controllable by the investigator to varying degrees, while a few, for now, remain outside the reach of human manipulation. We may not yet be able to predict the detailed physiologic responses of any organism to exogenous chemicals or environmental agents, but we can train ourselves and those who may provide pertinent technical services for us consistently to look for, describe, and analyze in an unbiased manner any and all changes apparent in an experimental system. The autopsy is the bridge between the experimental theory and fact, but frequently, it seems to be relegated to the status of a wearisome task that must be performed before we are allowed to know the answer to the experimental question. There are any number of references on the anatomy, physiology, husbandry, and microscopic pathology of laboratory animals (2–18), but comparatively few that deal with the autopsy as an integral and pivotal phase in animal studies.

The ability to perform a thorough autopsy is a necessary skill developed with time and experience. Additional prerequisites are a working understanding of the basic anatomy and physiology of experimental species in use and fluency in descriptive terminology. The manner in which tissues are removed, preserved, and prepared directly influences the relevance and quality of the slide specimen. The state of the animal before and at autopsy in turn modulates the dissection. The condition of the animal when it comes to the necropsy board is a result not only of treatment and genetics but also the environment in which it has been housed and handled. In this chapter we do not propose to teach the detailed anatomy of laboratory animals or to expound on specific pathologies; as noted previously, there are a number of sources on those subjects. One of the purposes of this chapter is to introduce investigators and technicians to the concept of the autopsy as a vitally important component in the experimental process, one that is fundamental to the accurate determination of disease (Fig. 1). If entrusted to the untrained, inexperienced, or totally mechanical, there will be some dilution of the inherent data (19–21). A second objective is to suggest some tested autopsy and tissue preparation procedures that can be modified to fit a wide variety of protocols and which may alleviate some common technical difficulties in tissue collection.

AUTOPSY PROTOCOLS

An autopsy protocol should do more than simply list tissues to be preserved. The necropsy is part of the total experiment and must be designed as such from the beginning of study formulation. It may go through several modifications in response to developments during the course of the study, but the investigator should think through the entire procedure and not leave the necropsy up to others who, while

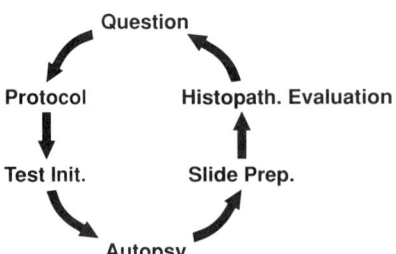

FIG. 1. Components of the experimental process.

they may perform numerous necropsies routinely, may not perform them in a way most relevant to the particular test.

Factors to consider in formulating the dissection protocol include historical records of previous studies using the same or similar chemical agents, which help to determine the appropriate endpoint as well as tissues to evaluate; experimental variables (including animal husbandry); the peculiarities of the animal species and strain selected; indirect as well as direct effects of treatment on tissues other than the "target" organ; the physical/chemical characteristics—known or suspected—of the agent(s) being tested; how the tissue specimens are to be handled; what preservative and histochemical stains will be used (19–29). The investigator may even decide to formulate an autopsy form specifically for the experiment. Examples of types of necropsy report sheets are shown in Fig. 2.

It is nearly impossible to design a study that will yield an isolated effect in one organ simply because an animal is an integrated system. However, for simplistic reasons, studies are often designed as if there will be only one or two effects of any treatment (e.g., the induction of liver tumors, with possible involvement of the lung as a preferred site of metastasis). In fact, disruption of proper liver function has profound consequences for certain other organs and several metabolic pathways; death can result from peripheral and secondary effects as well as from hepatic failure. Similarly, agents applied topically to the skin to induce dermal lesions can be absorbed and are often ingested during grooming. Thus topical applications often turn out to be more systemic in practice, and necropsies in such studies might do well to include at least an examination of internal organs, to include the entire GI tract from oral cavity to anus, in addition to the skin and subcutaneous tissues.

It is also extremely important to remember that not all animal species, strains, and even individuals within a supposedly identical population will respond in the same manner to a treatment. Another glossed-over fact in carcinogenesis and toxicological testing is that lesions other than tumors are frequently more common and may be just as significant. It is advisable to separate the two terms on paper as well as in the mind of the investigator.

Returning to the statement that the condition of the animals prior to sacrifice or death can influence the autopsy, the inclusion of clinical observations, which will be dealt with in more detail in a subsequent section, should be considered. Overall body weight and changes in organ-to-body weight ratios are indications of metabolic imbalances and possible disease states. Blood and urine values are important criteria in evaluating drug efficacy and general health. The amounts of food and water consumed and the rates of waste elimination may be useful parameters to record. Define the data to be collected well before the test is initiated.

A protocol should state the experimental endpoint, which is normally not the death of the animals, and also outline clinical conditions that would necessitate removal of animals before study termination for either palliative measures or euthanasia and necropsy. Any compromise in the health of an experimental subject, whether due to accidents in husbandry, handling, treatment or to naturally occurring disease, may confuse the interpretation of real test effects or undermine the integrity of the study (20–24,26–30).

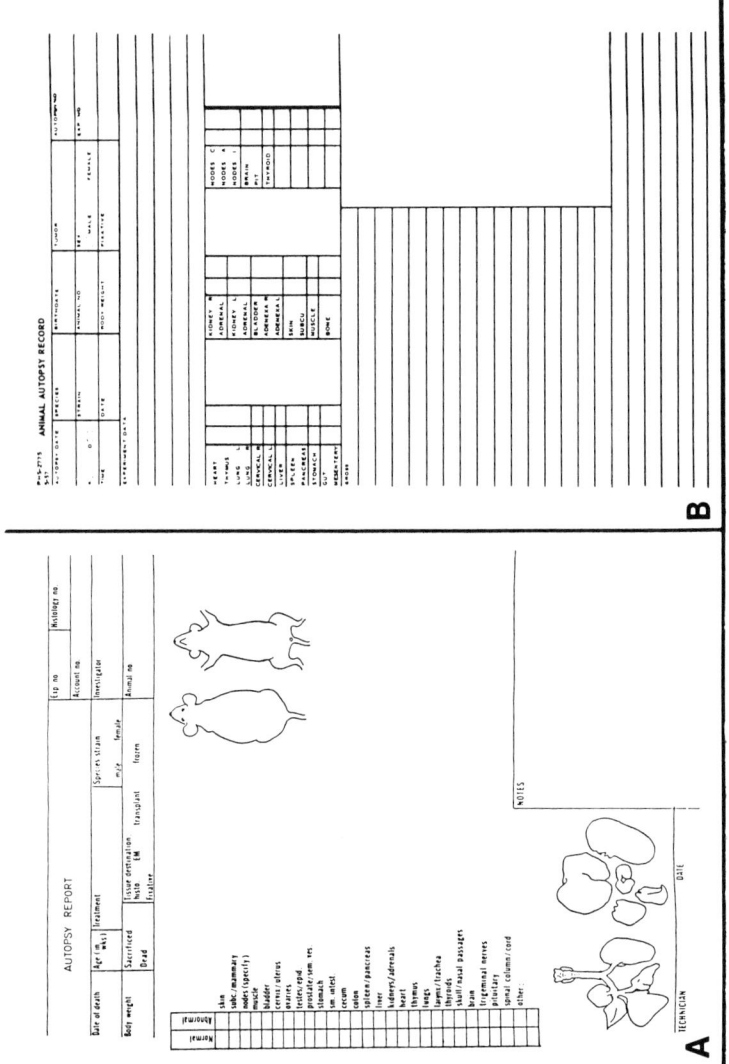

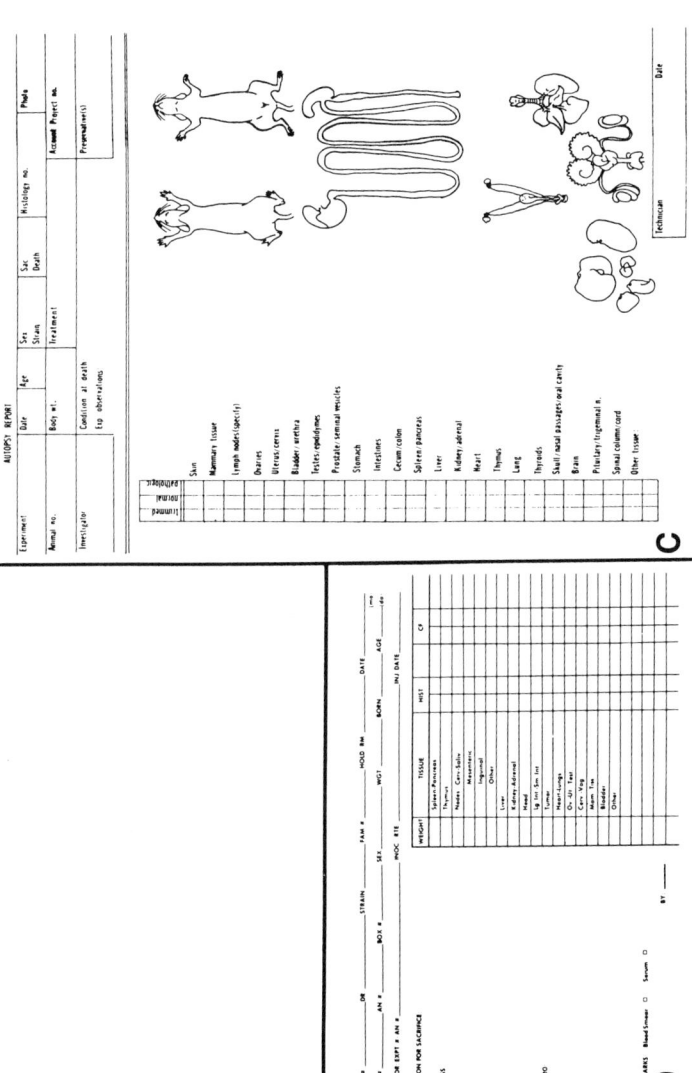

FIG. 2. Examples of autopsy forms. Note the variations in size and format. Inclusion of diagrams facilitates locating lesions. (Forms B and D courtesy of the Public Health Service.)

The method of euthanasia should also be taken into consideration as different methods produce different gross and histological artifacts (4,31,32). Depending on the expertise of personnel involved as well as the experimental purpose, some methods should be avoided altogether (31–33). For instance, pentobarbital solutions can be given intraperitoneally but are most effective and do less tissue damage administered intravenously (34,35). Smooth and humane i.v. injections, particularly in small animals, require a degree of skill that not everyone possesses or can even acquire. An intraperitoneal injection is easier; given incorrectly, however, internal organs may be punctured and ruptured. Because they are potential substrates and/or inducers of liver enzymes, use of barbiturates may not be desirable in studies concerned with hepatic biochemistry or cell morphology (35–38). Asphyxiation with CO_2 or overdose by some inhalation anesthetics can cause petechial lung hemorrhage, congestion, and changes in blood gas chemistry (31,32,38), factors that may interfere in diagnoses.

The investigator must also consider the eventual scope of the histopathological analyses. It is increasingly useful in modern pathology to augment conventional light microscopy with immunohistochemistry and molecular biology techniques. However, these protocols often require specialized tissue handling and processing procedures; autopsies may need to be done under RNAse-free conditions, for example, and utilize fixatives not commonly on hand. Organs and/or lesions may have to be equally divided among fixatives to satisfy all desired objectives and thus demand precise trimming and embedding to present equivalent sections. Will additional personnel be consulted or employed? Do arrangements have to be made to transfer materials? These types of details must be delineated early in the total experimental protocol, not as afterthoughts on the day of the terminal sacrifice.

INTERPRETING CLINICAL OBSERVATIONS

As in most animal experiments, important data are recorded long before the animal comes to the autopsy board in the daily observation of appearance and behavior (19,20,26,27). In many cases, animals show clinical signs of physiologic disease that allow the investigator to formulate an appropriate autopsy protocol or modify an existing one as the experiment progresses. These conscientiously recorded findings are relevant to the autopsy in that (a) organs and organ systems not specified in the protocol may be affected and thus deserve inspection; (b) latency, characterization, and progression of illness is annotated; and (c) accuracy and refinement of the diagnosis may be simplified. Changes in appearance and behavioral deviations, including changes in reaction to stimuli and in grooming habits, are relatively obvious (albeit subjective) observations that can be made without having to handle the animal physically and are reliable indicators of disease and adverse environmental conditions. Lethargy, kyphosis, body tremors, locomotor abnormalities, withdrawal from group activities, obsessive or repetitive movements, seizures, increased aggression, increased/decreased urination, diarrhea or constipation, changes in food and water consumption, anogenital soiling, changes in coat condition, abnormal postures—all are external signs of internal problems. All also require careful interpretation.

As examples, consider the following: "Respiratory distress" is a commonly reported phenomenon. Unfortunately, thinking only in terms of the lungs may result in missing the true etiology. Lesions of the areas of the brainstem regulating respiration or brain or pituitary tumors impinging upon those regions can also induce breathing abnormalities. Labored respiration combined with a relatively firm and immobile ribcage (abdominal breathing), in which the animal seems to be concentrating on the physical act of inhaling, is more frequently associated with intrathoracic tumor formation, obstruction, or some kind of consolidation process in the lungs and/or trachea, while an animal that chronically sneezes and paws at the nose—with or without abnormal respiratory patterns or a nasal discharge—is suspect for nasal cavity lesions. Audible respiratory efforts are indicative of fluid congestion, as found in pneumonia and pulmonary edema, and it can sometimes be felt via the ribcage or throat. A shallow, rapid respiratory pattern is usually compensatory for lack of full lung volume, but the reduction of that volume can result from compression of the thoracic cavity by enlarged abdominal organs, ascites, or masses as well as from thoracic or pulmonary causes. Cyanosis may result from any of the foregoing conditions or from the inability to fully utilize what is available due to pulmonary or cardiovascular failure or to disruption of biochemical systems.

Body weight may be the most frequently recorded clinical observation. Weight loss is a common finding in animals exposed to exogenous chemicals and stressful conditions. Interpretation of weight variations are not as straightforward as collection, requiring, among other things, knowledge of the growth characteristics of the particular species being used and the age at which weights are being recorded. Cachexia due to toxicity or tumor growth will certainly result in a weight decrease, but so will overgrown teeth; in rabbits and guinea pigs, malocclusions are a very common cause of weight loss (4,7,40). Adequate supply, palatability, and nutritional content of the food are other factors, as are dehydration and competition with cagemates. Conversely, excessive weight gain is unreported or ignored in studies. However, edema, ascites, and increases in organ as well as tumor mass are frequently marked by initial and unusual weight increase.

Routine palpations of experimental animals are occasionally necessary in studies, usually those that are concerned with organ-specific disease (e.g., lymphatic, renal, or hepatic syndromes). They are best performed by those anatomically knowledgeable and experienced; full stomachs have often been mistaken for enlarged spleens and ovarian, kidney, or liver masses. With very few exceptions (e.g., subcutaneous or intradermal transplantation studies), palpation alone should never be regarded as the sole means of determining tumor presence.

APPROACHES TO THE AUTOPSY

Two basic approaches to the performance of the autopsy are popular. One approach favors getting the tissues into a jar of preservative as quickly as possible and forwarding the reports and wet tissues to someone else considered more qualified to make evaluations. The advantage of this method is that it allows more autopsies to be done in a given amount of time, especially when performed as an assembly line operation with an invariable list of tissues to preserve. This method compensates for relatively unskilled personnel in that there is less need for judgment calls on gross pathology, and if enough animals are passed through the line, the general consensus is that, statistically, any real experimental result should still be apparent. The disadvantages lie in the attitude it conveys toward the autopsy itself, the emphasis placed on time, and the number of animals that may be needed to overcome deficits in technical quality.

The mechanical collection of tissues from large numbers of animals, which are then wisked away to the next workstation, by implication denies the importance of the purpose of the necropsy. Data on the subtle gross appearance of tissues are likely to be lost. All too frequently, routine processing and microscopy are carried out only if the organ is flagged on an autopsy report as spectacularly abnormal or overtly tumorous. Organs such as the liver are prime targets in toxicology/oncology studies; surface architecture and overall color can be crucial to routine pathological evaluation and to selection of proper stains for accurate differential diagnosis. Fixation tends to wash out true coloration and smooth out minor surface aberrations. If such findings are not recorded, the organ may well be passed as normal and not evaluated as stringently as might be appropriate.

Secondly, because of the emphasis on time and numbers, this system usually does not take full advantage of pertinent data that may have been gathered on test animals prior to the kill (Fig. 3A). Proper animal identification as well as observations of small lesions, unusual variations in weight, the presence of discharges, and so on, can easily be overlooked when time becomes the major factor in dissection. While some investigators will argue that inclusion of such data may introduce diagnostic bias, it must be remembered that in human diagnostics and treatment, clinical

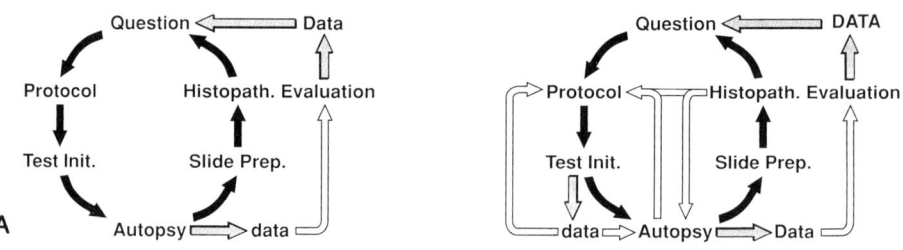

FIG. 3. Conceptualization of the potential of the autopsy.

history is imperative. If a bias is suspected in an experimental evaluation, adjunctive blind appraisals can be devised (19,21,23).

A third potential disadvantage is the numbers of animals that may be required to yield reliable data. In the current atmosphere against the use of animals in toxicology and carcinogenesis studies, as well as the rising costs of such studies, maximal utilization of minimal numbers of subjects would seem to be both prudent and practical (27,30,33,39).

An alternative approach to the assembly line method utilizes the autopsy as one more bank of information to correlate with clinical and microscopic evaluations, and as such, the quality, scope, and verbal/written report of every dissection becomes important (Fig. 3B). As can be seen from the figure, this second approach has the potential to yield a much more comprehensive picture of histogenesis and progression of disease.

When judiciously used, either approach to the autopsy may be legitimate, but the assembly line method lends itself more to an all-or-nothing bioassay than to a detailed carcinogenesis or toxicological study. The critical point, however, is that a quick mechanical dissection need not be so sloppy and a meticulous job so slow as to prohibit a routine application of either. One method to decrease time and inconsistency in necropsies is to establish a basic, systematic procedure for tissue examination and preservation (40,41) and to practice that procedure until it truly becomes second nature. Such a routine is here suggested in the following section, along with selected preservation and presentation techniques.

GENERAL AUTOPSY TECHNIQUES

Preparations

The proper instruments, rinses, and fixatives should be readily at hand before any animal comes to the autopsy board, as should the protocol and a means of recording the results. Data should be recorded on each animal at the necropsy and not relegated to memory for a more convenient time.

The size of the animal and the dexterity of the technician determine the instrument preference; instrument size, however, should be appropriate to the size of the specimen. Use small scissors and delicate forceps on small animals and organs such as the adrenals and pituitary. Toothed forceps are preferably used only for handling tough skin, connective or cartilaginous tissues, or bone, and even then should be used with some finesse. Ideally, an animal should be taken apart as if it had to be reassembled. Make sure that instruments are sharp, in good condition, and clean. The introduction of dried blood, feces, or other tissues or tissue exudates can easily confuse the histological appearance, as well as irretrievably compromise any molecular analyses performed for viral or genetic sequencing.

Tissues should never be rinsed in plain water or the fixative itself. Always use a physiologic saline solution or phosphate-buffered saline. In cases where tissues must be removed from the animal but not fixed immediately, place them in chilled rinse solution to retard autolysis. Putting tissues directly on wet ice has the same effect as rinsing in cold water; the differences in osmolarity between cells and external environment will cause cellular swelling and rupture. Rinsing in the preservative itself starts the fixation process, discoloring the tissues and retaining unneeded debris.

Sufficient volumes of fixative are imperative. Most histology texts recommend a 10:1 ratio of preservative to tissue for good fixation, with agitation and/or periodic changes of fluid if processing is not done right away. The thickness of the preserved tissue should not exceed 1 cm, and tissues that are not essential, including blood, should be removed, as they impede fixation and may prevent proper trimming and presentation of the slide specimen (42–45). Artifacts induced by extraneous debris, crushing and tearing, desiccation, and poor fixation of tissues detract from the ability to diagnose disease states with accuracy as surely as does failing to preserve the pertinent tissues at all.

Preliminary Examination of the Subject

Allow time to examine the animal before cutting. Confirm any individual or treatment identification and sex, and look for any visible abnormalities (confirming those previously noted), such as (a) the presence of blood or any other exudate from any orifice; (b) dermal lesions and aberrant hair growth; (c) the condition of the coat, to include a check for dehydration and subcutaneous fat loss; (d) the condition of the eyes and incisors; (e) external masses or swellings, including enlarged peripheral lymph nodes; and (f) body asymmetry and overall color and condition. Follow the visual examination with a palpation for subcutaneous and internal masses. These examinations can be performed in less than a minute and can save both effort and needless contamination of the autopsy field by such things as urine from an abnormally distended bladder, or purulent fluids from abscesses and masses that only appear to be solid. Abdominal distension caused by ascites or hemorrhage should be reduced prior to entry into the cavity; these fluids may be drained using a syringe and saved if they are of additional diagnostic value. All findings, including the body weight, should be recorded.

Preserving External Structures and Making the Initial Incisions

Hair should be shaved from any external tissues to be preserved, and this would include masses and other lesion types that may have invaded, adhered to, or originated from the skin (Fig. 4). Hair is nearly impossible to remove from tissues once in the jar. It does not cut well and will drag through tissues, introducing histological artifacts as well as causing problems in trimming and sectioning (42,45). For the same reasons, the surface selected for the opening incision should be thoroughly wet down with 70% ethanol to clump and flatten the hair and keep it out of the field of dissection. The incision area can also be shaved, if desired. Instruments will need to be rinsed or wiped frequently to remove adhered hair and other debris. Take measurements of masses and lesions before they are opened and/or drained. If a tumor is of such a size that it contributes significantly to the overall body weight of the animal, it should be weighed separately after excision. Since tumor invasion of adjacent tissues represents an important feature of neoplastic progression, a wide circumcision of such lesions should be practiced to preserve peripheral structures and make note of gross evidence of the effect of a neoplasm on normal tissues.

Skin

Normally, the initial incision is made ventrally, using scissors or scalpel, by cutting the skin of the abdomen and chest and reflecting it back away from the body wall. The skin of mice is readily pulled away from the underlying muscle using only the fingers, but a scalpel or razor blade is usually required on any larger species. There are a few organs that will adhere to the skin and adnexa (inguinal and axillary nodes, clitoral glands in females and preputial glands in males, scent glands, mammary glands, etc.). These organs, as well as the salivary glands and muscle itself, should be examined *in situ* while exposed.

Skin is most effectively preserved by flattening on paper to maintain the normal architecture, whether it be a very small section or the entire hide. Rinse the section thoroughly, blot, and place it subcutaneous side down on soft toweling, which is more flexible and permeable than stiffer backing; the edges will curl under but can easily be straightened out by alternatively stretching and gently pulling back the peripheries until flat. This is a necessary step if the sample is to remain flat and two-dimensional in the fixative. Let it set for a few seconds to a minute or so before placing it in preservative. The same procedure can be used for muscle and subcutaneous tissues, using less time to set them as they dry out much faster. Small organs or those that have a predominantly two-dimensional structure, such as the uterus, pancreas/mesenteric fan, and intestine, can also be flattened on paper to facilitate examination and trimming by supporting and immobilizing them.

Opening to the Body Cavities

It is advisable to examine the abdominal organs through the peritoneal wall before cutting into the cavity as it may avoid unnecessary damage to abnormal organs beneath (Fig 5). Scissors are preferentially used over a scalpel as they are easier to control. Open the abdominal cavity by cutting along the ventral midline and making subsequent lateral cuts at the groin, then following the lower edge of the ribcage to either side of the xiphoid process. Be aware, however, that the displacement or enlarged condition of one or more internal organs may make a routine midline incision impractical.

The *chest cavity* can be entered by lifting the xiphoid process with the forceps and bisecting either side of the sternum up to and through the cervical girdle (Figs. 5B and 6). Once the negative pressure in the cavity is released by puncturing the diaphragm, the lungs will collapse dorsally and allow further opening of the chest by cutting the ribs back to a greater degree. The pericardial sac may adhere to the sternum. Abnormalities of the sac itself, such as thickening due to inflammation or edema, accumulations of fluid around the heart, or depositions of tumor tissues become readily apparent as the sternum is removed. The thymus lies directly on top of the heart below the junction of the sternum and the collarbones (clavicles) and will also often adhere to the former as it is retracted. When this point is reached, slide the tips of the scissors gently over the thymus through the canal and snip the

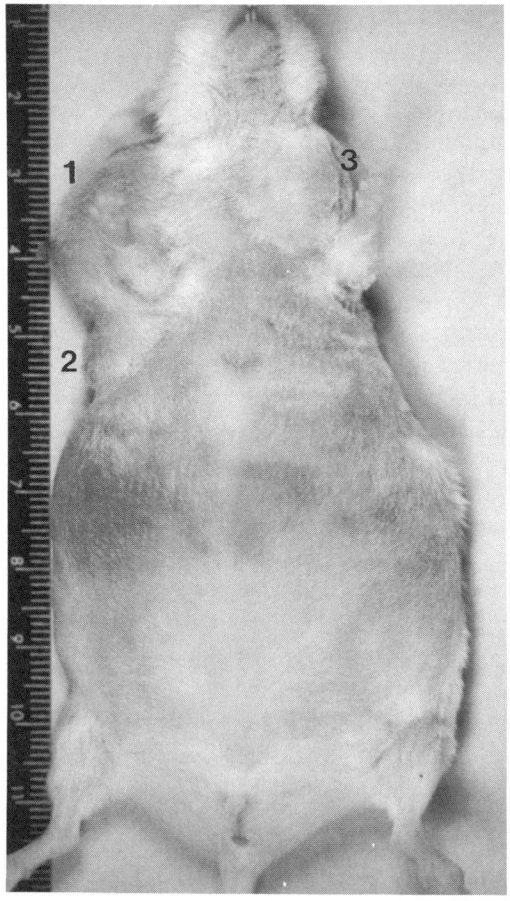

FIG. 4. A: Aged SENCAR mouse prepared for autopsy. Note masses 1, 2, and 3 and distended upper abdomen, somewhat darker on the right side. **B:** Same animal, turned over, with skin reflected to show masses. Mass 3 barely visible at this angle. Small mass 4 discovered below left shoulder. Note different appearances of tumors.

clavicles to finish removing the sternum. Precautions should be taken to avoid puncturing the trachea, which exits the chest cavity at this point and is protected only by a relatively thin muscle sheet.

Note should be made of any fluid or unusual solid contents in the abdominal and thoracic cavities. Make note of the color and textures of the organs and their size and anatomical relationships to each other. Provided that there have been no inadvertent punctures or tears of tissues or large vessels in the initial incision, there should be relatively little bleeding to blanch out the organs; the mesenteric tissues and fat will generally hold things together in a more-or-less normal arrangement.

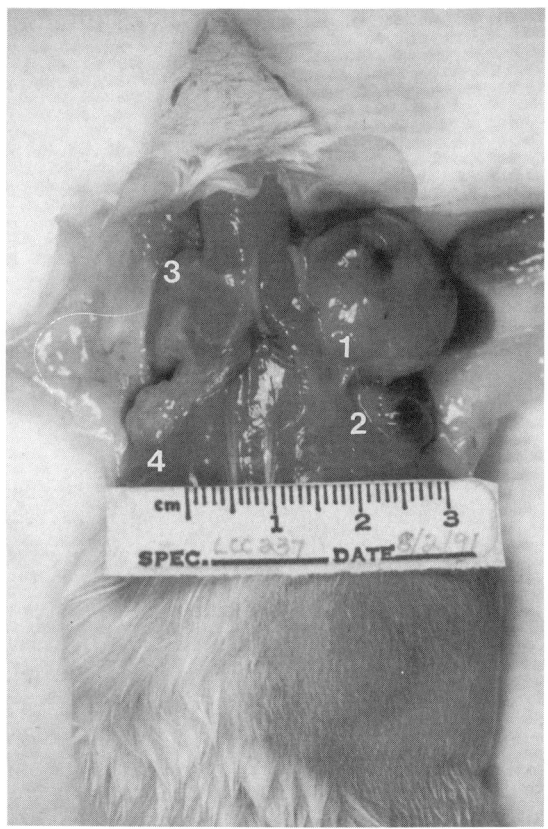

FIG. 4. *Continued.*

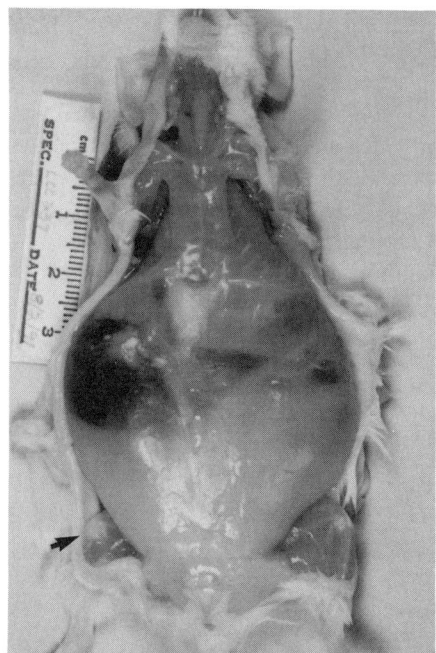 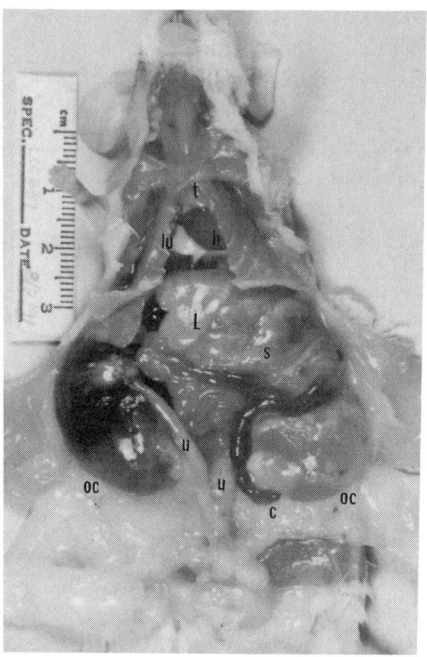

FIG. 5. A: Same animal with abdominal skin reflected. Note swelling of right knee (*arrow*) as well as confirmation of possible masses upper abdomen. **B:** Same animal, peritoneum opened. Abdominal masses prove to be ovarian cysts (oc), right shows bleeding. s, stomach (engorged); L, liver (blanched, possibly fatty); u, uterine horns; c, cecum (impacted). Sternum has been removed to check thoracic organs: t, thymus; h, heart; lu, lungs.

Internal Organs

Performing a complete autopsy involves scrutinizing all tissues, even in cases where not all tissues will be histologically preserved. This necessarily involves removing organs from the body to examine all surfaces, and removing capsules and connective tissues to ensure that one is truly seeing the organ and not a composite of several possibly unrelated tissues. Such procedures are advisable even in protocols specific for one or very few routinely preserved tissues, if for no other purpose than for the experience and knowledge in anatomical variations and relationships. However, peripheral data collected from nontarget tissues frequently enhances and broadens the original scope of the experiment beyond what was originally envisioned by the investigator. The easiest and most logical way to begin, therefore, is to start with organs and organ systems as they are presented anatomically.

Removing organs does not imply damage. Almost every structure in the body has a "handle" that can be used to maneuver the organ free with little or no injury. With practice and wide exposure, moreover, it will become apparent that each organ has a different consistency and strength which determines how much and what kind of

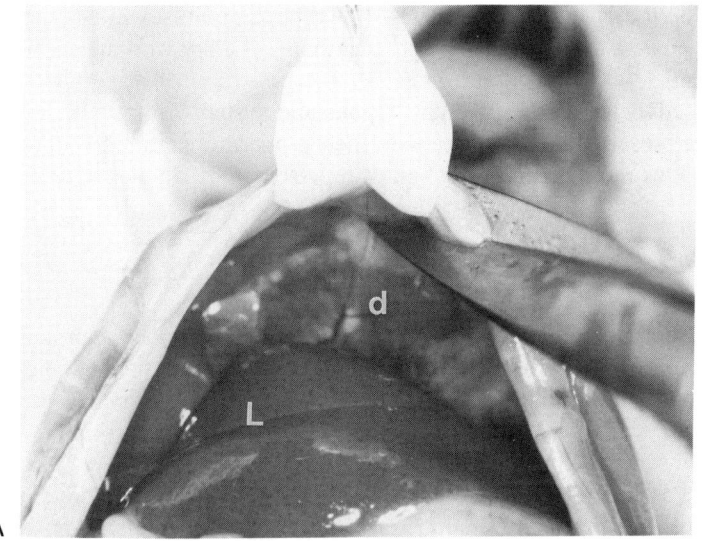

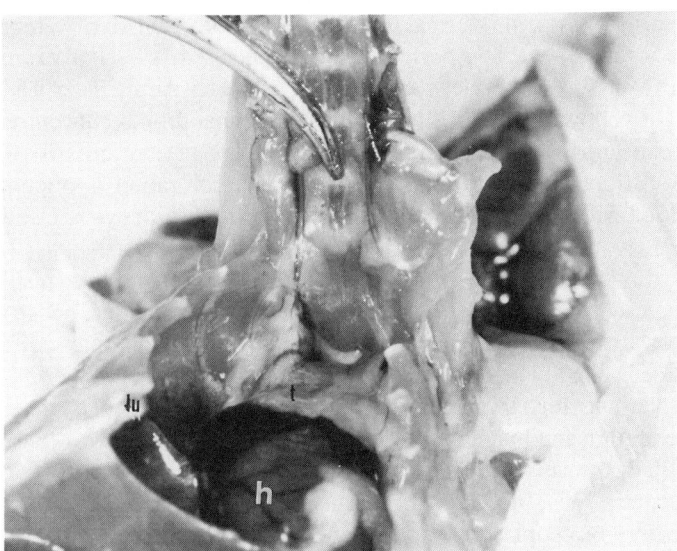

FIG. 6. A: Opening the chest. Lifting the xiphoid process away from the liver (L) to expose and puncture the diaphragm (d). **B:** Removing the sternum. Once the diagram is punctured, the lungs and heart fall back dorsally, allowing the sternum to be excised without damaging underlying organs. lu, lung; h, heart; t, thymus.

manipulation it can withstand. Tissues should be kept moist while being examined; a common error is to tear tissues by peeling them off a dry working surface to which they have stuck while being examined.

We also advocate removing entire organs and systems from the body. Doing so allows both preservation of tissues with their proper orientation to connected structures as well as more precise selection of representative samples of tissues.

Reproductive Organs and Urinary Bladder

In both males and females, the urinary bladder and reproductive organs lie ventral to the colon and must be removed if the underlying structures are to be exposed. [In cases where the gastrointestinal (GI) tract is the main objective of the study and must be dealt with first, the sex organs can be excised and placed in the physiological saline rinse until examination of the GI tract is completed.]

In most cases, it is advisable to remove the *bladder* and reproductive tract together. The bladder usually empties at death as the sphincters relax, but it is not unusual to have some urine retention; retained urine provides an indication of the state of the urinary system. Normal urine varies in color and clarity among different species; be aware of what is normal for the species in use. For example, in the mouse and rat it should be clear and yellow, while in the hamster it is milky and white to light yellow. Colorless fluid indicates an inability to concentrate the urine and can mean impaired kidney function even in the face of grossly normal-looking organs. Bright yellow to orange to brownish coloration is often due to pigments released with tissue breakdown or bleeding in the kidneys or elsewhere in the body (46).

Stones are calcareous deposits of variable white to green to brownish coloration, depending on their composition. They may be round to angular, occur singly or in multiples, or present as fine gravelly or sandy sediment. This fine sediment type of calculi can occasionally be detected as a granular deposition at the urinary orifice or in the surrounding fur. In female mice it is not unknown for stones to ulcerate through the urethra and lodge in the vaginal canal; large stones will cause a swelling and irritation of the vulva.

The presence of pus, blood, or soft tissue debris in the urine can also be indicative of inflammatory or neoplastic lesions in the urinary tract (46). Larger neoplasms of the bladder are usually conspicuous, but smaller papillomatous lesions or plaques may not be apparent in a contracted empty organ. Mild inflation with the preserving fluid and a detailed trimming protocol are required to demonstrate subtle abnormalities (Appendix A).

It is very common in male animals to see a whitish mass or plug in the neck of the bladder, intraurethrally, or free in the lumen. Produced by the seminal vesicles and coagulating glands, this hardened mix of seminal fluid is also responsible for the vaginal plug and should not be confused with a true calculus or stone (47,48). If removed and examined more closely, the plug will be white to off-white, firm but somewhat flexible, and often cylindrical or forming a cast of the urinary tract. Exactly when this plug is formed is still a topic of debate (47–50), but if the bladder is not overly distended, it would likely be a fairly recent event near or at the time of death.

Mouse urinary syndrome (also described as dysuria or obstructive uropathy) (Fig. 7), however, is a fairly common pathological finding in male mice and, to a lesser extent, in male rats as well. It is characterized by extreme distension of the bladder with or without abnormal urine, stones, or obvious plug formation. The phenomenon occurs more frequently in some strains than in others (49,50) and has been attributed to several as yet unconfirmed causes, including a deeper unseen obstruction in the lower urethra, inflammation or hyperplasia of the tract or prostate, or a possible neural defect affecting sphincter release. In all cases of pronounced bladder distension, the kidneys and ureters should be checked for backflow; if present, urine accumulation is likely to have been of some duration and not a consequence of death. Occurrence in females is rare compared to the male incidence. Distended bladders should be drained using a fine-gauge needle and syringe. Preservative can then be instilled for separation of the walls and proper fixation. Pinching the exit site of the needle as it is withdrawn usually controls leakage.

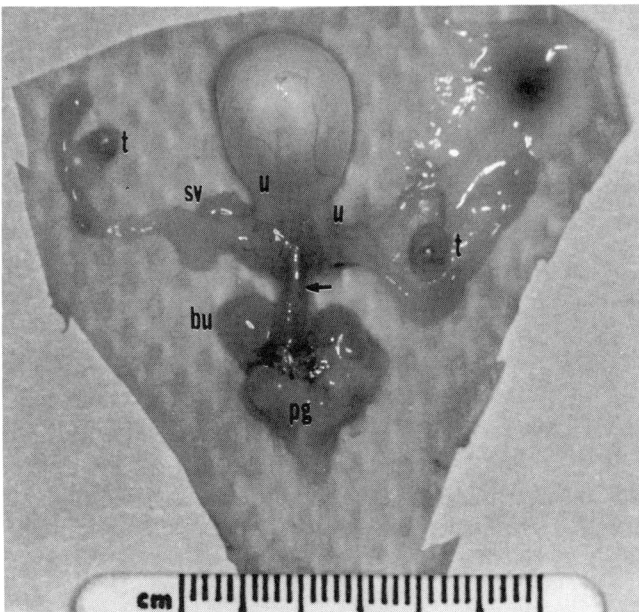

FIG. 7. Mouse urinary syndrome. In this case the bladder is not extremely distended, but the ureters (u) show distension at junctures. Urethral plug can be vaguely seen in upper urethra (*arrow*). Abscessing of preputial glands (pg) and cystic enlargement of bulbourethrals (bu). [Animal treated with DES and $CdCl_2$, resulting in degenerative atrophy of testes (t) and seminal vesicles (sv) as well.]

When removing the entire and intact reproductive tract from either sex, it is first necessary to expose and sever the pelvic arch (suspensory ligament in the pubic symphysis), spreading it carefully to allow the organs beneath to be pulled through. In the female, the *ovaries and uterine horns* are freed from their supporting fat and connective tissues and lifted away from the spinal column. Never attempt to clamp onto the ovaries themselves. They are extremely fragile and easily pulled from the Fallopian tubes and horns. Use the fat itself or the more muscular uterine horns as a handle. Once the ovaries and upper uterus are detached, shift to the denser and stronger body of the uterus to elevate the organ while the vagina is freed from the rectum beneath. Pull the entire complex through the pelvic arch until the external vulva is free. Rinse, blot, and allow the muscles to contract before flattening on paper to examine and/or preserve.

The *male genital system* is extracted similarly, with a few variations. The penis reflexes externally back over the pubis and should be straightened by cutting the ligamentous attachments. The testicles and epididymal capsules must be retracted and freed from the scrotum; if the organs have been withdrawn into the abdominal cavity, check to make sure that the scrotal attachment has been severed before attempting removal. The seminal vesicles and prostate are not as tough as the uterine body, and therefore more care should be taken when lifting the tract through the arch and off the rectum. Should the individual organs need to be separated, as when taking organ weights, do so carefully using the natural tissue boundaries.

In certain protocols, the external clitoral glands in the female and the male preputial and bulbourethral glands are also preserved. While these organs can easily be separated, it is best to leave them attached in their normal arrangement for identification and trimming purposes (Figs. 7 and 8). Especially when dealing with mice, it is recommended that the organs be flattened on paper—penis together with preputials and bulbourethrals, testes/epididymes with prostate and seminal vesicles.

Intestinal Tract, Spleen, and Pancreas

Excision of the liver and kidneys is much easier once the gut has been removed. The intestinal tract is removed together with the spleen and pancreas in a complex that includes the omentum, mesenteric fan, and lymph nodes.

With the minimal amount of force necessary, grasp the connective tissue beneath the ventral end of the spleen, lift until the connection to the dorsal peritoneum becomes apparent, and cut. Release the spleen and move to the stomach, which becomes the handle for the rest of the GI tract extraction. Grasp and lightly elevate the stomach. The two caudate lobes of the liver straddle the inner curve of the organ at the esophageal junction; cut the esophagus while maintaining the hold on the stomach and gently reduce the caudal liver connections. Still lifting the stomach, slide the scissors under the stomach and duodenum to sever the portal vein. The upper GI tract can now be raised up and out of the abdominal cavity to expose and free the colon from the spine all the way to the anus.

Once the entire tract is removed from the cavity, it can be spread out on moist paper and inspected closely. Note that the pancreas, which is normally easily distin-

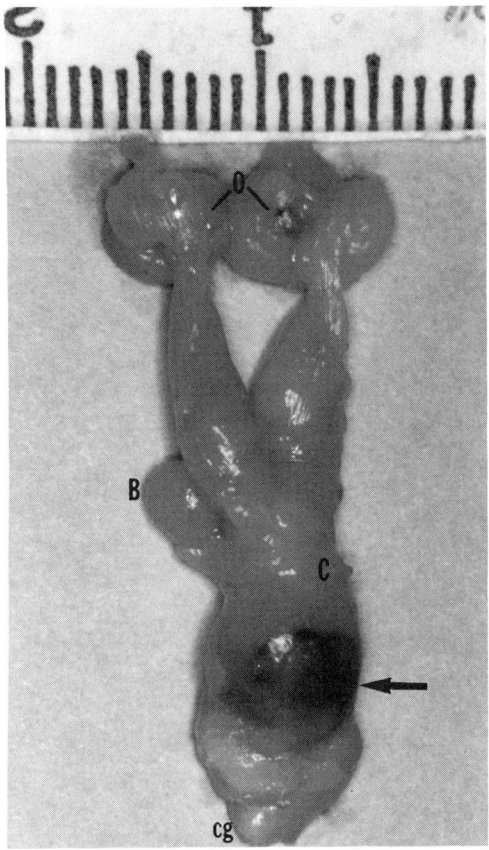

FIG. 8. Reproductive tract, mostly dorsal surface. Large polypoid mass (*arrow*) extending from lower right uterine horn through cervix (C) into vaginal canal. One of the clitoral glands (cg) can be seen distal to the vulva. B, bladder; O, ovaries. (Note bladder retains some urine, probably due, in part, to urethral compression by mass.)

guishable in color and consistency from the fatty membranous omentum and mesentery, attaches to the upper (ascending) colon (Fig. 9). Sampling the pancreas by preserving only that section directly beneath the spleen leaves at least half, if not two-thirds, of the organ unexamined. The line of mesenteric lymph nodes can be located in close proximity to the cecal junction and running parallel to the lower ileum and into the pancreas, forming the backbone of the mesenteric fan. With gentle tension and judicial snipping, the entire fan can be separated from the intestines intact with the pancreas and spleen.

There are several options in preserving the gut. The entire organ can be opened, rinsed, and flattened on paper for examination and fixation, or selected sections can be isolated and prepared in this way. The intestines may be left intact by segments and each segment cleared of ingested contents by rinsing with saline or preservative

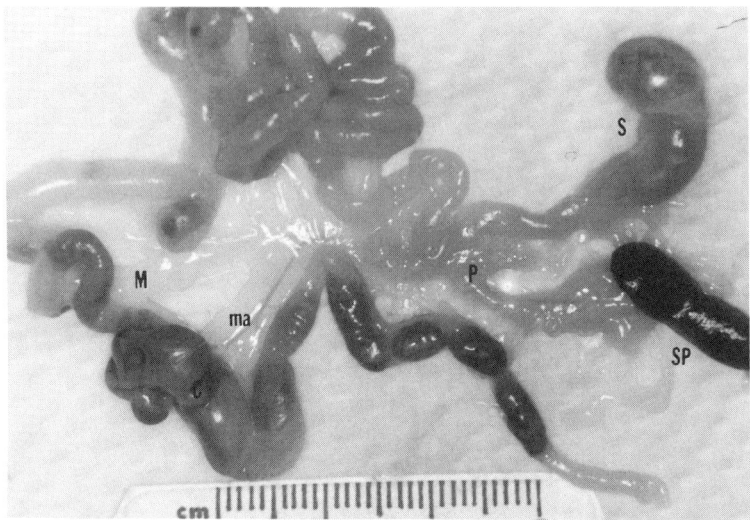

FIG. 9. Excised GI tract, including stomach (S), spleen (SP), and pancreas (P). Note the color and consistency of pancreas compared to fatty mesentery (M) and connections to duodenum and colon. Mesenteric nodes lie beneath the artery (ma). C, cecum. (Gaseous distension of ileum is not normal and spleen is enlarged.)

injected with a syringe prior to fixation. Gut rolls (Fig. 10), formed by winding the opened and flattened intestines, lumenal surface innermost, on a small-diameter wooden or cardboard cylinder or stick, are space-conserving methods of preserving the whole tract. Rolls can also be performed with the intestines unopened. Whatever method is chosen, it is recommended that the stomach be detached and treated separately. It can be opened and spread on paper as outlined above, but the strong muscle contractions and heavy ridging produce irregular angulated sections; it may, therefore, be preferable to inflate mildly with preservative and examine the organ after it has fixed a minimum of several hours. Fixative is instilled via the esophageal or duodenal openings; stomach contents will not interfere with fixation. The cecum may also be inflated in this fashion, using the ileal or colonic apertures. Cecal contents may have to be diluted or rinsed out if they are excessively tarry in consistency, as sometimes occurs in cases of intestinal bleeding or dehydration/constipation.

Liver

The liver is a large, turgid, ungainly organ. Normal livers are easily torn, punctured, and sliced both by autopsy instruments and not infrequently by incomplete reduction of connective membranes. By using the diaphragm for manipulations and blunt instruments for excision, however, removal of an intact organ is consistently feasible.

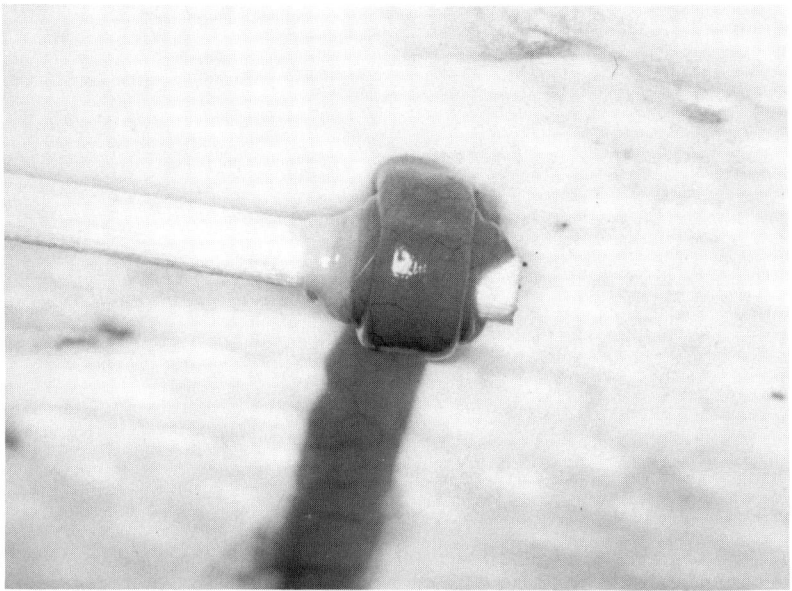

FIG. 10. Gut roll, in this instance, with intestines unopened.

Excise the liver from the abdominal cavity by first cutting the vena cava on the thoracic side of the diaphragm and pulling the esophagus (which was severed during removal of the stomach) through it. Being careful to avoid the adrenals, separate the diaphragm itself from the body wall down either side and behind the liver (Fig. 11), leaving it attached to the apical surface of the median lobe. Then, using the still-attached diaphragm as a handle, lift the liver up until a slight resistance is felt. The resistance comes from the vascular connections of the right lateral lobe of the liver and the major hepatic artery just above the right kidney. If this connection is not cut, the lobe is usually badly torn, as the muscle wall of the vessel is tougher than the hepatic membranes. Caution should also be exercised that the right adrenal is not accidentally caught in the cut. Remove the diaphragm before weighing or preserving the liver.

Since the liver is such a large and fairly dense organ, most fixatives penetrate slowly and incompletely if the fixation volume is insufficient or the fixing period is too short. To improve fixation, separate the lobes at the junctions, thoroughly rinse and drain of excess blood. Very large livers from the bigger rat strains, rabbits, dogs, primates, or larger farm animals may have to be scored across lobe surfaces to facilitate penetration, but scoring is not synonymous for mutilation. Think about how the organ will probably be trimmed and make the cuts in conjunction (i.e., do not score transversely if longitudinal sections are to be taken). In addition, it may not be necessary, or even possible, to preserve the entire liver for adequate representative sampling, but sampling must be accurately documented in the autopsy

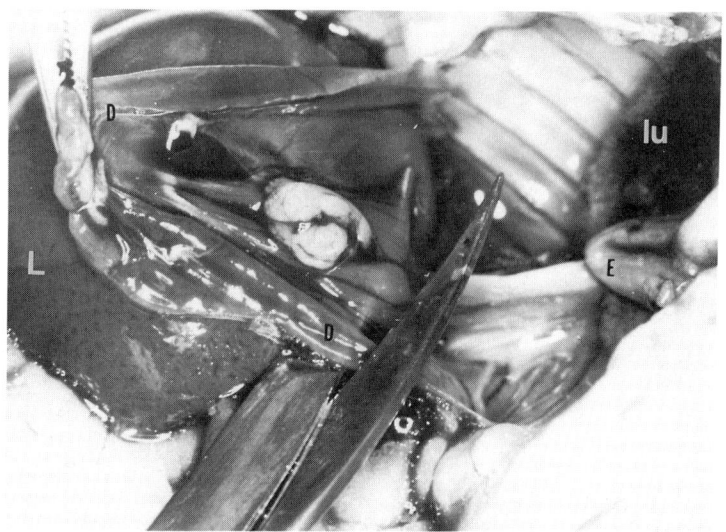

FIG. 11. Removing the liver by using the diaphragm. The diaphragm has been severed laterally from the peritoneal wall and left attached to the liver over the apical surface of the median lobe. Scissors are slid between the organ and the diaphragm, keeping the scissor points up off the hepatic surface. L, liver; D, diaphragm; lu, lungs; E, esophagus. (White nodule middiaphragm is a piece of fat pulled through with the esophagus.)

report (19,23,44). Appendix B illustrates a uniform method of representing the livers of small rodents histologically.

Kidneys and Adrenals

The kidneys and adrenals are retroperitoneal tissues, separated from the abdominal organs by a tough capsule that surrounds and holds them securely to the back of the cavity. The ureters are easily overlooked, as they are usually masked by body fat in a normal animal. They can be located, however, at the renal pelvis with the organs *in situ*, and exposed and removed by carefully teasing away peripheral fat while gently lifting. Each adrenal gland lies closely above its respective kidney, but at a distance that varies by species and individual. The renal lymph nodes usually lay in close proximity to the hilus near the vascular junctions. By clasping the renal vein at the hilus or getting a firm grip on the surrounding fat and sliding the scissors well beneath the organs, adrenals, nodes, and kidneys can be removed as a complex without damage.

Deposits of fat, disseminated tumor nodules, and encysted debris or fluid have all been described as lesions of the kidney when, in fact, they were adhered to or enmeshed within the renal capsule. In addition, discolorations and tiny lesions of the cortical surface are obscured by the membrane and surrounding fat (Fig. 12). To evaluate the kidney accurately, therefore, the renal capsule must be removed.

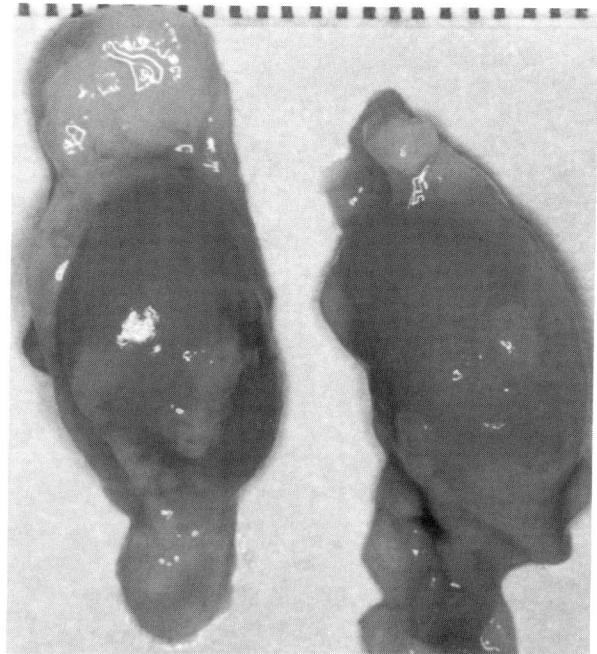

FIG. 12. A: Kidneys as they appear without capsules removed. These might be reported as nodular or tumorous. **B:** Left kidney from 12A with capsule removed. Note that surface nodules seen in the photo are part of the capsule, not the renal parenchyma. Also note the small hemorrhages (*arrows*) on the organ surface previously obscured by the capsule.

The kidney is immobilized at the hilus with forceps and the capsule nicked just above the forceps tips; insert the tips of closed scissors into the nick, keeping the points up and away from the cortical surface. Opening the scissors will spread the capsule and allow it to be peeled away from the cortex. If the adrenal glands were not previously dissected out of the fat off the apical poles of the kidneys, they can remain in this adnexal tissue adherent to the reflected capsules and the capsule left attached at the renal hilus (Fig. 13). When kidney weights are desired, cut off the capsular remains containing the adrenals and preserve separately. Kidneys from large animals may need to be scored for the same reasons as the liver, in the same manner, and under the same considerations. Organs from the smaller experimental species, however, usually fix well with removal of the capsule only.

Thoracic and Cervical Organs

Removing the sternum and opening the chest cavity was described earlier in the chapter. The lungs, heart, thymus, trachea, and thyroid are best removed as a unit, using the esophagus as a handle. The end freed when the gastrointestinal tract was dissected is lifted up and out of the thoracic cavity, reducing connective and mediastinal attachments as they become apparent. Care must be taken where the chest narrows at the cervical canal to ease the thymus and associated mediastinal nodes through without tears or separation. Also avoid sticking the scissors so far forward as to cut into the trachea. Once out of the cavity, the esophagus is pulled gently downward away from the head to expose the larynx. The trachea and esophagus are then cut above the larynx, as close as possible to the lower jaw, to leave the bilobular thyroid gland intact. To examine the *esophagus* itself, snip or gently pull it away from the pulmonary organs. Examine the white mucosal surface by slitting the organ carefully with scissors and flattening it, external surface down, on paper.

Unless there is a special need to remove it, the *thyroid* should remain *in situ* through trimming and embedding. Extraneous muscle and connective tissues should be removed from the trachea and larynx to facilitate inspection of the paired lobes of the gland and the thin connective isthmus lying on the ventral surface of the trachea just below the larynx. Against a white or illuminated background, thyroid abnormalities such as enlarged follicles, cysts, darker opaque areas, and possible hemorrhages may be seen (Fig. 14). Marginal increases in size are frequently more easily evaluated from the dorsal aspect. In the rat, each *parathyroid* may be seen as a small white nodule lying on the median lateral surface of each thyroid lobe, but in the mouse, these glands are usually embedded within the thyroid tissues and not grossly obvious.

The *thymus* is a white-to-translucent gland composed of two lobes and sits anterior to the heart, sometimes obscuring the atria. It is essentially absent in athymic nude strains and may decrease in size in conventional species and strains with age, under stress, and following lymphotoxic treatments (51–54). The mediastinal lymph nodes, found dorsolaterally to the thymus and heart, can enlarge and over-

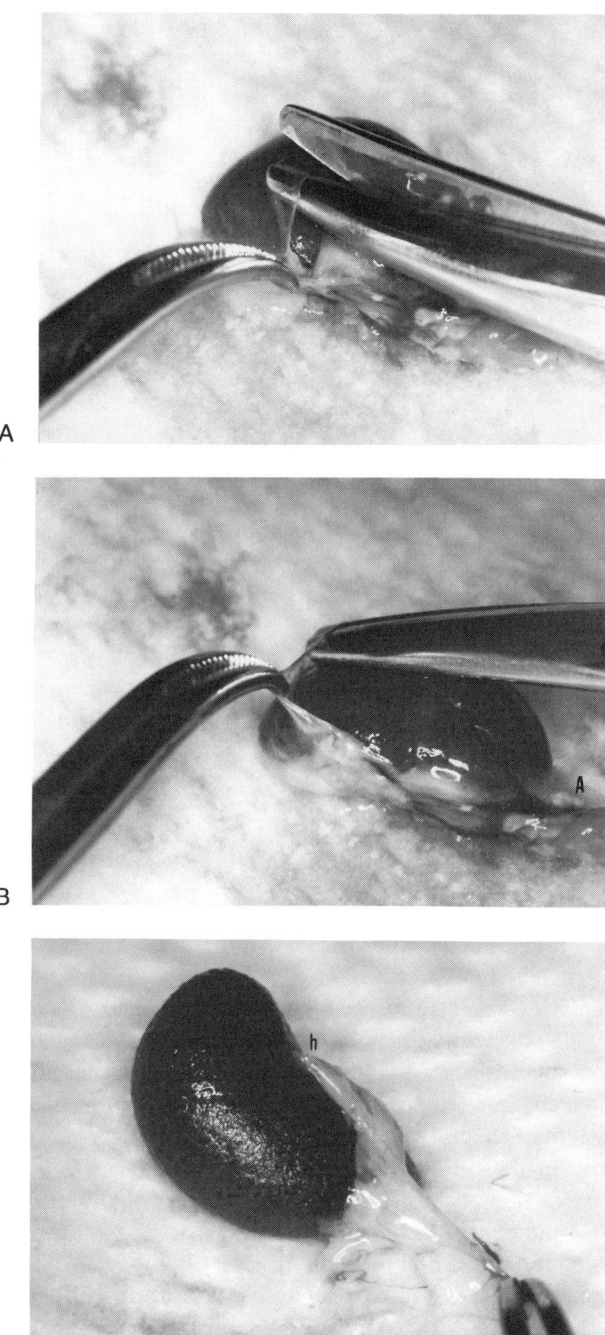

FIG. 13. A: Nicking the renal capsule at the hilus. (Note that blunt/blunt scissors are being used and tips are kept off the organ surface.) **B:** Slipping the capsule off one pole of the kidney. A, adrenal, still caught in membranes and fat. **C:** Capsule removed and still attached at hilus (h). Note true texture of renal surface.

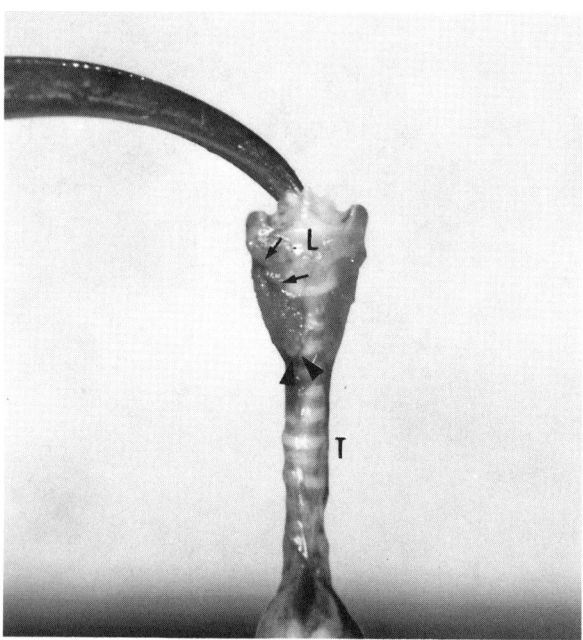

FIG. 14. Thyroid, mouse. Right lobe may be slightly enlarged with some darker tissue, possibly bleeding, apically (*arrow*) and enlarged follicles or cysts at distal edge (*arrowhead*). L, larynx; T, trachea.

grow the thymus, giving the appearance of a thymic neoplasm. Separation of the thymus from cardiac and mediastinal tissues can be done before or after fixation, depending on purpose and preference.

Inflation of the *lungs* with fixative via the trachea by means of a needle or catheter and syringe, helps to define the internal architecture better than processing in a deflated state and should be routinely performed when internal architecture/morphology is of prime concern (Appendix C). If the trachea or bronchi are mutilated or blocked, a needle may be inserted directly into the pulmonary tissue. However, inflation can mask small or subtle macroscopic lesions, and consequently, the lungs are best inspected in their natural state beforehand. To avoid artifacts, inflation should not be too rapid or with excessive volumes. It should mimic natural respiratory inflation, using the fixative in place of air.

The *heart* is a frequently overlooked organ because of the relatively uncommon occurrence of overt tumors or other macroscopic lesions, of either spontaneous or induced origin, in most small laboratory animal species (55,56). Dogs and swine are the most used species in cardiovascular research (57,59), but cardiovascular diseases and degenerative changes similar to those occurring in humans are not uncommon findings, especially in older rodents (>1 year) (57,58). Attention should be paid to the overall shape, size, and color of the atria and ventricles separately and in relation to each other. Normal hearts are a rich red brown; the atria are small and darker than the ventricles. The coronary vasculature is easily apparent without being overly prominent and there should be no white, gray, or yellowish streaks or spots indicative of scarring, mineral deposition, or necrosis. It should be mentioned, however, that mineralization of the heart is common in some rodent strains, notably in DBA and older BALB/c mice (29,60,61). Normally, there are no lumps or protuberances and no dark, thin-walled areas. Most hearts contract at death and are firm. Cardiovascular, pulmonary, renal, or hepatic disease may be responsible for cardiac hypertrophy, as seen in enlarged organs that are often flaccid and have a grayish tinge. Hearts of older animals, however, often show mild enlargement and loss of myocardial tone from normal aging processes. Atria that are enlarged and/or mottled may signal the presence of a mass or thrombus.

Spine and Organs of the Skull and Neural Tissues

The brain and spinal cord are arguably two of the most neglected organs as far as the autopsy is concerned (56). Because the tissues are so delicate and nature has, therefore, protected them well inside bony casings, the effort required to examine them thoroughly often seems excessive considering the usual incidence of abnormalities. In most cases, the only reason for opening the cranium at all is examination of the pituitary rather than the brain itself. The true incidence of neurogenic lesions may be much higher than recorded, but it requires greater attention to the nervous tissues to know with any certainty. The real secret to dissecting the brain and spinal cord is to find and work with the areas of give in thin areas or suture lines that virtually all bones possess.

Once internal organs have been removed from the carcass, the *spinal column and joints* should be inspected for bone spurs, degenerative changes, and malformations. There should be symmetry in the musculature of the limbs and in the large lumbar muscles of the spine. Large nerves, such as the brachial plexus in the cervical girdle and the major lumbar complexes innervating the pelvis and hind legs, should be white and smooth, without swelling or discolorations.

Dissection of the *spinal cord* is generally performed only when lesions are suspected from behavioral and locomotor abnormalities observed in the living animal. Preserving the spinal column is normally sufficient to sample the cord, but if the cord is to be excised completely from the canal, do so before fixing, as the cord is then more flexible and easier to handle. Neural tissue is an extremely soft and fragile tissue to work with, fixed or fresh, and requires an exceptionally gentle touch.

One method to expose the cord is to pin the carcass securely to the autopsy board, dorsal side down. Remove as much muscle and tendon as possible from the spine and snip the vertebral column medially down the ventral surface, pulling the edges apart as the cut progresses. The neural tissue is then retracted from the cranial end of the column. The two major disadvantages are that the cord lies a little closer to the ventral side, as do the spinal ganglia, and that the bone is thicker ventrally.

A second method entails cutting the spinal column, with or without the skull attached, free from the body altogether, trimming away all unneeded tissues, and approaching from the dorsal aspect. The vertebral bone is reasonably thin on the dorsum to either side of the dorsal processes; the net effect of repeatedly snipping through each vertebra lateral to the processes is to remove the strip of bone containing these projections down the length of the column. Having the entire column out of and unhampered by the remainder of the body also allows greater manipulation (Fig. 15). Use sharp/sharp scissors and keep the point up away from the spinal cord. Extreme care should be taken to avoid slicing the encasing meninges; the cord is under slight pressure within these membranes and will bulge out of any cuts or tears, thus producing some distortion artifacts.

Removal of the cord after exposing by either method above should, in most cases, be initiated from the cranial end. The cord actually ends in the first few lumbar vertebrae, separating into the large sacral and pelvic nerve tracts. While removal is possible beginning caudally, it is extremely difficult to maintain the integrity of the meninges and nerve bifurcations. A compromise is to preserve the caudal portions of the column intact, with the cord exposed or enclosed, disarticulating the hind legs at the hip joints. The bones of the pelvis can be cut away. The cord is examined histologically *in situ*.

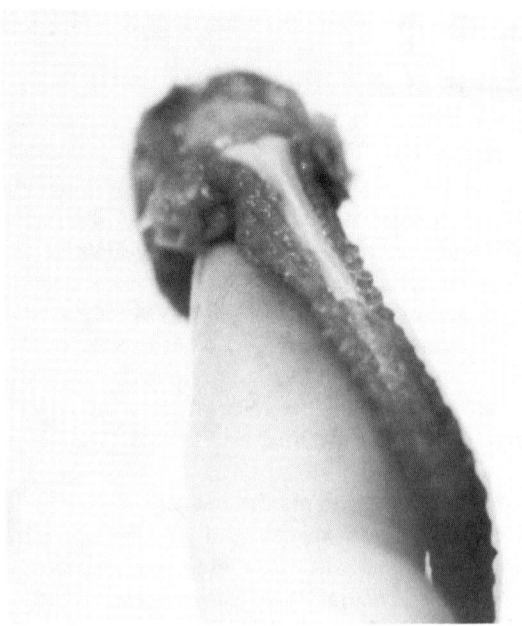

FIG. 15. Mouse skull and spinal column intact, cord exposed by dorsal approach.

To examine the *oral cavity and cranial organs*, the head can be detached from the spinal column at the occipital condyle, or, alternatively, left connected and the lower jaw detached (Fig. 15). Removal of the lower jaw can be accomplished by sliding the scissors into the oral cavity over the tongue until the points protrude out the back and cutting or disarticulating the mandibles. The condition of the hard and soft palates, the tongue, and the teeth can now be evaluated. The jaw does not have to be detached to examine the brain or nasal cavities, but in many cases, it is easier to manipulate the skull without it.

The *eyes* of rodents are subject to the same degenerative conditions seen in other species, notably cataracts and retinal lesions (57,62,63). Having no protective pigmentation in the eye, albino strains are especially susceptible to retinal damage that some pathologists link to exposure to the fluorescent lighting prevalent in animal facilities (57,63). Cataracts can be seen as opacities within the sphere, sometimes in crystalline patches and sometimes completely filling the lens. Looking at the eye from the side may reveal scars and abrasions from fighting or food/bedding lodged between the lids and the cornea. Some inbred strains are genetically prone to microphthalmia or anophthalmia. Certain viruses, bacteria, and parasitic infections are known to cause conjunctivitis or inflammation of the eyelids and glands (40). Optic nerve lesions and Harderian gland tumors (64) can force an eye completely out of the socket in severe cases, or cause ocular discharges or atrophy of the eyeball. Unless there is some specific reason for removing the eyes, they are best left in the skull through fixation.

There are two basic approaches to exposing the *brain*, both of which are contingent on the desired orientation of the nasal cavities. One approach is to split the skull from nose to hindbrain medially along the natural suture lines, in which case the nasal cavities usually divide into equal longitudinal halves readily amenable to gross observation (Fig. 16A). The second approach preserves the cavities *in situ* by removing only the top of the cranium for access to the brain (Fig. 16B).

Scissors can be used on mice initially to crack the brain case, but for larger species such as rats and hamsters bone cutters are required. Remove the skin and unneeded subcutaneous tissues from the skull and reflect the periosteum away from the medial suture line along the length of the head. Both of the approaches described above start with snipping the occipital and interparietal bones (Fig. 17) and pulling them off the hind brain and cerebellum. When the entire skull is to be split, make another shallow snip at the posterior end of the parietal suture, keeping the tips of the scissors or bone cutters up and off the brain. In many cases, this is enough to split the sagittal sutures over the cerebrum up to the frontal areas, but it rarely goes completely through the frontal sutures. Therefore, at a point roughly between the eyes, make a hole in the skull directly into the frontal suture line with the closed tips of sharp/sharp scissors. When the tips have penetrated the bone, turn them perpendicular to the suture and spread the points until the suture releases (Fig. 16A). Be aware that if the cranium is widened too far during the splitting, the pituitary, which remains on the cranial floor between the two thick trigeminal nerves, may be distorted or fragmented. The meningeal membranes will usually peel back laterally

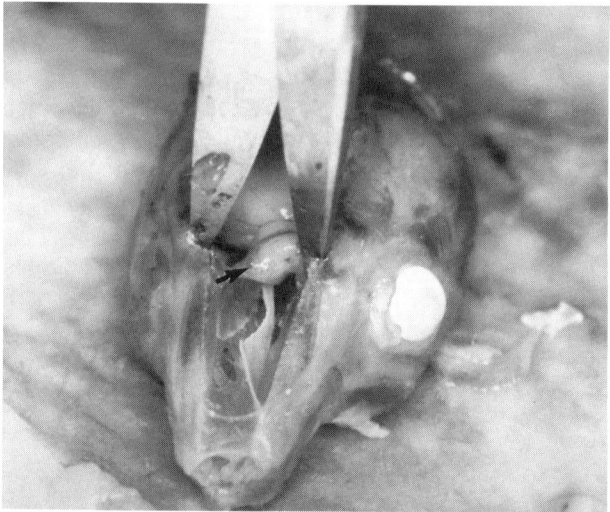

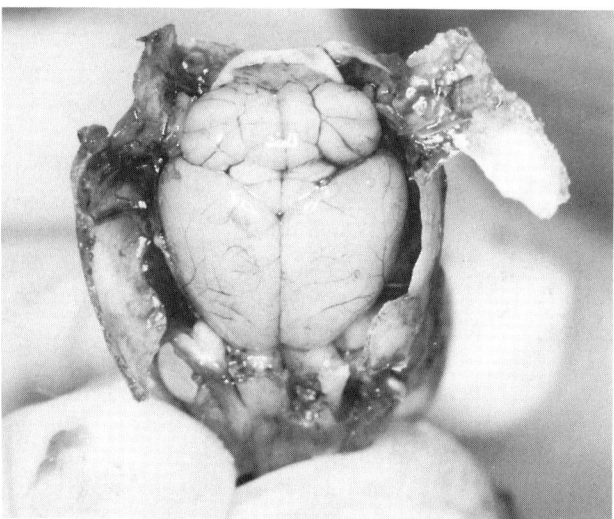

FIG. 16. A: Splitting nasal cavities longitudinally when exposing brain. Right olfactory lobe (*arrow*) and right cerebral hemisphere are visible just behind scissors. **B:** Brain exposed with nasal cavities intact. Cranial bones have been cut and reflected using natural sutures.

with the parietal bones, but vestiges may remain over the cerebellum and on the floor of the cranial vault and will have to be detached if the brain is to be removed without tearing or slicing. Lift the brain very gently from the cranium, severing the optic and trigeminal nerves as the organ is elevated, or alternatively, hold the skull with the oral cavity upward and let gravity pull the brain from its casing. The latter variation reduces the amount of manipulation on the delicate neural tissues, thus

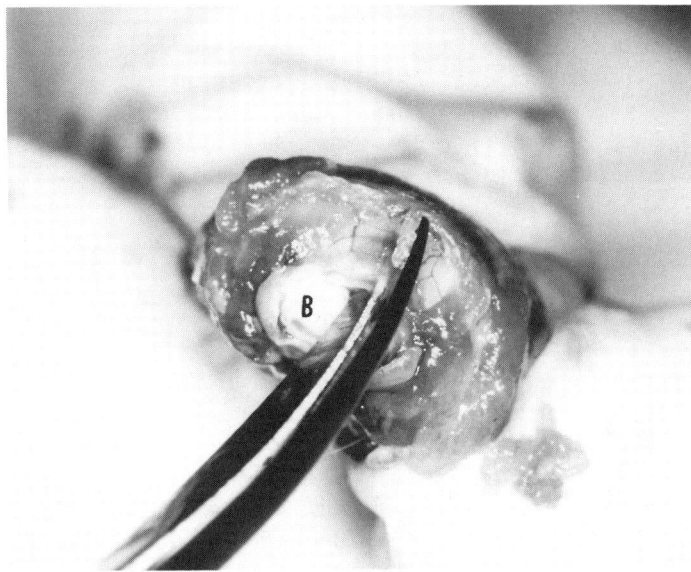

FIG. 17. Snipping the occipital bone at the base of the skull. Cerebellum lies directly below scissor tips, brainstem (**B**) projects at occipital condyle.

reducing pressure and puncture artifacts. The olfactory lobes can be left attached to the frontal lobes of the cerebrum or remain *in situ* with the nasal cavities. Similarly, the pituitary should be left in place in the skull for fixation; however, these softer tissues may show morphological and histological artifacts as a result of the chemicals used in decalcification and in being cut simultaneously with bone tissue (45,65). They are best removed from the cranium after fixing and before the skull is histologically processed.

To leave the *nasal passages* intact, the cranium is cut away laterally and peeled back off the top of the brain after the medial sutures have been split from the occipital end. Releasing the brain from the skull casing is done as described. This method increases the risk of damaging brain tissue, but is less disruptive to other structures if done with care. Adequate fixation of the nasal passages is achieved by injecting preservative via the nasopharyngeal duct. Obstructed outflow may indicate blockage as a result of malformation or abnormal tissue. The injected fluid may also wash out blood or purulent debris characteristic of tissue damage and/or infection.

APPENDICES

In carcinogenesis studies, quantitative evaluation of important and specified endpoints (e.g., preneoplastic foci, adenomas, carcinoma *in situ*) are often imperative. Concise gross descriptions of the tissues at autopsy, proper fixation and tissue trimming, consistently good processing and embedding are absolutely necessary for reliable histopathological evaluation of the effects of test agents or procedures. The following procedures for selected organs of significance in carcinogenesis/toxicologic studies may aid the investigator in presenting and evaluating his or her data. The methods presented here are by no means the only ones used or accepted, but are offered for consideration or modification according to purpose.

Appendix A: Urinary Bladder

After fixation is complete, the distended bladder is cut in half longitudinally. Each half can be embedded, cut side down, either in one block together or in two separate paraffin blocks (Fig. 18A). Representative sections, step sections at any desired interval, or complete consecutive sectioning can be requested.

In another method, followed by Ito et al. (66–68), four slices are cut from each half to yield eight sections. These sections are also embedded cut sides down for sequential evaluation of lumenal surface and basement membrane length using a color video image analysis system coupled with routine light microscope examination (Fig. 18B).

Appendix B: Liver

Since the liver is the major site of xenobiotic biotransformation and detoxification, it is a common target organ of the carcinogenic process (35,69–72). It is therefore an important source of data that can aid our understanding of the mechanisms involved in chemically induced tumorigenesis. The collection of data begins at the autopsy, where the color and general appearance of the liver should be noted. Grossly visible hepatic lesions should be counted, their locations noted, and their sizes measured.

The type of fixative used to preserve the tissue is related to the techniques utilized in the evaluation. For most cases, 10% neutral buffered formalin (NBF) is the fixative of choice; however, specialized protocols may dictate the use of other solutions. For instance, our laboratory has found the immunohistochemical detection of bromodeoxyuridine in DNA-synthesizing hepatocytes is best demonstrated in tissues fixed in 70% ethanol (unpublished data). Snap freezing in liquid nitrogen to preserve sensitive tissue antigens may be required for *in situ* hybridization and other immunological methods.

Typically, ethanol-fixed livers should be trimmed and embedded within 48 h of the autopsy. This will avoid overfixation, which causes the tissue to become brittle and impairs histological integrity. Tissues fixed properly in NBF can be held without serious side effects for months.

Proper trimming is also important. It is expensive, time consuming, and usually unnecessary to process the entire liver. Consistent sampling procedures should be established. For example, we cut two 2- to 3-mm sections from each liver lobe.

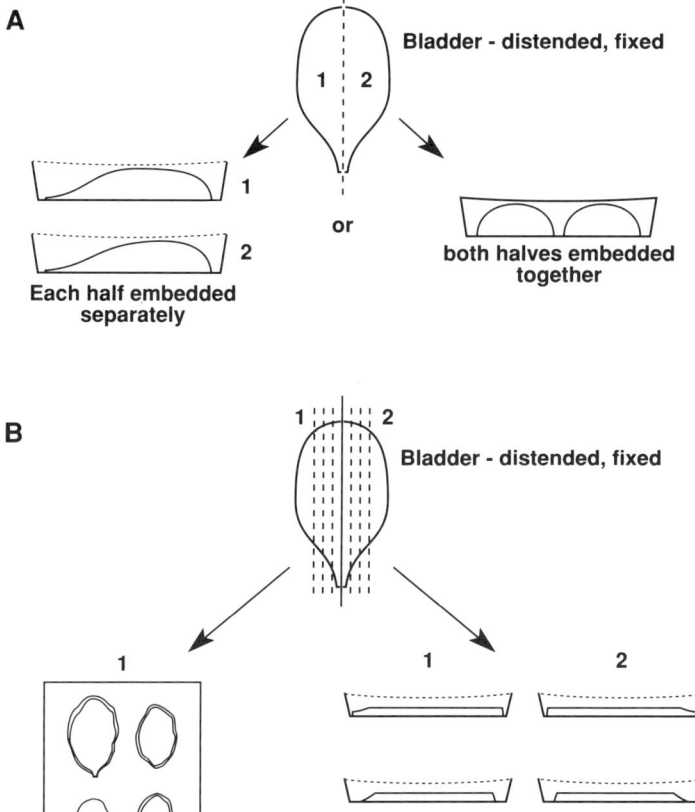

FIG. 18. A: Trimming and embedding urinary bladder, routine sections. **B:** Ito method, trimming and embedding bladder. Each half of the organ is sliced to yield four consecutive sections.

These sections are either embedded all in one block (mice) or in one lobe per block (mice, rats, or hamsters) (Fig. 19). Specific lesions not caught in the representative sections are placed in separate blocks for evaluation. The remainder of the liver is usually stored as wet tissue until no further need for it is determined. Standard H&E sections are cut for light microscopy and image analysis.

Appendix C: Lung

In the lungs, very small (<1 mm) lesions and tumors can easily be obscured by inflation; it is, therefore, extremely important to examine the organs carefully before they undergo further manipulation. However, some fixatives, such as Bouin's, cause areas of greater density to stand out with increased clarity if they are not too deep within the tissues.

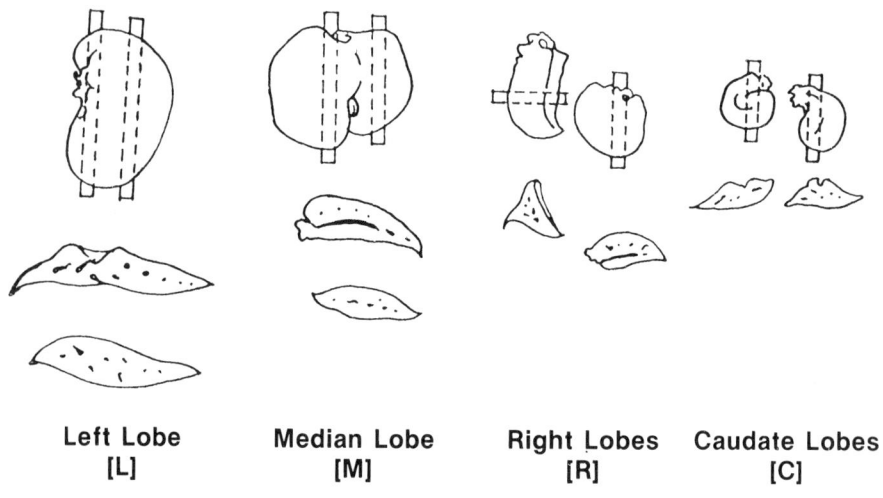

Left Lobe [L]　　Median Lobe [M]　　Right Lobes [R]　　Caudate Lobes [C]

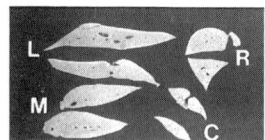

FIG. 19. Representative sampling of liver. Note that normal liver lobes have fairly characteristic shape and size if trimmed consistently to maintain orientation.

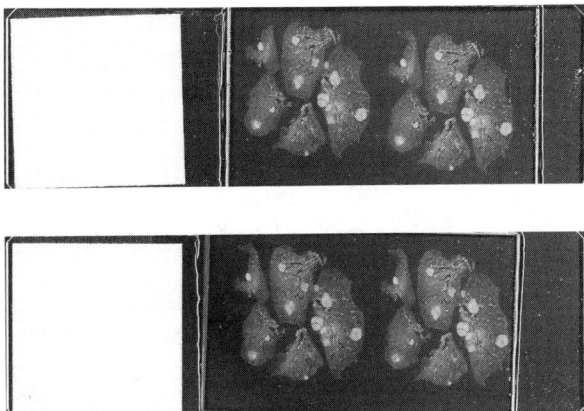

FIG. 20. Whole mount of lung for serial or step sectioning. Note that lung lobes also have characteristic shapes and sizes for orientation.

Some studies choose to report tumor data based on the gross numbers of nodules counted in fixed or unfixed specimens under a dissecting microscope; this method may also include sectioning through lung tissue to assess deeper lesions as well as to determine singularity or multiplicity. Gross assessment has the advantage that large numbers of animals may be evaluated relatively inexpensively in a short period. The disadvantages are that a great proportion of lesions, including nontumorous conditions, will be missed, and that this method cannot distinguish histogenesis. Some inflammatory responses and metastatic deposits will erroneously be classified as pulmonary tumors.

In a previous study (73), we documented in detail a feasible histologic method to evaluate lungs. In brief, inflated and fixed lung lobes are separated but embedded closely side by side in one paraffin block. Two sections from the block are mounted on one slide; individual lobes retain their identifying shapes, making orientation very easy (Fig. 20). Comparative analysis with serial sectioning shows that step sections of 10 (i.e., examining every tenth section) gives equally good results. At step sections of 20, lesions smaller than 100 μm may be missed. This method not only allows a correct evaluation of tumor frequency and progression, but also allows for a thorough pathological diagnosis of surrounding tissue and tumor type. Lesion size can also be approximated by measuring the perimeter of the largest section of a tumor. Embedding only the one or two largest lobes and mounting multiple sections on slides is a modification that might preferentially be used in a very large experiment.

ACKNOWLEDGMENTS

This work was supported in part with federal funds from the Department of Health and Human Services under contract NO1-CO-74102 with Program Resources, Inc./DynCorp. The contents of this publication do not necessarily reflect the views or policies of the Department of Health and Human Services, nor does mention of trade names, commercial products, or organizations imply endorsement by the U.S. government.

REFERENCES

1. Stedman TL. *Stedman's medical dictionary*. 24th ed. Baltimore: Williams & Wilkins, 1982.
2. Olds JR, Olds RJ. *A color atlas of the rat-dissection guide*. London: Wolfe Medical Publications; 1979.
3. Feldman DB, Seely JC. *Necropsy guide: rodents and the rabbit*. Boca Raton, FL: CRC Press; 1988.
4. Harkness JE, Wagner JE. *The biology and medicine of rabbits and rodents*. Philadelphia: Lea & Febiger; 1983.
5. Green EC. *Anatomy of the rat. Transactions of the American Philosophical Society.* New York: Hafner; 1963.
6. Gude ED, Cosgrove GE, Hirsch GP. *Histological atlas of the laboratory mouse*. New York: Plenum Press, 1982.
7. Wagner JE, Manning PJ, eds. *Biology of the guinea pig*. New York: Academic Press; 1976.
8. Hoffman RA, Robinson PF, Magalhaes M. *The golden hamster: its biology and use in medical research*. Ames, IA: Iowa State University Press; 1968.
9. Crispens CG Jr, Thomas CJ. *Handbook on the laboratory mouse*. Springfield, IL: American College of Laboratory Medicine; 1975.
10. Rugh R. *The mouse: its reproduction and development*. Minneapolis: Burgess; 1968.
11. Zeman W, Innes JRM. *Craigie's neuroanatomy of the rat*. New York: Academic Press; 1963.
12. Hebel R, Stromberg MW. *Anatomy of the laboratory rat*. Baltimore: Williams & Wilkins; 1976.
13. Farris EJ, Griffith JQ, eds. *The rat in laboratory investigation*. 2nd ed. Philadelphia: JB Lippincott; 1949.
14. Frith CH, Ward JM. *Color atlas of neoplastic and non-neoplastic lesions in aging mice*. Amsterdam: Elsevier; 1988.
15. Frith CH, Pattengale PK, Ward JM. *A color atlas of hematopoietic pathology of mice*. Little Rock, AR: Toxicology Pathology Associates; 1985.
16. Cotchin E, Roe FJC, eds. *Pathology of laboratory rats and mice*. Oxford: Blackwell Scientific; 1967.
17. Jones TC, Mohr U, Hunt RD, eds. *Monographs on pathology of laboratory animals*. Berlin: Springer-Verlag; 1984–1990.
18. Petter WL, ed. *Animals for research: principles of breeding and management*. New York: Academic Press; 1963.
19. Poole A, Leslie GB. *A practical approach to toxicological investigations*. Cambridge: Cambridge University Press; 1989:66–100.
20. Unwanted variables: preventing complicating factors. In: *Biomedical investigator's handbook for researchers using animal models*. 2nd ed. Washington, DC: Foundation for Biomedical Research; 1987:11–18.
21. Haseman JK, Huff JE, Rao GN, Eustis SL. Sources of variability in rodent carcinogenicity studies. *Fundam Appl Toxicol* 1989;12:793–804.
22. Goldberg L, ed. *Carcinogenesis testing of chemicals*. Cleveland, OH: CRC Press; 1974.
23. Gart JJ, Krewski D, Lee PN, Tarone RE, Wahrendorf J. *Statistical methods in cancer research*. Vol. III. *The design and analysis of long-term animal experiments*. IARC scientific publication 79. Lyon, France: International Agency for Research on Cancer; 1986:1–55.
24. Dayan AD. Are we ready for the future? Possibilities for laboratory animal science. In: Seamer JH, ed. *LASA silver jubilee 1988*. London: Royal Society of Medicine Services; 1988:36–42.
25. Williams GM, Weisburger JH. Chemical Carcinogens. In: Klaassen CD, Amdur MO, Doull J, eds. *Casarett and Doull's toxicology: the basic science of poisons*. 3rd ed. New York: Macmillan; 1986: 25–63, 99–173.
26. Jelinik V. Influence of the condition of the laboratory animals employed on the experimental results. In: *Defining the laboratory animal. Fourth symposium of the international committee on laboratory animals*. Washington, DC: National Academy of Sciences; 1971:110–120.

27. Rao GN, Huff J. Refinement of long-term toxicity and carcinogenesis studies. *Fundam Appl Toxicol* 1990;15:33–43.
28. *Animals for research: a directory of sources*. 10th ed. Washington, DC: Institute for Laboratory Animal Research, National Research Council, National Academy of Sciences; 1979.
29. Altman PL, Katz DD, eds. *Inbred and genetically defined strains of laboratory animals*, Vols. I and II. Bethesda, MD: Federation of American Societies for Experimental Biology; 1979.
30. Hewitt HB. Use of animals in experimental cancer research. In: Sperlinger D, ed. *Animals in research: new perspectives in animal experimentation*. Chichester, West Sussex, England: Wiley; 1981:141–174.
31. Feldman DB, Gupta BN. Histopathological changes in laboratory animals resulting from various methods of euthanasia. *Lab Anim Sci* 1976;26:218–221.
32. Messow VC, Fiolina A, Kaup F-J, Hackbarth H. Postmortal morphological changes in the rat lung. *Z Versuchstierkd* 1987;29:219–227.
33. *Guide for the care and use of laboratory animals*. NIH Publication 86-23. Washington, DC: US Department of Health and Human Services, Public Health Service; 1985.
34. Hughes HC Jr. Euthanasia of laboratory animals. In: Melby EC, Altman NH, eds. *Handbook of laboratory animal science*. Vol III. Cleveland, OH: CRC Press; 1976:553–559.
35. Borchard RE, Barnes CD, Eltherington LE. *Drug dosage in laboratory animals: a handbook*. 3rd ed. Caldwell, NJ: Telford Press; 1990:xv, xvii.
36. Maynert EW, van Dyke HB. Metabolism of barbiturates. *Pharm Rev* 1949;1:217–252.
37. Ariens EJ, Simons AM, Offermeier J. *Introduction to general toxicology*. New York: Academic Press; 1976:66–67.
38. Warren RG. Injectable anesthetic drugs. In: Warren RG, ed. *Mosby's fundamentals of animal health technology: small animal anesthesia*. St Louis, MO: CV Mosby; 1983:114–151.
39. Russell WMS, Burch RL. *Principles of humane experimental technique*. London: Methuen; 1959:105–153.
40. Porter JA, Port CD. Specific diseases of laboratory animals. In: Collins GR, ed. *Syllabus for the laboratory animal technician*. AALAS publication 72-7. Cordova, TN, 1972:333–368.
41. Diagnostic techniques. In: Stark DM, Ostrow ME, eds. *Laboratory animal technician*. Vol II. AALAS training manual series. Cordova, TN: American Association for Laboratory Animal Science; 1990:140–144.
42. Coolidge BJ, Howard RM. Procedures for submitting tissue to the pathological technology section for processing. In: Animal histology procedures. NIH publication 80-275. Washington, DC: US Department of Health and Human Services; 1979:23–31.
43. Humason GL. *Animal tissue techniques*. San Francisco: WH Freeman; 1962:11–12.
44. Thompson RG. *General veterinary pathology*. Toronto: WB Saunders; 1978:411–413.
45. Thompson WS, Luna LG. *An atlas of artifacts encountered in the preparation of microscopic tissue sections*. Springfield, IL: Charles C Thomas; 1978:13–106, 120–162.
46. Benjamin MM. Urinalysis. In: *Outline of veterinary clinical pathology*. 3rd ed. Ames, IA: Iowa State University Press, 1978:180–212.
47. Rapp JP. Terminal formation of urethral plugs in male mice. *Proc Soc Exp Biol Med* 1962;111:243–245.
48. Kunstyr I, Kupper W, Weisser H, Naumann S, Messow K. Urethral plug: a new secondary male sex characteristic in rat and other rodents. *Lab Anim* 1982;16:151–155.
49. Taylor DM. Urethral plugs and urine retention in male mice. *Lab Anim* 1985;19:189–191.
50. Bendele AM, Carlton WW. Urologic syndrome, mouse. In: Jones TC, Mohr U, Hunt RD, eds. *ILSI monographs on pathology of laboratory animals: urinary system*. Berlin: Springer-Verlag; 1986:369–374.
51. Kuper CF, Beems RB, Hollanders VMH. Development and aging, thymus, rat. In: Jones TC, Ward JM, Mohr U, Hunt RD, eds. *ILSI monographs on pathology of laboratory animals: hematopoietic system*. Berlin: Springer-Verlag; 1990:257–263.
52. Krueger GRF. Lymphoblastic lymphoma, mouse. In: Jones TC, Ward JM, Mohr U, Hunt RD, eds. *ILSI monographs on pathology of laboratory animals: hematopoietic system*. Berlin: Springer-Verlag; 1990:264–265.
53. Vos JG, Kranjnc-Franken MAM. Toxic effects on the immune system, rat. In: Jones TC, Ward JM, Mohr U, Hunt, RD, eds. *ILSI monographs on pathology of laboratory animals: hematopoietic system*. Berlin: Springer-Verlag; 1990:168–181.
54. Imai K. Atrophy of thymus induced by cytostatic chemicals, rat. In: Jones TC, Ward JM, Mohr U,

Hunt RD, eds. *ILSI monographs on pathology of laboratory animals: hematopoietic system*. Berlin: Springer-Verlag; 1990:293–295.
55. Strandberg JD, Goodman DG. Neoplasms of the cardiovascular system. In: Foster HL, Small JD, Fox JG, eds. *The mouse in biomedical research*. Vol IV. *Experimental biology and oncology*. ACLAM series. New York: Academic Press; 1982:540–546.
56. Altman NH, Goodman DG. Neoplastic diseases. In: Baker HJ, Lindsey RJ, Weisbroth SH, eds. *The laboratory rat*. Vol I. *Biology and diseases*. ACLAM series. New York: Academic Press; 1979: 334–377.
57. Anver MR, Cohen BJ. Lesions associated with aging. In: Baker HJ, Lindsey RJ, Weisbroth SH, eds. *The laboratory rat*. Vol I. *Biology and diseases*. ACLAM series. New York: Academic Press; 1979:378–399.
58. Fairweather FA. Cardiovascular disease in rats. In: Cotchin E, Roe FJC, eds. *Pathology of laboratory rats and mice*. Oxford: Blackwell; 1967.
59. Michaelson SM, Schreiner BF Jr. Comparative biology in the selection of experimental subjects for cardiac pathophysiologic investigations. In: *Defining the laboratory animal. Fourth symposium of the International Committee on Laboratory Animals*. Washington, DC: National Academy of Sciences; 1971:121–147.
60. Van Vleet JF, Ferrans VJ. Inherited dystrophic cardiac calcinosis, mouse. In: Jones TC, Mohr U, Hunt RD, eds. *ILSI monographs on pathology of laboratory animals: cardiovascular and musculoskeletal systems*. Berlin: Springer-Verlag; 1991:9–14.
61. Everitt JI, Olson LM, Mangum JB, Visek WJ. High mortality with severe dystrophic cardiac calcinosis in C3H/OUJ mice fed high fat purified diets. *Vet Pathol* 1988;25:113–118.
62. Saunders LZ. Ophthalmic pathology in rats and mice. In: Cotchin E, Roe FJC, eds. *Pathology of laboratory rats and mice*. Oxford: Blackwell; 1967.
63. Robison GW Jr, Kuwabara T, Zwaan J. Eye research. In: Foster HL, Small JD, Fox JG, eds. *The mouse in biomedical research*. Vol IV. *Experimental biology and oncology*. ACLAM series. New York: Academic Press; 1982:69–96.
64. Holland JM, Fry JM. Neoplasms of the integumentary system and Harderian glands. In: Foster HL, Small JD, Fox JG, eds. *The mouse in biomedical research*. Vol IV. *Experimental biology and oncology*. ACLAM series. New York: Academic Press; 1982:513–528.
65. Pearse AGE. *Histochemistry: theoretical and applied*. 2nd ed. Boston: Little, Brown; 1961:776–778.
66. Ito N, Shirai T, Fukushima S, Hirose M. Dose-response study of urinary bladder carcinogenesis in rats by N-butyl-N-(4-hydroxybutyl)nitrosamine. *J Cancer Res Clin Oncol* 1984;108:169–173.
67. Nakanishi K, Hagiwara A, Shibata M, Imaida K, Tatematsu M, Ito N. Dose response of saccharin in induction of urinary bladder hyperplasia in Fischer 344 rats pretreated with N-butyl-N-(4-hydroxybutyl)nitrosamine. *J Natl Cancer Inst* 1980;65:1005–1010.
68. Fukushima S, Imaida K, Sakata T, Okamura T, Shibata M, Ito N. Promoting effects of sodium L-ascorbate in two-stage urinary bladder carcinogenesis in rats. *Cancer Res* 1980;43:4454–4457.
69. Alvares AP. Oxidative biotransformation of drugs. In: Arias I, Popper H, Schacter D, Shafritz DA, eds. *The liver: biology and pathobiology*. New York: Raven Press; 1982:265–280.
70. Caldwell J. Conjugation reactions in the metabolism of xenobiotics. In: Arias I, Popper H, Schacter D, Shafritz DA, eds. *The liver: biology and pathobiology*. New York: Raven Press; 1982:281–295.
71. Sipes IG, Gandolfi AJ. Biotransformation of toxicants. In: Klaassen CD, Amdur MO, Doull J, eds. *Casarett and Doull's toxicology: the basic science of poisons*. 3rd ed. New York: Macmillan; 1986: 64–98.
72. McConnell EE. Mouse liver tumors: the problem. In: Stevenson DE, McClain RM, Popp JA, Slaga TJ, Ward JM, Pitot HC, eds. *Mouse liver carcinogenesis: mechanisms and species comparisons*. New York: Wiley-Liss; 1990:1–3.
73. Rehm S, Ward JM. Quantitative analysis of alveolar type II cell tumors in mice by whole lung serial and step sections. *Toxicol Pathol* 1989;17:737–742.

Subject Index

A

Acetaldehyde, in upper respiratory tract carcinogenesis, 215, 217, 243, 244, 245, 247, 248–250, 252, 256
2-Acetylaminofluorene (2-AAF), 9–10, 387
  in hepatocarcinogenesis, 46, 53
  in rodent urinary bladder carcinogenesis, 182–190, 192
Achalasia, 73
Acrolein, 253, 254
Acromegaly, 6
Acrylamide, 12
Acrylonitrile, 12, 370
Adenocarcinomas
  in celiac disease, 93
  nasal, 230–231
  renal, 124–125
  rodent olfactory mucosa, 247–249
  of small intestine, 91, 92, 93
  of upper respiratory tract, 235
Adenomas
  cholangiocellular, 43
  hepatocellular, 41, 47–48
  hepatocholangiocellular, 44
  renal, 124–125
  in rodent respiratory epithelium, 244–245
Adenosine diphosphate (ADP), 276
Adenosine triphosphatase, 40–41
  in preneoplastic lesions in hepatocarcinogenesis, 48–50
Adrenals, autopsy of, 450–452
Adriamycin, 192
Aflatoxins
  B1, 1, 12, 53
  in hepatocarcinogenesis, 53
  in renal carcinogenesis, 134
Age factors
  in neurocarcinogenesis, 304–305
  in prostate cancer, 374–375
  in rodent urinary bladder carcinogenesis, 190–191
Agent Orange, 344
AIDS, 422
Air pollution, 200
Alcohol
  in esophagus cancer susceptibility, 73–74
  gastric cancer and, 79
Aldehydes
  in cigarette smoke, 257
Aliphatic compounds
  one-carbon, 5–6

P450 oxidation of, 5, 6
  in renal carcinogenesis, 4
  sources of, 5
  three-carbon, 7
  two-carbon, 6–7
Alkalinization, intracellular, 95
Alkylating agents, in neurocarcinogenesis, 310–311
2-Amino-3-methylimidazo[4,5f]quinoline, 9
11-Amino-*n*-butyric acid (GABA), 90
Aminoazo dyes, 10–11
4-Aminobiphenyl (4-AB), 10
Amophilic cell foci, 41, 47
Androgens, in prostate carcinogenesis, 384–386
Animal research. *See also* Pathology procedures
  autopsy in, 430–434
  classification of hematopoietic tumors, 408–414
  complete experimental protocols, 265
  generalizability of, 26, 28–35, 33, 34, 253–255, 328–329
  individual differences in, 207
  methods of euthanasia in, 434
  nasal cavity epithelia, 217
  in neurocarcinogenesis, 302, 303–304, 328–329
  in prostate cancer, 375
  record keeping, 431, 434–435
  in respiratory tract cancer, role of, 200, 202, 206–211
  rodent laryngeal histology, 223–224
  rodent nasal histology, 217–223
  role of, 429–430
  in upper respiratory tract carcinogenesis, 215–217, 253–255
Anti-oncogenes, 424
Anticarcinogens. *See also* Inhibition/prevention
  in gastrointestinal tract, 69
  in rodent urinary bladder, 193
Antioxidants, 15, 69, 193, 276
Arachidonic acid, 104–105
Aromatic amines
  in bladder cancer, 1, 3
  metabolism, 9–10
Arsenic, 13
Aryl hydrocarbon hydroxylase (AHH), 71
  in skin carcinogenesis, 282
Asbestos, 13
Ascorbic acid, 75, 80

467

SUBJECT INDEX

Autocrine metabolism, 315
Autopsy
　approaches to, 436–437
　cervical-thoracic organs in, 452–455, 462–463
　determinants of effectiveness in, 430, 459–460
　examination of subject prior to, 438
　examining body cavities in, 439–441
　gastrointestinal tract complex in, 446–448
　handling of internal organs in, 442–444
　liver in, 448–450, 460–462
　materials preparation, 437–438
　opening incisions, 438–439
　protocols, 431–434
　reproductive organs in, 444, 446
　skin handling, 439
　spine-skull in, 455–459
　tissue handling, 437–438
　urinary bladder in, 444–445, 460
Aziridine, 2

B

Barrett's esophagus, 100
Basophilic cells
　as hepatocellular proliferative lesions, 40, 47
　in renal epithelial tumors, 126
Bay region diol-epoxide, 268
Bay region hypothesis, 9
Benz[a]anthracene, 267
Benzene, 417
　in early research, 1–2
　metabolism, 7–8
Benzo[a]pyrene, 9, 416
　DNA adduct of, 268
　in skin carcinogenesis, 267, 268, 282
　in upper respiratory tract carcinogenesis, 217, 245
Benzoyl peroxide, 276
Bile duct proliferative lesions, 42–44
Bile salts, 91
Biliary cysts, 42–43
Bioassay
　analysis of macromolecular adducts, 83–84
　medium-term liver carcinogenesis, 57–60
Bis(2-chloroethyl)sulfide, 2
Bis(chloromethyl) ether, 2, 215, 217, 256
Bladder. *See also* Urinary bladder
　carcinogenesis (rodent)
　aromatic amines in cancer of, 1, 3
　epigenetic carcinogens in, 5
Bone marrow. *See* Hematopoietic system
Brain. *See* Neurocarcinogenesis
Brush cells, intestinal M-cells and, 219
Bulbourethral gland, 387, 446

C

Cadmium, 346, 347, 349–350, 351, 353–355, 357, 371–372, 377
　metallothionein and, 382
Calcium
　in cell proliferation in renal carcinogenesis, 147
　in colorectal carcinogenesis, 94–95
　metabolism, 277–278
Cancer. *See also specific site; specific type*
　animal research, generalizability of, 26, 33, 34
　current understanding of, 25–26
　epidemiology, 25, 33, 199
　known causes of, 26–27
　lifestyle factors in, 34
　originating from aberrant tissue, 93
　suspected causes of, 27–35
Caprolactam, 27
Carbon tetrachloride, 5
　metabolism of, 6
Carcinogenesis. *See also* Mechanism of carcinogenesis
　chemical processes in, 16
　host factors in, 317
　individual response variables, 3
　inhibition-prevention, 15–16
　initiation-promotion concept, 14–15
　multistage, in rat liver, 53–57
　oncogene activation in, 16
　organ specificity, 302, 307
　tissue damage leading to, 250–251
Carcinogenic Potency Data Base, 188
Carcinogens
　chemical, 25–35
　classification of, 26–35
　colorectal cancer, 103–104
　dietary, in colorectal cancer, 94
　early research on, 1
　esophageal, 76
　gastric cancer, 89
　generalizability of animal research on, 26
　of hematopoietic system, 415–418
　implicated in gastrointestinal tract cancers, 68
　inorganic, 13–14
　kidney, 123
　liver, 58–60
　nasal cancer, 226–232
　naturally occurring, 12
　in neurocarcinogenesis, 302–303
　organic compounds as, 5–13
　preputial gland, 386–387
　prostate cancer, 376–377
　radiation-related, 99, 137–138, 328, 372, 377, 418–421
　renal, 132–138
　respiratory tract, 200–206
　site-specific chemicals, numbers of, 201–202

in skin carcinogenesis, 267–268
testicular cancer, 350
types of mechanisms of action, 2–5
of upper respiratory tract, 215–216, 254
urinary bladder, 182, 188–190
Carcinoids, small intestine, 91
Carcinomas
　in celiac disease, 93
　cholangiocellular, 44
　colorectal, precursors, 96–97
　esophageal, 75–76
　gastric, dysplasia with, 88
　hepatocellular, 42
　hepatocholangiocellular, 44
　neuroendocrine, 237
　renal pelvis, 127
　in rodent urinary bladder, 170, 173–178
　in small intestine, 91, 93
　upper respiratory tract, 233–235
a-carotene, 358–360
Celiac disease, 93
Chediak-Higashi syndrome, 69–70
Chemoprevention
　in colorectal carcinogenesis, 94
　direct acting carcinogens, 2
　indirect acting carcinogens, 2–3
　in inhibition of carcinogenesis, 15
　nerve growth factor, 320–323
　in neurocarcinogenesis, 315
　in skin tumor promotion, 275–281
Chloramphenicol, 418
Chlorination, 5
Chloroform, 5
Chocolate, 79
Cholangiocellular lesions, 42–44
Cholangiofibrosis, 43
Cholic acid, 104
Chromium, 13–14, 227
Chrysarobin, 274, 278
Cirrhosis, 48
Classification systems
　chemical carcinogen, 26–35
　hematopoietic lymphoma, 405
　hematopoietic tumor, 403
　leukemia, 404
　liver lesion, 39–46
　olfactory neuroblastoma, 235–237
　rodent hematopoietic tumor, 408–414
　rodent hepatocellular carcinoma, 42
　rodent leukemia, 410–411
　rodent lymphoma, 408–410
　rodent nasal epithelia, 217–223
　urinary bladder tumor, 181
Clear cell foci, 41, 47
Clofibrate, 49–50
Clusters of differentiation, 404
Cocarcinogens, 15
Colitis, 99

Colorectal cancer
　in animal model, 103–105
　carcinoma precursors, 96–97
　colon crypt in, 101–102, 103
　dietary risk factors, 94–95, 103
　disease states related to, 99–100
　field effect theory of, 102
　genetic risk factors, 95–96, 97–99
　hyperplasia in, and carcinogenesis, 251
　immune system in, 96
　intracellular alkalinization in, 95
　large intestine cancer, 67
　markers for high-risk, 100, 102–103
　protein kinase C in, 94–95
　risk factors, 94–96
　stages of, 100–102
Crohn's disease
　colorectal cancer and, 99
　intestinal cancer and, 92–93
Cryptorchidism, 341–342, 346, 347–348, 351–352
Cyclophosphamide, 2, 350, 417
Cyclosporine, 422
Cylindrical cell carcinoma, 235
Cysteamine, 90
Cytopenias, 408

D

Dehydroepiandrosterone, 58–59
Deoxycorticosterone acetate, 80
Diacylglycerol (DAG), 94–95
Diagnosis. See also Risk assessment
　analysis of macromolecular adducts, 83–84
　familial adenomatous polyposis, 97
　glycogen enzyme markers in hepatocarcinogenesis, 48–52
　of hepatocellular carcinomas vs. hyperplastic nodules, 42
　of hepatocellular hyperplasia vs. adenoma, 41, 47–48
　hyperplasia vs. neoplasia in renal carcinogenesis, 138–140
　of intrahepatic cholangiocellular lesions, 42–44
　of leukemia, 404–405
　medium-term liver carcinogenesis bioassay, 57–60
　nephroblastomas, 128, 130–131
　olfactory neuroblastomas, 235–237, 249–250
　preneoplastic lesions in hepatocarcinogenesis, 46–47
　renal epithelial tumors, 124–126
　renal mesenchymal tumors, 128–130
　rodent lymphomas, 408–410
Dialkyl-N-nitrosamines. See Nitrosamines

Dialkyltriazenes, 12
Dibenz[a,j]anthracene, 270
Dibenz[c,h]acridine, 270
1,2-Dibromethane (DBE), 6–7
1,2-Dibromo-3-chloropropane (DBCP), 7, 247
Dibutylnitrosamine, 11
o,p'-Dichlorodiphenyldichloroethane, 350
1,2-Dichloroethane (DCE), 6–7
Dichloromethane, 5
Diepozybutane, 2
Diet
  antioxidant sources in, 69
  cancer and, 33–34
  colorectal cancer and, 94–95, 104
  esophagus cancer and, 72, 73, 74–75
  fat in, 3, 95, 192–193
  gastric cancer and, 78–80
  gastrointestinal tract cancers and, 68
  hematopoietic carcinogenesis and, 423
  inhibitive effects, 79–80
  pickled foods, 74
  prostate cancer and, 356–360, 374–375
  rodent urinary bladder carcinogenesis and, 192–193
  salted fish, 215
  smoked foods, 79
  as variable in carcinogenesis, 3
Diethylnitrosamine, in hepatocarcinogenesis, 46, 50, 53–55, 57
Differentiation factors, 319–326
Diffusely basophilic cell foci, 40, 47
Dihydrodiols, 268
3,2-Dimethyl-4-aminobiphenyl (DMAB), 376, 381–382, 387
Dimethyl sulfate, 215
Dimethylamine, 253, 254
7,12-Dimethylbenz[a]anthracene, 265, 269–271, 416
Dimethylcarbamoyl chloride, 215, 245
Dimethylformamide, 344, 370–371
1,2-Dimethylhydrazine (DHM), 11–12
Dimethylnitrosamine, 53
Dinitrosopiperazine, 256
Diol-epoxides, 268, 270
Direct acting carcinogens, 2
Disulfiram, 7
Dose-related responses, in neurocarcinogenesis, 306–307
Dysplasia
  in Crohn-related intestinal cancer, 93
  esophagus cancer and, 75
  gastric cancer and, 77, 88

E

Enzyme function, in renal carcinogenesis, 140–141
Eosinophilic foci, 40–41, 47
Epichlorohydrin, 215, 217

Epidemiology
  brain tumor, 302
  cancer, 25, 33, 199
  esophagus cancer, 71–72
  gastric cancer, 77–81
  gastrointestinal tract cancers, 67–68
  intestinal metaplasia in gastric cancer, 88
  larynx cancer, 232–233
  male reproductive system, 339
  nasal cancer, 226–232
  prostate cancer, 339, 356
  renal carcinogenesis, 123
  respiratory cancer, 199–200
  small intestine tumors, 91, 93
  spontaneous upper respiratory tract tumors in rodents, 240–242
  testicular carcinogenesis, 339–346
Epidermal growth factor, 275, 278–281, 284
  in neurocarcinogens, 315
Epigenetic carcinogens, 4–5
  in hepatocarcinogenesis, 58, 59
  in renal carcinogenesis, 148
Epithelial cells
  in human upper respiratory tract, 224–226
  in rodent nasal cavity, 217–223
Epithelial tumors
  in renal carcinogenesis, 124–127
  rodent thymomas, 414–415
  in rodent upper respiratory tract, 242–246
  in upper respiratory tract, 233
Epstein-Barr virus, 421–422
Erionite, 13
Esophagus cancer
  animal models, 76–77
  epidemiology, 71–72
  epithelium in, 75
  food-related risks, 72, 73, 74–75
  predisposing medical conditions, 75–76
  susceptibility factors, 72–76
  trace minerals and, 74, 77
Estragole, 12
Estrogens
  in cryptorchidism, 341–342, 351–352
  prostate carcinogenesis and, 378–380, 385–386
  renal carcinogenesis and, 137
  testicular cancer and, 342–344, 345–346, 347–348, 351–353
Ethanol, 15
Ethyl acrylate, 253, 254
Ethyl carbamate, 12
Ethyl phenyl propiolate, 274–275
Ethylene dibromide, 215
Ethylene oxide, 2
Ethylene thiourea, 5
Ethyleneimine, 2
Ethylnitrosurea
  nervous system specificity, 307–309
  in neurocarcinogenesis initiation, 310–311

neurocarcinogenesis promotion, 312–314, 323–325
neurocarcinogenic potential, 302
species-dependent neurogenic effects, 303–304
Eyes, autopsy of, 457

F

Familial adenomatous polyposis, 97
Fat, dietary, 3, 95, 192–193, 357–358
Fiber, dietary, 104
Fiddlehead ferns, 13
Flexner-Wintersteiner rosettes, 235
N-(4-Fluro-4-biphenylyl) acetamide (FBPA), 133
Foci of cellular alteration, hepatocellular, 40, 46–47
Formaldehyde
  metabolism, 12
  occupational exposure, 231–232
  in upper respiratory tract carcinogenesis, 243–244, 252, 254, 256, 257
Furfural, 253, 254
Furniture makers, 230–231

G

Gardner's syndrome, 97
Gastric cancer
  animal models, 89–91
  blood type and, 80
  chemical carcinogens, 89
  epidemiology, 77–81
  genetic factors in, 77, 80
  intestinal metaplasia in, 86, 87–88
  intestinal-type, 81–82
  macromolecular adducts in, 83–84
  multifactorial etiology, 83
  N-nitroso compounds in, 81–83
  norepinephrine in, 80, 90
  oncoprotein expression in, 84–86
  precancerous histopathology, 87
  precursor conditions, 77
  promoters, 90–91
  protooncogene expression in, 84–86
  risk factors, 90
  salt hypothesis, 78–80
  socioeconomic factors in, 80–81
  sympathetic nervous system in, 80
  tumor suppressor gene mutations in, 86
Gastritis, 77
Gastrointestinal tract carcinogenesis. *See also* Esophagus cancer; Gastric cancer; Intestinal cancer
  autopsy procedures, 446–448
  cancer epidemiology, 67–68
  genetic factors in, 68–69, 70–71
  inflammatory reactions in, 68, 70, 92

risk factors, 68–70
susceptibility factors, 70–71
Gender differences
  in animal models, 207–208
  in neurocarcinogenesis, 306
  in respiratory tract cancer epidemiology, 199
  response to xenobiotics, 3
  in rodent urinary bladder carcinogenesis, 190
Genetic alteration
  in colorectal carcinogenesis, 95
  in free-radical promotion of skin cancer, 276–277
  in gastric cancer, 84–86
  in initiation of hepatocarcinogenesis, 53
  latency period, 312
  in neurocarcinogenesis initiation, 309–311
  in neurocarcinogenesis progression, 315–316
  in oncogenes in hepatocarcinogenesis, 56–57
  in promotion of carcinogenesis, 54
  in skin carcinogenesis, 265–266, 269–271, 283
Genetic risk factors
  colorectal carcinogenesis, 95–96, 97–99
  in esophagus cancer, 76
  in gastric cancer, 77, 80
  in gastrointestinal cancers, 68–69, 70–71
  intestinal cancer, 91–92
  in neurocarcinogenesis susceptibility, 328
  in prostate cancer, 362–363
  skin carcinogenesis, 281–283
Genotoxic carcinogens, 3–4
  cadmium as, nongenotoxic mechanisms in, 354–355
  in hepatocarcinogenesis, 58–59
  in renal carcinogenesis, 148
Gliomas, 307–308
  antigenic heterogeneity, 318–319
Glucose-6-phosphatase (G6Pase), in hepatocarcinogenesis, 48–50
Glucose-6-phosphate dehydrogenase (G6PDH)
  in hepatocellular lesions, 40–41
  in skin carcinogenesis, 277
γ-Glutamyltranspeptidase, 40–41
Glutathione S-transferase, 40–41
  in renal carcinogenesis, 141
Glycogen synthetase/phosphorylase
  in hepatocarcinogenesis bioassay, 57–60
  in hepatocellular lesions, 40–41, 48–52

H

H-*ras*, 16, 269–271, 283
Halogenated aliphatics, 5–7
Hand-Schueller-Christian disease, 405
Heart, autopsy of, 454–455
Hematopoietic system. *See also* Leukemias
  chemical-induced tumorigenesis, 415–418
  classification of rodent tumors, 408–414
  immune system and, 422–423

Hematopoietic system (*contd.*)
  leukemias of, 403–405
  lymphomas of, 405
  mechanism of carcinogenesis in, 423–424
  nutrition and, 423
  radiation-induced tumors of, 418–421
  thymomas of, 408
  viral-induced tumors in, 421–422
Hepatoblastoma, 44–46
Hepatocellular adenoma, 39
  vs. hepatocellular hyperplasia, 41, 47–48
Hepatocellular carcinomas, 42
Hepatocholangiocellular lesions, 44
Hexamethylphosphoramide, 215
Histiocytosis, 405
Hodgkin's disease, 405
Homer Wright rosettes, 235
Hormonal system
  androgens in prostate carcinogenesis, 384–386
  in inducing prostate tumors, 378–381
  prostate cancer and, 367–370
  in renal carcinogenesis, 137
  in testicular cancer risk, 342–344, 345–346, 347–348
  vasectomy and prostate cancer, 341, 363–364
HTLV-I,II, 421, 422
Human papilloma virus, 76
Hydrazines, 11–12
N-Hydroxy derivatives, 9–10
Hyperplasia
  definition, 146
  hepatocellular, 41, 47–48
  leading to carcinogenesis, 250–251
  in nephropathy, 147
  renal carcinogenesis and, 138–139, 146–148
  rodent nasal, 243
  in rodent urinary bladders, 165, 166, 167–170, 182–186
  in skin tumor promotion, 273–275
Hyperplastic nodules vs. hepatocellular adenomas, 41, 47–48
Hypolipidemic drugs, 4

I

Immune system
  anticarcinogenic role of, 69–70
  brush cells in, 219
  in colorectal carcinogenesis, 96
  in gastrointestinal cancer susceptibility, 71
  hematopoietic tumors and, 422–423
  leukemia cell antibody phenotyping, 404
  in neurocarcinogenesis, 317–319
Indirect acting carcinogens, 2–3
Inhibition-prevention, 15–16
Inhibition/prevention

  antioxidant action, 69
  ascorbic acid in, 75, 80
  gastric cancer, food consumption in, 79–80
  hyperprolactinemia in, 348
  immune system response, 69–70
  lung cancer, strategies for, 200
  of prostate cancer, vitamins in, 357, 358–360
  in rodent urinary bladder carcinogenesis, 193
  vitamin A in, 79–80
  zinc effects in, 354
Initiation-promotion-progression, 14–15. *See also* Multistage carcinogenesis; Promotion of carcinogenesis
  in gastrointestinal carcinogenesis, 68
  genetic alteration in, 53
  in hematopoietic carcinogenesis, 424
  hepatocarcinogenesis, 53–57
  of neurocarcinogenesis, 311–314
  skin carcinogenesis initiation, 265–271
Injury
  cell, and renal carcinogenesis, 143–148
  in esophagus cancer susceptibility, 73
  in gastrointestinal cancer susceptibility, 70
  skin-tumor promotion and, 284
  tissue damage in carcinogenesis, 250–251
  in tumor promotion, 271–272
Inorganic carcinogens, 13–14
Inositol hexaphosphate, 69
Inositol triphosphate, 94–95
International Agency for Research on Cancer, 26–27, 32, 202–203
Intestinal adenocarcinomas of the nose, 231
Intestinal cancer. *See also* Gastrointestinal tract
  celiac disease and, 93
  Crohn's disease and, 92–93
  inherited predisposition, 91–92
  large intestine. *See* Colorectal cancer
  small intestine, 91–93
Intestinal metaplasia, in gastric cancer, 86, 87–88
Iron deficiency, 74–75
Isopropyl alcohol, 229

K

K-*ras*, 16, 269–270
  in colorectal carcinogenesis, 95, 97, 102
  in renal carcinogenesis, 149
Kidney. *See* Renal carcinogenesis
Kiel classification, 405

L

Larynx. *See also* Upper respiratory tract carcinogenesis
  cancer epidemiology, 215, 217, 232–233
  human, histology, 225

rodent, histology, 223-224
spontaneous tumors in rodents, 240-242
tumors of, 250
Latency period, 312
Leimyosarcomas, of small intestine, 91
Letterer-Siwe syndrome, 405
Leukemias, 403-405
  as antitumor treatment side effect, 417
  chemical-induced, 415-417
  immunologic phenotyping of, 404
  lymphoblastic, 404-405
  radiation-induced, 418-421
  rodent, types of, 410-411
  viral-induced, 421-422
Leydig cell tumors
  cadmium induction of, 354-355
  estrogen and, 353
  inhibition of, 348, 349
  in testicular cancer, 339, 341, 346, 347-351
  zinc inhibition of, 354-355
Lifestyle factors, 34
Liver
  autopsy procedures, 448-450, 460-462
  cell proliferation in carcinogenesis, 56
  cholangiocellular lesions in, 42-44
  cirrhosis, 48
  classification of lesions in, 39-40
  dichloromethane carcinogenicity in, 5
  epigenetic carcinogens of, 4
  genetic factors in carcinogenesis in, 56-57
  glycogen marker enzymes in carcinogenesis in, 48-52
  hematopoietic carcinogenesis and lesions of, 423
  hepatoblastoma in, 44-46
  hepatocellular proliferative lesions of, 40-42
  hyperplasia in, and carcinogenesis, 250-251
  multistage carcinogenesis in, 53-55
  preneoplastic lesions in, 46-53, 57-60
  in vivo assay system, 57-60
Lukes-Collins classification, 405
Lung. See Respiratory tract carcinogenesis
Lymphomas. See also Hematopoietic system
  in celiac disease, 93
  Hodgkin's disease, 405
  immune system and, 422-423
  non-Hodgkin's, 405
  rodent, types of, 408-410
  in small intestine, 91, 93
  of upper respiratory tract, 237-238
Lynch syndromes, 96, 98

M

Macromolecular adducts, 83-84
Magnesium, 423
Male reproductive system. See also Testicular carcinogenesis
  bulbourethral gland, 387
  preputial gland in, 339, 386-387
  seminal vesicle tumors, 387
  tumor epidemiology, 339
Malocclusion, 252
Marital status
  prostate cancer and, 366-367
  testicular cancer and, 341
Mast cell tumors, rodent, 411-412
Mechanism of carcinogenesis
  antioxidants and, 69
  cadmium, 354-355
  direct acting, 2
  epigenetic, 4-5
  genotoxic, 3-4
  in hematopoietic system, 423-424
  indirect acting, 2-3
  inhibition-prevention in, 15-16
  multistage model, 14-15
  mutagenesis-mitogenesis in, 423-424
  nerve growth factor and, 321-323
  in promotion stage, 312
  tissue damage in, 250-255
Melanoma, upper respiratory tract, 238-239
Melphalan, 417
Mercury, 146
Mesenchymal tumors
  renal, 128-130, 136
  rodent urinary bladder, 178
Metallothionein, 354, 382
3'-Methyl-4-dimethylaminoazobenzene, in hepatocarcinogenesis, 53-54, 56
Methyl methane sulfonate, 2
N-Methyl-N-benzylnitrosamine, in esophagus carcinogenesis, 76-77
N-Methyl-N'-nitro-N-nitrosoguanidine (MNNG), 89-91, 270
7-Methylbenz[a]anthracene, 270-271
Methylcholanthracene, 416
Methylcholanthrene, 350
Methylene chloride. See Dichloromethane
Methylnitrosurea, 270
  in bladder cancer, 317-318
  in neurocarcinogenesis initiation, 310-311
  neurocarcinogenesis promotion, 314
  neurocarcinogenic potential, 302
  species-dependent neurogenic effects, 303-304
Metronidazole, 350
Milk, 357
Mitomycin, 192
Mixed cell foci, 41
Müllerian inhibiting substance, 352
Multistage carcinogenesis. See also Initiation-promotion-progression
  colorectal, 100-102
  DNA adducts in, 309-310
  hematopoietic system, 424

Multistage carcinogenesis (*contd.*)
  in intestinal-type gastric cancer, 81–82
  model, 14–15
  in rat liver, 53–57
  renal, 132
  skin, 265–267, 283–284
Mustard gas, 229
Myasthenia gravis, 408
Mycotoxins, in pickled food, 74

N

N-*myc* amplification, 314–315
N-*ras*, 311
Nasal cancer. *See also* Upper respiratory tract carcinogenesis
  epidemiology, 226–232
  spontaneous tumors in rodents, 240–242
Natural killer cells, 69–70
  in colorectal carcinogenesis, 96
  impairment in, 71
Neoplasia
  hepatocellular, vs. hyperplasia, 48
  immune system response in, 317
  in latent neurocarcinogenesis, 312
  in rodent urinary bladder, 166–167, 170–172, 186–190
Neoplastic nodules
  vs. hepatocellular adenomas, 41
Nephroblastomas, renal, 130–131, 136
  vs. mesenchymal tumors, 128
Nephrotoxicity, renal carcinogenesis and, 123, 144–149
Nerve growth factor, 319–326, 329
neu gene, 311
Neuroblastomas, upper respiratory tract, 235–237
Neurocarcinogenesis
  age as factor in, 304–305
  autopsy procedures, 455–459
  chemicals associated with, 302–303, 328–329
  differentiation/growth factors in, 319–326, 329
  dose-related responses, 306–307
  early neoplastic proliferation in, 312
  epidemiology, 302
  gender-related differences in, 306
  generalizability of animal studies, 328–329
  host factors in, 317
  immune mechanisms in, 317–319
  initiation, 310–311
  models for, 301
  N-*myc* amplification in, 314–315
  organ specificity in, 307–309
  progression, 314
  promotion, 311–314
  protooncogenes in, 314–316

  risk factors, 328–329
  species-dependent differences, 303–304
  tumor suppressor genes in, 316
Neuroendocrine carcinoma, 237
Nickel, 227–229
  carcinogenicity, 14
Nitrates/nitrites
  in gastric cancer, 81–83
5-Nitrofurans, 416
Nitrogen mustard, 2
Nitrosamines, 346
  carcinogenesis inhibition, 15, 16
  carcinogenicity of, 11
  in esophagus cancer susceptibility, 73, 76
  excretion inhibited by ascorbic acid, 80
  in hematopoietic system carcinogenesis, 416
  in nasopharyngeal cancer, 215, 217
  in renal carcinogenesis, 133
  in rodent nasal tumors, 243
  in rodent urinary bladder carcinogenesis, 190
N-Nitroso compounds, in gastric cancer, 81–83
N-Nitrosobis(2-oxopropyl)amine (BOP), 346–347, 376
Nitrosodiethylamine, 245
N-Nitrosodimethylamine (DMN)
  in renal carcinogenesis, 133, 134, 135, 136
N-Nitrosomethylallylamine, 256
N-Nitrosomethylurea, 416
N-Nitrosomethylvinylamine, 256
Nitrosureas, 11
Non-Hodgkin's lymphomas, 405
Nongenotoxicity. *See* Epigenetic carcinogens
Norepinephrine, in gastric carcinogenesis, 80, 90

O

Obesity, 361
Occupational risks
  nasal cancer, 227–232
  prostate cancer, 370–372
  renal carcinogenesis, 123
  testicular cancer, 344–345
  upper respiratory tract carcinogenesis, 215, 251–252
Okadaic acid, 278
Olfactory cells, 225–226
  neuroblastomas of, 235–237, 249–250
  rodent tumors of, 246–250
Oncogenes
  activation of, 16
  anti-oncogenes, 424
  definition, 16, 424
  genetic alterations in hepatocarcinogenesis, 56–57
  in hematopoietic carcinogenesis, 424
  neu, 311
  in renal carcinogenesis, 149

SUBJECT INDEX

Oncoproteins, in gastric cancer, 84–86
Organ transplants, 422
Organic compounds, classes of, 5–13
Oval cell hyperplasia, 43
Oxygen radicals
 in gastrointestinal tract carcinogenesis, 68
 in skin cancer, 276
 source of, 69

P

P450
 in benzene metabolism, 8
 in genetic susceptibility to gastrointestinal cancer, 71
 in genetic susceptibility to skin carcinogenesis, 282
 in nitrosamine metabolism, 11
 in oxidation of aliphatic compounds, 5, 6
 in oxidation of tetrachloroethylene, 6
 in oxidation of trichloroethylene, 6
 in skin carcinogenesis, 268
 system, 3
Palytoxin, 278
Papillomas
 esophagus, in animal models, 76
 in rodent urinary bladder, 172
 skin, T-cell growth factor in, 280
 in skin tumorigenesis, 267
Pathology procedures. See also Autopsy
 interpreting clinical observations, 434–435
 method of euthanasia, 434
 necropsy report sheet, 431
 in toxicologic research, goals of, 429–430
Perchloroethylene, 149
Pesticides, 344, 371
Petroleum hydrocarbons, 134
 in renal carcinogenesis, 123, 148, 149
Phenylglycidyl ether, 215, 243
Phenytoin, 418
Phorbol esters, 271, 275
Physical activity, 360–361
Pickled foods, 74
Pituitary metabolism, 349
Platelet-derived growth factor, 315
Plummer-Vinson syndrome, 74–75
Polycyclic aromatic hydrocarbons, 3
 bay region hypothesis, 9
 metabolism, 9
 in skin carcinogenesis, 265, 268–269, 282
 vegetables and, 80
Polymyositis, 408
Polyoma virus, 136–137
Polyposis
 familial adenomatous, 97
 juvenile, 98
Preneoplastic lesions
 in hepatocarcinogenesis, 46–53, 57–60

 in renal carcinogenesis, 138–143
Preputial gland, 339, 386–387, 446
Prevention. See Inhibition/prevention
Progression of carcinogenesis. See Initiation-promotion-progression
Promoters
 of colorectal cancer, 94
 definition, 15
 experimental role of, 265
 gastric carcinogenesis, 90–91
 renal carcinogenesis, 132, 135–136
 in rodent urinary bladder, 191
 of skin carcinogenesis, 271–272, 282–283
Promotion of carcinogenesis. See also Initiation-promotion-progression; Promoters
 definition, 54
 in nervous system, 311–314
 in skin, 266–267, 271–278, 282–284
a-Propiolactone, 2
Propylene oxide, 215, 250
Prostaglandins
 in colorectal cancer, 104–105
 E2 in gastric carcinogenesis, 90
 H synthase system, 9
Prostate cancer
 androgens in, 384–386
 cadmium and, 371–372, 377
 cell proliferation in, 377–378, 383
 chemical carcinogens, 376–377
 dietary factors in, 356–360, 374–375
 epidemiology, 339, 356
 experimental induction, 375–381
 genetic factors in, 362–363
 hormonal system and, 367–370, 378–381, 386–387
 latency of, 374
 marital status and, 341, 366–367
 occupational risks, 370–372
 physical activity and, 360–361
 prostatitis and, 365
 race as risk factor, 373–374
 smoking and, 361–362
 socioeconomic factors in, 372
 target-organ-specific mechanisms of, 381–386
 vasectomy and, 341, 363–364
 veneral disease and, 365
Protein kinases, 424
 C, 15, 94–95, 275, 277, 284
 in colorectal carcinogenesis, 94–95
 in skin carcinogenesis, 275, 277, 284
Protocols, autopsy, 431–434
Protooncogenes
 definition, 16
 in gastric carcinogenesis, 84–86
 in hematopoietic carcinogenesis, 424
 in hepatocarcinogenesis, 56–57

Protooncogenes (contd.)
  in neurocarcinogenesis, 314–316
  role of, 84
Ptaquiloside, 12–13
Pthalate ester plasticizers, 4
Puetz-Jeghers syndrome, 91–92, 97–98
Pyrolizidine alkaloids, 12

Q
Quinones, 268
Quinoxaline-1,4-dioxide, 247

R
Radiation
  hematopoietic cancer induced by, 418–421
  prostate cancer and, 372, 377
  in renal carcinogenesis, 137–138
  therapy, 99, 328, 421
Rappaport classification, 405
Reed-Sternberg cell, 405
Renal carcinogenesis
  autopsy procedures, 450–452
  cell injury in, 143–148
  chemical induction, 132–136
  chemical promoters, action of, 135–136
  embryonal tumor morphology, 130–131
  enzyme function in, 140–141
  epidemiology, 123
  epigenetic carcinogens, 4
  epithelial tumor morphology, 124–127
  experimental models, 135–136, 149
  genotoxic vs. epigenetic effects in, 148
  hormonal induction, 137
  hyperplasia vs. neoplasia in, 138–139
  medical risk factors, 137–138
  metastases from, 136
  nephrectomy and, 138
  nephrotoxicity/nephrocarcinogenicity and, 123, 144–149
  nonepithelial tumor morphology, 128–130
  preneoplastic lesion in, 138–143
  tumor-associated antigen, 141–143
  viral induction, 136–137
Reproductive organs. *See also* Male reproductive system
  autopsy procedures for, 444, 446
Reserpine, 350
Respiratory tract carcinogenesis. *See also* Upper respiratory tract carcinogenesis
  autopsy procedures, 452–455, 462–463
  chemical carcinogens, 200–206
  epidemiology, 199–200
  relevance of animal models, 200, 202, 206–211
  risk-reduction strategies, 200
  route of exposure, 201–202
Restriction fragment length polymorphism, 85
Retinoids, 193, 359–360

Rhinitis, 252
Risk assessment
  colorectal cancer marker, 100, 102–103
  for direct-acting carcinogens, 2
  hepatocarcinogenesis, 57–60
  indirect acting carcinogens, 2–3
Risk factors. *See also* Genetic risk factors; Occupational risks
  antitumor treatments as, 417, 422
  cancer, 25–35
  colorectal cancer, 94–96, 97–100, 103–104
  esophagus cancer, 72–76
  in gastrointestinal tract cancers, 68–70
  lung cancer, 199–200
  medical, in renal carcinogenesis, 137–138
  physical activity as, in prostate cancer, 360–361
  prostate cancer, 356–370, 372–375
  renal carcinogenesis, 123
  testicular cancer, 341–346
  in upper respiratory tract cancer, 215
  upper respiratory tract carcinogenesis, 253–256
Rosettes, olfactory neuroblastoma, 235
Rubber industry, 370

S
Safrole, 12
Salt, in gastric cancer, 78–80, 90–91
Salted fish, 215
Schistosomiasis, 100
Selenium, 74, 104, 357
Seminal vesicle, 387
Sexual behavior, prostate cancer and, 366–367
Shoemakers, 231
Silica fibers, 272
Sinusitis, 252
Skin carcinogenesis
  animal stock/strains sensitivity, 283
  biochemical mechanisms in promotion of, 275–278
  chemicals associated with, 267–268
  in complete experimental protocol, 265
  DNA adducts in, 268–269
  epidermal growth factor in, 275, 278–281, 284
  experimental protocols, 265
  genetic alteration in, 268–269
  genetic factors in susceptibility to, 281–283
  handling of autopsy specimens, 439
  initiation, 265, 267–271, 283
  multistage model, 265–267, 283
  necropsy procedures in study of, 431
  premalignant papillomas in, 267
  tumor promotion, 266–267, 271–278, 283–284
  tumor types, 267
Skull, autopsy of, 457–459

Smoked foods, 79
Socioeconomic factors
  in gastric cancer, 80-81
  in prostate cancer, 372
  in testicular cancer, 345
Sodium chloride, in gastric cancer, 78-80, 90-91
Sodium saccharin, 192
Soy sauce, 80
Spinal column, autopsy of, 455-456
Spindle cell carcinomas, 233-234
Surfactants, in carcinogenesis promotion, 89
Sympathetic nervous system, in gastric carcinogenesis, 80

T

T-cells
  in carcinogenesis immunosuppression, 71
  growth factor, in skin carcinogenesis, 278-281, 284
  human T-cell leukemia virus, 421, 422
  in leukemia assessment, 404
Tanning industry, 226
Testicular carcinogenesis
  cadmium-induced, 349-350, 351, 353-354
  chemicals associated with, 350
  cryptorchidism and, 341-342, 346, 351-352
  estrogen and, 342-344, 345-346, 347-348, 351-353
  hormone exposure in, 342-344, 345-346, 347
  Leydig cell induction of, 346, 347-351
  low birth weight and, 344
  non-Leydig cell induction of, 346-347
  occupational risk factors, 344-345
  pituitary factors in, 349
  race as risk factor, 345
  socioeconomic factors in, 345
  target-organ-specific mechanisms in, 351-355
  tumor epidemiology, 339-341
  tumor types, 340
Testosterone
  prostate carcinogenesis and, 367-370, 384-385
  prostate tumors induced by, 378-379, 380-381
Tetrachloroethylene, P450 oxidation of, 6
Tetradecanoylphorbol-13-acetate (TPA)
  as carcinogenesis promoter, 15, 271-274, 312
  in skin carcinogenesis, 276-278, 279, 284
Thapsigargin, 277-278
Thymectomy, 421
Thymomas, 408
  rodent, 413-415
Thyroid, autopsy of, 452-454

Tigroid basophilic cell foci, 40, 47
Tissue damage, in upper respiratory tract carcinogenesis, 250-255
Tobacco
  aldehydes in cigarette smoke, 257
  4-aminobiphenyl in, 10
  in esophagus cancer susceptibility, 73-74
  gastric cancer and, 79
  identification of carcinogenicity of, 208-209
  laryngeal cancer and, 215
  nitrosamine derivatives, 11, 16
  prostate cancer and, 361-362
  renal adenocarcinomas and, 123
  respiratory cancer and, 199-200
Transitional cell tumors
  renal, 127, 136
  in rodent urinary bladder, 173-178
  upper respiratory tract, 234-235
Trichloroacetic acid, 4
Trichlorobutene, 247
Trichloroethylene, 6
Trihalomethanes, 5
Tumor suppressor genes, 68-69
  in neurocarcinogenesis, 315-316
  p053 mutations in gastric cancer, 86
Turcot syndrome, 98
Two-stage carcinogenesis, in rodent urinary bladder, 186, 191
Tyrosine methyl ester, 90

U

Ultraviolet light, 271
Upper respiratory tract carcinogenesis. *See also* Respiratory tract carcinogenesis
  adenocarcinomas with glandular differentiation, 235
  chemical carcinogens in, 215-217
  epidemiology, 227-233
  exposure patterns in, 255-256
  generalizability of animal research, 215-217, 253-254, 255, 257
  handling autopsy specimens, 459
  histopathology, 233-239
  malignant lymphomas in, 237-238
  malignant melanoma in, 238-239
  of nasal respiratory mucosa, 242-246
  neuroblastomas, 235-237
  normative histology of human, 224-226
  normative histology of rodent, 217-224
  occupational risks, 215
  role of tissue damage in, 250-255
  spindle cell carcinoma, 233-234
  spontaneous tumors in rodents, 240-242
  squamous cell carcinomas of, 233-235
  transitional cell carcinomas, 234-235
  tumors of rodent olfactory mucosa, 246-250
  tumors of squamous epithelium, 242-246
  verrucous carcinoma, 233

Uracil, 192
Ureterosigmoidostomy, 99–100
Urethane, 12, 267, 270
Uric acid, 69
Urinary bladder (rodent)
    2-Acetylaminofluorene carcinogenesis, 182–190, 192
    autopsy procedures, 444–445, 460
    calculi in, and carcinoma, 192
    cancer promoters in, 191–193
    carcinogens, 182, 188–190
    cystitis, 166, 167
    diverticuli in, 171
    generalizability to humans, 181
    gross anatomy, 161–162
    hyperplasia during carcinogenesis, 182–186
    induced lesions in, 167–178
    metastases, 181
    methylnitrosurea in cancer of, 317–318
    microscopic features, 162–163
    modulating factors in carcinogenesis in, 190–193
    neoplasia during carcinogenesis, 186–190
    pleomorphic microvilli in, 170–171
    preparation for microscopic evaluation, 163–166
    spontaneous lesions in, 166–167
    transitional epithelium in, 161, 162, 163, 170

V
Vasectomy, 341, 363–364
Vegetables, 80

Veneral disease, prostate cancer and, 365
Verrucous carcinomas, 233
Vinyl chloride, 32, 328
    metabolization, 6
    nasal cancer and, 215, 247, 248
Viruses
    in hematopoietic system tumorigenesis, 421–422
    in renal carcinogenesis, 136–137
Vitamins
    A, 79–80, 104, 357, 358–360
    C, 193
    a-carotene, 358–360
    D, 357
    in esophagus cancer, 75
    in prostate cancer, 356, 357–360
    rodent urinary bladder carcinogenesis and, 193

W
Wilms' tumor, 130
Wood dust, 230–231, 251–252, 254
Working Group classification, 405

X
Xenobiotics. *See also* Carcinogens
    gender differences in response to, 3

Z
Zinc, 354, 357
    esophagus cancer and, 74, 77